The Late ALMA NEMIR, M.D.
Formerly, University of Utah

and WARREN E. SCHALLER, H.S.D.
Professor and Chairman
Department of Physiology and Health Science
Ball State University

Fourth Edition

The School Health Program

W. B. Saunders Company
Philadelphia, London, Toronto

W. B. Saunders Company: West Washington Square
Philadelphia, PA 19105

1 St. Anne's Road
Eastbourne, East Sussex BN21 3UN, England

1 Goldthorne Avenue
Toronto, Ontario M8Z 5T9, Canada

Library of Congress Cataloging in Publication Data

Nemir, Alma.

The school health program.

Bibliography: p.

Includes index.

1. School hygiene. I. Schaller, Warren Edward. II. Title.
[DNLM: 1. School health. WA350 N434s]

LB3405.N36 1975 371.7′1 74–4582

ISBN 0–7216–6748–1

The School Health Program ISBN 0-7216-6748-1

01234 147 987

To the memory of Alma Nemir
and to
Jean Elizabeth and John Frederick Schaller

PREFACE

The third edition of this textbook was based on the philosophy expressed in the following two paragraphs taken from its Preface:

> This book is written primarily for teacher candidates in colleges and universities and for teachers in service. All teachers are expected to have competencies in detecting and handling the health problems of school-age youth and they must understand their own roles in the school health program. Many institutions and state departments of education require a course in this area for certification.
>
> Other personnel interested in the health of the school child will find valuable resource material in this book—superintendents and principals, school physicians, school psychologists, school nurses and social workers, consultants in health and physical education, speech correctionists, audiologists, and educators in special education.

The same fundamental beliefs form the foundation for this fourth edition. Teachers and other school personnel have an unparalleled opportunity to assist the school-aged child in having a positive learning experience. An understanding of the health problems of school children and the school's responsibility will contribute greatly to this objective.

This text integrates the discussion on the health problems of the school-aged child with the role health services, health instruction, and healthful environment play in working with the child. A general updating of content, resources, and references has, of course, been made. In addition, there has been an expansion of material on the health instruction program, incorporating instructional strategies. The inclusion of discussion questions at the end of each chapter should help promote class interaction.

Much progress has been made in improving school health programs over the past 150 years. It is comforting to recognize past accomplishments, but it is to the future that we must direct our energies. Our greatest need in education is for dedicated teachers, administrators, and other school personnel. There is a tremendous need for personnel, properly prepared insofar as the school health program is concerned.

The many problems that exist provide extraordinary challenges. Our success in meeting these challenges will be determined by the health status of school children. Concerned professionals—well prepared, self-confident, self-motivated—and sensitive human beings are needed. Won't you be one?

Finally, I would be remiss if I did not recognize the major contributions Dr. Alma Nemir made to the previous editions. She certainly met the challenges, as well as the criteria, mentioned in this Preface, for school health program personnel. Dr. Nemir was a major contributor to the health of school children, and she will be missed.

WARREN E. SCHALLER, H.S.D.

CONTENTS

Chapter 1

RESPONSIBILITIES OF A TEACHER IN THE SCHOOL HEALTH PROGRAM 1

Part One – THE SCHOOL CHILD: HIS NORMAL HEALTH STATUS AND COMMON HEALTH PROBLEMS 11

Chapter 2

PHYSICAL GROWTH AND DEVELOPMENT 13

Introduction 13
Physical Growth and Development 14

Chapter 3

NUTRITIONAL STATUS – NORMAL AND ABNORMAL 39

Nutritional Requirements 39
Standards of Good Nutrition 49
Malnutrition 50
Underweight 56
The Fat Child 57
Nutrition Education Program 59
School Food Services 61

Chapter 4

POSTURE AND FEET 70

Posture 70
Feet 76
Role of the Teacher 78

Chapter 5

HEALTH PROBLEMS OF THE EYES 81

Introduction 81
Physiology of Vision 81
Common Problems of the Eye 83
School Health Program 98

Chapter 6

HEALTH PROBLEMS OF THE EARS, NOSE, THROAT, MOUTH, AND TONSILS 115

Ears 115
School Health Program for Hearing Problems 122
Nose 134
School Health Program 139
Throat (Pharynx) 140
Mouth 141
School Health Program 147
Disorders of Speech 148

Chapter 7

PROBLEMS OF DENTAL HEALTH 153

Anatomy and Physiology of Teeth 153
Growth and Development of Teeth 153
Incidence of Dental Defects 157
Common Dental Problems 158
Dental Health Program 175

Chapter 8

COMMUNICABLE DISEASES 183

Definition 183
Methods of Spread and Entry into the Body 183
Progress of a Disease 185
School Health Program in Handling Communicable Diseases 186
Descriptions of Individual Diseases 197

Chapter 9

ALLERGIES IN CHILDREN AND YOUTH 220

Introduction 220
Basic Explanation 221
Channels of Entry of Allergens 222
Types of Allergy 223
Effects of Allergies on Children and Youth 226
Management of the Individual with Allergy 226

Chapter 10

HEALTH PROBLEMS OF SKIN 229

Introduction 229
Common Bacterial Infections 231
Common Viral Infections 232
Fungal Infections 234
Infections Caused by Animal Parasites 238
Allergies 240
Rashes in Communicable Diseases 240
Acne Vulgaris 240
Seborrheic Dermatitis (Dandruff) 243
Other Health Problems 243

Chapter 11

PROBLEMS OF THE DIGESTIVE SYSTEM 247

Significance of an "Upset Stomach" 247
Emotional Disturbances 248
Appendicitis 248
Injuries 249
Ulcers 249
Gastroenteritis 250
Management at School of a Child with Abdominal Pain 252

Chapter 12

HEART PROBLEMS OF CHILDREN AND YOUTH 254

Growth of the Heart 254
Heart Function in Health and Disease 254
Common Causes of Heart Diseases in Childhood 257
School Health Program 261

Chapter 13

JUVENILE DIABETES MELLITUS 270

Physiology 270
Detection 272
Management of the Juvenile Diabetic at School 273

Chapter 14

EMOTIONAL PROBLEMS 277

Introduction 277
Developmental Patterns at Various Levels of Growth 278
Mental Health Program at School 283

Chapter 15

SOME SPECIAL PROBLEMS WITH SIGNIFICANT EMOTIONAL IMPLICATIONS 298

Introduction 298
Hyperactivity 301
Epilepsy 307
Cerebral Palsy 319
Mental Retardation 320
Learning Disabilities 322
Superior Intelligence 324
Headaches in Youth 325
The Battered or Neglected Child 331
Management at School of the Child with a Malignant Neoplasm 333

Part Two—THE SCHOOL HEALTH PROGRAM 339

Chapter 16

DEVELOPMENT OF THE SCHOOL HEALTH PROGRAM 341

Growth of the Public Health Program 341
Development of the School Health Program 346

Chapter 17

ORGANIZATION AND ADMINISTRATION OF THE SCHOOL HEALTH PROGRAM 353

Introduction 353
Health in the Home 354
Health in the Community 354
Health in the School 355
Community-School Relationships 370

Chapter 18

HEALTHFUL SCHOOL LIVING 376

Definition and Philosophy 376
Healthful Physical Environment 376
A Healthful School Day 393
Health of Personnel 406

Chapter 19

SCHOOL HEALTH SERVICES 412

Objectives 412
Health Appraisal 413
Health Counseling and Follow-Up 431
Other Health Services for the Child 434
Health Services for School Personnel 449

Chapter 20

SCHOOL HEALTH EDUCATION 457

What Is School Health Education? 457
The Need for School Health Education 458
The Health Education Curriculum 461
Implementing the Health Education Program 504
Evaluation of School Health Education (See Chapter 21) 505

Chapter 21

EVALUATION OF THE SCHOOL HEALTH PROGRAM 509

Evaluation—Benefits, Scope, and Procedures 509
Evaluation of Healthful School Living 516
Evaluation of School Health Services 517
Evaluation of School Health Education 518
Evaluation of Knowledge 519
Evaluation of the Total School Health Program 522

Appendix A

RESOURCES 527

Resources for Printed Materials 527
Resources for Audiovisual Materials 531
Journals, Newsletters 533

Appendix B

SCHOOL HEALTH RECORDS AND FORMS 535

Appendix C

CHECK LISTS 552

INDEX 561

Chapter 1

RESPONSIBILITIES OF A TEACHER IN THE SCHOOL HEALTH PROGRAM

In the preparation of a classroom teacher emphasis is placed upon understanding the child as a whole person. His emotional, social, intellectual, and physical needs must be brought into focus. A teacher should develop a health awareness, should perceive needs which may otherwise be unnoticed. This awareness uses professional skills for the promotion of a child's emotional and physical well-being.

A school brings together individuals of various skills and perceptions. When they work together and make their contributions to promote this well-being, the result should be an efficient school health program.

This school health program not only involves personnel within the school but reaches out for the cooperation of the family and those in the community who are vitally interested in the health of the school child.

This text is written primarily to acquaint every teacher with his role in the school health program. The objective is to promote and conserve the health of children and youth. More and more responsibility is being placed upon *every* teacher as the first line of defense in such a program. He is in a strategic position to assume this responsibility because of his daily observation of those in his classroom. Teacher education institutions recognize this phase of preparation by including content in the preservice curriculum which will promote competencies and skills in the area of school health.

A competent teacher appreciates his part in a well-organized school health program. He understands the growth and development of boys and girls. He has had courses in health education, educational psychology, and related areas. He participates in workshops and in-service training which will increase his understanding of his pupils. If a teacher understands a health problem, whether it be asthma, epilepsy, or some other handicapping condition, he can anticipate any possible repercussions in the classroom and find ways to meet a special child's needs. He himself should be in good health and emotionally stable. He is sincerely interested in the physical, mental, and social welfare of his pupils. Every teacher, whether he teaches in elementary or secondary schools:

1. Should see the child against his family background. A child of any age is himself plus his family. The strengths of the home must be preserved and made stronger; at the same time the child's strengths and potentials must be protected.

2. Should be familiar with the duties of other people in the school and with his own role in the school health program.

3. Should serve as an example where health attitudes and practices are concerned. A healthy, happy teacher is more likely to have contented pupils.

4. Ascertains the findings of the school medical and nursing staffs and uses them in guidance and often in the instruction of children with health problems.

5. Gives valuable assistance to physician and nurse about his charges. He works with the physician and nurse.

6. Maintains continuous supervision to meet a child's needs as outlined by a physician.

7. Teaches health education as an organized subject or incidentally in daily living at school. Every teacher is a health teacher.

8. Accepts responsibility in many ways for the environment of the school plant and for safety measures.

9. Observes the deviations from normal in health patterns. For instance, he observes the posture, the position of the head when listening or writing, the mannerisms, the expression, the appearance of illness, the suggestions of emotional disturbances. Emotional factors will be the most subtle. He makes it his business to follow through on his suspicions. A good teacher influences the lives of his students by his alertness in detection of health problems—a pair of glasses secured to improve vision, a change of classroom seats, a word to the school nurse or social worker concerning the eating habits or nutrition of a student, the early discovery of an acute depression. These are the deeds which live long after a date in history or the conjugation of a verb is forgotten.

10. Seeks opportunities to meet parents. A special effort is made to create an environment in which parents will feel free to visit their child's classroom periodically. Parent-teacher conferences are routinely scheduled and not solely reserved for problem situations. The teacher supports the parent-teacher association through attending its meetings, serving on committees, and participating in its activities. Involves parents in the instructional process by encouraging parents (with an extra-special invitation to fathers) to share their experiences with the entire class, e.g., travel experiences, hobbies, and occupational specialties. Other ways to provide service and

involvement include librarian activity, assistance with safety patrol program, lunchroom supervision, and field trip transportation and supervision. Provides opportunities for helping to plan, prepare, and execute special parties such as at Christmas, Halloween, and Easter. These are, of course, merely a few suggestions on ways to involve parents which will foster mutual respect. This respect for one another will be of great value when working together toward the health of their school-aged child.

11. And must appreciate the role of the community in the school health program. A child moves and has his being in his school, his home, and his community. He must understand the health interests of the community in the individual, as well as the health problems of the community itself. For example: since the leading cause of death in his age group is accidents, the community is vitally interested in a safety program. Consequently, police often go to schools and give instruction on bicycle regulations. Public and private health agencies play a dominant role in the health of the school child of all ages. They work with the teacher and all other school personnel.

The need for a teacher's active cooperation in the school health program is great. The Head Start program has demonstrated that the most prevalent of health problems in the preschool group are defective teeth, poor nutrition, and emotional problems. Many children start kindergarten or first grade with health handicaps. More chronic conditions are accumulated through the school years, including high school. Authorities state that about 12 per cent of youngsters in school suffer from physical, mental, or emotional disabilities. Consider these facts: 80 per cent of the nation's children live in 40 major cities; enrollment is high throughout the nation; our school population comprises one of our largest groups today. Therefore, the school health program will be under pressure in its effort to be efficient. The building and physical environment are on the whole greatly improved. However, health services and health education will be dependent to a great extent upon teachers.

To delimit one's interest in health problems of children to one age group is a mistake. The elementary teacher needs to know what happens to pupils before they come to his classroom and after they leave his school. Growth and development does not stop with the sixth or seventh grade. There should be a feeling of continuity. A junior or senior high school teacher needs to know what happened to the adolescent before he reached the higher grades and what happens as he grows older. There is no line of demarcation on diseases and defects. Impetigo and mumps look the same at any age. Methods of detection of defects are the same at any age. Even though environment and curriculum are altered to meet the needs of the growing child, the objectives are the same—conservation and promotion of good health of our school population.

The whole child comes to school, not just his mind. His needs are the concern of every teacher as he progresses through the grades.

The pattern of the school health program will vary in the elementary and secondary schools. Emphasis shifts with the growth and development of the child. Physical, mental, and social needs must be met in every aspect of school living.

The Elementary Teacher. Everyone recognizes and assumes that the teaching day of the elementary teacher is intimately associated with health procedures—in the school environment, in the health services which are performed, and in health education, or health science instruction. Most teachers measure the weights and heights of their pupils and use these measurements as an educational experience. They participate in screening tests, such as vision and hearing. Most of them accept responsibility for follow-up services, for teacher-nurse and teacher-parent conferences, and for health guidance at school. The many hours of teacher observation in a classroom should be fruitful in promoting and conserving the good health of pupils. In health education the elementary teacher exercises ingenuity in planning living-learning experiences which motivate a child to acceptable health attitudes and practices.

The Secondary Teacher. Secondary teachers should be familiar with screening tests and know how to interpret the results. A high school teacher should be able to read the cumulative health record on an individual student. What about vision? Or hearing? Is there some physical or emotional problem to account for poor academic achievement?

Adolescent students are the neglected students, as far as health is concerned. They are expected to be more responsible for their own health. There is not as much immediate need to work through parents. There are difficulties, however, in detecting deviations in behavior in this age group. Unless a problem is quite flagrant, it will probably not be noted. As a student goes through the day's schedule, he is in contact with each teacher for less than an hour. Moreover, a teacher sees too many students during the day to notice any one particularly. Yet, secondary teachers do have a responsibility, just as much as elementary teachers, to be alert to health problems. The student is a human being who becomes tired and upset, stoops, squints, worries about his complexion, becomes depressed, and may even commit suicide. Although a teacher has specialized in some particular academic area, modern concepts of education dictate that a teacher teaches more than subject matter. He is concerned with the person who sits before him, is trained to appraise him from day to day, and his observation should lead him to detect or suspect emotional, mental, or physical problems. And there are plenty.

Health education at the secondary level is more often a separate discipline, taught in the classroom. Many teachers correlate health information with their subject matter specialty. Most teachers in their daily contacts with students offer a certain amount of health guidance. Every teacher is a health teacher, either through classroom discussions or individual associations.

Hence, every secondary teacher should be competent to observe the health of students from a well-prepared background of information in school health. He should know the avenues offered for follow-up. High school students need health counselors and more help on emotional problems.

NEW DEFINITIONS: REPORT OF THE 1972–1973 JOINT COMMITTEE ON HEALTH EDUCATION TERMINOLOGY[1]

The new definitions listed below were prepared by representatives of the:

American Academy of Pediatrics (AAP)
American Association of Health, Physical Education and Recreation (AAHPER)
American College Health Association (ACHA)
American School Health Association (ASHA)
Public Health Education Section, American Public Health Association (PHE, APHA)
School Health Section, American Public Health Association (SHS, APHA)
Society for Public Health Education, Inc. (SOPHE)

These were based on earlier defintions prepared by the Joint Committee on Health Problems in Education (AMA and NEA) and the 1962 Joint Committee on Terminology. The process of formulating definitions is difficult at best, but necessary in order for effective dialogue to take place.

Definition of Health Education

A process with intellectual, psychological, and social dimensions relating to activities which increase the abilities of people to make informed decisions affecting their personal, family, and community well being. This process, based on scientific principles, facilitates learning and behavioral change in both health personnel and consumers, including children and youth.

Other Health Education Definitions (Listed in Alphabetical Order)

Community Health Education. That health education process utilizing intergroup relationships, value patterns, and communication resources in a specific social system.

Community Organization **(for health).** That process or method of health education in which the combined efforts of individuals and groups are designed to generate, mobilize, coordinate and/or redistribute resources to meet unsolved or emergent health problems.

Consumer Participation **(in health planning).** A specific health education application of the principle of involvement in learning which is intended to increase "provider" (health per-

[1]Lawrence W. Green (Ed.), *Health Education Monographs,* Society For Public Health Education, Inc., 1973, Number 33, Pages 63–70. Abridged and reprinted with permission.

sonnel) learning and to make program plans more relevant to the needs perceived by consumers.

***Group Process* (in health education).** The application of educational and communication principles in group situations designed to facilitate problem-solving and decision-making, through mutal stimulation of creative and critical thinking, or to increase the credibility and attractiveness of recommended health practices.

Health Education of the Public. A process designed for improvement and maintenance of health directed to the general population as contrasted with education for the preparation of a health professional.

Health Education Program. A planned and organized series of health education activities or procedures implemented with: 1) an educational specialist assigned primary responsibility; 2) a budget; 3) an integrated set of objectives sufficiently detailed to allow evaluation; and 4) administrative support.

Health Education Resources. All of the assets, human and material, that may be enlisted in the school or community to enrich the health education experiences of individuals and groups.

Healthful Environment. The promotion, maintenance, and utilization of safe and wholesome surroundings, organization of day-by-day experiences and planned learning procedures to influence favorable emotional, physical and social health.

Health Information. The communication of facts about health designed to develop the cognitive base for health action.

Health Instruction. The process of providing a sequence of planned and spontaneously originated learning opportunities comprising the organized aspects of health education in the school or community.

Health Science.[2]

Health Science Educator. Same as *School Health Educator.* This term also is sometimes used in life sciences, medicine, or the allied professions to denote instructors who prepare various health professionals or teach other than applied science.

Health Science Instruction. Synonymous with *Health Instruction.*

***Mass Communications* (in health).** The transfer of health information to a large and usually heterogeneous population, usually by means of such media as direct mail, newspapers, magazines, radio, television, and motion pictures.

Patient Education. Those health experiences designed to influence learning which occur as a person receives preventive, diagnostic, therapeutic and/or rehabilitative services, including experiences which arise from coping with symptoms, referral to sources of information, prevention, diagnosis and care, and con-

---

[2]Health Science has many connotations. It is used to describe a broad complex of disciplines concerned with the observation and classification of facts, concepts, generalizations, principles, and laws pertaining to the life process of growing and developing, interacting, and decision making. It also includes facilities such as a health science center encompassing professional schools for health personnel and health services for students and others.

In addition, it is used to refer to a college or university department offering health science instruction and professional preparation of health personnel. Health Science Education as a process may be defined synonymously with Health Education.

tacts with health institutions, health personnel, family and other patients.

Private Health Agency. A non-governmental agency concerned with health, organized as one of three types: 1) a non-profit incorporated (voluntary); 2) a non-profit unincorporated (voluntary); 3) a proprietary (commercial). (See also *Voluntary Health Agency.*)

Public Health Agency. An official governmental tax-supported organization mandated by law and/or regulation for the protection and improvement of the health of the public.

Public (Community) Health Educator.[3] An individual with professional preparation in public health and education including training in the application of selected content from relevant social and behavioral sciences used to influence individual and group learning, mobilization of community health action, and the planning, implementation and evaluation of health programs.

School Health Education. That health education process associated with health activities planned and conducted under the supervision of school personnel with involvement of appropriate community health personnel and utilization of appropriate community resources.

School Health Education Curriculum (**also *School Health Education Program).*** All the health opportunities affecting learning and behavior of children and youth in the total school curriculum. These health experiences are gained in both school and community settings as the individual interacts with his environment, including other students, school personnel, parents, and community members.[4]

School Health Education Curriculum Guides **(including Instructional Guides or Teaching-Learning Guides).** The plans or framework for the curriculum. The plans are developed and implemented cooperatively by health personnel, teachers, administrators, students, parents, and community representatives, preferably under the leadership of a qualified health educator.[5]

---

[3]The specific educational methods in which the public health educator is trained include community organization, communications, group work and consultation. Also included in his preparation are the public health sciences of epidemiology, biostatistics, environmental health, microbiology and health administration.

[4]The health content in a comprehensive health education curriculum includes such areas or concepts, both interdependent and interrelated, concerned with: health as a quality of life; the human organism (growth and development); nutrition; safety; disease control, including venereal disease; drug use and abuse, including alcohol and tobacco; family health or family life education (human sexuality); mental health; consumer health; personal health practices; health careers; and community health, including environmental health factors and ecology.

[5]The guides indicate the type of curriculum pattern or patterns used to organize content and student activities; i.e., health through *integration* or *core* commonly used K–6, with some experimentation in secondary schools; health as a subject-centered curriculum plan, a *separate course*; or a *separate course* and *natural correlation* with related fields, i.e., with social studies, science, physical education. (The latter is highly recommended for secondary schools to assure a comprehensive health education program.) *Correlation* as a single pattern is not recommended.

The guides also include the components for developing the teaching-learning process; long-range goals; behavioral objectives; health content; methods of teaching, including learning opportunities; health materials and media; and evaluative procedures.

School Health Educator.[6] An individual with professional preparation in health education or health science who is qualified for certification as a health teacher and for participation in the development, improvement, and coordination of school and community health education programs.

School Health Program. The composite of procedures and activities designed to protect and promote the well-being of students and school personnel. These procedures and activities include those organized in: school health services, providing a healthful environment, and health education.

School Health Services.[7] That part of the school health program provided by physicians, nurses, dentists, health educators, other allied health personnel, social workers, teachers and others to appraise, protect and promote the health of students and school personnel. Such procedures are designed to (a) appraise the health status of pupils and school personnel; (b) counsel pupils, teachers, parents and others for the purpose of helping pupils obtain health care, and for arranging school pro-

---

[6]Preparation of the school health educator is based on the health, biological and behavioral sciences, education, and includes health education history, principles, curriculum, methodology, administration, coordination, research, and evaluation.

[7]Based upon Joint Committee on Health Problems in Education of the National Education Association and the American Medical Association, *Health Appraisal of School Children,* 4th edition, American Medical Association, 1969.

Other activities directly related to health services include health appraisal, health observation, and screening tests, as defined in *Suggested School Health Policies* or *Health Appraisal of School Children,* Joint Committee on Health Problems in Education, NEA-AMA.

Cumulative School Health Record. A form used to note pertinent, consecutive information about a student's health status.

Dental Examination. A procedure conducted by a dentist to determine all oral conditions including the normal as well as abnormal. It may include the use of X-rays.

Dental Inspection. Observation and a limited evaluation of the oral structures to determine the presence of obvious defects, to be followed by referral to a dentist. The dental inspection provides an educational opportunity to encourage good oral practices including periodic visits to a dentist. (Revised from previous report and approved by ADA representatives.)

Health Examination. Used synonymously with *Medical Examination.*

Medical Examination. The evaluation by a physician of the medical status of an individual. Based on earlier definitions of the Joint Committee on Health Problems in Education (AMA and NEA) and the 1962 Joint Committee on Terminology.

Physical Examination. Used synonymously with *Medical Examination.*

School Medical Adviser. A physician who counsels and assists with those school procedures that influence the health and well-being of students and school personnel.

School Nurse. A professional nurse who has preparation in community health nursing and education, whose work focuses on improving, protecting, and maintaining the health of pupils, their families, and school personnel. The services are performed to emphasize prevention and early detection of health problems, and to provide health experiences for health counseling and health education.

Public Health Nurse. See American Nurses' Association, *Functions and Qualifications in the Practice of Public Health Nurses.*

grams in keeping with their needs; (c) help prevent and control communicable disease; (d) provide emergency care for injury or sudden illness; (e) promote and provide optimum sanitary conditions and safe facilities; (f) protect and promote the health of school personnel; and (g) provide concurrent learning opportunities which are conducive to the maintenance and promotion of individual and community health.

Voluntary Health Agency.[8] Any non-profit association organized on a national, state or local level, composed of lay and professional persons, dedicated to the prevention, alleviation and cure of a particular disease, disability, or group of diseases and disabilities. It is supported by voluntary contributions, primarily from the general public, and expends its resources for education, research and service programs relevant to the disease and disabilities concerned. (See also *Private Health Agency.*)

[8]*The Directory of National Voluntary Health Organizations,* 1971 edition, American Medical Association, 535 N. Dearborn Street, Chicago, Illinois, 60610, 1971.

SUMMARY

All teachers need to be familiar with the health problems of children and youth. They need to have the same background information in health. Emphasis will shift as the child grows to adulthood. Our teachers are the first line of defense in the school health program. They should accept this responsibility regardless of grade level and subject matter taught.

Part I

THE SCHOOL CHILD: HIS NORMAL HEALTH STATUS AND COMMON HEALTH PROBLEMS

Chapter 2

PHYSICAL GROWTH AND DEVELOPMENT

INTRODUCTION

Parents and teachers are immediately concerned with the growth and development of children in all their aspects—physical, emotional, social, and mental. Each individual, whether a child in elementary school or a high school student, is a whole being living at a particular time in a particular environment and society. He must fulfill two obligations: develop and maintain his own individuality and potential, and learn to live in a society.

Many children grow up under adverse home conditions, with poor medical care, poor nutrition, and general negligence, both physical and emotional. These are the ones who swell the statistics of rejections from military services. These often become welfare problems and burdens on society. They pass on to the next generation their own inadequacies. Others grow up to achieve good adjustments to themselves and to their culture. The welfare of all children is important to themselves, their parents, the schools, the community, and the nation. It follows that the growing child is the focus of attention and understanding of many groups—the anthropologist, school administrator, educator, physical educator, home economist, mental hygienist, psychologist, educational psychologist, physician, dentist, school nurse, social worker, public health official, and last, but not least, the parents.

The parents' influence is the first and most impressive throughout a child's life. A teacher can also influence a child's health and his attitudes towards himself and society. Every teacher must appreciate the simple facts of physical growth from year to year, the psychological characteristics of each period, and the changing needs of children and youth. The whole educational program from kindergarten through high school with its attention to physical and emotional environment, architectural planning, curriculum development, and approaches or techniques of teaching is based upon current knowledge of growth and development.

PHYSICAL GROWTH AND DEVELOPMENT

The term "child growth and development" is often used glibly without understanding of terminology. The word "growth" is used to indicate the actual increase in size of either a part of the body or the whole organism in terms of multiplication of cells. "Development" has a more subtle interpretation, since it refers to the function of a part and may be more difficult to evaluate or measure. Consider that growth may be measured in terms of pounds and inches, but nothing so concrete can be offered where function is concerned. Progress in function may parallel growth or may continue long after growth has ceased. For example, the size of the brain may be estimated from the increasing size of the head from birth to six or seven years of age, when the brain has reached 90 per cent of adult size. It then grows slowly for a few more years. The functions of the brain, however, continue development for many years thereafter. Another example is the development of small-muscle coordination in the fingers. Although the nerve supply to the skeletal muscles is provided early, skill in using the fingers for precise work in writing, drawing, and sewing is slowly developing at ages six and seven. Some six-year-old children find it difficult to tie their shoe laces. Development may also refer to emotional and social behavior. The combined words "growth and development" suggest a broader scope than the use of one word alone. The term "maturation" is sometimes used to connote development. "Adolescence" indicates the broad span of transition from childhood to adulthood when physical, emotional, and psychological changes are quite apparent. "Pubescence" or "puberty" refers to the specific phase of this transition in which changes occur in the reproductive systems.

How a Child Grows

A child's principal business is to grow and develop toward his optimum in health—in mental and physical fitness and social and emotional maturity. Physical growth occurs continuously from conception to adulthood, not with a uniform smoothness of the whole body and all of its parts, but with a certain overall pattern and "growth innings" of the parts which can be predicted. There will be plateaus and spurts of growth and infinite variations within this pattern. A description will be given of the usual characteristics in a group level, but each child still may differ from his peers in his growth and in his response to his environment. Children vary within the same family. Because of the differences among children, one child should never be compared to another in his age group. In any one year an individual may grow very little and be "normal," even though his classmates pass him on the scales. The large child is not necessarily as mature as he looks, yet a teacher will demand more of him. Each child can be stimulated to appreciate his progress from his own past record. This record will be followed not only in pounds and inches but by observation of his emotional, social, and intellectual development as well.

One is accustomed to think of growth in terms of something specific, something to be measured and recorded on paper, such as height and weight. Actually, these are only outward indications of growth. The organs within the body are also increasing in size and developing their unique functions at their own speed (Figure 1). For convenience, and because outward manifestations are presumed to mirror inner maturation as well, the immediate discussion will dwell upon height and weights as indices of growth and normal well-being. The interpretation of the measurements and the standards applied will be criticized later.

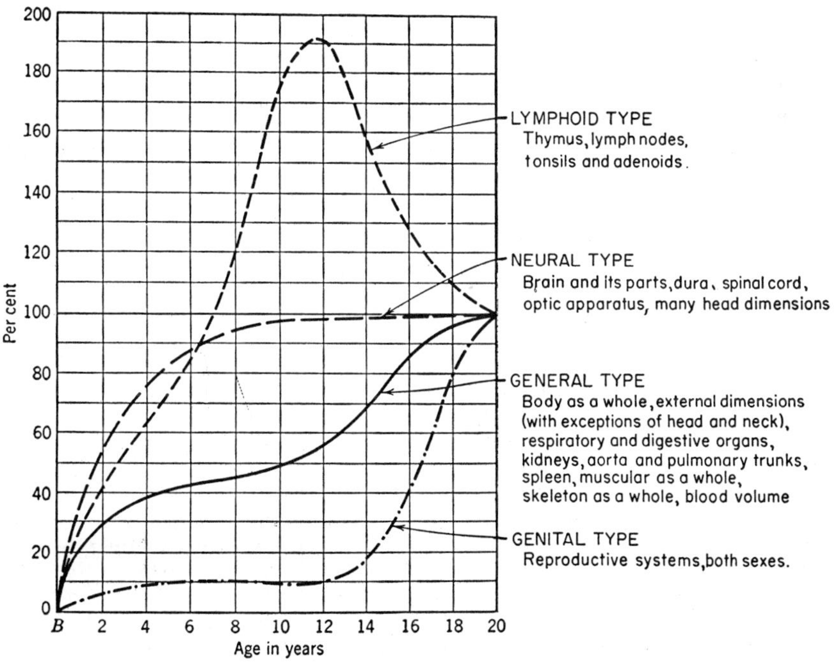

Figure 1 Graph showing growth of various organs of the body. (Scammon: "The Measurement of the Body in Childhood" in Harris, Jackson, Paterson, and Scammon: *The Measurement of Man.* University of Minnesota, 1930.)

Growth of the Whole with Variations

There are two periods of rapid growth in a child—just before birth and at the beginning of pubescence. The slowest rate is between ages two and four and again between six and eight, when a child seems to be marking time. Weight increase averages 5 pounds a year until the age of six and averages 4½ to 8¾ pounds from then until 16 years of age. A child averages an annual increase of 2 inches or better in height. It is not unusual, however, for a boy during adolescence to grow 6 inches in six months to one year, literally growing out of his clothes. Large, well-developed children are likely to reach maturity earlier than the average. The reverse is true for small-sized children. Moreover, a child who is accelerated in skeletal development is more likely to enter puberty at an earlier age. He tends to continue at approximately his original rate of growth, unless it is altered by factors to be discussed later. Children who are tall in preschool days tend to be tall at 18 years. The speed of growth slows up in late adolescence. Generally speaking, the earlier maturity occurs, the earlier the rate of deceleration of growth and final cessation. Increase in weight is noticed more in late summer and autumn, and continues at a reduced rate in spring and early summer.

As for height, another measurable index of growth, boys are generally taller than girls from ages three months to ten years. Then there is a short period from ages ten to 14 years when the girls exceed the boys in height. The early teenage is the time in junior high school when matinee dances cause such agony to a tall girl who is being piloted by a short boy. At this age she favors the tall boys in senior high. Girls at this time are also heavier than boys. At no other period do the girls exceed the boys in these measurements (Figure 2).

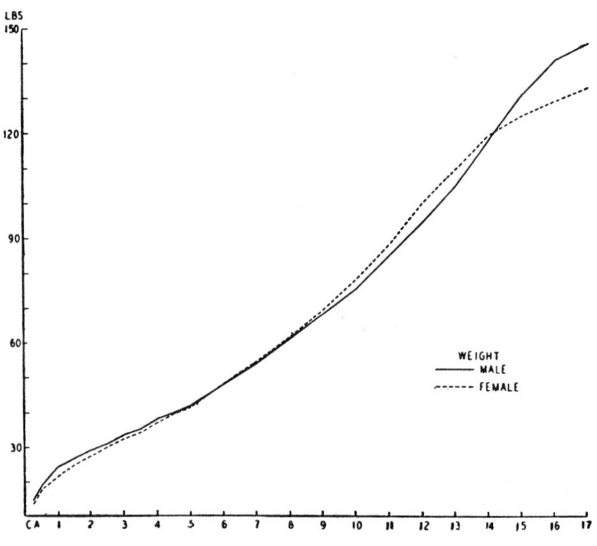

Figure 2 Curves showing the growth in weight of boys and girls from three months to 17 years of age. (From Brush Regular Series. Simmons, K.: The Brush Foundation Study of Child Growth and Development. II. Physical Growth and Development Monogr. 9[1]. Washington, D.C. Society for Research in Child Development, National Research Council, 1944.)

Girls have their adolescent acceleration of growth in height from about ages ten to 12 or 13; boys in general start two years later. "The average boy reaches puberty at about age 15."[1] Pubescence is indicated in girls by the menarche (first menstrual period). This occurs normally between nine and 16 years. The average is 12 to 14 in this country. "After the menarche a girl is not likely to grow more than 3 inches in height."[2] This is a rule to which there are exceptions. A sudden spurt in height and genital growth serves as a notice of beginning of adolescence in boys. The weight increase in girls is caused, to a great extent, by the fatty tissue deposits which characterize feminine contours. The increase in weight in boys is caused by muscular development. The transition to adulthood is completed in girls at about 18 to 19 years of age, and in boys shortly thereafter.

It is interesting to observe the changes in outward proportions as a child grows (Figures 3, 4, and 5). At birth, his head measures about one fourth of his total length. The legs are short but continue to lengthen over the years, proceeding more rapidly than the trunk, especially during early adolescence. Girls at this stage are characterized as leggy, and boys as gangly. The trunk and legs then grow at an equal pace for a while, after which the trunk continues to lengthen in the post-pubescent period. At last the awkward adolescent appears well-proportioned. After the trunk has reached full length, it widens. The stripling becomes broader chested during the last year of senior high school and for a while afterward. Girls, who reach their

[1]Children's Bureau, *Your Child From 6 to 12,* U.S. Department of Health, Education, and Welfare, 1966, p. 14

[2]Ernest H. Watson and George H. Lowrey: *Growth and Development of Children.* Fourth edition. Chicago: The Year Book Medical Publishers, Inc., 1962, p. 88.

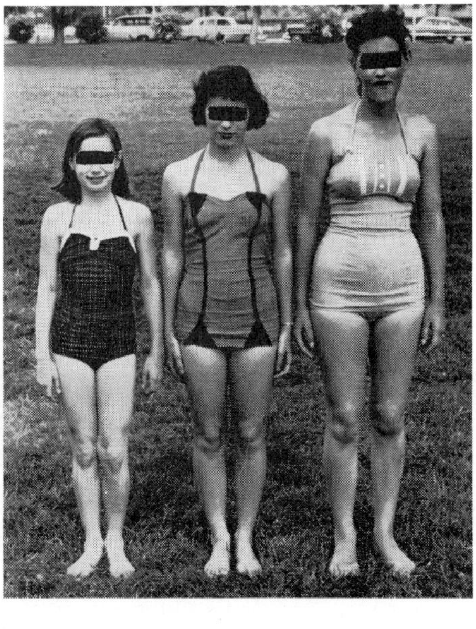

Figure 3 Representative body builds in junior high school girls – seventh, eighth, and ninth grades. Note evidence of maturation processes – widening of pelvic girdle and adult development. Note the increase in growth of the extremities and the trunk.

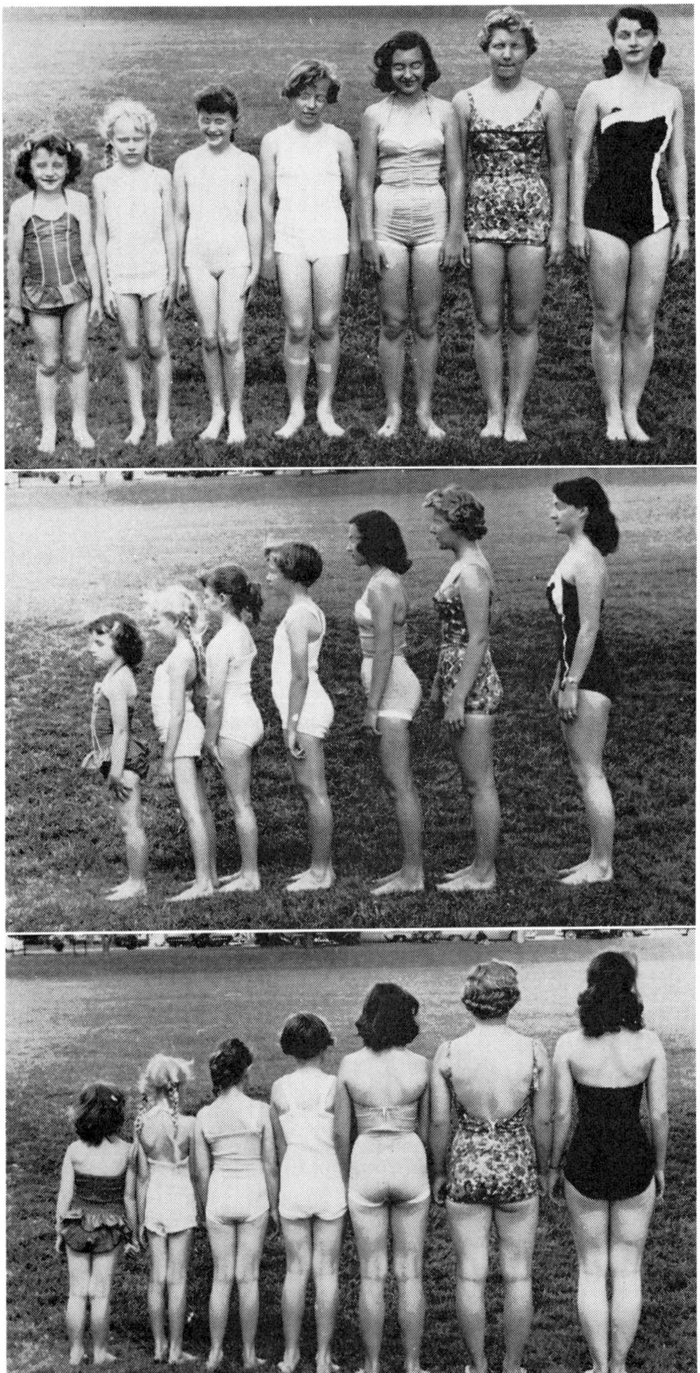

Figure 4 Growth and development. Ages 5-7-9-11-13-15-18. Note figures in side view—the protruding abdomen and prominent scapulae (shoulder blades) are normal up to 13 years of age. There is not too much growth from foot to knee; the increase is from knee to hip.

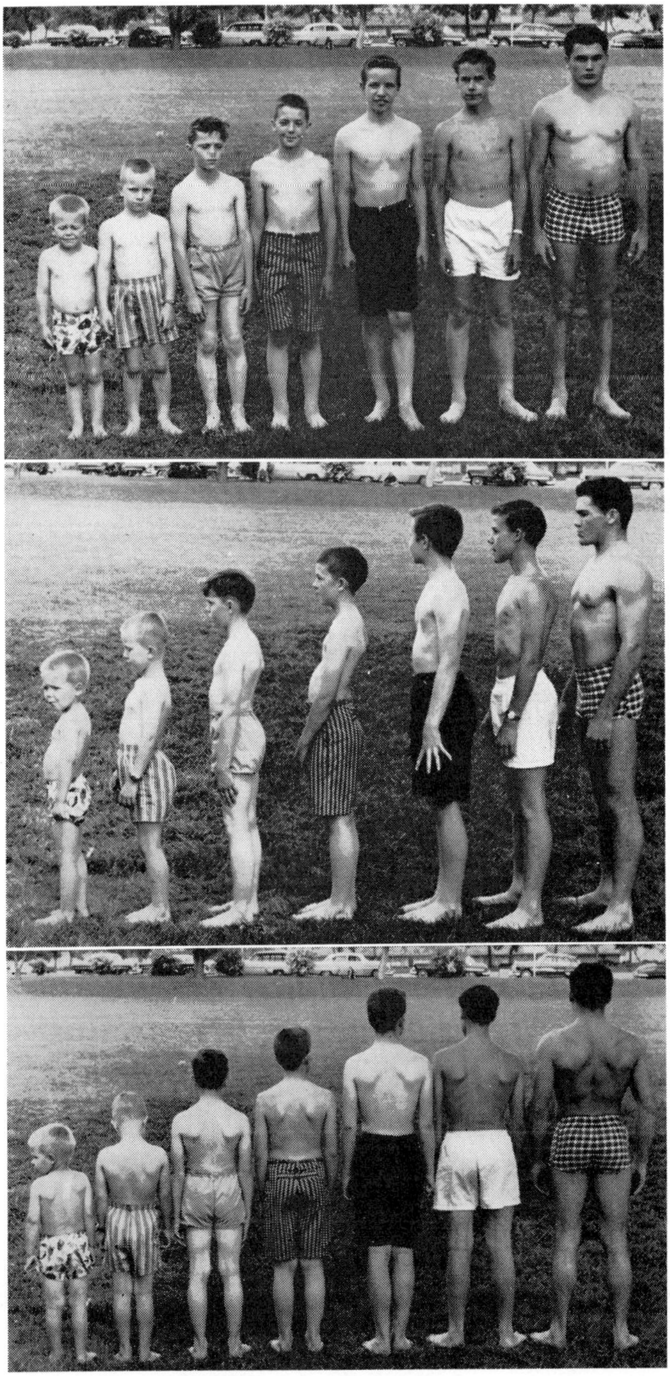

Figure 5 Growth and development. Ages 5-7-9-11-13-15-18. Note gradual increase in height. Shoulder girdle development is prominent.

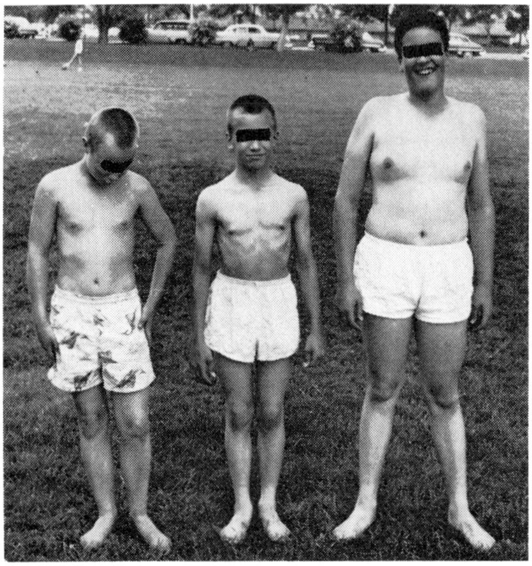

Figure 6 Seventh and eighth grade boys—same chronological age—each maturing at his own rate.

full height earlier than boys, become wider in the hips as well as broader through the shoulder girdle.

Unfortunately, we think in terms of chronological rather than physiological age. Variations may be striking in any classroom, especially in junior high school (Figure 6). Here, a slender, small, baby-faced boy sits next to a robust youth who has already started to shave. A flat-hipped, flat-chested little girl is contrasted to a more developed, more mature classmate. Various physical, emotional, and psychological patterns are represented. The speed of growth and development is not important. What is important is the progress from one stage to another without blocking.

Growth in Individual Organs

Knowledge of growth of the individual organs promotes an understanding of a child and the intelligent management of his daily living. As teeth, eyes, heart, lymphoid tissue, and other parts of the body are discussed in later chapters, references are made to their development at the various age levels. For instance, lymphoid tissue is increased in amount in the first decade of life, as will be observed in the amount of tonsils and adenoids and in the size of lymph nodes. Enlarged tonsils and adenoids create health problems. In later years, lymphoid tissue tends to shrink.

The *heart* grows slowly during the early years. Its adequacy in performing the many functions imposed upon it must be considered in planning physical activity and in protecting the child against infection. It is only after the growth spurt and puberty that the heart grows rapidly, doubles its weight, and reaches adult size in the middle and late teens (Chapter 12); yet, in the early years, during the growth in size of the whole body, the heart must supply the needs of normal metabolism, rapid growth, and physical activity. Youth tires easily. Vigorous physical activities must be interspersed with periods of rest. The excitement of competition, which in itself will increase the heart rate, must be controlled. Physical educators in junior high schools must keep the above facts in mind.

The process of growth of the skeletal system must be understood, as well. In early childhood, bones are largely cartilaginous and soft. As growth proceeds, cartilage cells ultimately are replaced by bone. Then growth ceases. Different bones ossify in their own growth patterns. Vertebrae grow most rapidly from 11 to 15 years of age. Many of the bones of the feet do not become completely ossified until the middle or late teens. Until a bone is completely ossified, injury to cartilage can affect its ultimate size and function.

The growth of a *long bone* occurs at the ends. The *epiphysis* is a piece of bone separated in early life from the shaft of the long bone by a plate of cartilage cells, the epiphyseal plate. These cells are gradually transposed into bone cells and with their continued growth and ossification, the shaft increases in length. Eventually, growth ceases with the disappearance of the plate. The final appearance is a long bone with rounded ends which fit into joints. The area of the epiphyseal plate is well-demarcated, can be observed readily by x-ray, and is quite vulnerable to injury. The epiphysis and the epiphyseal plate can be knocked out of place or fractured. These should be returned to their original positions as soon as possible. Even with the replacements, injury to the plate may result in a growth disturbance of the long bone. It may be shortened or deformed. Hence, injury must be detected early.

This detailed description of the growth of a long bone should serve to emphasize two facts: first, in planning the physical activities of both boys and girls in the elementary and junior high grades, there must be close supervision to detect any complaint of injury to any bone or joint. When young people are participating in organized games, in addition to close supervision, there must be excellent protective equipment.[3]

During periods of rapid growth, children enjoy voracious appetites, and should be supplied with ample amounts of nutritious foods. Because of hormonal change and good appetites, adolescents tend to become overweight. Care must be taken to meet their growth and activity needs without excessive calories. This is easier said than

---

[3]National Committee on School Health Policies of the National Education Association and the American Medical Association, *Suggested School Health Policies*, Joint Committee on Health Problems in Education of the NEA and the AMA, 1966, pp. 32–40.

done, because this is the age when the refrigerator is being raided at all hours and when stacks of sandwiches vanish like magic.

Factors Which Affect Growth

It has been the usual practice to distinguish between the hereditary and environmental, or intrinsic and extrinsic, factors which affect growth. As a matter of fact, except for a few recognized hereditary attributes, such as sex, color of eyes, some developmental defects, body build, height, and characteristic growth patterns, there is no clear line of demarcation between hereditary and environmental factors. Interrelationships between these influences are common. Obviously, an acquired disease of an endocrine gland, particularly during the growth period, may alter impressively the physique of an individual. Tall parents tend to have tall children, yet prolonged severe malnutrition as seen in war-torn countries may cause permanent stunting in height. Is it possible that a favorable environment permits the genes to achieve their potential?

Erroneously, we associate certain body types with so-called nationalities; for instance, the tallness of the Nordic is contrasted with the short stature of the southern Italian. Actually, variations are found in all politically designated populations. To some degree there has been a common ancestry in a locale; but the intermingling of chromosomes over the centuries prevents a rigid concept of race and nationality, or even of particular distinguishing characteristics. Supposed racial traits are seen to be modified by environment.

"Growth is a result of the response which the individual makes to his environment with the hereditary equipment he is given at the time of conception. Few if any traits—intellectual, emotional, physical, social—can be said to be either hereditary or environmental."[4] Except for a few health conditions to be described, no attempt is made here to separate hereditary and environmental factors.

Hereditary Factors. These account for some mental deficiencies and some diseases of the central nervous system, e.g., deafness and blindness. Various skeletal and organic disorders may be present at birth, such as cleft palate and harelip. All of these abnormalities will surely influence intellectual, emotional, and, in most instances, physical development. Heredity seems to influence sexual maturity. A high correlation has been noted between the appearance of menarche (onset of menstruation) in mothers and daughters and between sisters.[5]

Endocrine Glands. The endocrine glands provide the most potent and dynamic influence upon physical and mental characteristics at all ages in life, and especially so during the growth and

---

[4]Harold W. Bernard: *Human Development in Western Culture.* Second edition. Boston: Allyn and Bacon, Inc., 1966, p. 97.

[5]J. M. Tanner: *Growth at Adolescence.* Second edition. Springfield, Illinois: Charles C Thomas, Publisher, 1962, p. 113.

development of an individual. Their function is to a great degree directed by heredity. These glands—pituitary, thyroid, parathyroid, adrenal, pancreas, and gonads—secrete hormones which are powerful in influencing health. The gradations in amounts of secretions, particularly during the growth period, produce interesting variations which characterize a person, his physiognomy, body build, weight, height, general physiological balance, and many other features.

Study of the endocrine glands has produced voluminous information which can only be suggested here. Their function is determined by heredity but can be altered by various disturbances before or after birth. The interrelationship between the glands is so fine that dysfunction in one may result finally in the altered physiology of another. The various hormones may be produced in normal, lowered, or increased amounts. Low function is designated as *hypo*-function, excessive as *hyper*function. Marked deviations in secretion produce fairly typical clinical pictures. There may be delayed growth or permanent stunting (dwarfism) produced by hypothyroidism or by reduced amounts of the growth hormone of the pituitary gland. A disproportionate overgrowth in height (gigantism) is usually caused by hypersecretion of the latter hormone just before and during adolescence.

As has been stated, deviations in hormone production may be caused by heredity or by acquired disorders. Injudicious "dieting" (insufficient nutrients) can affect the ovaries and cause severe menstrual disturbances. Nutritional deficiencies, as seen with low intake of iodine, can influence the physiology of the thyroid gland. Diseases, both acute and chronic, may produce damage. An early nerve or bone injury may cause retardation of growth of bone and muscle in an extremity regardless of hormone activity. Diabetes is usually considered to be hereditary in tendency, but there are occasions when a specific acquired causative factor is known.

Congenital Defects. These may affect embryonic or postnatal growth. Some congenital heart anomalies definitely alter the growth pattern; but with modern surgery many of these defects are corrected early.

Environmental Factors. Environmental factors may be complex and interrelated. No one circumstance will explain the whole picture. Discussion of one major factor, the *socioeconomic status* of a family, must encompass all of the aspects of family living to which a child is exposed. Families with good income can afford better housing, medical care, food, and education. With more living space, sick children can be isolated so that others in the family may be protected. Hygienic rules for rest and sleep and diet are better observed, particularly in a child's earlier years. Studies show that children from families in the higher socioeconomic bracket tend to have greater average height and weight than those less privileged, although many of both groups are identical in height and weight.

Climate. Climate and seasonal variations seem to have a slight influence upon the pattern of growth. In temperate climates children usually acquire more height in the spring and gain more weight in the fall. How much these observations can be explained by diet, winter sicknesses, and amount of exercise is problematical. When children return to school in the fall, their activities are somewhat curtailed and their diet will usually contain more starches and fewer vegetables. Perhaps this type of living will account for gain in weight. Respiratory infections and childhood communicable diseases occurring later in the school year can cause a retardation in weight gain or actual loss of pounds.

Nutrition. This is manifestly a major factor in growth and development. Weight is more affected than height. During growth the long bones and nervous system will secure any nutritives which may be present in the body at the expense of all the other organs; therefore, height will not be much affected unless malnutrition is prolonged and severe. Malnutrition can delay growth and may retard the adolescent spurt. Adequate nutrition, particularly in the early years, also influences intellectual development. More discussion on nutrition in relation to growth follows in a later chapter.

Activity and Exercise. These are necessary to some extent for muscular and motor development, for good muscle tone, and for finer coordination. Exercise must be based on age, sex, physical condition, and individual reaction to activity. Not every child can execute a set number of sit-ups to indicate physical fitness, nor should he be downgraded on this basis.

Illness. Particularly if extended or severe, illness may directly alter the developmental pattern of an organ or part of the body, and as a consequence, alter growth in general. Rheumatic fever may cause damage to the heart and affect its function. Acute illness, such as whooping cough, streptococcal infections, or kidney infections, may delay growth for a while; but usually the lag is overcome. Normal children who have frequent minor ailments suffer no permanent impairment of growth. A child who has been absent from school for some time with an illness may on his return show a loss of weight and mark time for a while before again gaining either in weight or height.

In the wealthier countries, with progress in medical knowledge, health education, child psychology, and better care, children are maturing earlier and growing taller and heavier with each generation. In the period from 1850 to 1950 the average age for pubescence in the female decreased from 17 to 13.5 years of age. In the United States one study reveals that in 1900 the menarche occurred at about 14.5 years of age but now occurs at an average of 13 years in the same region. The adolescent growth spurt seems to begin sooner, and the final stature is reached at an earlier age than in previous generations.[6]

Comparison studies of heights and weights of our young people

---

[6] Ernest H. Watson and George H. Lowrey: *Growth and Development of Children.* Chicago: The Year Book Medical Publishers, Inc., 1962, pp. 33–34.

made with an urban group in the years 1885 to 1900, and 1935 to 1953 show that young men of 15 to 16 years are 1.8 inches taller and 10 pounds heavier; at ages 17 to 19 they have gained 1.6 inches and weigh slightly less than the older generation. Girls of 15 to 16 years are 0.6 inch taller and 1.3 pounds heavier, and in ages 17 to 19 are about 0.4 inch taller and have decreased 3.2 pounds in weight. The smaller gains in girls in the late teens can be explained by early attainment of final height and the current emphasis on slenderness.[7]

On the whole our current generation of well-nourished children is fulfilling its maximum growth potential.

Evaluation of the Progress of Growth and Development

Measurements of height and weight are commonly employed in estimating the progress of growth. Since growth is dependent to a great extent upon good nutrition, the same measurements are also used, with limitations, to judge the nutritional status of an individual. All the standards or scales for evaluation of the height and weight of a particular child are subject to criticism.

The Height-Weight-Age Standards. For years charts have been used which give standards based upon the height, weight, and age of a child. In general these charts are acceptable if he has average build, but they do not take into account variations in stature. Most of our weight is bone and muscle. Naturally, the child who has small bones and slight build will always appear underweight, according to these standards; conversely, the husky, broad, heavily muscled, big-boned youngster will be recorded as overweight. In both instances, the standards will be inaccurate. To make allowances for this apparent discrepancy, it is customary to permit a leeway of 10 per cent below the accepted average before considering a child underweight, and 20 per cent above before considering him overweight. There is a tendency on the part of children and adults, however, to feel that weights must conform exactly to the average indicated and to ignore the wide margin.

Height-Weight-Age-Width Standards. Because of the inadequacy of the long-used height-weight-age scales, attempts have been made to formulate others which consider body build. Standards are available which consider pelvic and chest width, and, in some studies, knee and leg circumferences. These various measurements all attempt to assay physique in order to reach more reasonable norms. The slender child and the broad child receive merited consideration with these criteria, and their averages will differ from those recorded on the usual height-weight-age scale. If a youngster is average in build, the norms from various scales will approximate each other. If one is

---

[7]Metropolitan Insurance Company: "Growth Trends in the Teen Ages." *Statistical Bulletin,* October, 1960.

not well-proportioned, as noticed at times in older girls with average chests and hips, and short, heavily muscled thighs, then no formulated standards will apply. These girls need reassurance that they are not overweight and that, with their type of muscular development, they do not need to conform to the usual norms.

In the final analysis, the numbers on a weight chart are not conclusive as far as estimation of a child's growth is concerned. Anyone with an experienced eye, who has been observing a child in a classroom over a period of time, can evaluate his progress. As long as he is healthy and is gaining in height and weight, he does not need to fit into a category. He competes with his own past performance and with no one else.

Growth Chart. A simple procedure of evaluation is to keep a "growth chart" on each child, something comparable to Figure 7, and record the height and weight at frequent, regular intervals. The child watches the ascent of the connecting lines between the plotted points. Children want to grow taller and larger, and this chart serves as a teaching device. A youngster should be eager to participate in periodic measurements of his height and weight, and will find satisfaction in his achievements. Any alterations in rate of progress or any loss of weight can be discussed with the child himself. The growth chart offers a springboard for investigation of health problems.

Various printed forms have been used by school systems. Physical growth records for boys and girls were developed by the Joint

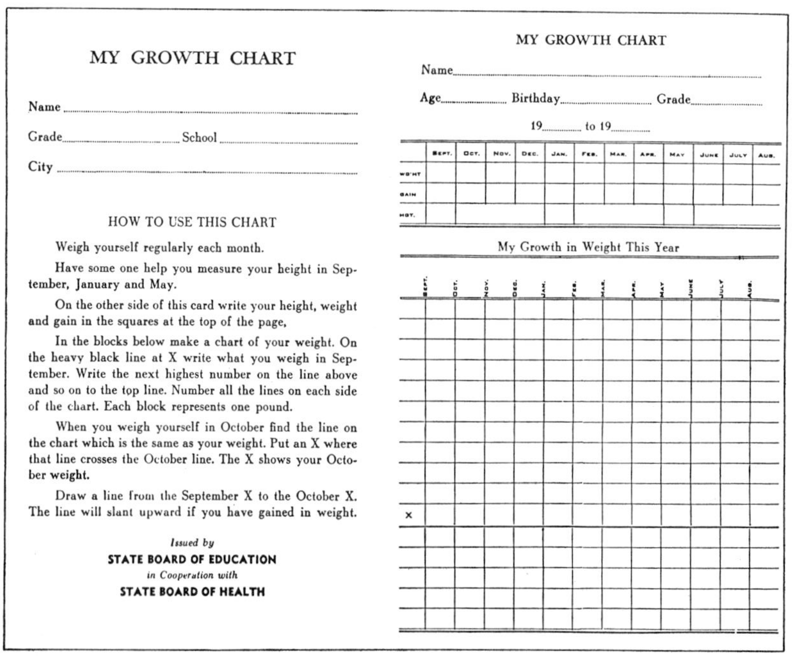

MY GROWTH CHART

Name ....

Grade .... School ....

City ....

HOW TO USE THIS CHART

Weigh yourself regularly each month.

Have some one help you measure your height in September, January and May.

On the other side of this card write your height, weight and gain in the squares at the top of the page.

In the blocks below make a chart of your weight. On the heavy black line at X write what you weigh in September. Write the next highest number on the line above and so on to the top line. Number all the lines on each side of the chart. Each block represents one pound.

When you weigh yourself in October find the line on the chart which is the same as your weight. Put an X where that line crosses the October line. The X shows your October weight.

Draw a line from the September X to the October X. The line will slant upward if you have gained in weight.

Issued by
STATE BOARD OF EDUCATION
in Cooperation with
STATE BOARD OF HEALTH

MY GROWTH CHART

Name ....

Age .... Birthday .... Grade ....

19.......... to 19..........

	SEPT.	OCT.	NOV.	DEC.	JAN.	FEB.	MAR.	APR.	MAY	JUNE	JULY	AUG.
WG'HT												
GAIN												
HGT.												

My Growth in Weight This Year

Figure 7 My growth chart. (Prepared by the Utah State Board of Education.)

Committee on Health Problems in Education of the American Medical Association and the National Education Association (Meredith Physical Growth Records, reproduced in Appendix B). These indicate normal zones for gradations of stature and weight. Instructions for their use accompany the forms.

Wetzel's Grid.[8] (Appendix B.) Using the simple information on height, weight, and age, Wetzel devised a grid which provides an objective method of evaluating a child's trend in growth and development according to body build and physical status. Copies of the Wetzel grid and of modified forms with instructions for use are available.

Wetzel's grid is not commonly used in schools, but is used more in institutions and for research purposes. One study on 134 boys, covering a ten-year span from the grades 3 through 12, had the objective of discovering the relationship between their growth and scholastic achievement. The latter was evaluated by teachers' marks, periodic intelligence test scores and profile ratings, and achievement test results. Physical growth was evaluated twice a year on the Wetzel grid. The data revealed that poor directions of growth were accompanied by scholastic underachievement which grew worse as the years of poor growth persisted. The conclusion reached was that steady scholastic achievement, consistent with a student's intellectual capacity, cannot be expected from those whose physical growth is demonstrated to be under par by Wetzel's grid standards.[9]

In using these various standards for evaluating growth, a teacher must remember that they are not substitutes for the periodic health examination. However, since less than one third of school children are seen at least every two years for medical checkups from their own physicians, it is good for nurses and teachers to have a growth chart of some type on every child. It is only one more tool for evaluation. Constant observation by the teacher in the classroom to detect defects is still most important in preserving and promoting the health of a child. Another reminder is that emotional development is not evaluated to any extent by these measurements. Only insofar as emotional disturbances affect general health and nutrition will deviations be noticed.

Since the height and weight measurements on a child provide valuable health history, they should be available for the examining physician.

Technique of Measuring Height and Weight. Instructions on actual technique in securing these data may seem superfluous; nevertheless, it is surprising to note the number of children whose height is taken inaccurately (Figure 8).

---

[8]Norman C. Wetzel: "Physical Fitness in Terms of Physique, Development and Basal Metabolism, with a Guide to Individual Progress from Infancy to Maturity. New Method for Evaluation." *J.A.M.A.* *116*:1187–1195, 1941.

[9]H. H. Hopwood and S. S. Van Iden: "Scholastic Underachievement as Related to Sub-Par Physical Growth." *J. Sch. Health* 35:337–349, 1965.

Height can be measured by any standard, such as the one attached to beam scales, or by a ruled strip of metal, wood, or paper applied to a wall. The child should have his back to the standard with chin in horizontal position; the feet should be parallel and close together (shoes removed); heels, buttocks, and shoulders should touch the wall. Whatever object is used as a cross-arm should press through the hair and just clear the crown of the head.

Weight should be taken at the same time of day with the same amount of clothing on, or with the child disrobed. The beam type of scales is preferable to the spring type.

Sliding calipers with instructions for measuring hip and chest widths can be purchased. Standards are secured with them.

The attitude of the teacher toward this whole project of weighing and measuring is important. He can make it an ordeal to be dreaded by the large and the tiny people, or he can instill anticipation and pride. No derogatory comparisons or embarrassing comments should ever be made.

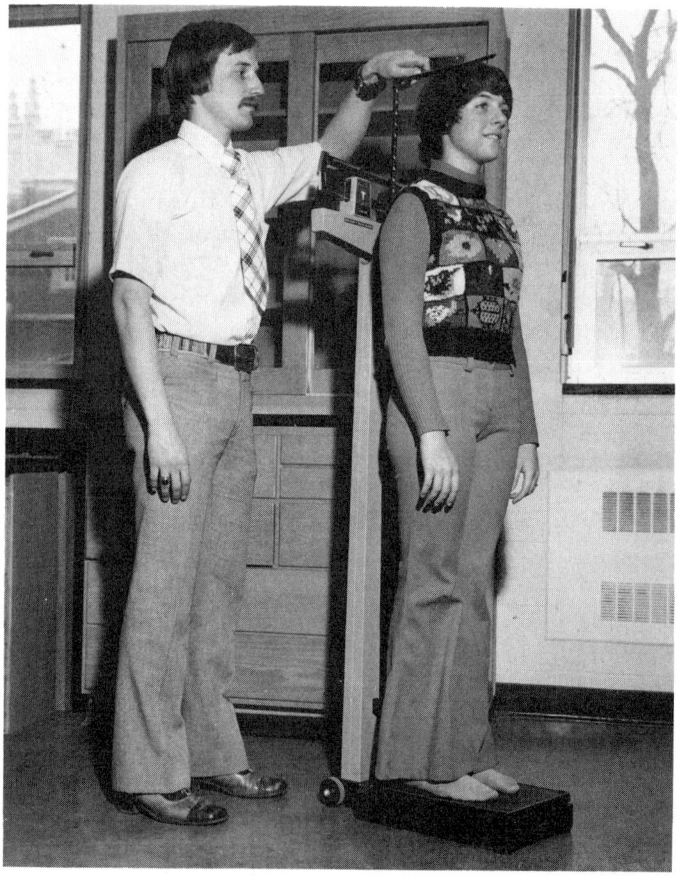

Figure 8 Measuring height–chin horizontal, back to the standard, no shoes.

Physical, Emotional, Social, and Intellectual Changes

Just how important to an educator is an understanding of growth and development in children? The answer is simple. The whole fabric of education is based upon this knowledge. Because of the need for understanding the characteristics and needs of a child as he progresses from birth to high school graduation, the tables on the following pages were formulated. Curriculum planning and methodology of teaching rely upon these observations. In the selection of content for health education and in the determination of methods for presentation of this content, the teacher takes into account such factors as the physical growth of a child, his intellectual interests, his attention span, his need for rest, and his interactions with peer group, family, and society. The various needs of this child must be met at each level, whether it be physical, emotional, social, or intellectual.

Study the following tables. As the eyes scan the charts horizontally, the planning of a progressive, continuous program in many aspects of education is unfolded—physical education, health education, family life, and mental health education. Physical defects are more prominent at certain ages. Age levels for satisfaction of curiosity, optimum mental stimulation, appeals to idealism, and the needs for social adjustments are designated. As the eyes move down each column, one gets a picture of the child in his age group. The opportunities for improving every facet of a child's development are many and challenging.

The whole school health program is based upon our knowledge of the growth and development in children. Even the architectural planning of a school varies from elementary to junior high to senior high schools, because the physical beings of children, their learning experiences, and the curricula differ. The same can be said for school health services and health education at different ages.

SUMMARY

Young people are in better health, are taller, and mature earlier than previous generations. Good food, plenty of play and rest, early detection and correction of defects, protection from disease, prompt and adequate medical care, and a wholesome emotional climate promote favorable growth and development and enable a child to reach his genetic potential. Teachers not only must understand the process of growth and development from kindergarten through high school, but must understand that each child is an individual who has his own pattern of growth. *There is no normal, average child.*

Tables 1 and 2 on the following pages present in outline form the characteristics and needs of school-age children. The changes in growth and development from one age level to the next are apparent.

Emotional Development. Physical growth and development

(*Text continued on page 36.*)

TABLE 1 Physical, Emotional, Social, and Intellectual Characteristics of School-Age Youth*

	PRESCHOOL AGES 3 THROUGH 5	KINDERGARTEN THROUGH GRADE 3 AGES 5 THROUGH 8	GRADES 4 THROUGH 6 AGES 8 THROUGH 11	GRADES 7 THROUGH 9 AGES 11 THROUGH 14	GRADES 10 THROUGH 12 AGES 14 THROUGH 18
PHYSICAL	Rate of growth slows. Disproportion in size of trunk to short arms and legs, and trunk to head. Still developing balance, falls easily.	Growth relatively slow.	Growth slow and steady. Girls begin to forge ahead of boys in height and weight. Extremities begin to lengthen toward end of this period.	Accelerated, uneven growth. Individual differences most prominent; girls continue rapid growth, are taller and heavier than boys in early period.	Rapid growth nearing end of physical maturity by graduation time. Increase in height of trunk, then widening of shoulder and pelvic girdles.
	Large muscle development. Locomotor and manipulative play enjoyed. Physically more stable in circulation, respiration, and body temperature. Body functions and habits fairly well established.	Increase in large muscle coordination, beginning of development of small muscle control. Bones growing. Nose grows larger.	Muscle coordination improving. Continued small muscle development. Bones growing, vulnerable to injury.	Muscular growth toward adult size begins toward end of period. Variable coordination. Bones growing, vulnerable to injury.	Gradual increase in adult muscular development. Posture approaches adult stance. Bone growth gradually reaches completion.
	Primary teeth erupted.	Permanent teeth appearing or replacing primary teeth. Lower part of face more prominent. Hungry at short intervals. May overeat and become fat.	Permanent dentition continues. Malocclusion may be a problem. Appetite good. Increasing interest in food.	Dental caries common. Permanent dentition – 28 teeth. Malocclusion may be present. Appetite ravenous but may be capricious.	Dental caries common. Malocclusion may be present. Voracious appetite. Develops food fads.
	Restless, active. Fatigue displayed by crossness, possibly heightened activity.	Enjoys active play – climbing, jumping, running. Susceptible to fatigue and limits himself.	Boundless energy. Tires easily.	Enjoys vigorous play. Tires easily (girls especially).	Vigorous play satisfying. Still tires readily in early period.
	Visual acuity approaches normal.	Visual acuity reaches normal.	Visual acuity normal.	Visual problems increase.	Visual problems increase.
	Highly susceptible to communicable diseases.	Susceptible to respiratory and communicable diseases.	Menarche possible towards end of this period.	Variations in development of secondary sexual characteristics. Menarche. Skin problems, voice changes, etc. Reproductive organs growing.	Approaches and completes adult maturation.

*See footnote to Table 2.

(*Table 1 continued on the opposite page.*)

EMOTIONAL	Self-centered—just learning to share. Wants to do things himself. Resents interference with play or possessions. May show off, yet shy of strangers. Periods of negativism in effort to exert self-determination. Few inhibitions, frank expression of emotion; may bite, scratch, fight, or cry to get what he wants. Shows affection freely. Accepts self as an individual. Increasing individuality. Strong attachment to mother.	Self-centered, desires immediate attention to his problem—wants to be first. Sensitive at being left out. Sensitive to ridicule, criticism, or loss of prestige. Easily aroused emotionally. Can take responsibility but needs adult supervision. Parent image strong, also identifies with teacher. Expresses likes and dislikes readily.	Seeks approval of peer group. Desire to succeed. Enthusiastic, noisy, imaginative, desire to explore. Negativistic—early part of period. Begins to accept responsibility for clothing and behavior. Increasingly anxious about family and possible tragedy.	Emotional instability—sudden and deep swings in mood. Strong feelings of like and dislike, negative and positive attitudes. Sensitive, self-critical but cannot take criticism. Overanxious about health—thinks he has a gruesome disease. Over-concerned about physical and emotional changes. Striving for independence from adults. Hero worship. Searching for sensational emotional experiences. Self-conscious.	Intensely emotional, labile, volatile, gradually settles down. Sensitive to economic and social status of family and self. Sensitive to own inadequacies and incompetencies—may be expressed as antisocial or childish behavior. Concerned about future. Intensely loyal to an individual or group with whom he identifies. Still striving for independence from parents and others, but often wants adult support. Self-conscious.
	Curious about sex organs.	Questioning attitude about sex differences.	Increasing self-consciousness. Sex hostility. Becomes "modest" but not too interested in details of sex.	Shows growing restraint in expressing feelings. Unique sense of humor.	
SOCIAL	Will cooperate in play but likes to be "bigger than." Cooperative play and parallel play intermixed. Begins to initiate play with several other children. Beginning sense of ownership, but more willing to share.	Lack of interest in personal grooming. Engages in imitative play. Friendly, frank, sometimes aggressive, "bossy," assertive. Generally tolerant of race, economic status, etc.	Learns to cooperate better. Group planning and group play, and abides by group decisions. Interested in competitive activities and prestige. Competition keen. Begins to show qualities of leadership.	Interested in competitive sports as participant and spectator. Developing good sportsmanship. Socially insecure. Peer-conscious—very much so. Desires freedom with security. Argues against authority but wants it.	More mature adjustments in social groups. Sense of fair play in games. Concerned about justice, moral code, right and wrong. Responds well to group responsibility and group participation.
	Responsive to cultural pressures.		Developing interest in appearance.	Sensitive to appearance, clothes, skin. Imitative fads in clothing, speech, etc.	Regards possessions as evidence of social prestige. Imitative fads.
		Gradually more socially oriented and adjusted.	Strong sense of fair play. Belongs to a gang or secret club. Loyal to group.	Wishes to conform to clearly defined pattern of good school citizenship. Assumes responsibility for personal and group conduct. Beginning to discriminate right from wrong	Tends to challenge traditional customs, values, and procedures. Tends to identify with an older, admired friend. Wants to be accepted by gang, clique, or social group.

(Table 1 continued on the following page.)

TABLE 1 Physical, Emotional, Social, and Intellectual Characteristics of School-Age Youth* *(Continued)*

	Boys and girls play together. Similar interests.	Boys and girls play together as sex equals, but aware of sex differences.	Close friendships with members of own sex. Separate play for boys and girls.	Aware of opposite sex, chivalry, rivalry, teasing. Separating into groups by sex – boys into large groups, girls into small groups – then gradually to mixed groups.	Interested in opposite sex, gradually, consciously or unconsciously, seeking a mate.
INTELLECTUAL	Imaginative play. Learns to distinguish between real and fantasy.	Varied intellectual growth and ability of children.	Likes to talk and express ideas.	Eager to learn. Curious, alert, exploring.	Wider range of differences in mental abilities of students.
	Beginning interest in stories, music, art work. Laughter and nonverbal forms of communication are frequent.	Interested in things that move, bright colors, dramatizations, rhythmics, making collections.	High potential of learning – in science, adventure, the world. Eager to acquire skills.	Reads widely. Wider range of abilities and interests. Wants to succeed. Wants precise assignments and meaningful experiences.	May tend to subordinate intellectual drives to social and emotional. Is trying to establish a degree of independence – intellectually, socially, and economically.
	Growing interest in world around him, what makes things "work." Developing initiative and language communication.	Interested in the present, not the future. Learns best through active participation in concrete, meaningful situations. Can abide by safety rules. Wants to know "why."	Wide range of interests. Curious, wants to experiment. Goals are immediate. Demands consistency. Generally reliable about following instructions.	Skeptical, demands facts. Unrealistic in passing judgment. Overconfident in own information.	Searching for ideals – developing a philosophy of life. Planning future role. Extending interest to world situation, citizenship, scientific progress.
	Easily distracted.	Attention span short.	Attention span short.	Increasing span of attention and concentration.	Long periods of concentration possible.

TABLE 2 Physical, Emotional, Social, and Intellectual Needs of School-Age Youth*

	PRESCHOOL AGES 3 THROUGH 5	KINDERGARTEN THROUGH GRADE 3 AGES 5 THROUGH 8	GRADES 4 THROUGH 6 AGES 8 THROUGH 11	GRADES 7 THROUGH 9 AGES 11 THROUGH 14	GRADES 10 THROUGH 12 AGES 14 THROUGH 18
PHYSICAL	To have wide variety of activities for use of large muscles – running, climbing, hanging.	To develop large muscle control through motor skills.	To develop and improve coordination of both large and small muscles.	To have adequate nourishment for growth spurt and daily energy.	To have plenty of nutritious foods and establish good habits of food selection – to avoid food fads.
		To have play space and materials.			
	To use equipment for developing muscle control – wagons, tricycles, hammer, nails, blocks, dolls, sand.	To use instructional tools and equipment geared to stage of development.	To have plenty of activities and games which will develop body control, strength, endurance, and skills – stunts, throwing, catching, running, "it," bicycles, skates.	To understand developmental changes of adolescence.	To understand body growth and development of own and opposite sex.
				To recognize wide physical differences as normal.	To accept individual differences without feeling inferior or superior, knowing that differences are desirable.
	To develop independence (self-help) in toileting, washing, dressing, eating.	To establish basic health habits – toileting, eating, covering nose and mouth with cough, etc.	To have careful supervision of games appropriate to strength and developmental needs – protective equipment.	To have good protective equipment in games.	To have help in accepting or improving own stature, muscular development, complexion, visual defects, etc.
		To have snack time and opportunity to develop social graces.	To have competitive activity with children of comparable size.		
	To have guidance in establishing habits of cleanliness, sleep, and rest.	To have plenty of sleep and rest, and exercise interspersed with rest.	To have sleep, rest, well-balanced meals.	To have physical activity interspersed with rest.	To have adequate rest.
	To have health examinations and follow-up.	To have health examinations and follow-up.	To have health examinations and follow-up.	To have health examinations and follow-up.	To have health examinations and follow-up.
	To have visual and auditory checks.	To have visual and auditory checks.	To have visual and auditory checks.	To have visual and auditory checks.	To have visual and auditory checks.
	To have dental attention.	To have dental attention.	To have dental attention.	To have dental attention.	To have dental attention.
	To discover emotional satisfactions with companions of own age group.	To receive encouragement, recognition, ample praise, patience, and adult support.	To begin seriously to gain a realistic image of self and appreciate uniqueness of personality.	To express volatile emotions, grief, anger, disappointments, likes, dislikes.	To have relationships with adults who invite confidence and give moral support and security.
	To begin independence from parents yet maintain security of parental protection.	To express inner feelings, anxieties, and fears.	To be recognized for individual worth, to feel self-assurance and self-esteem.	To assume responsibility for own conduct.	To achieve success.
	To have freedom to explore, try new ideas, extend environment, "to do," "to help."	To feel secure, loved, wanted, accepted (at home and at school).	To receive encouragement and affection, to be understood and appreciated.	To achieve more independence.	To have a family solidarity as an escape from the confusion of the world.
		To be free from pressure to achieve beyond capabilities.		To feel secure, wanted, loved, trusted, adequate, capable.	

(Table 2 continued on the following page.)

TABLE 2 Physical, Emotional, Social, and Intellectual Needs of School-Age Youth* (Continued)

	PRESCHOOL AGES 3 THROUGH 5	KINDERGARTEN THROUGH GRADE 3 AGES 5 THROUGH 8	GRADES 4 THROUGH 6 AGES 8 THROUGH 11	GRADES 7 THROUGH 9 AGES 11 THROUGH 14	GRADES 10 THROUGH 12 AGES 14 THROUGH 18
EMOTIONAL	To have adult support individual needs of acceptance and love.	To have a consistent, cooperatively planned program of classroom control. Must have guidance.	To exercise self-control.	To have privacy respected.	
			To talk out problems, receive reasonable explanations, to have questions answered.	To exercise self-discipline.	To exercise self-control.
	To have affectionate personal interests of adults.	To develop self-confidence.		To experience success, receive individual recognition.	To be accepted, receive approval and recognition.
	To accept authority.	To have some immediate desirable satisfactions.		To identify with a friendly adult – teacher, parent, older friend.	To understand one's self and others.
	To learn to identify with parents, siblings, and others.	To know limitations within which he can operate effectively.		To be alone occasionally.	To have group acceptance and identification.
		To develop realistic expectations of self.		To feel the support, firm guidance, and assurance of an adult.	
				To differentiate between reality and fiction, fact and fiction.	
SOCIAL	To have companionship and play with other children of same age.	To have satisfactory peer relationships, to receive group approval.	To be recognized and accepted by peer groups – receive social approval.	To see one's self as a socially accepted, important person.	To feel adequate in associations with the opposite sex.
	To take turns and share – cooperative and loosely shared play with one or at times several children.	To learn the importance of sharing, planning, working, and playing together – both boys and girls.	To have relationships with adults which give feelings of security and acceptance.	To relate to members of the same and opposite sex.	To have a wide variety of social activities and competencies, including social dancing.
	To enjoy active play.	To have help in developing socially acceptable behavior.		To receive recognition from and acceptance by peers.	To be increasingly independent.
	To have help in gaining social skills.		To assume responsibilities, have increased opportunities for independent actions and decisions.	To work and play with different age groups.	To talk, to communicate freely with others on any topic.
	To accept children who are "different."	To learn to assume some responsibility, to have opportunities to initiate activities, to lead.	To develop appreciation for others and their rights.		To increase wholesome relationships with people of all ages, races, creeds, and cultures.

*Material for Tables 1 and 2 was gleaned from many sources. One valuable source was "Curriculum Framework for Utah Schools – A Guide to Curriculum Planning," which presents (1) the summarized reports of teachers who met in the school districts and worked in groups, concentrating upon the age levels in which they were interested, and (2) suggested changes made by administrators at a conference.

(Table 2 continued on the opposite page.)

	To note sex differences and cultural roles of the sexes.	To work independently and in groups. To accept sex role. To develop an appreciation of social values, such as honesty, sportsmanship, etc.	To learn to get along with others and accept those different from self.	To recognize the importance of leadership as well as being a follower. To have congenial social settings.	To receive fair and consistent treatment. To have respect for authority.
INTELLECTUAL	To have first-hand experiences—to see, feel, touch, taste, smell. To have explanations repeated while learning new concepts. To have time and opportunity to explore. To have answers to "why." To be treated with patience and courtesy and listened to and talked to by accepting adults.	To experience frequent success and learn to accept failure when it occurs. To have concrete learning experiences and direct participation. To be in a rich, stable, challenging environment. To have time to adjust to new experiences and new situations. To learn to follow through to completion. To develop a love for learning. To learn without developing feelings of hostility. To communicate effectively.	To experiment, explore, solve problems, be challenged, use initiative, select, plan, evaluate. To receive individual help in skill areas without harmful or undue pressure. To have opportunities for creative self-expression. To have a rich environment of materials and the opportunity to explore it. To participate in concrete, real-life situations. To be able to accept one's self with strengths and weaknesses.	To determine individual motives, goals, standards, and ideals. To satisfy curiosity, desire to know, to experiment. To express one's self orally, manually, and through activities such as dance, music, clubs, debate, etc. To appreciate the value of work and products of work. To know the satisfaction of achieving to the extent of one's ability.	To set realistic goals in terms of interest and ability. To receive vocational guidance. To assume responsibility for own acts and decisions. To understand values of achievements and behavior. To develop own interests, personal skills, and talents. To have direction in critical thinking. To develop a wholesome philosophy of life. To develop leisure-time resources and cultural interests. To develop a respect for work.

cannot be separated from emotional development. The two aspects of the whole being are completely interrelated and should be discussed together. However, because the subject of mental health is so broad, and a description of the school and community programs for handling mental health problems of children should be quite detailed, and also because there are a number of health problems with prominent emotional implications, the discussion of emotional development is presented in a later chapter after problems which are more physical in nature have been presented.

DISCUSSION QUESTIONS AND ACTIVITIES

1. Define growth. Define development. How are they different and how are they interrelated?
2. Describe "normal" growth and development characteristics. Why is it important to know these characteristics?
3. Discuss the growth parameters of individual organs. How do some school programs hamper normal growth?
4. What external factors affect growth? How?
5. What are the advantages and disadvantages of the various methods for evaluating progress of growth and development?
6. How valid are age-height-weight tables? When and how should they be used and interpreted?
7. Discuss the use of the Wetzel grid.
8. Discuss the use of the physical growth records developed by the Joint Committee on Health Problems in Education of the American Medical Association and the National Education Association.
9. Learn the technique for measuring height and weight and try it out on several people.
10. Discuss the relationships between growth and development and the learning process.

ADDITIONAL SOURCES OF INFORMATION

READINGS

Birch, H. G.: "Symposium; Nutrition, Growth, and Mental Development. Eightieth Annual Meeting of the American Pediatric Society." *Am. J. Dis. Child.* 120:395–397, November, 1970.

Dugdale, A. E. et al.: "Patterns of Growth and Nutrition in Childhood." *Am. J. Clin. Nutr.* 23:1280–1287, October, 1970.

Eisner, V. et al.: "Health Assessment of School Children VI. Height and Weight." *J. Sch. Health* 42:164–166, March, 1972.

"Growth Patterns and Sex Education, A Suggested Program Kindergarten through Grade Twelve." Special issue. *J. Sch. Health* 37, No. 5a, May, 1967.

Hansman, C.: "Physical Maturation in the Teenager." *J. Sch. Health* 42:509–512, November, 1972.

Smart, M. S., and Smart, R. C.: *Children—Development and Relationship.* New York: Macmillan Co., 1967.

Thomson, A. M.: "The Evaluation of Human Growth Patterns." *Am. J. Dis. Child.* 120:398–403, November, 1970.

Thomson, A. M.: "Hypoglycemia in Children. Relationship Between Adrenocortical Function and Growth." *Am. J. Dis. Child.* 121:10–14, January, 1971.

U.S. Department of Health, Education, and Welfare: National Institute of Child Health and Human Development. Write for catalog.
"Your Child from One to Six." Publication 30 (Revised 1962), 105 pp.
"Your Child from Three to Four." Publication 446 (1967), 22 pp.
"Your Child from Six to Twelve." Publication 324 (1966), 98 pp. U.S. Government Printing Office, Washington, D.C.

Curriculum guides which detail the characteristics and needs of the growing child, with educational implications, are available from state and local departments of education.

AUDIOVISUAL AIDS

And So They Grow
28 min. — Campus Films Productions, Inc.*
Documentary.
Highlights the variety of approaches in meeting children's ever-widening interests. Suitable for teacher education.

Changing Voice
45 min. — Color — International Film Bureau
Demonstrates nature and uses of voices of seventh and eighth grade children. Concert presented as illustration.

Child Development Series
13–22 min. — Black and White — McGraw-Hill
"Child Care and Development"
"Children's Emotions"
"Children's Fantasies"
"Development of Individual Differences"
"Each Child is Different"
"Physical Aspects of Puberty"
"Principles of Development"
"Sibling Relationships"
Somewhat old but still good.

The Time of Man
54 min. — Color — Metromedia Producers Corp.
Describes the natural history of our world.

They Grow Up So Fast
27 min. — Color — Association Films, Inc.
Designed to interpret physical education to the public, to educators, and to parents.

U.S. Department of Health, Education, and Welfare.
"Selected Films on Child Life." Publication 376 (1965).
Children's Bureau. Annotated listing of 480 films.

MATERIALS FOR TEACHERS' USE IN SCHOOLS

AUDIOVISUAL MATERIALS

Recommended grade levels are designated *pri, int, jh, sh.*

About the Human Body
15 min. — Color — *int, jh* — Churchill Films
A boy's physical examination gives an occasion to discuss parts of the body with the doctor. Animated with live action.

---

*See Appendix A for addresses of film companies.

Boy to Man

17 min. Color *int, jh* Churchill Films

Designed primarily for boys entering adolescence. Describes physiological and physical changes of maturation.

From Sociable Six to Noisy Nines

20 min. Black and White McGraw-Hill

Shows the typical behavior and sensible parental guidance of several children of six to nine years of age.

From Ten to Twelve

26 min. Black and White McGraw-Hill

Shows that ten- to 12-year-olds are no longer little boys and girls, but instead young, independent individuals. Presents the problems of discipline, guidance, and understanding that confront most parents. Shows that much of the conflicting behavior of preteens is a normal part of their growth and development.

Girl to Woman

16 min. Color *int, jh* Churchill Films

Designed for girls just entering adolescence. Stages of female maturation, variations in body structure, comparative differences in growth rate of boys of comparable age. Animated.

Human Beginnings

22 min. Color *pri* Association Films, Inc.

Includes the drawings of a group of first graders showing their ideas about how life begins.

Human Growth

20 min. Color *int, jh* Purchase
University of Oregon Medical School
Portland 1, Oregon

A group of seventh-grade children discusses a film on reproduction.

Human Reproduction

20 min. Black and White *jh, sh* McGraw-Hill

Excellent film on reproductive system. Also, revised in color.

These last two films, taken in schoolrooms where children are learning about the part sex plays in life, provide an excellent background for parents' exploration of how they feel about their ability to develop their children's attitudes on this subject, and what they feel is the school's share of the responsibility. Excellent aid for teachers.

It's Wonderful Being a Girl

22 min. Color *int, jh* Modern Talking Picture Service

The psychological and physiological aspects of growing up presented through the experiences of two teen-age girls. Classroom scene with discussion on menstruation. 1966 edition.

World of a Girl

18 min. Color *int, jh, sh* Modern Talking Picture Service

Describes menstrual process and hygiene.

Your Body During Adolescence

10 min. Black and White *jh, sh* McGraw-Hill

Eighteen young people from 13 to 15 are shown to vary widely in size and shape, although all are changing to adulthood. Discussion of endocrine glands and reproductive systems.

Chapter 3

NUTRITIONAL STATUS–NORMAL AND ABNORMAL

NUTRITIONAL REQUIREMENTS

The subject of nutrition is always of paramount importance to those interested in the health of a child. "A sad irony of the current popular interest in better nutrition is that often it is warped by misinformation—and results in an unhealthful kind of eating for our children. Much of what the nation sees, hears, reads, and believes about nutrition is not only untrue but can actually be destructive."[1] Good nutrition forms the basis of good health for all the organs of the body. Whether it is a question of helping the healthy child to maintain the good nutrition necessary for growth and activity, or the sick child who must have nutrients for good recovery, the fundamentals of nutrition remain the same. Food is necessary for: (1) building and rebuilding tissues, (2) providing energy, and (3) regulating metabolic functions. Food is taken into the body through the digestive tract.

A discussion of the daily recommended nutritional allowances of the child leads to the following considerations: caloric needs and the nutrients—water, proteins, fats, carbohydrates, minerals and vitamins. Daily requirements are presented in Table 3.

Calories

A calorie is a unit used to measure the amount of energy available from foods. Practically every food supplies calories. Tables have been

[1]Ronald M. Deutsch: "The Nutrition Boomerang." *Sch. Health Rev.* 5:4:2, May/June, 1974.

TABLE 3 Food and Nutrition Board, National Academy of Sciences – National Research Council Recommended Daily Allowance (Designed for the maintenance of good nutrition of practically all healthy people in the U.S.A.)*

						FAT SOLUBLE VITAMINS			WATER SOLUBLE VITAMINS				MINERALS	
	Age Years	*Weight (lbs.)*	*Height (in.)*	*K calories*	*Protein gm.*	*Vitamin A Activity I.U.*	*Vitamin D I.U.*	*Vitamin E Activity I.U.*	*Ascorbic Acid mg.*	*Niacin mg. equiv.*	*Ribo-flavin mg.*	*Thiamine mg.*	*Calcium gm.*	*Iron mg.*
Children	1- 2	26	32	1100	25	2000	400	10	40	8	0.6	0.6	0.7	15
	2- 3	31	36	1250	25	2000	400	10	40	8	0.7	0.6	0.8	15
	3- 4	35	39	1400	30	2500	400	10	40	9	0.8	0.7	0.8	10
	4- 6	42	43	1600	30	2500	400	10	40	11	0.9	0.8	0.8	10
	6- 8	51	48	2000	35	3500	400	15	40	13	1.1	1.0	0.9	10
	8-10	62	52	2200	40	3500	400	15	40	15	1.2	1.1	1.0	10
Males	10-12	77	55	2500	45	4500	400	20	40	17	1.3	1.3	1.2	10
	12-14	95	59	2700	50	5000	400	20	45	18	1.4	1.4	1.4	18
	14-18	130	67	3000	60	5000	400	25	55	20	1.5	1.5	1.4	18
	18-22	147	69	2800	60	5000	400	30	60	18	1.6	1.4	0.8	10
	22-35	154	69	2800	65	5000	–	30	60	18	1.7	1.4	0.8	10
	35-55	154	68	2600	65	5000	–	30	60	17	1.7	1.3	0.8	10
	55-75+	154	67	2400	65	5000	–	30	60	14	1.7	1.2	0.8	10
Females	10-12	77	56	2250	50	4500	400	20	40	15	1.3	1.1	1.2	18
	12-14	97	61	2300	50	5000	400	20	45	15	1.4	1.2	1.3	18
	14-16	114	62	2400	55	5000	400	25	50	16	1.4	1.2	1.3	18
	16-18	119	63	2300	55	5000	400	25	50	15	1.5	1.2	1.3	18
	18-22	128	64	2000	55	5000	400	25	55	13	1.5	1.0	0.8	18
	22-35	128	64	2000	55	5000	–	25	55	13	1.5	1.0	0.8	18
	35-55	128	63	1850	55	5000	–	25	55	13	1.5	1.0	0.8	18
	55-75+	128	62	1700	55	5000	–	25	55	12	1.5	1.0	0.8	10

*Adapted from revised edition, 1968.

formulated which estimate individual caloric needs on the basis of age and weight. The highest needs per kilogram of body weight are those of the infant. In periods of rapid growth and development, as before and during puberty, caloric requirements are also high. In general, the indices for judging adequate caloric supply are growth, hunger, and general well-being. Restriction of calories for some time, if the essential nutritive components are present, may not necessarily be serious. It must be emphasized, however, that if calories are curtailed, the essential nutrients must be maintained at needed levels. The greatest danger from excessive intake of calories is obesity. Experience has shown that the caloric needs of children can be distributed about as follows: protein, 15 per cent; fat, 35 per cent; carbohydrates, 50 per cent.

Water

Water is necessary for every cell of the body, for every chemical process, for the spaces between cells where interchanges of chemicals occur, for the transportation of oxygen and nutritive products to the cells, and for the removal of carbon dioxide and waste materials—in effect for every metabolic process. Its ability to vaporize on the skin is utilized in temperature regulation of the body.

Insufficient intake of water interferes with good metabolic function, and the resulting dehydration may be serious. Water is eliminated through the lungs, skin, intestinal tract, and kidneys. With normal function of the kidneys, excessive intake of water is not harmful. Children need a great deal of water, since their metabolic activities are proportionately heightened to care for growth and activity. It is probably safe to make the observation that children do not drink their required amounts during the hours of school. Usually there are not enough drinking fountains. A child who is anxious to play will not stand in line very long for a few swallows of water. Mild deprivation can result in a dry, itchy skin, lessened urinary output, and thirst.

Proteins

Proteins form a large part of the protoplasm of every cell in the body. They constitute about one fifth of the body weight. Complex protein structures are taken into the gastrointestinal tract where they are reduced by enzyme action to simple amino acids. These are absorbed from the tract into the blood stream and carried to all the tissues of the body. There are approximately 21 different amino acids in the body, ten of which are considered essential for children (eight for adults). Their metabolism is related to that of fats, carbohydrates and vitamins, particularly the B-complex group. They are present in most body fluids and secretions.

Proteins are involved in practically all physiological processes of the body and are necessary for the manufacture of enzymes, hormones, antibodies, and hemoglobin.

With the increase of new cells in the growing child, and with the need for repair of cells used in activity, an amply supply of protein is essential daily. Comparatively little is used for energy. There is no substitute for protein; excessive amounts cannot be stored; hence, a protein of high quality, one that has most of the essential amino acids, should be eaten at each meal.

Mild restrictions of protein can result in lassitude, inadequate growth, and lack of stamina; extensive deprivations are serious.

Protein foods differ in their content of amino acids; therefore, a variety of sources, both animal and vegetable, is necessary in order to secure a complete supply. Protein in the American diet is found in such animal products as meat, fish, poultry, milk, eggs, and cheese, and in such vegetable sources as legumes (dried beans and peas, soy beans, lentils, and peanuts), cereals, and nuts. Meats, milk, and eggs offer the most concentrated amounts of protein and are useful in supplementing the protein in cereal and vegetable foods. Examples of such combinations are bread and milk, macaroni and cheese, and baked beans and pork.

Fats

The principal and most concentrated source of energy is fat stored in the body. It is derived from ingested fat and is also synthesized from the products of carbohydrate and protein metabolism. As a source of energy it is particularly valuable when caloric demands are high for increased work. It forms cushioning pads for organs, blood vessels, and nerves, and is depositied as an insulating layer beneath the skin. It also serves as a vehicle for the fat-soluble vitamins A, D, E, and K. Fat gives flavor to foods and makes them more palatable. It also produces satiety because of delayed digestion which fends off hunger pains.

The principal dietary sources of fat are: (1) animal fats found in cream, whole milk, bacon, butter, cheese, fats around meat, and fish liver oil; (2) vegetable oils, used principally for cooking and salad dressing, and oleomargarine; and (3) nuts and nut products.

Carbohydrates

About 50 per cent of the caloric needs of a child should be provided as carbohydrates, a quick source of energy. Digestive enzymes in the mouth and gastrointestinal tract reduce carbohydrate foods to simple sugars—fructose, glucose, and galactose. These are absorbed through the intestinal wall into the blood stream and distributed to various tissues of the body, especially the liver. In the latter organ the sugars are converted into glycogen and stored. Glycogen furnishes a ready source of energy by being rapidly reconverted into glucose, the oxidation of which produces energy. Only a small amount of glycogen is stored at one time. Excessive amounts of ingested carbohydrates are converted into fat and stored in the body, later to be used as energy.

Sources of carbohydrates are: sugars and sweets of all kinds, including fruits and the lactose in milk; foods with high starch content, such as cereals, potatoes, breads, dried beans and peas; and vegetables.

Minerals

The word "mineral" is used to indicate those inorganic elements necessary for structure and function of the body. These elements are numerous—calcium, magnesium, potassium, sodium, phosphorus, sulfur, chlorine, iron, and iodine. Traces of other elements are also used—fluorine, copper, zinc, manganese, cobalt, silicon, selenium, boron, nickel, aluminum, bromine, and arsenic.

The role of minerals is understood to some extent by the manner in which they occur in the body. Their presence in bone produces hardness of this tissue; as an element in organic compounds they form a part of cells and of many hormones and enzymes; and as inorganic compounds and dissociated ions circulating in the body fluids, they assist in maintaining osmotic equilibrium and acid-base balance, influence the contractibility of muscle and irritability of nerve tissue, and help in control of coagulation of blood.

Reserve stores of some of the minerals are found in the body. Bone as a calcium reserve is a good example. However, most mineral salts are continuously being excreted and must be supplied constantly in the diet. A child's requirements are relatively higher per kilogram weight than the mere maintenance requirements of an adult. He needs an additional amount for the construction of new tissues and fluids. A number of foods are fortified by the addition of minerals, and, although the mineral intake of different children varies greatly, the well-balanced diet will ordinarily furnish the necessary elements in sufficient amounts. Those which are most likely to be deficient in amounts and need to be provided in the diet are calcium, iron, iodine, and possibly fluorine.

Iron. Iron forms part of the hemoglobin molecule so necessary for gaseous interchange of oxygen and carbon dioxide in the tissues. Deficiency produces varying degrees of anemia with its characteristic symptomatology: fatigue, air-hunger, and lack of stamina. Excessive amounts produce no deleterious effects. A well-balanced diet should contain adequate amounts of iron. Common sources are: (1) all meats—meat, fish, poultry, and shell fish, especially oysters; (2) egg yolk; (3) dark green leafy vegetables; (4) enriched and restored whole grain cereals, bread and flour; (5) dried beans and peas; (6) dried fruits; and (7) molasses. The cause of anemia must be carefully determined. Iron deficiency anemia often is produced by grossly apparent or unsuspected blood loss rather than by dietary insufficiency.

Iodine. Iodine is another element necessary for normal metabolic processes. It is incorporated into each molecule of thyroxin, the hormone produced by the thyroid gland. This hormone is essential in regulation of energy metabolism in the body. In addition, iodine is stored in the thyroid gland.

A deficiency of this mineral may result in a compensatory diffuse, uniform enlargement of the thyroid gland in its attempt to produce sufficient effective hormone. It is natural for adolescents to have a little uniform fullness of the thyroid gland, and no fuss should be made over a normal physiological phenomenon. Quite an increase in size (simple goiter) may be the result of iodine insufficiency. About 1963 the Department of Defense found in a survey of 18-year-old boys only two in 1000 with simple goiters. This finding is in marked contrast to the observations in 1918 of one in 50 boys, a dramatic drop credited to the addition of iodine in the diet, particularly with the use of iodized salt.

In areas of the country where the soil and water contain iodine, supplement of this mineral as a medication by mouth is not usually necessary. Vegetables and fruits grown in coastal areas contain a supply of iodine. Sea foods are also good sources. Large areas of the country, however, do not have sufficient amounts in the soil. These are the so-called "goiter belts," found especially around the Upper Mississippi Valley Basin and Rocky Mountain regions.

Whenever iodine is lacking in the diet, iodized salt is recommended. The latter was introduced in 1924. It provides a cheap, easy and simple insurance against a deficiency. The amount of iodine in iodized salt is too low to produce harmful effects. In individual cases iodine in either organic or inorganic form is prescribed by the physician. Excessive amounts are probably of no clinical significance. Most authorities believe that if all salt used for seasoning food were iodized, everyone would obtain sufficient iodine to satisfy the natural demands of his thyroid gland. Occasionally, a physician may limit intake of iodine.

Calcium. Calcium is another of the major essential minerals. Ninety-nine per cent of the calcium in the body is found in bone (calcium phosphate) and teeth (calcium carbonate). The concentration, excretion, and fine balance of calcium and phosphorus are regulated by the parathyroid hormone and vitamin D. Calcium is involved in the normal behavior of heart muscle and nerves, in coagulation of blood, and in some enzyme actions. Large amounts of calcium are required during the growth spurts. A deficiency can result in sponginess and weakening of the bony structure or even in retardation of growth. Excessive amounts of calcium-containing foods evidently produce no harmful results, unless excessive amounts of vitamin D are taken also. Principal sources of calcium are milk, dried skimmed milk (less expensive), milk products, and leafy vegetables, among them mustard, turnips, and broccoli. Dried peas and beans provide a fair amount.

Fluorine. The function of fluorine will be discussed under dental health.

Vitamins

One of the thrilling chapters in the development of the science of nutrition is the unfolding of information about vitamins. The complex role of vitamins in the metabolism of other nutrients, in the formation and activation of enzymes and hormones, in antibody formation, in the release of energy within cells, in relation to the genetic substance in cells, and in relation to each other is fascinating. Because of the complex role of each vitamin, it should not be viewed merely as serving a distinct and isolated function to prevent some specific disease. For example, vitamin C does so much more than prevent scurvy. The trend now is to designate many of the vitamins by their chemical formulas rather than by the alphabet. The interweaving and interlocking of their influences can only be suggested in this text, with the purpose of creating an appreciation of their significance and the need for them in a well-balanced diet. The very latest research by scientists must be scrutinized to keep step with the most recent information. The crudest and most fallacious interpretation possible is to consider them as "pep pills."

Vitamins are chemical compounds in foods. Some are synthesized in the laboratory; a few are formed within the body. To understand their roles fully is to know every biochemical reaction in the body in which they participate. We need vitamins but cannot live on vitamins alone. By eating a variety of foods, we secure the necessary ones. In addition, physicians usually prescribe vitamins A, C, and D or C and D to children under two years of age, and occasionally to those during the adolescent growth spurt.

Many foods are enriched, fortified, or restored by supplementing vitamins, sometimes because of legal requirements. Examples are: milk with extra vitamin D, flour enriched with some B vitamins, and oleomargarine with vitamin A.

Vitamin A. Vitamin A occurs in several forms, all of which apparently function the same way. A deficiency seldom develops in children since the vitamin is present in all foods containing animal fats or yellow pigment. Severe and prolonged deprivation may produce a special type of blindness involving the cornea (xerophthalmia). Vitamin A keeps mucous membranes moist and skin supple. The functional and structural integrity of all epithelial cells of the body is maintained by this vitamin. It is necessary for normal growth of bone and is involved in the production of adrenal hormone. Night blindness results from a deficiency of pigments in the retina necessary for night vision, pigments consisting of proteins attached to vitamin A. Large amounts of the vitamin do not prevent colds or infection. This fat-soluble vitamin is found in fish liver oils and in animal fats, including cream and butter. Other important sources are liver; egg yolk; yellow vegetables, such as sweet potatoes, carrots, and yellow squash; leafy green vegetables, such as kale, spinach, beet and mustard greens; and some fruits, particularly apricots, cantaloupes, and tomatoes. Vitamin A is not found naturally in the vegetable oils; hence it is added to commercial oleomargarine. Prolonged intake of excessive amounts of this vitamin may produce toxic or harmful effects.

Vitamin B-Complex. The B-complex vitamins, a group which contains more than a dozen water-soluble factors, are easily found in sufficient amounts in the ordinary diet in most parts of this country. The factors niacin, riboflavin, and thiamine (B_1) are extremely important for good nutrition of infants and children. They maintain good health of cells, organs, and of the nervous system of the body. Pantothenic acid, pyridoxine, and folic acid seem necessary in antibody formation to produce immunity. Fat protects the body from thiamine and protein deficiency, which in turn permits efficient use of carbohydrates. Vitamin B_{12} combines with folic acid to assure healthy functioning of the blood. "Deficiency perpetrates a particular kind of anemia occasionally due to abnormal absorption of the vitamin and now believed to be related to a malfunction of the pancreas."[2] Thiamine deficiency can cause inflammation of nerves and heart failure, a combination of which in advanced stages produces beriberi. Some of the B vitamins, especially biotin, are necessary in the conversion of carbohydrates to fats. At least five, including thiamine, biotin, and niacin, are necessary in processes which unlock energy from sugar and fat. This brief description of the multiple functions of the B-complex group gives an idea of the intensive research being done.

Principal sources of the three outstanding members of the B-complex group are listed below. If these are included in sufficient quantities in diets, the other factors will be also.

Thiamine: lean pork, poultry, fish, and other meats, dried peas and beans, nuts, whole grain and enriched breads and cereals, milk, eggs, potatoes, green peas.

Niacin: liver, poultry, fish, good amounts in tuna and salmon, eggs, peanuts, whole grain and enriched breads and cereals.

Riboflavin: milk, liver, meats, salmon, green leafy vegetables, whole grain and enriched breads and cereals.

Vitamin C. Vitamin C (ascorbic acid) was one of the first vitamins studied. Its deficiency results in a disease observed for centuries, namely scurvy. Ascorbic acid is essential for the intracellular substance in which cells are imbedded and cemented together. This is particularly true of the fibrous tissue in bone, coverings of bone, dentin of the teeth, cartilage, and the lining of blood vessels. Thus,

[2] Dod: Schultz, "The Verdict on Vitamins." *Today's Health* 51:57, January, 1974.

the clinical picture of scurvy with the bleeding gums and pain with movement of joints or pressure on bone can be explained. Not only may a deficiency produce scurvy, but defective formation of teeth may occur. This vitamin assists in the absorption of iron and enables every cell in the body to utilize folic acid. Excessive amounts of ascorbic acid produce no abnormal symptoms. Ascorbic acid is readily destroyed by heat or by fairly long exposure to air. It is found in adequate amounts in citrus fruits, tomatoes, berries, dark green leafy vegetables, green peppers, raw cabbage, and potatoes. The frozen juices of citrus fruits and canned commercial juices from citrus fruits and tomatoes contain large amounts of vitamin C.

Vitamin D. Vitamin D is ingested by mouth, absorbed through the intestinal tract, and stored in the liver and other organs of the body. It can also be manufactured from the irradiation of the sterols (fats) under the skin by sunlight or ultraviolet light.

The several forms of vitamin D serve the same purpose. Mention has been made of the relationship of this vitamin and parathyroid hormone to the regulation of calcium and phosphorus metabolism. A deficiency can cause poor tooth development and faulty growth of bone with softening and bone deformities. Rickets, a disease seldom seen in this country, may develop. Vitamin D is more likely to be deficient in diets of children in which animal fats are low or absent. Very young children usually need to supplement the natural supply of vitamin D with preparations of fish liver oils, usually cod or halibut.

Prolonged use of excessive amounts of vitamin D may be manifested by decreased appetite, loss of weight, nausea, vomiting, weakness, and apathy.

Principal sources of vitamin D are some animal fats, fish liver oils, fortified vegetable oils, irradiated milk, and irradiation of the skin by ultraviolet light or sunlight.

Well-Balanced Diet

It is not necessary to review the components item for item in choosing a meal or planning a menu. A well-balanced diet contains all the nutritious foods required for healthy growing children. Studies show that the body makes better use of nutrients when a variety of foods is eaten. Choice of foods from each of the following groups will usually provide the necessary nutritives: (1) meat, fish, poultry, and eggs; (2) milk and milk products; (3) fruits and vegetables; and (4) cereals, breadstuffs, and miscellaneous foods (Figure 9). Daily selection from these four basic groups promotes good eating habits, and these habits should be formed very early in childhood.

Teachers must remember that all mothers do not cook the same foods; so in addition to selection of foods from the various groups, there must be adjustments to national habits of eating. It would not be amiss for teachers to take a course in nutrition in order to acquire

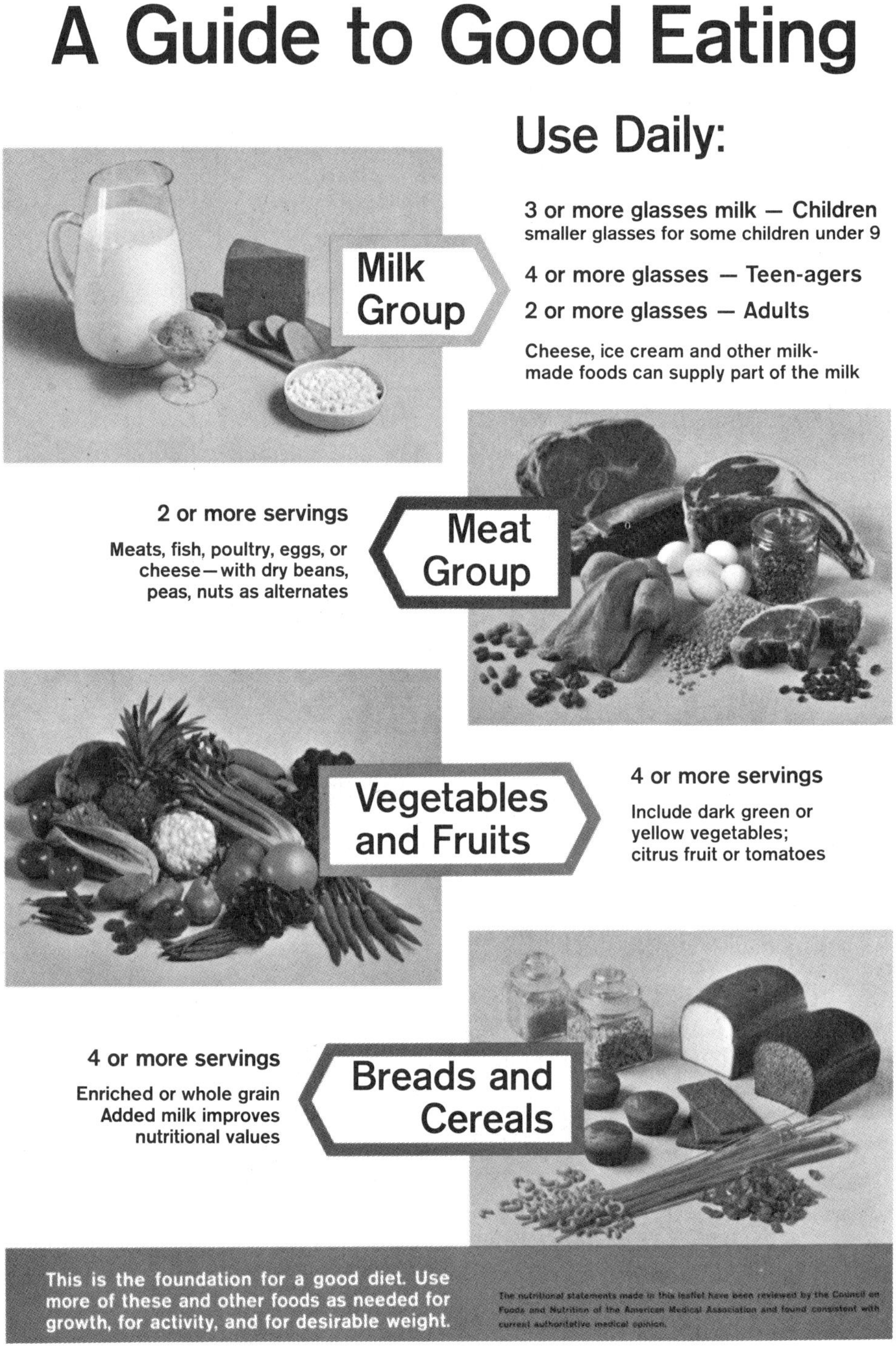

Figure 9 Note the four groupings of food. (Courtesy National Dairy Council.)

basic information and learn how to stimulate interest in good eating practices.

STANDARDS OF GOOD NUTRITION

What is good nutrition?

Good nutrition of all systems of the body establishes the basis for their good function. Proper food is necessary in children and young adults for maintenance of good health, for continued growth, and for reasonable physical activity. A *well-nourished* child grows and develops at an acceptable pace. He is brimful of energy and life, interested in play, and appears relaxed. His eyes shine, his hair is glossy, his skin feels good and elastic, his coloring is normal, and he holds himself in good posture for his age. He is poised and self-confident, eats and sleeps well, gains weight and height and has fat under his skin—he is a robust, healthy individual (Figure 10). If he remains healthy, he reaches puberty in average time, grows to maturity, and achieves his potential. After some exposure to them, a

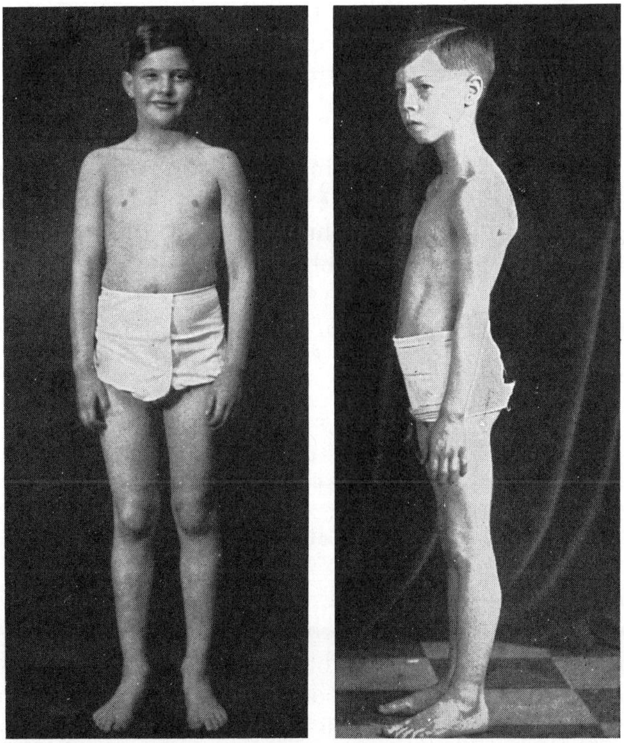

Figure 10 *Left,* A well nourished ten-year-old boy who has practically all the characteristics of good nutrition listed in the text. The ten-year-old boy at the right is stunted both in height and weight and has the posture and expression of a little old man. (Roberts: *Nutrition Work with Children.* University of Chicago Press.)

teacher usually becomes quite a connoisseur of healthy children. In brief, the criteria used by a teacher in judging nutritional status are *weight, appearance,* and *activity* or performance.

In evaluating weight, comparison of a child's progress in height and weight with his own past record is desirable. The growth charts should be used and kept up to date with interval measurements. As long as there is some gain, no anxiety is indicated. Failure to gain weight may occasion some speculation and an early recheck. Any loss in weight should have an explanation and an investigation, if necessary. A recent illness or emotional upset can explain many of the losses. Progressive loss of weight is serious and should be discussed with the school nurse and the family. On the other hand, a child who lives mostly on peanut butter and jelly sandwiches and carbonated beverages may well maintain average or excessive weight and still be malnourished. This does not mean that the usually accepted standards should not be used. Rather, there should be an appreciation of their interpretation. The parents whose child is labeled as healthy according to weight standards only may be given a false sense of security. Evaluation of these standards for growth and development and for nutritional status has been discussed under Growth and Development.

It is sometimes difficult to make a decision concerning a child's nutritional status. A complete health examination may be necessary. There may even be disagreement among physicians. A good deal of information may be necessary before a conclusion is reached. The various factors which affect nutrition (Causes of Malnutrition) must be taken into consideration.

An expert eye can size up a youngster and watch his daily performance. Does the child look thin and pale and have prominent ribs? Does he have rolls of fat? Even if every rib can be counted, is the child healthy, active, and full of good humor? Even if the child appears to have an average weight, is he flabby, listless, slumped in posture, and does he have circles under his eyes?

A study of the weight line on his growth chart, inspection of the child himself, and observation of his activities should be guides in the evaluation of good nutrition.

MALNUTRITION

Causes

Malnutrition means poor nutrition or that the body lacks one or more essential foods. The underlying causes usually stem from the very pattern of family living and are interlinked and complex. Each family has its own eating practices, influenced by health knowledge and surrounded with racial, religious, sectional, and personal prejudices, likes and dislikes. All of the habits of living within the home as well as the attitudes toward discipline in regulating them affect the diet of a child from the time he is born. His own health, both physical and psychological, will determine his hunger pattern. The money available for food is a big factor. Even in our own country, we are confronted with hunger and poverty. One elementary teacher noticed for several months that a child did not bring any lunch to school. Finally, a social worker was sent to the home for an explanation. He learned that the father had deserted the family and there simply was not enough to eat.

If it will be kept in mind that the underlying causes of malnutrition cannot be placed in distinct categories but are interwoven, a better understanding of malnutrition is possible. From this understanding, a better follow-up can be undertaken.

CAUSES OF MALNUTRITION—OUTLINE

I. The family pattern.

A. Poor emotional tones in the environment may be responsible for a child's attitude toward foods and eating. A contented, well-adjusted child accepts food with pleasant anticipation.

B. Poor emotional tones at eating time influence a child's eating habits. Overanxiety for fear the child will not eat enough or eats too much and too much focusing upon the child as he eats not only disturbs his immediate well-being, but may show up as complex psychological reactions later in life. The "clean-up-your-plate" philosophy can be physiologically unsound. Surely, a child with allergies can be harmed; moreover, this formidable, rigid discipline can foster emotional turmoil.

C. Ignorance of nutritional needs will determine not only the selection of foods and planning of menus but the establishment of health attitudes and practices within the home. Parents need to be better informed on child nutrition.

D. Inadequate financial resources will govern the kinds and amounts of food bought. With correct health information this handicap can be overcome to some degree. Malnutrition is not necessarily associated with poverty, however. It occurs in all economic levels; children from the high income groups tend to eat more nourishing foods. More children have good diets and fewer have poor diets in communities of higher income levels.

E. Poor eating practices and personal dislikes may influence the selection of foods in spite of good educational background in nutrition and adequate income. A mother and father may have a revulsion against eating meat, yet appreciate the fact that their child should eat this food for growth. Coaxing and bribery will have little effect if the parents do not eat meat themselves. Another example: if a parent eats just enough food to justify the bounteous dessert at the end of dinner, young people will gather that the latter is the most important part of the meal. Or, they will consider the dessert a reward. No food should be a reward, and it does not matter when specific foods are eaten during a meal.

F. Cultural and religious practices may account for the

avoidance of certain foods. Proper nutritional substitutes must be made for them.

II. The individual pattern.

A. Poor eating practices.

1. Personality disturbances which the child may develop from the emotional climate of his home may be identified symptomatically in feeding problems of infancy and childhood.

2. Inadequate intake of nutrients.

a. Insufficient intake of food.

(1) Poor breakfast.

Mother may not get up to prepare breakfast or may have gone to work already and left the child to prepare his own. He may be hurried, tired, too sleepy, or not hungry.

(2) Poor lunch.

b. Poor selection of foods.

The diet may contain the calories but not provide the nutrients.

(1) Too little milk

(2) Too few vegetables and not enough variety.

(3) Too few vegetables and fruits rich in ascorbic acid (vitamin C).

(4) Scanty amount of proteins.

(5) Too much candy and sweets.

(6) An overuse of soft drinks.

3. Hurried meals.

"Hurry has already been considered as a factor in poor breakfasts. The problem extends to other meals of the day—hurried school lunches during a limited lunch period, hurried home lunches to get back to school on time, hurried evening meals to get out to the playground, to follow favorite radio and television programs, to start homework, or just to escape an unpleasant mealtime atmosphere. The outcome is serious when the nutritive quality of the diet is materially affected, that is, when the hasty meals routinely consist of foods which contribute little in nutrient or safety value and the total food intake for the day is thereby rendered inadequate. . . . It is well known that meals eaten unhurriedly in happy, peaceful surroundings, with friendly companionship, not only create the most favorable conditions for social and emotional development, but for the digestion and utilization of the food as well."[3]

4. Eating between meals.

This practice may not only produce overweight, if the caloric intake is too high but can destroy desire for later well-balanced meals.

5. Dietary fads.

Fads in diet do promote faulty practices, such as too little milk and meat, expensive sugars and wheat preparations, and indiscriminate use of laxatives. Weight-reducing fads impress the consciousness of the whole family. Children receive poor education and attitude toward nutrition.

---

[3]Ethel Austin Martin: *Roberts' Nutrition Work with Children.* Chicago: The University of Chicago Press, 1954, p. 151.

B. Poor health practices.
   1. Too little sleep.
   2. Lack of outdoor play.
      Children need sunshine, fresh air and exercise.
   3. Overexercise and chronic fatigue.
C. Poor health.
   1. Impaired physical health. Sick children are usually not hungry.
      a. Chronic infections, as seen with diseased tonsils and adenoids.
      b. Poor condition of teeth, caries, malocclusion and missing teeth.
      c. Acute infections with loss of appetite and weight.
      d. Heart disease.
         Children with organic heart damage tire easily, are less active, and demand less food. With enforced rest some may eat too much and gain too much weight.
      e. Chronic diseases, such as:
         (1) Allergies to various foods which may restrict food intake. Substitutions of equally nutritious foods must be made.
         (2) Diabetes with its dietary restrictions.
         (3) Crippling conditions.
             Those which restrict activity may result in boredom and decreased desire for food or in overweight from excessive eating. Cleft palate, if uncorrected, causes mechanical difficulties in eating.
   2. Some psychological aspects of illness.
      Sick children develop finicky appetites and whims. One little girl who suffered an afternoon fever daily for six months during an episode of acute rheumatic fever would eat very little except tuna fish sandwiches. Solicitude and hovering anxiety of members of the family may lead a child to use eating as a weapon for attention or for fulfilling various demands. Sick children often find satisfaction in being favored in diet over others in the home.

A great deal of attention must be devoted to solving the problem of malnutrition in an individual child. Questions ranging from specific ones on finances and food intake to general ones concerning family customs are asked. The child, teacher, school nurse, social worker, doctor, and parent eventually may be involved.

Effects

Effects of poor nutrition may or may not be discernible, depending upon the severity and length of deprivation. Lack of essential foods for short periods, such as during acute illness, can be overcome. Whether the deficiency is in the absence of one or more essential foods or in caloric intake, some disturbances usually follow. The child who will not drink milk or eat milk products may not only have trouble with his teeth, but may be extremely nervous and irritable because of restricted calcium intake. Lack of iron may result in anemia, with symptoms of pallor or a sallow complexion, and fatigue. Regardless of how much candy, carbonated beverages, and snacks are eaten, all of which supply calories, and regardless of weight, the nutrients required for the body's needs must be supplied. Otherwise, health will be impaired, susceptibility to infections increased, and energy lessened.

Malnourished children tend to be underweight; at times, however, overweight may predominate. The child who fills up on desserts and soda pop may be of average weight, or even fat, and still be poorly nourished. People who subsist on potatoes and starchy diets in an emergency or because of poverty may appear well-nourished, but they still lack essential foods. Their endurance is poor. *The weight of an individual, therefore, is not necessarily an index of nutrition.*

Except in underprivileged areas, a teacher will rarely meet a child suffering from severe malnutrition. Prolonged deprivation of adequate food elements, as found in war-torn countries and in some sections of our own country, may occur, however. And there will be at least one child in practically any classroom whose nutritional status is below par. Malnutrition has been a problem among the youngsters in the Head Start program.

Because of food taboos, religious beliefs, and poverty, 60 per cent of the population in under-developed countries is malnourished. There are millions who are always hungry. Teachers who serve in these areas see children with marked nutritional deficiencies. One disease produced by prolonged protein deficiency, *kwashiorkor*, is found throughout most of Africa, Latin America, and southern Asia, where people subsist mostly on starchy foods. It is characterized by reddish discoloration of skin and hair, stunted growth, bulging abdomen, flabby musculature, swelling of arms and legs, sores, apathy, fatigue, and susceptibility to disease.

With *pronounced or prolonged malnutrition*, an individual tires easily, limits his activity, is inattentive, learns slowly or not at all, has difficulty in memorizing, and is retarded in progress at school. Scholastic performance may be better in the morning than in the afternoon. Many of these children are phlegmatic, sit quietly in their seats, and cause no trouble. Some, however, are nervous, restless, irritable, and throw temper tantrums. Physically, the body may be stunted in growth in both height and weight. The scapulae (shoulder blades) and bony landmarks of the chest may be unusually prominent. Posture may be slumped because of poor muscular tone and fatigue; the abdomen will protrude; the expression of the face is strained; the eyes will look dull with dark circles underneath, and the child has the appearance of old age (Figure 10).

It is also of interest to note that prolonged deprivation of food affects sexual maturity. Lowered birth rates in countries whose living standards have fallen during and in the aftermath of war have a physiological basis. The gonads respond quickly to malnutrition by failing to develop at an average rate (retarded maturity), or in some instances failing completely to function. The latter results in sterility. The ovaries may fail to develop or may shrink in size, or, more usually, carry on irregular and lowered function. The common fad among our young girls for slim figures, which occasions injudicious dieting, has not only influenced their health in general but definitely has caused menstrual irregularities, pain, and even complete cessation of menstrual periods.

Management

Malnutrition may be a continuation of an existing condition from infancy and preschool years, or it may be acquired at any time thereafter. Management of a child suffering from malnutrition is always an individual problem and depends upon the causes. If malnutrition is caused by ignorance or poverty, correction is not too difficult; when caused by faulty parent-child relationships, finical eating patterns set by other members of the family, overanxiety of parents concerning eating habits of children, or by chronic disease, the problem presented is more complex.

The customs of the gang are important. Girls in intermediate and secondary grades who have a phobia against gaining weight will throw away the lunches prepared at home and adopt the current dietary fads. Reasoning is futile arrayed against prejudices and the dictates of fashion. Eating between meals of such foods as peanuts, candies, and sweetened soft drinks, or dropping in for a snack at a rendezvous, is traditional in the older groups, and these customs will prevail. Many a teacher has noticed how children rush through their lunches in order to have more time for play. A child will take the time to peel a banana; but after the lunch period is over, oranges will be found tucked into corners of stairways and corridors. No time for peeling!

If a child is suffering from malnutrition, he needs medical supervision. The underlying causes should be ascertained and corrected as fully as possible. Teachers should maintain close observation over the months, and work closely with parents, school nurse, physician, and social worker. The child may need to take time out for rest on a cot at school. Extra milk and crackers and lunch, and in some schools, a breakfast, may be provided—at no cost, when indicated.

Some school districts have been operating breakfast programs, and others have tried to determine the need. A survey in Indiana revealed the following:

1. A significant number of students do not eat breakfast at home.
2. The students seem to have a highly favorable attitude toward

the social aspects of eating breakfast with friends after the morning rush to school is over, and they have had sufficient time to develop an appetite.

3. Many breakfasts eaten at home could be made adequate if the student would purchase fruit juice or milk when he arrived at school.

4. A significant number of students surveyed indicate that they would participate in the breakfast program if one were available.[4]

This study appears to indicate that a breakfast program in a secondary school is one positive alternative to solving nutritional problems for this age group.

UNDERWEIGHT

Underweight sometimes presents a more difficult problem than overweight. Some of the following factors should be considered. Hereditary influences, as manifested by the stature of other members of the family, may be dominant. Some children tend to be thin. Or, physical examination may reveal a chronic infection. A recent acute debilitating illness can cause extensive weight loss. Many children are in so many activities outside of class that they do not have time to eat, or they may be too tired to eat. The emotional climate in the home may not encourage much pleasure in eating. The boy who receives a 15-minute lecture at breakfast because he reached in front of his father for a piece of toast will not only leave the table in disgust but may be emotionally upset for the remainder of the day. Parents' habits of scolding at mealtime breed resentments in youngsters. Sometimes the record made of daily food intake will produce revealing information. It is surprising how many adolescent girls, despite a desire to gain weight, simply do not eat sufficient food for their daily requirements. Their protests of eating to satiety soon turn to expressions of consternation if the daily record of food is calculated. Some youngsters have poor appetites and do not become hungry.

It is apparent that each case of underweight must be approached as an individual problem with attention to psychological as well as to physical implications. The school has a role to play. Between-meal lunches and plenty of rest at school should help to correct the problem. For the convalescent child a cot should be provided for a regular rest period. Careful and repeated checkups by the physician are necessary, and a weight record can be kept at school for the satisfaction of the teachers. The parent, child, teacher, school nurse, and physician cooperate in their attention toward the underweight child.

---

[4]Stewart, Roberta, "The Feasibility of Establishing a Breakfast Program in the Middle Class Secondary School." *J. Sch. Health* April, 1973, pp. 239–40.

THE FAT CHILD

A great deal of concern can be aroused over the child who is labeled "fatty" at school; and the present obsessive, neurotic attitude of adults toward overweight and "dieting," coupled with teasing, can make a child miserable. A fat girl can become morose, isolate herself from her classmates, grieve because she has no dates, refuse to change her dress for gymnasium activities, and assume a bitter, hostile attitude in all her human relationships. Boys tend to cover up feelings with a laugh or a semblance of good humor. Because of the psychological scars which may occur, a teacher should have an understanding of the physiological basis of obesity (excessive fat deposition).

The three ages in childhood when overweight may be prevalent are: infancy, prepuberty (ages eight to 11 years), and adolescence. With interval spurts of rapid growth, the child usually gains more normal proportions and at maturity should assume average weight.

In evaluating overweight the following questions may be asked: Is this individual truly fat? Does he have rolls or pads of fat? Or does he have a big bony frame with heavy muscles? Much has been written about the obese adolescent. Obesity may be difficult to determine. In general, an individual who weighs over 20 per cent more than the average for his height, age, and body build is considered overweight or obese.

Very few cases of overweight are caused by endocrine disturbances. Nevertheless, some are. Low thyroid function, diabetes, or pituitary dysfunction can be ruled out by a physician's examination. Most children are fat because of overeating; more food is ingested than can be burned for energy. The excess is transformed into fat and is deposited in the body, especially under the skin. Fat children tend to grow into fat adults more often than children who have average weights. Those who are relatively inactive because of crippling conditions still have good appetites and tend to put on fat. Obesity is not particularly a hereditary trait; it is more a family characteristic explained by good foods, foods high in calories, and enjoyment of eating. Mother is usually a good cook, and desserts are popular. Fifty per cent of fat children have one or both parents who are overweight. The similarity is probably on an environmental basis. Often a change in the entire family's eating habits is essential for control of the child's eating habits.

In some cases a more profound and significant explanation of obesity is offered. Unhappy, poorly adjusted youngsters, as well as adults, derive a great deal of satisfaction from eating. A child who feels frustrated, insecure or inadequate in various aspects of his life gets great pleasure from eating or can secure attention from overeating. A fat girl who feels unattractive seeks refuge in eating as a compensatory gratification, gains more weight, feels more unattractive and eats more; the cycle is vicious. Many people under emotional or mental tension gravitate toward the refrigerator. One must be careful not to place too much emphasis upon the psychological and emotional factors in producing obesity, however, and keep in mind that eating can be a pleasurable experience.

A younger child who is placed under a strict "reducing" dietary regimen has no motivation and may feel deprived. The mother of a second grader was advised at school that her son was overweight, and she proceeded to place him on such a diet. He began to suck his thumb and wet the bed at night, which he had not done since preschool days. His pediatrician advised that a return be made to the old dietary with a mild restriction in calories but not nutrients. Soon after, the regressive behavior disappeared. Adolescents are interested in grooming and appearance, which should stimulate a positive emotional response. They do need reassurance, particularly the maturing fat boys, that they will be normal. An attempt is made to prevent a gain in pounds and await the natural growth which will permit the growing youth to become better proportioned and assume a more average weight. With extremely excessive weight, of course, a child should be placed under medical supervision.

An unrelenting obsession with overweight is deplorable. The mother who considers giving her child pills to reduce his desire for food, the father who never fails to admonish his son before each meal to take it easy on food, and the parents, relatives, and friends who call attention even in jocular fashion to a child's overweight are stupidly doing irreparable harm. Consider the emotional damage which has been done a chubby third grader who, with a recently acquired stutter, holds a morsel of food and haltingly asks, "Will this make me fat, Mother, will this make me fat?"

At the same time that a well-balanced diet is followed, the home, school, and social contacts should be gratifying and offer security and acceptance. Overprotection and anxiety in the home should be avoided and the teacher's constant encouragement over the long road back to normal weight builds up the morale of the obese person.

The secret of success in handling obesity of children is not just weight loss. The emotional stability of the child and his home are factors. Reducing weight does not solve a child's problems. He needs to build up his self-esteem, and to develop independence and a strong sense of identity.

"Since their peer relations are often poor, it is helpful to involve teenagers in school and church activities, encouraging them to participate in clubs, craft classes, volunteer work programs, and service committees. These outlets can provide the means for attaining some degree of success and a feeling of achievement and thereby help to bolster the adolescent's poor self-image."[5]

One effective way of helping fat adolescents has been through group projects, supervised by a school nurse or a health or home eco-

---

[5] S. L. Hammar: "The Obese Adolescent." *J. Sch. Health.* 35:246–249, 1965.

nomics teacher. By discussion of their mutual problems and reactions, a group of girls ceases to be isolated and withdrawn. Studies on nutrition, selection of foods, and meal planning can form the basis for practical application. Selection of clothing and emphasis upon good posture will be other considerations. In order to assure success of a project of this type, the interest and cooperation of the mothers and families concerned must be enlisted. Self improvement will be a powerful stimulus for more intensive nutrition education. With loss of weight a better figure assures a more attractive appearance. Many psychological and emotional benefits should accrue to the girls who participate in this plan, and those instructors who have attempted such group therapy have found satisfactory rewards.

These weight control group projects are being conducted in some high schools.[6] Since causes of overweight do vary in the participating individuals, and because the supervisor is accepting responsibilities which do have some medical implications, a wise procedure to follow is to require that each person have a physical examination from her physician first. A letter outlining the objectives of the undertaking and the plan to be followed should be taken by her to her physician. His written consent for her to participate should be filed. Such a measure serves several purposes. The physician decides whether his patient really needs to lose weight; possible harm is being anticipated; the individual's physician is giving approval; and if supplementary medical therapy is indicated, the benefits to the students will be more effective. If a girl needs to see her physician at intervals, this must be done. Psychological support may be necessary. When a school system profits from having a school physician, he should be a consultant.

NUTRITION EDUCATION PROGRAM

Detection of Nutrition Problems

Deviations should not be too difficult to detect in a child who is watched a number of hours each day, whose eating habits and diet are observed, whose height and weight are recorded at regular intervals, and whose growth and physical performance are watched. A teacher can check upon the types of lunches brought from home or selected in the cafeteria.

For the older student the same observations should prevail. This group tends to be the neglected group. The home economics teacher, the health educator, the guidance counselor, the physical education instructor, and the coach particularly should be alert.

[6] A. Joyce Kline, Jewell Barron, and Margaret M. Roberts: "Comprehensive Self-Improvement Program for Inner City Obese Teenage Girls." *J. Sch. Health* 29:21–28, 1969.

Follow-up

As has been stated under management of malnutrition, the follow-up is strictly a matter of individual study and investigation. A consultation with the family physician is often a first requirement. The school nurse can assist by counseling with the youngster and his parents. A discussion of dietary needs with the mother may produce desired improvement. Such an interview must be conducted with infinite tact, however, for a housewife and mother is jealous of her prerogatives in the kitchen. Needless to say, procedures in follow-up are based upon causes of malnutrition.

A social worker can provide liaison with the home. His services are particularly valuable where socioeconomic factors explain a child's nutritional status. Education of parents in selection and preparation of food, provisions for welfare assistance, and the offerings of free meals at school are usually in order.

Health Education

Emphasis is placed both upon promotion of good nutrition and upon prevention of malnutrition. These objectives are achieved by instruction of the individual, group, family, and community.

Instruction is both formal and incidental. Teachers themselves should set examples in their eating habits at school. A teacher who prepares to eat his own lunch and sends a student to buy him a soft drink should not expect the student to drink milk under the same circumstances. A teacher who expresses dislike for certain foods as he carries his tray along the cafeteria line can expect imitation from the children who immediately follow him.

Formalized class instruction in nutrition may be presented in health, biology, home economics, or physiology classes. Elementary teachers spend quite a bit of time in nutrition education. Curriculum planning in a school and in a school system should insure an integrated program which avoids boring repetition. Surveys show that students of all ages have been "vitaminized" to a negative attitude.

Nutrition Education

A. Aim—to establish good food habits which will result in intelligent food selection throughout life.
   1. Attained through knowing the actual food habits of children—how they learn at different age levels; and an appreciation of the joint responsibility to be assumed by the school and the home.

B. An effective program of Nutrition Education will have the following characteristics:
   1. It is planned cooperatively by administrators and teachers.
   2. It is adapted to conditions in local community.
   3. Help of specialists is made available to the teacher.

4. Teachers have practical training in foods and nutrition.
5. Teacher, rather than a specialist from outside the school, is responsible for the teaching in her classroom.
6. It is designed to reach the parents.
7. Information about foods is taught through many educational activities.
8. It is an integral part of the curriculum within each grade level.
9. *Nutrition Education is a continuous program for grades Kindergarten through 12.*

C. Today's teacher who finds time in her schedule to include nutrition learning experiences based upon real-life needs and interests of boys and girls contributes not only to their health but also their learning readiness. This in turn lightens her load and adds to the joy of teaching.[7]

SCHOOL FOOD SERVICES

The school food services should fulfill the objectives of a good nutrition education program because of its potential educational aspects; in addition, these services provide nutritious foods and prevent malnutrition. The last observation has been amply demonstrated in underprivileged areas of this country where the national school lunch program has been in existence. Participating children have improved not only in health, but in academic achievement. In needy districts where a free breakfast of cereal and milk is provided, absenteeism is definitely decreased.[8]

Where children attend a neighborhood school, those living within a certain area are permitted to go home for lunch. Hopefully, one expects prepared nutritious meal and time to eat it. Secondary schools usually have cafeterias which offer their own menus or participate in the federal school lunch program. Children should have at least a 30-minute lunch period, 20 minutes of which should be spent in consuming the lunch.

Growing children get hungry and thrive and learn when their stomachs are stoked with nutrients. Arrangements should be made for nutritious foods, including milk, to be available at other than meal time. Some children can pay; others get it at no cost. An effort should be made to discourage the use of carbonated beverages, which have no food value except for a few calories in the sugar content. Nutritious foods should be substituted. Here is an opportunity for nutrition education.

School lunch time should be supervised. Children who bring lunches should be invited into the cafeteria or eating-room. The contents of a sack lunch should be observed in casual fashion by a teacher. A child may not be bringing an adequate lunch. His needs may be

[7] The Utah State Board of Education: *School Lunch News:* 1968, p. 6.

[8] Mary M. Hill: "The National School Lunch Program—Its Contribution to Child Health and Nutrition Education." *Clin. Pediatr. 10*:651–655 November, 1971.

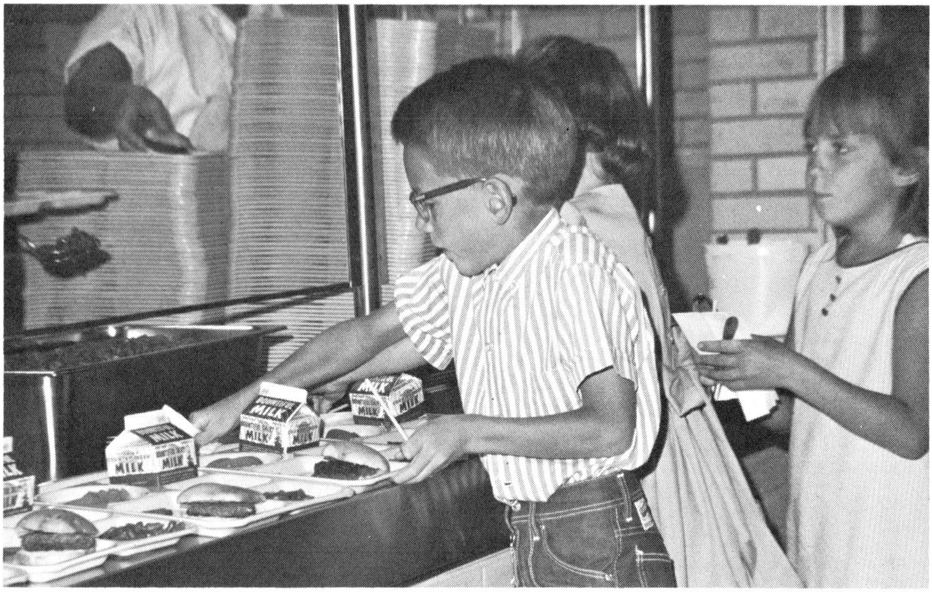

Figure 11 School lunch. (Courtesy Utah State Board of Education.)

supplemented at school. Perhaps his family needs help, and the aid of a school nurse or social worker may be engaged. The type of food selected by a student from the lunch offered at school, if there is a selection, should be the subject of critical observation. Occasionally, a child may not like certain foods or may have an allergy. Allowances and understanding are necessary.

Teachers and school lunch supervisors should also be aware of the cultural and religious practices of the school population. For instance, Navajo children have a taboo against eating fish at any time. Alternate selection of foods should be available to those who need it. No child should be permitted to go hungry or suffer because of apparent nonconformity to dietary habits of the majority.

If possible, a glass barrier should be placed between children and food waiting to be served, to avoid handling and to avoid contamination of food by respiratory discharges.

Pupils can share in directing and carrying on the lunch program. They may be given realistic experiences in preparing foods and in selecting meals. They learn which foods offer greatest nutritive values and share in deciding whether candy, carbonated drinks, packaged cookies and the like are to be placed on sale. They come to understand problems in running a lunch room. Teachers of health education, physical education, nutrition, social problems, and many other important aspects of public health find the school lunch kitchen and dining room, as well as planning and financial activities of the program, a valuable laboratory experience.

The Federal School Lunch Program

This program was first established in the 1930's to get rid of surplus food and make work for needy women who might prepare it. The project was successful, and its results could be measured in the better health and scholarship of satisfied children. In 1943 standards were set up by the government for a full Type A meal designed to give a child one third to one half of his daily nutritional requirement. In 1946 the National School Lunch Act was passed, and the program is now under supervision of the Department of Agriculture. State departments of instruction receive federal aid in both money and commodities and administer the program on state levels. Participating schools are obligated to offer lunches to all children and to serve lunches to students not able to pay. Breakfast, supplementary food items, and in some places a late afternoon meal may be supplied, depending upon need and agreements.

Objectives of the Program

A. To provide nutritionally balanced and well-cooked school lunches.
B. To develop desirable food and eating habits in children and youth, and indirectly to improve food habits of all members of the family.

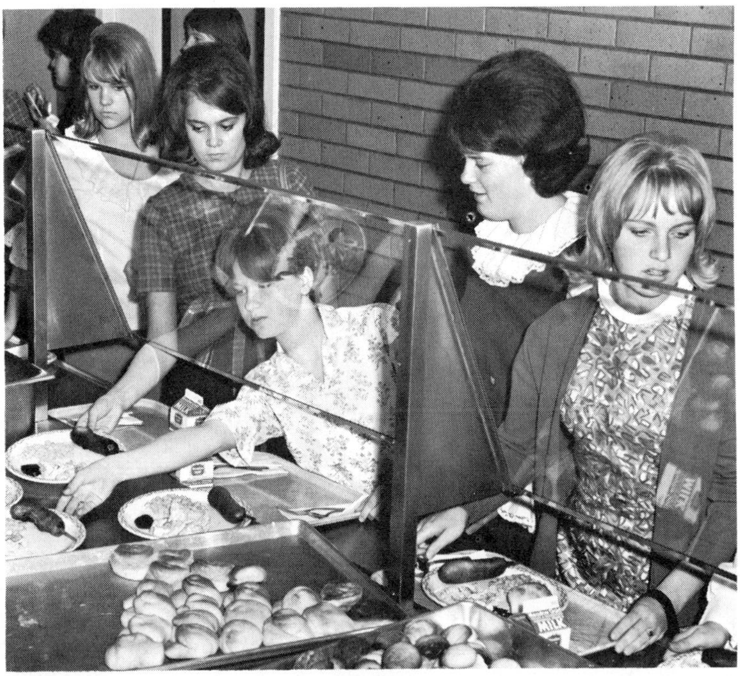

Figure 12 School lunch. Senior high school. Tray and individual dish service. Note the glass barrier. (Courtesy Utah State Board of Education.)

C. To develop an appreciation and understanding of nutritional needs of varying ages of individuals.
D. To develop habits and appreciation of cleanliness and knowledge of the matter of selecting, storing, preparing, and serving food.
E. To improve the general health of the school-going population through such measures as can appropriately be taught.
F. To provide, through the eating of food, a learning situation by which the child gains educational and social experience.
G. To provide for the child such school lunchroom facilities as are necessary to create and develop an appreciation for a quiet, clean, happy, and peaceful environment while eating.

Type A Lunch (provides 1/3 to 1/2 recommended daily dietary allowance)

A. One-half pint of whole milk to drink.
B. Two ounces of meat, poultry, cheese, or fish, or one egg, or one-half cup dried peas, beans or soybeans, or four tablespoons of peanut butter.
C. Three-fourths cup of vegetables and/or fruit.
D. One or more slices of bread or muffins or other hot bread made of whole grain cereal or enriched flour or meal.
E. Two teaspoons of butter or fortified oleo-margarine.

In high school a choice is usually offered daily within one of the component parts of the lunch, between two entrées or two salads, etc. Sometimes this is done in elementary schools.

Need for School Lunches

A. A hungry child is unable to learn. Studies indicate that poor nutrition during early childhood has an effect not only on physical growth but on the mental functioning of the child.
B. Increased need for the School Lunch Program becomes more evident during or after war years. Both in this country and in Europe the number of young men found unfit for military service has brought into sharp focus the need for better nutrition.
C. Nutrition education is as important in America, where food is in abundance, as in those areas of the world where nourishing food is woefully scarce. While severe nutritional deficiencies have practically disappeared here during the last decade, borderline deficiencies are evident and other serious nutritional problems have developed.
D. It is commonly accepted that a large proportion of adolescents, especially teenage girls, in the United States today have poor food habits and consume diets which do not provide all of the essential nutrients. The biggest single problem facing today's teenagers, said a young man at the White House Conference, is "knowing the value of good nutrition and eating good, nutritious food."[9]

About 20 million children are fed a subsidized school lunch every day under the federal school lunch program. The pupil pays about one-half of the actual cost; about two million indigent children

[9] *Ibid.*, p. 5.

receive a free lunch or one below average cost. Another 100,000 are receiving free breakfasts; these are being served in "underprivileged" areas. Educators are enthusiastic with the results. Also, free (or very lost cost) milk is provided daily for 17 million youngsters.

The Joint Committee on Health Problems in Education of the National Education Association and the American Medical Association affirms:

> The school lunch, contributing as it does to the child's nutrition, is a fundamental factor in the general health of that individual and, therefore, necessarily becomes a part of the school health program and of the educational program as a whole.

The above material summarizes concisely the values to be found in the lunch program. Whether arrangements exist to participate in the federal- and state-sponsored affair or to plan a school's own cafeteria activities, the ultimate benefits should be the same. Every child should have a nutritious midday meal. When a child cannot pay for it, he should receive food without cost.

The school lunch project involves all phases of the school health program: (1) the physical facilities (environment); (2) the services which require medical examinations of food handlers and utilize the lunch for preservation and improvement of the health of children; and (3) the use of this facility as a teaching experience. One of the evaluation instruments in health instruction is the achievement of the objectives of the school lunch program.

SUMMARY

The essential nutrients—water, proteins, fats, carbohydrates, minerals and vitamins—their functions, and their usual sources in foods have been discussed. These are necessary for a well-balanced diet which assures growth, energy, maintenance and repair of tissues, and good function of all the metabolic processes. Measurements and evaluation of a child's nutritional status, both normal and deviant as shown by malnutrition, underweight, and overweight should be understood by teachers. Causes of malnutrition are delineated to cover practically every possibility. Such an outline is invaluable in handling a nutrition problem.

The nutrition education program is one of the most vital in a school. It involves detection of individual problems in nutrition with the proper follow-up, a vigorous effort to teach the scientific facts of nutrition appropriate to each grade level, and motivation of children and youth to pay close attention to their eating habits, and health. The school lunch program is valuable in such education. The cooperation of teachers, lunchroom supervisors, administrators, parents, school nurses, social workers, and specialists from various agencies is necessary to promote good nutrition of our school population.

DISCUSSION QUESTIONS AND ACTIVITIES

1. Discuss the dangers—both physical and emotional—of obesity in children.
2. Discuss what you think should be included in a well-balanced diet and why.
3. Obtain a menu for one day from a school food service and analyze its nutritional value.
4. Make a picture collection of persons with malnutrition and analyze the effects of each dietary deficiency.
5. Learn the method of counting calories and keep a calorie intake count for two days. Then, try to estimate your average daily caloric expenditure and correlate it with intake.
6. Relate Abraham Maslow's theory of needs to nutrition. At what level does nutrition fit?
7. Discuss some reasons why children become obese. What could be done to remedy each of these problems?
8. Find out what a nutritionist's education consists of and what job possibilities are open to them.
9. Discuss how this unit can be an interdisciplinary course. In what other fields can nutrition play a part?
10. Explain the use of the "basic four." What is the purpose of this food group?

ADDITIONAL SOURCES OF INFORMATION

READINGS

Adams, R. C.: "Natural Foods." *New Eng. J. Med.* 283:1058, November 5, 1970.

American Association for Health, Physical Education, and Recreation: "Nutrition Resource Unit for Primary Grades." 1967, 16 pp.

Arlin, M.: *The Science of Nutrition.* New York: The Macmillan Co., 1972.

Bogert, L. J., Briggs, G. M., and Calloway, D. H.: *Nutrition and Physical Fitness.* Ninth edition. Philadelphia: W. B. Saunders Co., 1973.
Useful as a reference book for teachers who need to refresh their information. Excellent appendix which includes data on nutritive value of foods in average servings.

Bowden, N. J.: "Food Patterns and Food Needs of Adolescents." *J. Sch. Health* 43: 114–115, March, 1973.

Cameron, A.: *Food—Facts and Fallacies.* London: Faber & Faber Ltd., 1971.

Cordaro, J. B., and Levinson, F. J.: "A Curriculum for the Nutrition Programmer." *Am. J. Clin. Nutr.* 24:1352–1353, November, 1971.

Dugdale, A. E.: "Patterns of Growth and Nutrition in Childhood." *J. Clin. Nutr.* 23: 1280–1287, October, 1970.

Guthrie, H.: *Introductory Nutrition.* Second edition. St. Louis: The C. V. Mosby Co., 1971.

Hiemstra, S. J.: "Nutritional Standards in School Food Science." *J. Sch. Health* 42: 317–319, June, 1972.

Howe, P. S.: *Basic Nutrition in Health and Disease.* Philadelphia: W. B. Saunders Co., 1971.
Joint Committee on Health Problems in Education of the National Education Association and the American Medical Association: "Health Aspects of the School Lunch Program." Second edition. Washington: N.E.A., 1962.
Katz, M.: *Vitamins, Food and Your Health.* New York: Public Affairs Committee, 1971.
Mata, L. J.: "Infection and Nutrition of Children of a Low Socioeconomic Rural Community." *Am. J. Clin. Nutr.* 24:249–259, February, 1971.
Osman, J.: "Nutrition Education: Too Much, Too Soon, or Too Bad?" *J. Sch. Health* 42:592–596, December, 1972.
Paige, D. M.: "School Feeding Program: Who Should Receive What?" *J. Sch. Health* 41:261–263, May, 1971.
Paige, D. M.: "The School Feeding Program: An Underachiever." *J. Sch. Health* 42:392–395, September, 1972.
Taylor, C. M.: *An Annotated International Bibliography of Nutrition Education: Materials, Resource Personnel, and Agencies.* New York: Teachers College Press, 1971.
Watson, George: *Nutrition and Your Mind: Psychochemical Response.* New York: Harper & Row, 1972.

AUDIOVISUAL AIDS

Why Tommy Won't Eat

17 min. Color *adult* National Film Board of Canada

Deals with problem of children who refuse to eat. Traces background of his home atmosphere as basis of the difficulty. (Produced in 1948 but still very good.)

MATERIALS FOR TEACHERS' USE IN SCHOOLS

RESOURCES (partial list)

Local and State Departments of Health
U.S. Department of Agriculture
  Write Consumer and Marketing Service.
U.S. Department of Health, Education, and Welfare
Professional Associations
  American Association of Health, Physical Education, and Recreation
  American Dental Association
  American Dietetic Association
  American Home Economics Association
  American Medical Association
    *Department of Health Education
    Council on Foods and Nutrition
Trade Associations and Commercial Companies
  American Institute of Baking
  Cereal Institute
  General Mills
  John Hancock Mutual Life Insurance Company
  H. J. Heinz Company
  *Metropolitan Life Insurance Company
  *National Dairy Council
    State and some City Branches
  *National Livestock and Meat Board
  Sunkist Growers
  Wheat Flour Institute

A variety of excellent materials can be secured from these resources in the form of pamphlets, teaching plans and materials, posters, exhibits, bulletins, kits and packets of teaching material for various grade levels, reports on research, and in some instances audiovisual aids. Write for catalogs. Addresses are in Appendix A. Those above marked with an *asterisk* will place names of teachers on a mailing list for regular reports or bulletins. No attempt is made here to list reprints or pamphlets because they may become outdated, out of print, or replaced.

State and City Departments of Health have divisions of Health Education and Nutrition. Nutritionists, public health nurses, and other public health personnel are glad to serve as resource persons.

AUDIOVISUAL MATERIALS (partial list)

Recommended grade levels are designated *pri, int, jh, sh.*

These may often be secured for use from the film libraries of state and local departments of health, schools, and universities free or for nominal loan charges and from the distributors indicated after each film.

They may be purchased or rented from the latter source.

Assignment Children

10 min. Color *int, jh, sh* Association Films, Inc.*

Gives account of Danny Kaye's world tour on behalf of United Nations' Children's Fund. In fun making, he advises how to avoid disease.

Bill's Better Breakfast Puppet Show

13½ min. Color *pri* Cereal Institute

Food, Color of Life

22½ min. Color *sh* National Dairy Council

Objective – to motivate people towards better diet and to emphasize individual responsibility for intelligent food selection. 1968 film. Excellent.

Food and Nutrition

12 min. Black and White *sh,* teachers Encyclopaedia Britannica Educ. Corp.

Animated diagrams indicate amounts of food elements necessary. Presents dietary experiments with rats. Explains metabolism.

Foundation Foods

10 min. Color *pri* Avis Films, Inc.

Emphasizes necessity of eating slowly, chewing well, and eating all foods served to you.

Four Food Groups

11 min. Color *pri, int* Avis Films, Inc.

Uses charts and narration to explain needs of foods for building a strong "base" or body foundation.

It's All in Knowing How

14 min. Color Grades 7 – 12 Association Films, Inc.

Challenges teen-agers to use their knowledge of food and to recognize that eating can be pleasant and profitable. For boys.

Something You Didn't Eat

9 min. Color Grade 6 and up Walt Disney Productions

Shows historical developments of knowledge of certain foods and how the meal-planner may select a balanced diet by using the "basic seven" food groups as a guide.

Stanley Takes a Trip

10 min. Color *pri, int* National Film Board of Canada

Two dimensional "cut-out animation" to impress importance of balanced diet on youngsters.

*For addresses of film companies see Appendix A.

Uncle Jim's Dairy Farm

11 min. Color Grades 1–4 Association Films, Inc.
National Dairy Council

Shows wholesome daily living on a dairy farm.

Understanding Vitamins

14 min. Color *int, jh, sh*
Encyclopaedia Britannica Educ. Corp.

Explains what vitamins are, how they work, and why they are necessary for good health. Tells of sources of vitamins and the effect on the body of lack of vitamins.

You and Your Food

8 min. Color *int, jh* Walt Disney Productions

Shows value of food and well-balanced diet.

Young Mother Hubbard

9 min. Color *pri* Avis Films, Inc.

Stresses what to eat, when to eat for good health. Uses specified grouping charts attractive to young students.

Chapter 4

POSTURE AND FEET

Good growth of the skeleton involves gradually laying down a strong bony structure which is shaped for optimum function. When a child is born, the bones are largely cartilaginous and soft. As growth proceeds, cartilage cells increase in number and are gradually replaced by osteoid tissue which is subsequently calcified or ossified. Increase in length of the long bones occurs at the ends. Once ossification is complete, growth ceases. After a bone is completely ossified, its contours are altered only by injury or disease. The shape of a bone and its articulations with others influence its function. It is for this reason that the weight-bearing structures, the vertebrae and the bones of the feet, deserve particular attention during the years of childhood.

POSTURE

Posture involves the alignment of parts of the body to achieve balance in sitting, standing, walking, or physical activity. The bony skeleton and muscles govern balance, which varies with age, occupation, type of activity, physique, and health. There has been a tendency to neglect emphasis upon good muscle balance and alignment of the spinal column. Perhaps this attitude represents a swing to the opposite direction from the time when parents and teachers nagged and pleaded with youngsters to sit up and stand up straight and "throw their shoulders back."

Good posture promotes an attractive appearance with its accompanying psychological benefits, both for the individual and in the favorable impression made upon others. This is worthwhile and should offer prime motivation to adolescents as an objective.

Development of Good Posture

The spinal column is not a straight rod. The vertebrae are aligned one above the other to form a straight line when viewed from the back; but when viewed from the side there are mild natural curves in the neck (cervical), chest (thoracic), low back (lumbar), and pelvic (sacral) regions. Exaggerations of these curves produce what is commonly termed "poor posture." An angulation forward of the vertebrae, usually in the upper thoracic region, is referred to as *kyphosis* (hunchback, humpback). This occurs at times because of organic or structural changes and commonly from posture. An increased inward curve, ordinarily in the low back, is labeled *lordosis* (sway back). The spinal column may also present a deviation laterally (side-to-side-curve), producing *scoliosis*.

Children do not assume the same stance as adults, nor should they be expected to do so. Their postures must not be judged by adult standards. From the crawling position the infant learns to stand erect and to place stress on the vertebrae with their supporting muscles and ligaments. Weight bearing and proper balance of the body, which alter as the body proportions change in the growth to adulthood, determine the spinal curvatures at different ages. The spinal column is extremely flexible in children. The center of gravity in a small child is in the upper part of the trunk. His head is large and he tends to drop his head and chest forward. To compensate for the forward weight, he throws his trunk back upon the pelvis and develops lordosis. As he grows older, the center of gravity gradually drops toward the umbilical and pelvic regions; the pelvis rotates upward; the abdominal and back muscles become stronger and better coordinated; and a proper erectness is attained during adolescence.

Observe Figures 4 and 5 carefully. Note the early lordosis and protuberant abdomen, the gradual changes in the pelvic tilt, gradual flattening of the abdomen owing to increase in strength of the abdominal muscles, and the proper erectness assumed by 13-year-olds. Parents and teachers should realize that exaggerations of spinal curvatures are normal in the early years.

The period of most rapid growth of vertebrae is from 11 to 15 years of age. They are shaped as ossification continues to completion. This shaping and response to weight bearing is naturally affected by posture. The key to good posture is the lumbosacral joint in the low back. It carries the weight of the trunk, head, and upper extremities, and permits flexibility of the upper part of the body on the pelvis. It is a weak joint and is liable to injury. Most backaches later in life are caused by strain in this region. If good balance of this joint is maintained during the growth period, if it is well-centered while the vertebrae are being shaped, much future discomfort will be avoided. A good alignment of the lower vertebrae should be maintained during the ages of six to 17 years.

To promote a good position of the lumbosacral joint, exercise of the abdominal muscles and a correct pelvic tilt are necessary. In the first few grades of school not much can be done about posture except to maintain an environment which will encourage a proper sitting position and to give exercises which will strengthen the abdominal muscles. The physical education teacher can help here.

As the vertebrae begin to grow, more exercises can be undertaken. The basic activity involves strengthening the lower abdominal muscles and rotating the pelvis as these muscles pull it in. A good exercise to accomplish this result is the properly executed sit-up. This should be started in the later elementary grades and continued through high school.

With the lower back in good balance, the upper part will assume fairly good position of its own accord. Shoulder girdle exercises are recommended for all ages. In children they may be achieved by climbing and by use of playground apparatus, such as the jungle gym, parallel ladder, and chinning bag. Rope jumping when the youngster swings his own rope is excellent exercise for the shoulders and upper back. Once the shapes of the vertebrae are fully molded, belated acquisition of good posture becomes a problem of muscle balance and maintenance of good sitting habits. It is better, therefore, to develop satisfactory posture in the early years when the vertebrae can be shaped properly.

Perhaps some mention should be made here concerning the knees and legs. Up to 1½ years of age the infant is bow-legged. Then a transition is made toward knock-knees. From two to 12 years knock-knees are the common pattern. With adolescence the balance becomes normal, although a few bow-legs and knock-knees may persist.

Examination of Posture

Who examines the posture of a child? Marked deviations from normal do not need much of a trained eye. Parents observe deviations and may comment upon them to a teacher. Elementary teachers, indeed all teachers, can readily observe the marked kyphosis or scoliosis beneath a blouse, shirt, or sweater. Physical education teachers notice undressed students in the dressing rooms and showers. They should also make it a project to examine carefully the posture of each student. This is too often a neglected part of class procedure because the importance of good posture is not appreciated.

Posture is evaluated by inspecting a child from the front, rear, and side views. The levels of the shoulders, the heights of the hips, and the possibility of a pelvic tilt are observed. Alterations in curvature from front to back are detected easily.

To detect early *scoliosis,* the examiner observes the child, *undressed,* from the rear, marks the spinous processes of the vertebrae with a pencil and observes the alignment. If any side-to-side devia-

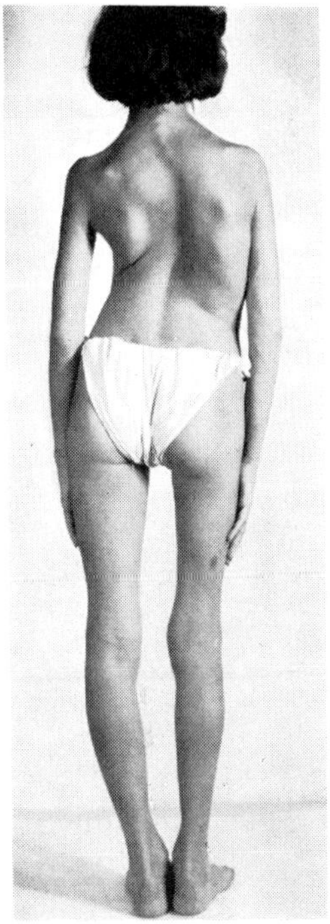

Figure 13 Scoliosis in a girl ten years of age, showing the tilt of the pelvis and shoulders and deformity of the chest.

tion (scoliosis) is noticed in a student (Figure 13), consultation with an orthopedic surgeon is indicated. Early recognition of scoliosis is important. It becomes more prominent and increases in severity during the period of rapid growth of the vertebrae. Some cases of scoliosis are explained on a postural basis; others result from structural defects. The orthopedist makes the differentiation. Therefore, a student with scoliosis should be placed under medical supervision so that a diagnosis can be made. With progression of a structural deformity, the child can become a cripple. Parents and teachers need to understand the importance of this problem.

Kyphosis also is important. Although much of it is on a postural basis, a certain number of children have a disturbance of the epiphyses in the vertebrae. The condition is called Scheuermann's disease. The result is pain. A teacher or parent will complain: "He won't stand up straight. He's round-shouldered. He looks hunchbacked." *It hurts to straighten up.* In contrast to a child with a postural problem, the one with vertebral disease cannot straighten up. As time goes on, the pain becomes worse. As compensation for the kyphosis in order to maintain balance, he develops a lordosis. The result eventually is pain in both upper and lower back. Kyphosis is not normal. It is not outgrown. If there is pain with the attempt to assume a good posture, there will most likely be an accompanying bony deformity of vertebrae. A child deserves most urgently an orthopedic consultation.

As a part of a postural fitness program, in the spring of 1968 the

Medical Services Branch of the Denver Public Schools conducted individual posture inspections on 3327 seventh grade girls, enrolled in 17 junior high schools. Fifty-two girls needed further orthopedic evaluation. Seventy-eight girls were given specific individual posture instructions, to be followed outside the physical education classes. Their postural deviations were not serious enough for medical referral. School nurses and women physical education teachers assisted in the project.

Causes of Poor Posture

Good posture cannot be forced upon a child. Any factors, either of health or environment, which weaken muscular strength or encourage exaggerations of spinal curves, will produce poor posture. Children need more exercise to counteract sedentary habits. Good health and strength are reflected in bearing. Chronic fatigue, malnutrition, illness, and psychological feelings which motivate an attempt at self-effacement affect posture. Other causes may be poor adjustment of seats and desks, poor lighting, poor vision, impaired hearing, careless habits of sitting, walking, and standing, and poorly fitted shoes and clothes. Postural fads which develop in high school, such as throwing the trunk back on the pelvis, produce poor posture. A postural alteration of vertebral alignment during the growth period could become permanent in time. Tall students tend to throw the head too far forward and develop "round shoulders." Congenital anomalies or diseases of the vertebrae, involvement of their cartilaginous surfaces as in rheumatoid arthritis, spasm of supporting muscles to the spine caused by a slipped disc, or weakness of the supporting muscles themselves all have produced poor posture.

Children do complain of *backaches*. This pain is not exclusively the privilege of adults. The pain from disease of the epiphyses of the vertebrae, mentioned in the description of scoliosis, may occur as early as nine or ten years of age. Adolescents can suffer injuries of the back. Rheumatoid arthritis can cause variable amounts of disabilities in joints, including those in the back. Recurrent or persistent backache must be diagnosed. Teachers should listen to the complaints.

Promotion of Good Posture

How can a teacher promote good posture? Attention must be paid to environment. The classroom must be correctly lighted so that children do not stoop forward in an attempt to see better, or so that they will not need to twist the body in order to avoid glare. A good adjustment of seating equipment for each young person, regardless of age level, should encourage him to a good sitting position.

Not only is a comfortable adjustment made, but a child should be taught how to sit properly. He needs changes of activities so that he will not sit for too long periods. He should use playground equipment to make his activities and exercises pleasurable. He should be made posture-conscious, without being nagged. Teaching methods should be used which will motivate a youngster at each age level to adopt good postural practices. Good practices of sitting, standing, and walking develop good posture in the growing child.

A teacher should be alert to a child's health problems and to environmental situations which cause fatigue and slumping. An elementary teacher inspects the posture of her pupils. She should not expect adult posture but should be familiar with the desirable body alignment at various ages (Figures 4 and 5).

Every teacher in a junior or senior high school should be concerned about posture. One can hardly fail to observe the tall adolescent who slumps down and sticks out his feet, or who bends forward so that his eyes are a few inches above the paper as he writes. Good posture is particularly emphasized in such classes as physical education, speech, music, art, health education, sewing, typing, and accounting, or wherever good grooming and good carriage are essential for comfort and appearance.

One way to promote good posture is to arouse interest and pride in maintaining a good posture. Los Angeles city schools sponsor a Posture Contest annually. The year 1966–67 found 165,000 pupils

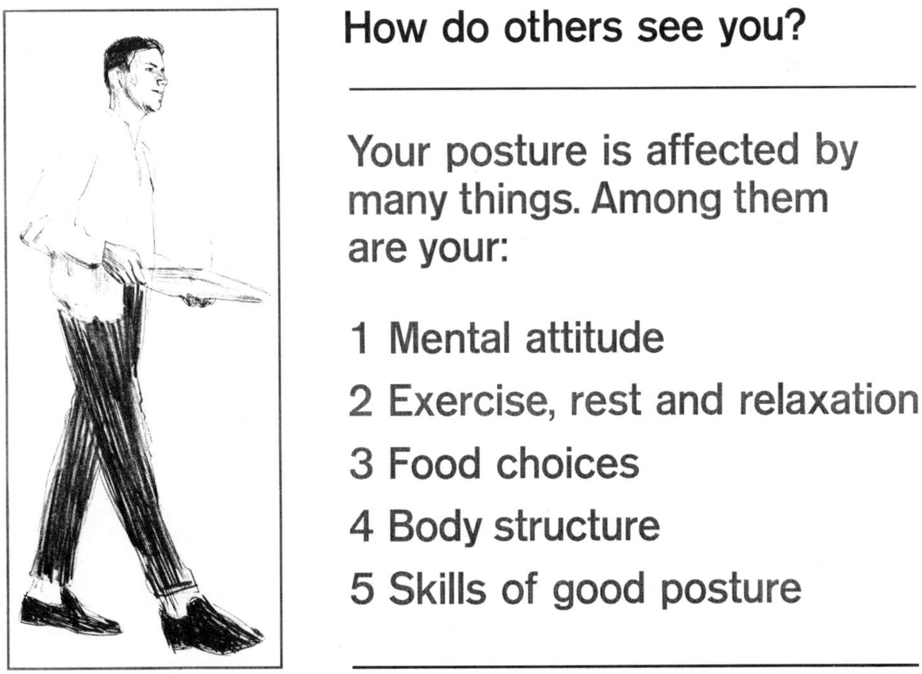

Figure 14 (Courtesy National Dairy Council.)

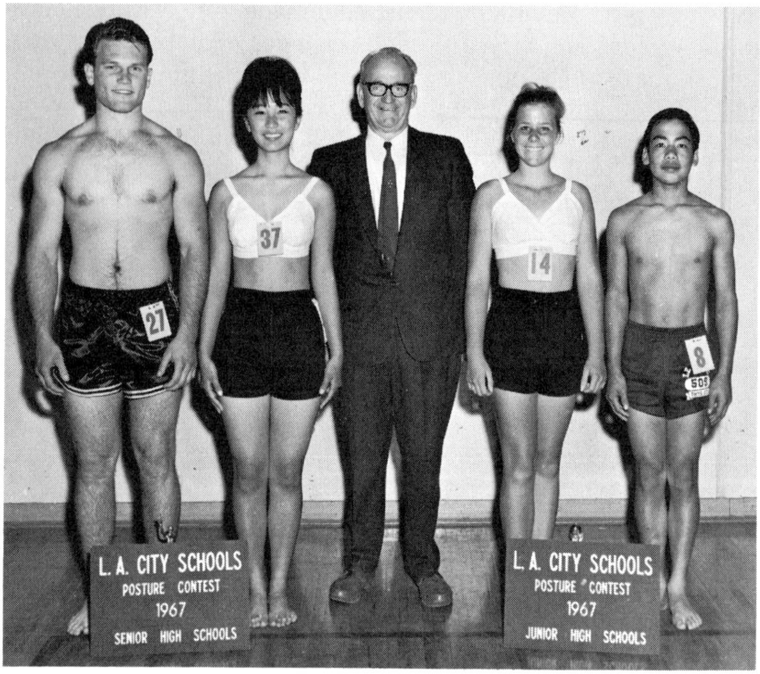

Figure 15 Good posture winners. (Photographer–L. Lee Hansen.)

in the contest from 72 junior and 42 senior high schools. The physical education departments were directly involved. Trophies were awarded. In addition, the Health Services Branch of the Los Angeles City Districts is closely associated with the Corrective Physical Education and Posture Education programs for all grade levels and arranges for orthopedic consultations. (See Figure 15.)

Parents need to be educated so that they can provide an environment at home which enables a child to sit and study properly. Above all, they need to know what constitutes normal posture in a young child.

FEET

Growth

A small child is mildly flat-footed. As he begins to walk, the arches of the feet gradually form. At first the bones of the feet are cartilaginous and incapable of bearing much stress. Gradually they become stronger as the cartilage is replaced by bone. The time of complete ossification varies with the different bones.

By five to six years the feet are 65 to 75 per cent of adult size. Growth usually ceases in girls about the age of 14 and in boys a couple of years later.

Since cartilage can be molded and is not as strong as bone, properly fitted shoes which permit growth of the feet and provide support for weight bearing are necessary. The heel bone must be kept in firm position in the shoe and enough room provided for free movement of the toes. Exercise to develop good musculature for support of the bones and arches and instructions on proper position of the feet while standing or walking may be advised in some cases. One foot exercise involves walking on the outer border of the foot with the toes pulled in. Once the bones of the feet are fully grown, their structure is usually not changed. Exercises after this period serve only to develop muscle balance and relieve strain.

The flexibility of the foot is not as well-developed as of the hand. If balance is not good, the foot tends to pronate, or roll inward, and the forefoot tends to twist to the outside. Such a deviation may become a permanent deformity and disability because a flat foot and strain usually develop.

Children often complain of leg pains. These have been erroneously labeled "growing pains." Growing is not painful. Leg pains may be caused by overexertion or bruising or injury. Pains in the knees with no external signs are exceedingly common in children. Such pains, especially if they occur at night or late in the day and disappear in the morning, even if fairly severe, are generally not significant unless persistent.

Some parents in rural districts may buy or order shoes without fitting them on the child. The outline of the foot may be traced on paper and be used as a basis for selection of footwear. Some parents have the attitude encountered by one third-grade teacher who noticed that a little boy who sat on the front row was immobile, unresponsive, and appeared to be in pain. She happened to look down at his shoes and noticed that they were obviously too small. A phone call to the parent elicited the following vehement response, "I paid good money for those shoes, and he is going to wear them until he wears them out." Fortunately, most parents do give close attention to the proper fitting of their children's shoes, at least in the early years. They appreciate the rapidity of growth of the feet and the importance of frequent changes in size.

Teachers in elementary grades and physical education teachers need to understand how shoes should be fitted. This can be explained to parents and children. The foot is fitted from the heel through the ball of the foot, with room forward for toes. Too tight a shoe across the ball of the foot, with squeezing together of the toes, will produce a bunion. Bunions are observed on both boys' and girls' feet. Children up to the age of 12 should be encouraged to wear shoes which can either be buckled or laced. Otherwise, the shoes will have to be tight, in order to stay on. If strapped or laced, they can be fitted large enough and will not fall off. Children should wear well-fitted shoes, particularly in the early stages of growth of their feet.

ROLE OF THE TEACHER

Teachers in the elementary grades and physical education teachers should be on the alert for abnormal attitudes of the head and neck, bowed legs, knock-knees, pronated feet, deformed feet and toes, deviations of the spine, or an abnormal gait, and should call such defects to the attention of parents or the physician. Such deviations should not be considered normal or hereditary. If the deviation is detected early, correction is possible in most instances. The physical educator may act as consultant to elementary teachers on problems of posture and feet.

SUMMARY

The preceding discussion on posture and feet is by no means comprehensive. More detailed information can be secured from texts in the field, from orthopedists, from those interested in corrective therapy, and from physical educators. Enough discussion is presented to bring the attention of teachers to problems with which they can assist.

Good posture is the arrangement of parts of the bony skeleton and the use of muscles to maintain a comfortable, functional body balance. The spine and the feet are involved. Good posture varies with the growth of the child and does not achieve the adult position until adolescence. During the growth phase, attention is focused upon an environment which promotes good position of the vertebrae, particularly in sitting and studying. Teachers should be alert to detect moderate or severe deviations from normal and request consultation. Complaints of pain should be heeded.

Observations of feet and shoes during the growth period will prevent many permanent deformities and subsequent discomforts.

Teachers have a role to play in all classes in promoting good posture, but they must first appreciate the need.

DISCUSSION QUESTIONS AND ACTIVITIES

1. With the help of a partner, obtain a standard posture test and evaluate the posture of your partner. Did you find any abnormalities?

2. Discuss the implications of administering a posture test in the elementary school. Is it a wise thing to do? Why or why not?

3. Discuss the reasons for bad posture, including factors such as physical, emotional, and social influences.

4. Why should a mother be particularly careful when buying her children shoes? Discuss factors influencing the malformation of the feet.

5. Discuss how organic function could be affected by unhealthy posture.

6. Discuss the importance of being physically fit with regard to posture.

7. Compile a reference bibliography in the areas of posture and feet. You may wish to obtain samples of a few posture tests and compare them.

8. Organize a "posture team" and arrange to evaluate the posture habits at a public school in your area.

ADDITIONAL SOURCES OF INFORMATION

READINGS

American Medical Association: Department of Health Education. Pamphlets.

Greenspan, S. B.: "Effect of Children's Nearpoint Lenses upon Body Posture and Performance." *Am. J. Optom.* 45:982–990, October, 1970.

Lecerof, H.: "Influence of Body Position on Exercise Tolerance, Heart Rate, Blood Pressure, and Respiratory Rate in Coronary Insufficiency." *Brit. Heart J.* 33:78–83, January, 1971.

Lowman, C. L., and Young, C. H.: *Postural Fitness: Significance and Variances.* Philadelphia: Lea & Febiger, 1960.

Reiter, M. J.: *Dynamic Posture and Conditioning for Women.* Minneapolis: Burgess Publishing Co., 1970.

Schulman, D.: "Body Posture and Thinking." *Percept. Motor Skills* 32:27–33, February, 1971.

Stern, F. M.: "The Reflex Development of the Infant." *Am. J. Occup. Ther.* 25:155–158, April, 1971.

Yahraes, H. C., Jr.: "Caring for Your Feet." New York: Public Affairs Pamphlets, 1963.

AUDIOVISUAL AIDS

Dynamic Posture

24 min. For teachers Association for the Aid of Crippled Children

Also a four-part version in color—40 min.

MATERIALS FOR TEACHERS' USE IN SCHOOLS

AUDIOVISUAL MATERIALS

Recommended grade levels are designated *pri, int, jh, sh*

Beginning Good Posture Habits

11 min. Color *pri* Coronet Films*

Care of the Feet

12 min. Black and White *jh, sh* Encyclopaedia Britannica Educ. Corp.

Discusses anatomy and disorders of feet. Foot hygiene. Properly fitted shoes.

*See Appendix A for addresses of film companies.

Healthy Feet

11 min. Color Coronet Films

Discusses structure of feet, causes of foot trouble, and their prevention and cure.

On Your Feet

11 min. Color *int, jh* Avis Films, Inc.

Compares one's feet to a cowboy's mount. The old adage "Take care of your mount and he will take care of you" is used. Includes a list of ideas for foot care.

Posture in Action

20 min. Black and White *jh, sh,* adults Iowa State University

Emphasizes importance of reasons for preferred ways of performing posture and body mechanical skills. Explains body mechanics and principles of posture of particular interest to young women.

Posture Pals

10 min. Color *pri, int* Avis Films, Inc.

Four elementary grade children learn that they have poor posture. Because they wish to improve, they have special instruction from the teacher. Parents cooperate.

Your Body Speaks

12 min. Black and White Center for Mass Communication Columbia University

Relation of posture to muscular tension, exercises for developing good posture in walking, sitting, standing, and climbing stairs are illustrated.

Your Posture

10 min. Black and White *int, jh* Young America Films

Demonstrates posture and factors which affect it.

Chapter 5

HEALTH PROBLEMS OF THE EYES

INTRODUCTION

Good vision and proficiency in learning are closely correlated. Defective vision can account for some cases of retardation in scholastic achievement and for some emotional problems. The child who cannot measure up to the standards of his classmates becomes discouraged, loses interest, and soon finds other avenues for his attention. Some of these avenues may be antisocial or lead to disciplinary problems. The cross-eyed child who is keenly aware of his appearance can develop complexes which linger throughout his lifetime. The nearsighted child who cannot see well enough to bat an approaching ball is soon left off the team. The earlier a defect is noticed and compensated for, the greater the child's promise of a normal life. The teacher who watches the conduct and mannerisms of children in the classroom and on the playground and is alert to detect defects of vision can influence a child's whole future life.

PHYSIOLOGY OF VISION

The eye is frequently likened to a camera, for it has a lens system, a variable aperture system, and a retina comparable to film. The eye itself, however, represents only one part of the whole process which ends with the perception of an image. A brief description of the known mechanism of vision will lend a more comprehensive understanding of the complexity of the problem of investigating a visual defect.

Light rays pass through the transparent cornea, the fluid anterior chamber (aqueous), the lens, and the clear gelatinous mass (vitreous) in the posterior compartment, and are focused upon the retina (Figure 16). The amount of light admitted is regulated by the iris, the colored part of the eye. The muscle fibers in the ciliary body regulate the

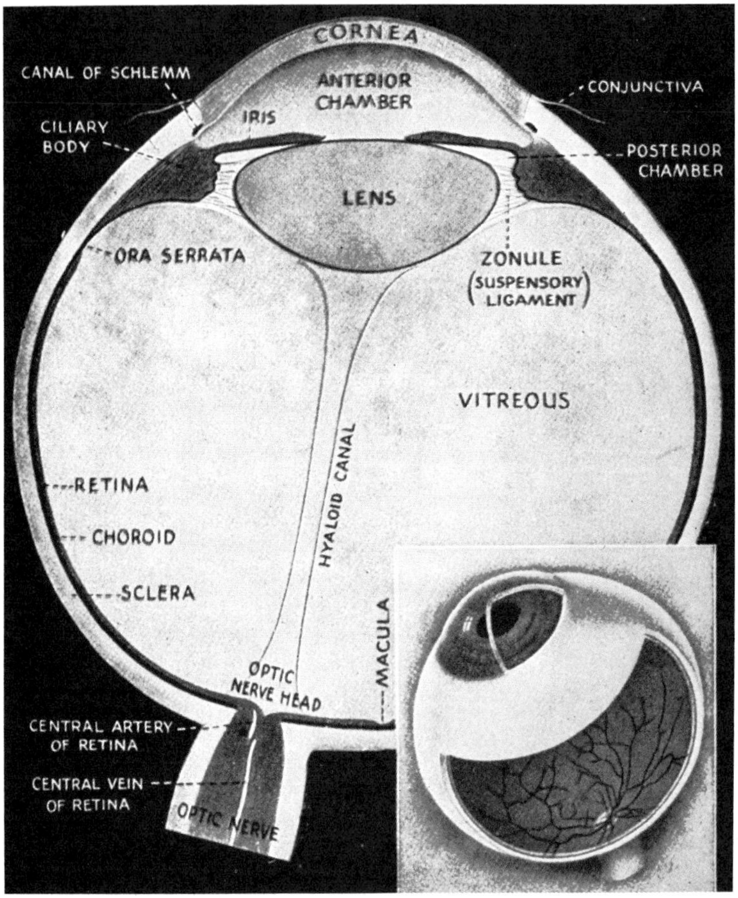

Figure 16 Horizontal section of the eye. (James H. Allen, ed.: *May's Manual of Diseases of the Eye.* The Williams and Wilkins Co., 1968.)

shape of the lens which alters the angle of light rays so that they can finally focus upon the retina. This process of adjustable focusing is referred to as *accommodation.* The outermost portion of the retina consists of a layer of pigment cells which absorb excess light and prevent dazzling. Special cells in the retina designated as rods and cones because of their characteristic appearance receive the light rays, and this radiant energy is converted to electrical energy. Electrical energy is then conveyed through the attached nerve fibers, via the optic nerve, optic tract, and optic radiations, to the back of the brain in the occipital area where the image is finally perceived.

Any disturbance anywhere along the system can result in impairment of vision. For example, if an opaque white scar on the cornea is placed in a position where it blocks light rays, defective vision will result. An opacity in the lens, referred to as a *cataract,* can disturb passage of light rays. Tumors, hemorrhages, or scars in

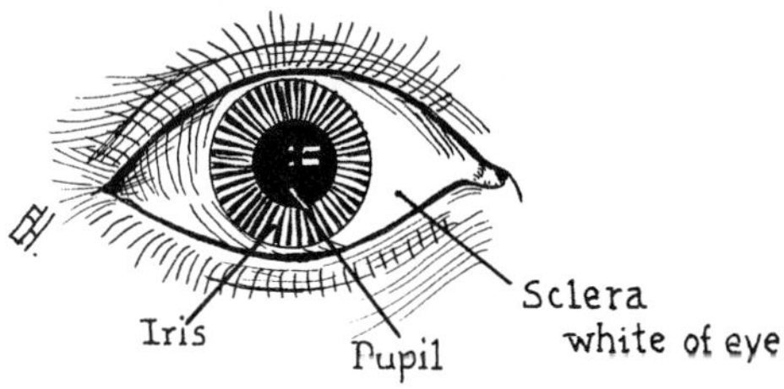

Figure 17 Schematic drawing of the eye.

the retina can prevent reception of good images. Other causes of impaired vision may be a tumor of the pituitary gland pressing upon the optic nerves; infections or inflammations of the nerve; concussion; a fractured skull; or tumors, hemorrhages, or brain damage anywhere along the optic tract, the optic radiations in the brain, or the occipital lobe. Impairment may vary from a slight amount to blindness in one or both eyes.

With any defect of vision a thorough examination should be made, not only for the purpose of measuring vision, but with the idea in mind that deep-seated changes may be present, either beyond the eyeball, in the extended nerve tract, in specific areas of the brain, or in other parts of the body. The specialist who diagnoses and treats a defect of vision should have ample specialized training to detect the cause or causes of the defect. On occasion, delay in recognition of the causative factor and the employment of palliative treatment, such as glasses or medication, have resulted in blindness.

COMMON PROBLEMS OF THE EYE

The Refractive Errors

The eye without refractive error is so constructed that parallel light rays from a theoretical far point at infinity are brought to a focus upon the retina. With the eye at rest, with no use of the mechanism of accommodation, objects at a great distance, as far as size permits, should be seen distinctly. Practically, it is found that objects at a distance of 20 feet project rays that are so nearly parallel that they focus upon the retina without any accommodating effort on the part of the eye; hence, this distance measures the practical far point of the eye.

DESCRIPTION

An ideal refraction exists if parallel rays of light are brought to a focus upon the retina when the eyes are at complete rest. The eye is labeled as *emmetropic* and the condition is known as *emmetropia*. Such an eye enjoys distinct vision without effort or fatigue, particularly for distance. Incidence of pure emmetropia is low.

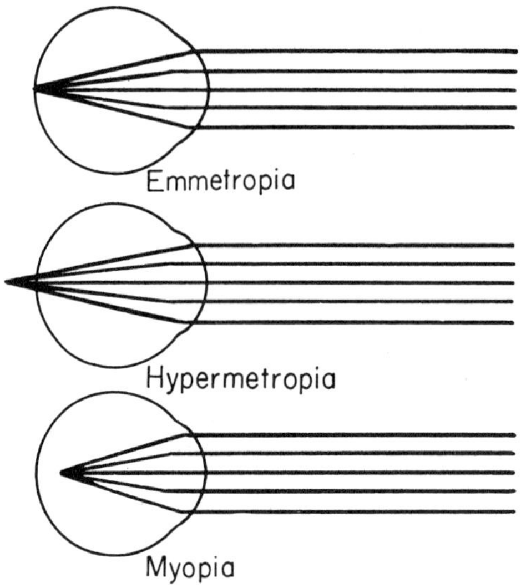

Figure 18 Emmetropia, parallel light rays focus upon the retina; hypermetropia, parallel light rays reach the retina before coming to a focus; and myopia, parallel light rays focus in front of the retina. (Guyton, *Textbook of Medical Physiology.* Fourth edition. W. B. Saunders Co., 1971.)

Variations in refraction are referred to as *refractive errors* (Figure 18). The most common causes of these errors are: (1) variations of the axial length of the eye, or (2) less commonly, variations in corneal or lens refractions. If parallel rays come to a focus before reaching the retina, the axial length is relatively too great for the refractive powers of the eyes and the condition is called *myopia.* On the other hand, if the rays reach the retina before comming to a focus, the axial length is relatively too short, and the condition is called *hyperopia.*

Development of Normal Visual Acuity

The development of normal visual acuity is slow, although the newborn child has a well-developed eye and visual system. Images are fuzzy, about 20/960. By eight months of age a baby sees detail. Thereafter the sequence is approximately:

one year	20/100
two years	20/70
five years	20/30
six years	20/20

Coordinated use of the two eyes to form a single fused image in the brain is present by the sixth month. The eyeball is small and shortened in the anterior-posterior axis in the infant. It grows as the bony orbit grows in childhood and reaches adult size at age seven to eight. The cornea is full size at two years of age. Most of the growth after that is in the back part of the eyeball. The eye may become emmetropic and then proceed to elongate beyond average length and become myopic.

Almost 80 per cent of children are born with hyperopia; almost 5 per cent with myopia and about 15 per cent with emmetropia.[1] About five of every 100 preschool children have visual problems, whereas statistical studies show that 25 per cent of children of school age may have some eye difficulty which may require professional care.[2] The refractive status of the eye is constantly changing and junior and senior high school teachers must be alert.

HYPEROPIA (Hypermetropia, "Farsightedness")

Hyperopia results when the eyeball is short in the anterior-posterior axis. Theoretically, parallel light rays would focus back of the retina (Figure 18), so that a blurred image does occur on the retina. A hyperopic child compensates and forms a sharp image by accommodating unless the hyperopia is extreme. If hyperopia is excessive, the use of glasses is indicated. Hyperopia decreases a little from about the ages of eight to 25. Most adults in the United States remain slightly hyperopic.

One or both eyes may be hyperopic. The hyperopic eye cannot see objects clearly without accommodation, either distant or close. Hence, the eye is never in a condition of rest when distinct vision is being obtained. As a result, the muscles of accommodation are constantly in use; but this is tolerated without symptoms unless hyperopia is extreme.

The mere existence of hyperopia does not necessarily indicate need for glasses. Competent advice by a specialist is required in handling each individual case. Refraction is certainly indicated in children with poor vision.

Farsighted people are proud of their distant vision and consider themselves as eagle-eyed. Actually, they perceive details in the distance with the same clarity as those with emmetropic eyes.

MYOPIA ("Nearsightedness")

During the growth from ages six to 25 years, and particularly during the teens, the increase in length of the eyeball is relatively rapid. If the eyeball is too long in the anterior-posterior axis, light rays from a distance will focus in the vitreous and diverge again to form diffusion circles on the retina. The resultant image is blurred (Figure 19). Such a condition is called *myopia* or *nearsightedness*. The amount of error depends upon the length of the eyeball. Myopia

---

[1]Daniel Vaughan, Robert Cook, and Taylor Asbury: *General Ophthalmology*. Los Altos, California: Lange Medical Publications, 1965, p. 13.

[2]Joint Study Committee of the American School Health Association and the National Society for the Prevention of Blindness, Inc.: *Teaching About Vision*. The Associations, 1972, p. 20.

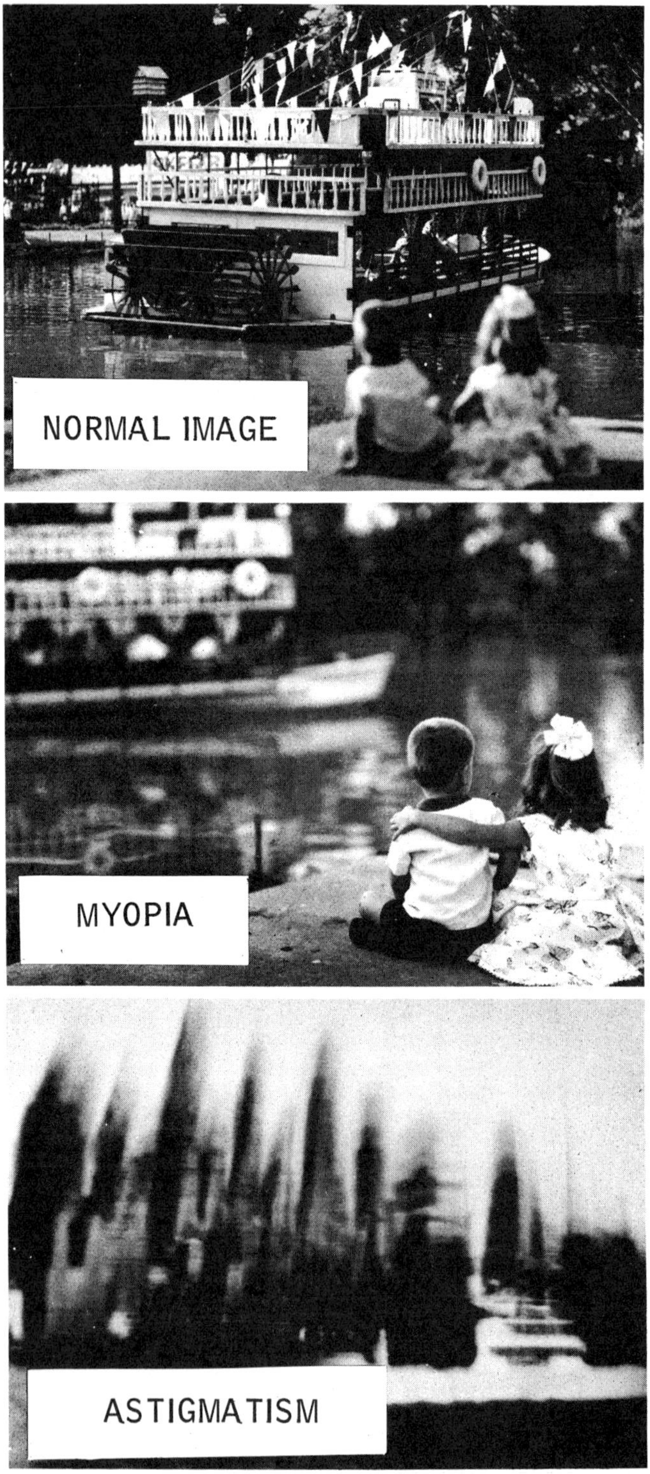

Figure 19 Images as seen in myopia and astigmatism. (Eubank: *When Your Child Needs Glasses*. Courtesy American Medical Association.)

may progress, and sometimes it regresses; no exact explanation for these phenomena has been offered. Contrary to some opinion, *excessive reading or study neither promotes nearsightedness nor causes it to progress.* Some cases of myopia may be caused by too much power in the lens system of the eye.

The fact remains that the myopic eye cannot focus distant objects distinctly upon the retina, but near objects are sharply focused. The habit of holding objects close to the eyes has produced the term "nearsightedness." Myopic children do not usually complain of discomfort with near work. They can sew and read with ease. Distant images are blurred or may not be perceived at all. One or both eyes may be myopic, or one may be myopic and the other hyperopic.

Myopia occurs more frequently in older children, in junior and senior high school, and its more rapid progress ceases about the age of 25. Myopia is expected to increase during the teens, regardless of eye exercises, vitamins, near work, lighting, or rest. Younger children may be myopic; and some youngsters have been found, who, when standing up, can barely see an object upon the floor at their feet. These are extreme cases and should be detected early. A child with extreme myopia may be considered feeble minded or retarded. Wonders in scholastic accomplishment can be gained once the defect is found and proper glasses fitted. Many times it is the teacher who makes the first correct observations. In order to perceive distant objects more clearly, the myopic squeezes the eyelids together. The word "myopia" means "I squeeze." The result is squinting or frowning.

Single vision lenses should be prescribed for the myopic child, to be worn for both distance and near vision; this places the eyes under normal conditions of vision and accommodation. *Children should be unrestricted in their reading.* They should be examined at intervals.

ASTIGMATISM

Astigmatism is a refractive condition of the eye in which the curvature of the cornea or lens or both varies, so that light rays from the different meridians will be refracted differently. The result is a blurred image upon the retina, the degree of blurring depending upon the amount of variation (Figure 19). The accommodative powers of the eye can only partially compensate for this defect. Astigmatism may occur alone or combined with hyperopia or myopia. With slight astigmatism vision may not be affected; with a greater degree there is a diminution in acuteness of vision, both distant and near. The person with astigmatism tends to frown and hold work near. Slight degrees of astigmatism may not need correction; mild degrees may necessitate the use of glasses for such activities as reading, movies, television, and driving; severe cases require constant use of glasses. Most astigmatic errors remain fairly constant throughout life.

Strabismus
(Squint, Cast, Wall-eyes, Cross-eyes)

Definition and Description

Strabismus exists when one eye looks in a different direction from the other eye. The extraocular muscles are the muscles attached to the outside of the eyeball which enable the eye to move in different directions in the eye-socket. Six muscles attached to each eye enable it to turn in, out, up, down, and obliquely. Yet the 12 muscles of both eyes should be so beautifully coordinated in action as to permit a single image at all times. Any imbalance of nervous stimulation to the muscles can result in a situation where one eye does not look in the same direction as the other.

Slight "crossing" may not be noticed on an inspection of the eyes, since both eyes will appear to be in normal position. It may be noticeable with fatigue or with emotional disturbances. Some specialists instruct a parent to bring a child in for examination toward the end of the day when he is tired, irritable, and fussing. Sometimes the eye may be seen to wander to an obviously different position from its mate. Close and persistent observation on the part of the teacher may be helpful to confirm a suspicion of strabismus.

In severe cases, when neuromuscular effort no longer brings the visual axes to bear upon the same point, a strabismus can be observed at all times. If an eye turns "in," the term used is *internal* or *convergent strabismus* (Figure 20); the opposite is *external* or *divergent strabismus* (Figure 21). The eye may become drawn occasionally into other positions because of neuromuscular weakness. Internal strabismus is the most common. About 1.5 per cent of children in this country have eyes that are not "straight." Strabismus appears most frequently at two and one half to three years of age.

With strabismus a single fused image is not possible if both eyes are used, so the child favors the image from the clearer eye and ignores the other. The result is one-eyed central vision with loss of three-dimensional vision, but retention of the depth perception which one eye can provide. If the habit of using only one eye continues over a long period of time, the child will suppress vision in the

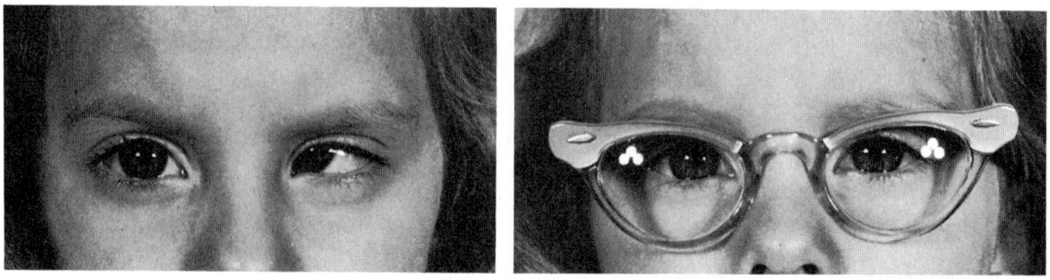

Figure 20 Accommodative convergent strabismus straightened by corrective lenses. (From Nelson, McKay, and Vaughan: *Textbook of Pediatrics.* Ninth edition. W. B. Saunders Co., 1969.)

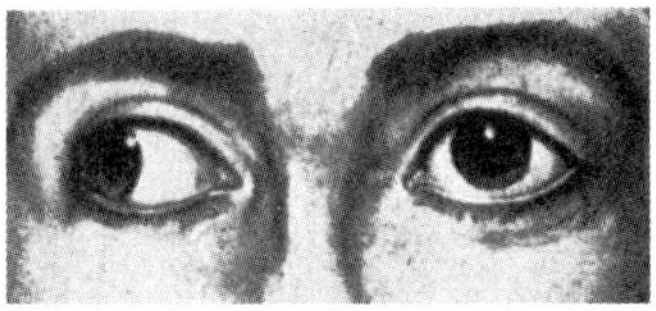

Figure 21 Divergent strabismus. (James H. Allen, ed.: *May's Manual of Diseases of the Eye*. The Williams and Wilkins Co., 1968.)

other. In some instances an alternating fixation may exist, in which the youngster alternates fixation of the eyes and maintains adequate vision in both. One-eyed vision still results, however, since the image from the non-fixated eye is ignored.

Causes

Many times the cause cannot be established. Strabismus may be *hereditary,* with more than one member of a family's being affected. Mention has been made of *impairment of nervous stimulation* to extraocular muscles, causing an imbalance. This is probably the greatest single factor. The problem is usually in the central nervous system and is usually hereditary. *Injury* to an extraocular muscle or to its nerve supply may weaken or paralyze it. A boy of 15 rammed a sharply pointed pole into the lower muscle attached to one eye. The resulting weakness caused the eye to be pulled upward out of normal position. Since surgery and glasses were not corrective, he has repressed the image from the affected eye.

Strabismus may follow a *severe illness.* The eyes may be observed to cross for the first time after a child recovers from an illness. Usually, except with neurological problems, the squint is not attributable to the illness. The interpretation is that the potential to develop the squint was there, and the illness precipitated it.

Refractive errors may produce strabismus. A refractive error in one eye only, or greater in one eye than the other, causes the child to favor use of one eye. One of the most common errors is *uncorrected hyperopia.* Most small children are hyperopic but in severe cases an extreme accommodation is necessary for focusing upon near objects and a convergent or internal strabismus may develop. The condition frequently appears at ages two to four. If the hyperopia is treated immediately with appropriate glasses and other remedial measures as prescribed by the specialist, the strabismus may gradually be corrected over the years of childhood.

Loss of vision in one eye from disease, such as a tumor, may result in strabismus. *Accentuation factors* are excitability, fatigue, drowsiness, or an emotionally wrought reaction causing a child to be angry or upset.

Results

Amblyopia. Neglected strabismus produces sad results. The child learns to ignore the vision from one eye. This process is called *suppression.* If suppression continues, *amblyopia* ("lazy eye," decreased vision) develops. Amblyopia can be defined as decreased visual acuity in one eye without organic eye disease. Its vision may measure as poorly as 20/200 or 20/400. The child does not see "double" because he learns to ignore the image coming from the crossing eye. Vision in the other eye may be normal unless an optical defect is present. If the good eye is lost later in life, the amblyopic eye will not produce satisfactory vision. If the good eye is lost before the age of five to seven, vision in the amblyopic eye may become normal. If strabismus develops after the age of eight, a persistent double image occurs.

Psychological. Children are called nicknames in school. Their appearance is unprepossessing. A child may become shy, inhibited, and withdrawn, or display overt behavior patterns.

Corrective Procedures

Parents should never be told to wait until a child starts to school before starting treatment, usually interpreted by many people as a simple correction with the fitting of glasses. Nor should they be told that time alone will correct crossed eyes. Nor should they be led to believe that the use of glasses will completely cure the condition. *Corrective procedures are indicated the moment the strabismus is noticed,* even in infancy. Good functional results "are obtained in 80 per cent of children up to two years of age, in 60 per cent of children from two to four years, and in only 40 per cent of those from four to seven years of age."[3]

The usual remedial measures are special lenses in glasses, forced use of the squinting eye by the use of patches over the better one, and training in binocular vision through fusion exercises. Various types of strabismus are treated differently; in some types, exercises and patches are of little value. Each case presents an individual problem; what may be effective for one child may be ineffective for another. Needless to say, close cooperation between parents, child, and specialist is required over many years. The results are worthwhile, for the eyes will likely become straight and fusion of the images in the brain will develop. (See Figure 20.)

At the discretion of the eye physician and surgeon (other titles—ophthalmologist, oculist), surgery is performed upon the extraocular muscle or muscles in order to produce "straight eyes." This goal is usually achieved, but more than one operation may be required. Surgery is occasionally undertaken with an infant. If surgery is indicated, it is usually done at an early age, while fusion is possible, and before a child starts school and suffers psychological trauma. Not infrequently older people elect operative procedures for cos-

[3]Waldo E. Nelson, editor: *Textbook of Pediatrics:* Eighth edition. Philadelphia: W. B. Saunders Company, 1964, p. 1489.

metic improvement only; generally speaking, surgery will not produce fusion of vision if a person is older than five to seven years because the image from one eye has been too long suppressed. There are exceptions.

The goals of treatment for strabismus are good vision in each eye, good cosmetic appearance, and binocular vision.

The Role of the Teacher and of the School

Early detection of strabismus and amblyopia is the key to this visual problem. These should be observed, in many instances, long before a child starts school, by the parent or physician. The school often conducts preschool vision testing. *A test for visual acuity* (using the E Snellen chart) *should be done about the age of four* (some say between the ages of three and four) while amblyopia can still be treated. This may be a school undertaking or a project of other interested groups. Since there are approximately 8,000,000 children in this country between the ages of three and four, the taks of detecting amblyopia is great. To reach those in urban, suburban, and rural areas means that intelligent assistance must come from many sources. The American Academy of Pediatrics is sponsoring a parent-administered project, using a chart that has imprinted upon it the image of a hand with outspread fingers. When a child is brought to a physician's office for a consultation, the parent is given this chart with instructions in its use and is asked to return the results.[4]

A teacher should be alert to the problem in the classroom. Many children with amblyopia do not have noticeable deviation of the eyes and usually look straight ahead. One teacher in the third grade had a hunch that one of her pupils suffered from a squint and watched him closely for two weeks before she finally decided that one eye tended to drift occasionally. When she discussed her observations with the parents, an immediate appointment was made for medical consultation. The child soon began to wear glasses, and the teacher certainly felt that her alertness was rewarded.

A good deal of space has been allotted here to the topic of strabismus and amblyopia (with technical explanation) in the hope that the message of early detection and treatment will be widely disseminated and save the vision of many children.

Use of Glasses

In addition to the special lenses used in the treatment of amblyopia and strabismus, there are two other indications for wearing

[4]Edward Press and Caroline Austin: "Screening of Preschool Children for Amblyopia." *J.A.M.A.* *204*:767–770, 1968.

glasses—better vision and comfortable vision. The indistinct images caused by refractive errors can usually be sharpened by the use of glasses. In cases of myopia appropriate lenses spread the light rays so that they finally meet on the retina (Figure 22). The lenses used in hyperopia have the opposite effect. Cylindrical lenses are prescribed for astigmatism and special ones for strabismus. Combinations of these are used when complex defects are present. Bifocal lenses are reserved for older people who gradually develop the typical changes in their own lenses which come with age, an immobility due to a hardening of the lens which limits accommodation for near work. This condition is referred to as *presbyopia.* Younger people do not need one set of lenses for distance and another set for near vision since their own power of accommodation is adequate. Occasionally, however, bifocal lenses are prescribed for internal strabismus.

Correctly fitted glasses do not make the eyes weaker. It is often stated that a person comes to depend upon his glasses as upon a crutch. The actual explanation is that an individual sees much better or is more comfortable with glasses which provide normal vision. When they are not worn, the resulting poor vision is more noticeable by contrast. The eyes are actually not weaker.

Safety lenses are considered by many sight-saving experts to be a necessity for all children's eyewear.[5] Ordinary glass lenses can shatter into dangerous slivers under slight impact. Three types of safety lenses are on the market:

1. Dress safety or tempered glasses are ground of ordinary glass, then subjected to a high temperature followed by quick cooling. They do not break easily; and if broken, they tend to fracture into small granules instead of slivers. The thinnest part of the glass measures 2.1 mm.

[5]*Ibid,* pp. 47–49.

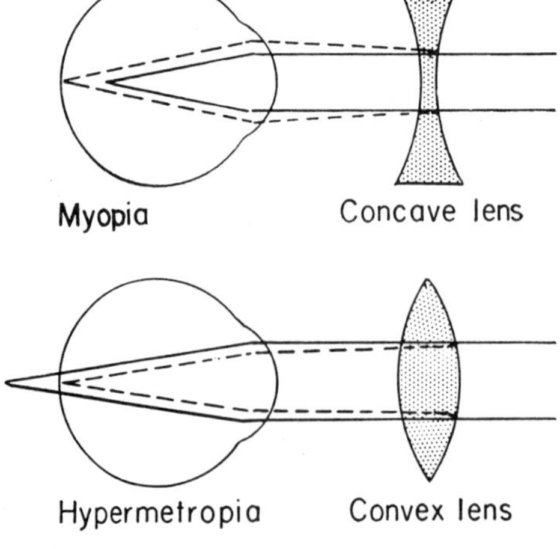

Figure 22 Correction of myopia with concave lens, and correction of hypermetropia with convex lens. (Guyton: *Textbook of Medical Physiology.* Fourth edition. W. B. Saunders Co., 1971.)

2. Industrial safety glasses are also tempered glasses, used in hazardous areas, including shop work. They measure 3 mm. in the thinnest area.

3. Unbreakable resin-plastic lenses offer protection but scratch readily. Since they are lighter than glass, they are often used by those who must wear thick prescription glasses. They can be used by older children who have learned to take care of their glasses.

The nominal additional cost of safety lenses is most worthwhile in preservation of vision against accidents, not to mention the elimination of the cost of new glasses every time a lens is broken. On occasion, safety lenses are prescribed without correction when an eye is to be protected, as in one-eyed vision with normal visual acuity.

Contact lenses are being widely used. They are made of plastic and rest on the cornea, kept in position by capillary attraction. The fitting of a contact lens is a delicate procedure which should be placed only in the hands of the most skilled. There are no refills or substitutes for eyes, and the finest care must be taken of them. Contact lenses should not be worn until a person accepts responsibility for their care and follows explicit instructions on their use.

When the use of spectacles is impractical, contact lenses are fitted. Athletes often wear them in contact sports. Myopic students who are self-conscious about their thick lenses find comfort in the use of contact lenses. Their use is not necessary in mild myopia when near vision is not handicapped, and spectacles are worn only part time for distant vision. Contact lenses give trouble sometimes until the individual becomes accustomed to them. After all, they are foreign bodies placed under the lids. A nervous person tends to contract and tighten the lids and press the lenses against the cornea, producing discomfort. On a windy day, when dust and pollen enter the eyes, or with inflammation of the conjunctiva (see Conjunctivitis), or with hay fever and allergies, often the lenses cannot be worn. Sometimes the cornea is scratched when a lens is inserted, causing pain and possible infection. Sometimes the lenses are interchanged, with the right one in the left eye and vice versa. Sometimes they become so oily that vision is poor. If they are painful to use, they should be checked. Saliva should not be used as a wetting agent, because it is not sterile and may cause infection. Complications may also come from wearing them for too long a period or from sleeping with the lenses in place.

Deficient Color Perception
(Color Blindness)

The trend to avoid the term "color blindness" is gaining favor.[6] Everyone can see color, but the interpretation can differ from that of

[6]Eleanor M. Grunberg: "Color Deficient Versus Color Blind." *J. Sch. Health* *43*:2, February, 1973.

an individual with normal color perception. Defective color vision is a disorder in which the ability to perceive one or more of the three basic colors, blue, green, or red, is impaired or absent. The red-green impairment is most common. An occasional person is said to be "blue" or "blue-yellow" color blind. In rare instances one may be totally lacking in response to colors.

Aside from a few acquired color vision problems based on nervous system involvement, defective color perception is hereditary. It is a sex-linked, recessive characteristic. Two per cent of all men are red color blind; 6 per cent are green color blind.[7] Approximately one woman in 1250 has faulty color perception, mostly with red-green colors.

Detection of color blindness can be done rapidly in a screening test, using spot charts in which spots of several colors are arranged so that various figures or numbers may be traced by a person with normal color vision. The use of such charts enables an examiner to determine color blindness within a few seconds. They are used routinely by the armed forces and by many industrial concerns. The Ishihara and Pseudoisochromatic Plates (American Optical Company) are examples. Women are usually not tested for color vision in mass examinations because the incidence is so low that the procedure is not considered feasible.

Formal tests with charts are not the only methods of checking color vision. Simple, rough tests are at hand for quick screening—matching yarns, using a duplicate set of colors (maybe color charts from the paint store), identifying the colors of book bindings or other objects in a room or in a picture.

Tests for color vision should be given in primary grades. Colorful devices—maps, charts, and pictures—are used for effective teaching. The color-defective child has gaps in his learning. In some industries which require an interpretation of color signals, such as employment with a railroad system, normal color vision is important. Color coding in electronics (wiring, etc.) and color changes in chemical reactions may confuse the color-deficient individual. Traffic signals may not be clear. Selection of colors in clothing will be unconventional, unless supervised. There is some indication that color-defective individuals may develop self-consciousness and social problems. The whole field of psychological use of colors is important—the use of those which are restful or stimulating, or those which suggest coolness or warmth. Certainly one's appreciation of the environment and the visual arts is enriched by a normal perception of colors.

Since defective color vision can be a handicap in some educational and vocational activities, early detection and counseling have been worthwhile. This problem must be considered in driver training.

---

[7]Arthur C. Guyton: *Textbook of Medical Physiology*. Fourth edition. Philadelphia: W. B. Saunders Co., 1971.

Common Infections of the Eye

Blepharitis

Blepharitis ("granulated eyelids") is a very common, chronic inflammation of the margin of the eyelid, characterized by white scales or yellow crusts at the bases of the lashes, redness and thickening of the lid, and falling out of the lashes. The latter occurs more on the lower lids. The lashes may or may not be replaced. The child may even complain of itching and soreness of the lids and sensitivity to light. The condition is common in children, is often resistant to treatment, and should be under the care of a physician.

Sty

A sty is an infection of a hair follicle in the margin of the eyelid, and is characterized by localized swelling, pain, tenderness, and redness. In most cases it gradually develops a core of pus. When the pus is evacuated, healing usually follows. Stys occur at all ages, but are most common in children and young people, and may come in crops. One or two are barely healed before others appear. These sufferers should consult their physicians.

Conjunctivitis

The conjunctiva is a thin mucous membrane lining the eyelids and deflected over to the eyeball. In health it is transparent with a few noticeable blood vessels coursing through it. With irritation or infection the blood vessels become congested and prominent; there may be tearing and discomfort; sometimes a thin mucoid secretion forms; or, in acute severe infections, a discharge of pus may be so profuse that it glues the lashes together during sleep. In the morning a mother may have to wash the lids to remove the discharge before the eyes can be opened. The lids may feel heavy, hot, gritty, and the lashes are sticky. There may be sensitivity to light, and a blurring of vision may result from the secretion lying on the cornea.

The acute *epidemic conjunctivitis (bacterial conjunctivitis),* characterized by a heavy discharge of pus and "bloodshot eyes" is popularly known as "pink eye." It occurs most often in spring and autumn. It may occur in one eye only, but commonly spreads to the other. It is highly contagious and spreads rapidly from one child to the other by indirect contact. Since the eyelids smart or itch, the child tends to rub them, gets discharge on his fingers, later handles doorknobs, pencils, books, and other articles which are handled subsequently by a classmate whose hands then become contaminated. The latter in turn touches his own eyes and transfers the infection. Towels, wash rags, and handkerchiefs can be common carriers.

Other infections can occur in the conjunctiva or on the cornea. *Trachoma* is an infectious disease of the conjunctiva and cornea caused by a virus. It is highly contagious in its early stages and is usually found among the poorer people living under poor sanitary conditions. About 15 per cent of the world's population suffer from this affliction, a major cause of blindness in Asia, Africa, and the Middle East. It is rare in the United States. Trachoma can spread from the conjunctiva to the cornea, causing redness, congestion, ulceration, scarring on the cornea, and ultimately, reduced vision. Both eyes will be affected. Mild itching and irritation are the most common complaints. This disease responds to the use of antibiotics; hence, early detection and treatment are of utmost importance.

Redness of the conjunctiva, either transitory or chronic, is frequently observed. The transitory form is caused by irritation from such factors as smoke, dust, foreign bodies, excessive glare from sun, snow, or bright light; or it may be associated with colds or hay fever. The chronic form may be caused by chronic infections or allergies.

The Role of the Teacher

Any teacher can inspect the eyes of children noting their appearance and any deviation from normal. *Any child with a discharge of pus in his eyes should be sent home with a recommendation to see his physician* and not be allowed to return until the infection has cleared.

Injuries

First Aid

Injuries to the eye occur frequently at school—injuries of any type from the presence of a minute foreign body to severe ones which threaten blindness. Blindness has resulted from the flick of a rubber band or a paper clip fired from a rubber band.

In first aid to injuries of the eye, the following practices should be observed:

1. Foreign particle on the transparent tissue covering the inner surface of the eyelid or the white of the eye: Do not rub. Let tears wash out. Or touch particle lightly with moistened cotton swab or moistened corner of a clean handkerchief. Do not touch the clear cornea. If removal is successful and person is comfortable and sees well, no further management is indicated. If there is any difficulty whatsoever in removal, the child needs medical attention.

2. Particles imbedded in cornea or scratch on cornea: Usually painful. Tearing. Leave alone. Should be seen by an ophthalmologist.

3. Penetrating wound into the eyeball: Do not touch the eye. If a child must be transported any distance, cover both eyes, avoiding pressure to wounded eye. Should be seen by an ophthalmologist *immediately.*

4. Bleeding from eye or eyelids: Let bleed. Otherwise pressure

may compress eyeball, which may have been injured, and cause damage. Should have medical attention.

Cut of eyelid with separation of edges needs fine plastic surgery.

5. Chemical eye burns (caustics, acids, poisons): *Wash immediately* with plain water at room temperature for at least 15 minutes. Pour water into the opened eye from a glass or other container or, if possible, hold head under a faucet. Do not use an eye cup. Do not go to a doctor or anywhere until eye has been washed thoroughly for at least 15 minutes. Do not try to neutralize with another chemical. Then, get medical attention. This procedure may mean the difference between vision and blindness.

6. With a blow to the eye (frequently from a ball or fist), the child should have medical attention. *Watch for* (a) blood back of the cornea, (b) complaint of double vision, (c) inequality in size of the pupils, and (d) pain and prominence (bulging) of the eye upon blowing the nose.

There may or may not be much discoloration of surrounding tissue.

7. "Black eye" or "shiner" may be important. Watch for above warnings. Child should see a physician to make sure eyeball or cheekbone or nose has not been damaged.

8. Any complaint of seeing a shadow or having a "curtain" in the eye, even if vision is 20/20, should be investigated by an ophthalmologist. Retinal detachment is a possibility.

9. Do not keep an eyewash or eye "drops" in first aid cabinet.

If a child is hit in the eye and complains of blurred vision, an ophthalmologist is contacted immediately. A *detached retina* sometimes follows a blow to the eye or jarring; and if this serious injury is not detected and treated quickly, blindness usually follows. The blow may cause a laceration of the cornea, which will produce severe pain. A "black eye" or "shiner" is caused by hemorrhage into the soft tissue around the eye. Sometimes the white part of the eyeball is hemorrhagic also. A "black eye" should not be taken lightly. It should be seen by an ophthalmologist or personal physician.

EYE SAFETY

In junior and senior high schools most eye injuries occur in the laboratories and industrial shops. The high incidence of these injuries and the increasing number of lawsuits against teachers for negligence (see Legal Responsibility), with damage awards running into six figures, have prompted the development of eye protection programs in schools. The first state law for eye protection in schools became effective in Ohio in August, 1963:

> Every pupil and teacher in any public school participating in any of the following courses:
>
> A. Vocational or industrial arts shops or laboratories involving experience with:
>
> 1. Hot molten metals;

2. Milling, sawing, turning, shaping, cutting, or stamping of any solid materials;
3. Heat treatment, tempering, or kiln firing of any metal or other materials;
4. Gas or electric arc welding;
5. Repair or servicing of any vehicle;
6. Caustic or explosive materials;

B. Chemical or combined chemical-physical laboratories involving caustic or explosive chemicals or hot liquids or solids; is required to wear industrial quality eye protective devices at all times while participating in such courses or laboratories. A board of education may furnish such devices for pupils and teachers, and shall furnish such equipment for all visitors to such classrooms or laboratories. A board of education may purchase such devices in large quantities and sell them at cost to pupils and teachers.

"Industrial quality eye protective devices," as used in this section, means devices meeting the standards of the American standard safety code for head, eye, and respiratory protection, Z2. 1-1959, promulgated by the American Standards Association, Incorporated.

Maryland and Massachusetts adopted similar legislation in June, 1964. Other states have followed.

Note that the quality of eyewear is specified. Each student has safety spectacles or goggles for individual use exclusively. He applies the eye protector before entering the shop or laboratory. Such mandatory regulations relieve the teacher and school of some responsibility and should reduce the number of eye injuries.

SCHOOL HEALTH PROGRAM

Detection of Eye Problems

Mannerisms or Conduct of Child

An observant teacher may detect visual defects by watching a child's actions. Symptoms, signs, and behavior patterns which may make a teacher suspect difficulties are in the following list; a child will not display all of these patterns, nor does it follow that children who manifest some of the abnormalities suffer from poor vision. This list serves as a guide. A child may:

Rub his eyes in an attempt to clear vision.
Favor one eye or turn or tilt head to one side.
Bend forward in an attempt to see better.
Have difficulty seeing the writing on chalkboard.
Ask to sit in front of the room.
Tend to squint, scowl, frown, or widen the lids.
Hold his eyes too close to his work in reading or writing.
Complain that letters or lines are blurred or "run together."
Tend to stumble over small objects.
Fail to see a distant object or oncoming ball while at play.

Inspection of Eyes

The teacher or examiner stands in front of the child, who is looking straight ahead. The eyes should look clear and normal. A cataract is sometimes seen as an oval or round gray or white opacity in the pupil. Conjunctivitis, discharge of pus, or a bloodshot appearance of the conjunctiva is easily observed. The pupils of both eyes should be aligned straight ahead, also.

Tests for Visual Acuity

Visual acuity refers to the sharpness of details and contours which are perceived. Screening tests can be readily done by a teacher or anyone trained to do them. They may be done on individual suspected cases or routinely for a group, whether in a preschool round-up, nursery school, elementary classroom, or a health or physical education class. The National Society for the Prevention of Blindness suggests that screening for visual acuity, hyperopia, and phoria take place every two to three years.[8]

Snellen Test. The Snellen test for distant vision is excellent and is the most commonly accepted of all screening tests. Visual acuity is usually measured by the familiar Snellen chart on which the letters in each line are smaller than those in the preceding line (Figures 23 and 24). If viewed from a distance of 20 feet, accommodation is not needed.

[8]Mildred E. Doster: "Vision Screening in Schools—Why, How and When." *Clin. Pediatr.* *10*:1:664, November, 1971.

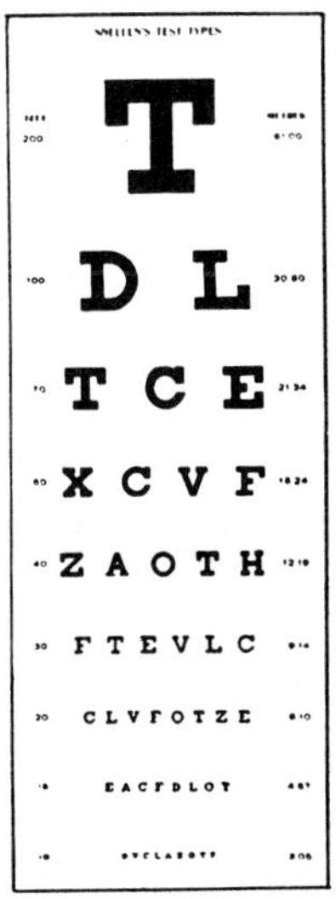

Figure 23 Snellen's test. Usual style of chart. All charts do not present same letters.

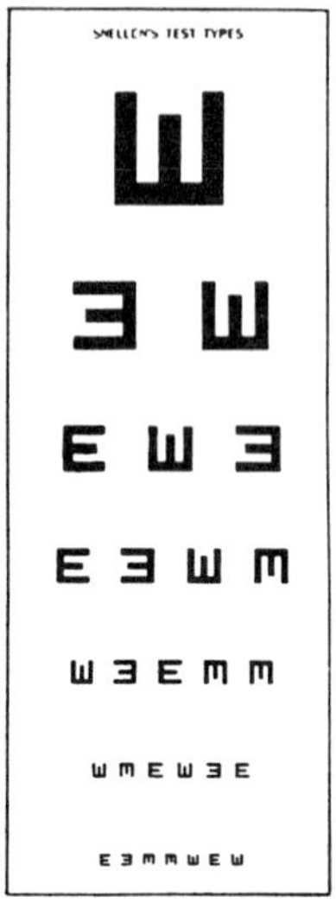

Figure 24 Test type for illiterate. E chart. (James H. Allen, ed.: *May's Manual of Diseases of the Eye.* The Williams and Wilkins Co., 1968.)

> "If at 20 feet the individual reads the letters of the line marked 20 feet, visual acuity is stated as 20/20 and is considered normal. If an individual can read only the line marked 100 (which a normal eye can read at 100 feet), his visual acuity is given as 20/100. Lines of test type smaller than the 20/20 line are provided and are rated 20/15, 20/13, and 20/10. Such ratings mean that the individual has better than normally acute vision and *do not mean that the individual is hyperopic.* The hyperope does not see better than the emmetrope at a distance. To reduce the visual acuity to a fraction by saying that a person with 20/40 vision has 50 per cent normal visual acuity is like saying that a temperature of 80 degrees is twice as hot as 40 degrees. In some Snellen test charts, the lines of type are labeled in percentage of useful vision."[9]

The actual technique of performing the test is simple. The chart is easily obtained and is cheap. It should be placed where a light can shine upon it, preferably opposite a window. Artificial illumination will give a more uniform and consistent light. The chart is placed at eye level. One eye is examined at a time; a card is placed before the other eye. The covered eye should not have any pressure on the eyeball. If so, there will be difficulty in reading the letters accurately. The child is instructed to read slowly and firmly. Little children require more time because of slow reading ability. Speed of reading is not an objective here. It is well to have only one child in the examining room at a time, since there is a tendency to memorize the letters. Moreover, such a procedure lends dignity and meaning to the test.

E Chart. For an illiterate person (including preschool children) the E Chart is used to test visual acuity. A series of E letters is used, corresponding to the Snellen types, with the limbs or "fingers" of the

---

[9]Theodore C. Ruch and Harry D. Patton, editors: *Physiology and Biophysics.* Nineteenth edition. Philadelphia: W. B. Saunders Company, 1965, p. 431.

E pointing up, down, to the right, and to the left (Figure 24). A child stands next to the chart and places his fingers on the letters to indicate the "fingers" of some of the E's; he is then placed 20 feet away and proceeds to indicate which way the "fingers" point by extending his own in the same direction. Tests for determination of visual acuity are fairly accurate in children over three and one half years. For children who are unable to read, pictures of familiar common objects the size of the Snellen types are used. This determination may not be too accurate.

Emphasis must be placed upon the preschool vision check. *Every child should have his vision checked at age four,* and must have a compensated 20/20 vision in both eyes before the age of six. (See Strabismus.)

The Department of Health Services, Denver Public Schools, reports the following screening survey made in 1967–1968:

> Preschool vision screening tests were done by 54 volunteers of the Delta Gamma Sorority on 1436 three- and four-year-old youngsters (most were four years old).
>
> Total referred to school nurse for rechecks was 83.
>
> Nurse reports on these children:

Normal	34
Referred to medical care	33
Already on medical care	3
Unable to be tested adequately	13

> By June 1st, the eye specialists had reported these findings on the first 17 children to get further care:
>
> 4 have been fitted with glasses
> 3 were normal
> 3 had amblyopia
> 1 had mild astigmatism
> 1 is scheduled for surgery
> 2 more have refractive errors and are being watched
> 1 has astigmatism and myopia
> 1 other was noted, needs "watching"
> 1 has mild myopia and will be rechecked in six months.

Modifications of the Snellen test are sometimes used. Several types of machines are available. In a school they are used for screening—not diagnosis. They are much more expensive and offer no advantages over the Snellen chart in checking visual acuity.

Criticism of All Screening Tests at School. The several methods of screening can be made by teachers, nurses, technicians or parents. All of these tests provide only rough screening. The Snellen test combined with careful observations by teachers is recommended. Some cases will be screened out who actually need care; on the other hand, the findings on some children will be falsely interpreted as indicating visual defects. This is unavoidable. And, interestingly enough, the proportion of unnecessary referrals to specialists varies little with the screening test used or the experience of the person performing the test.[10] To make a positive statement concerning a child's visual defect is not always justified on the basis of a screening test at school. A complete investigation, including a refraction, a check for strabismus, and an examination of the inner structure of the eye by ophthalmoscope are necessary for a conclusive diagnosis.

Follow-up

Once a visual defect is suspected, the next step is a more thorough examination by a specialist. It is estimated that more than 12 million school children require eye care. Parents should be notified and strongly advised to seek expert consultation. (See Figure 25.) Because of the possible error in interpreting results, a child is referred without information on the findings at school. A parent is simply informed that there are grounds for suspecting that further investigation is indicated. The manner of contact with the parents must be tactful and wise. They must be made to feel that the school wishes their child to be normal and healthy and is alert to make sure that he does not suffer from neglect. Also, these parents should be made to realize that the screening methods used at school to detect defects of vision may subject some normal children to the inconvenience and expense of a specialist's examination.

The prejudice against placing glasses upon a small child is fading, and more and more bespectacled youngsters can be seen. Sometimes this prejudice has to be combated with a great deal of persuasion and reassurance. Most parents wish to do right by their children. The cost of glasses is quite a problem for some families, and various communities provide different means of caring for this need. Welfare and PTA groups and various civic organizations may offer assistance; funds raised from social events at school, or those provided by boards of education may provide some of the money required for examination and glasses.

All efforts must be made to give attention to the child with impaired vision. *He should be encouraged to wear his prescribed glasses.* These glasses should be protective.

It is not necessary to stress that the visually impaired should be detected early, and that those who need special education should be started on a regimen as quickly as possible. Conceivably, a family feels so keenly the stigma of possessing a blind child that its presence will be concealed from others. It is difficult to appreciate the behavior of a so-called intelligent professional couple who finally bring their blind child, age nine, to a school and ask for advice.

---

[10] Franklin M. Foote and Marion M. Crane: "An Evaluation of Vision Screening." *Exceptional Children* 20:153–161, 1954.

DENVER PUBLIC SCHOOLS
Health Service Department

HOME REPORT ON VISION SCREENING

Date____________________ School__________________________

Recently, ____

was given a vision screening test at school and seemed to have some visual difficulty. Although glasses may not be needed, we urge you to have an examination to recheck this condition. Would you please take this report to an eye specialist to be completed so that it may be returned promptly to the school nurse.

Thank you,

__________________________ (Principal)

__________________________ (School Nurse)

Report From Eye Specialist

I have examined the above pupil on __________________ and found the following eye condition:__________________________________

____

____

My recommendations are:______________________________________

____

____

____________________ (Date)

__________________________ (Signature of Examiner)

STOCK NO. 10719
FORM 819 DSP 6-66-200 PADS D-587-57243

Figure 25 Sample of referral form on vision screening.

Management of the Visually Handicapped

Definitions

A partially sighted person has best corrected vision in the better eye of 20/70 to 20/200 with correcting lens. This is an arbitrary standard. About one in 1000 to 1500 children in school needs special attention in studies because of defective vision. These children are not considered blind, but their defective vision cannot be improved to normal with glasses. These individuals are eligible for special services.

Only one in four blind persons suffers complete loss of vision; the others are handicapped by a visual defect which prevents them from carrying on the usual activities of life in the normal way. Technically, the definition drafted by the Committee on Statistics of the Blind, recommended by the Federal Security Board and adopted by most state agencies serving the blind, is as follows: (1) visual acuity of 20/200 or less in the better eye with correcting lens or (2) any degree of visual acuity when there is a visual field of 20 degrees or less in the better eye.

Visual Field Loss. A loss of visual field may impose severe limitations and still go undetected. For this reason teachers need to understand the characteristics of this visual defect:

Most of us have a visual field of 180 degrees. This means that if we hold both of our arms out horizontally, with hands as far apart as possible making our arms form a straight line with the body profile, we should be able to look straight ahead and still detect by sight the finger movements of both hands at once. As the two hands are brought slowly together, we should be able to see the fingers of both hands moving at every point. When the visual field is restricted to 20 degrees, the person sees only straight ahead, and he is considered legally blind; yet he may still pass the Snellen test with a 20/20 measurement. The field loss may be (1) peripheral (outside edges), (2) macular (in the center), (3) spotty and irregular, or even (4) one sided, right or left. Any one of these will make reading, sports, and numerous other school tasks much more difficult.

The behavior of children varies with the degree and the position of the loss. A teacher may point to a word and the child will see only the ones around it. He may see an approaching object only intermittently or tilt his head to follow it better. He may not see an object in his path in time to avoid it. Two children may have 20/20 vision but differ in functional visual acuity.

The best rule to follow when working with a low vision student is: When in doubt about a pupil's ability to perform a particular task, the teacher should observe his attempts and determine realistic expectations.

Statistics on the incidence of blindness are unsatisfactory. It is estimated that there are more than 400,000 blind individuals, more in the older age groups. Probably not more than 10 per cent are under 20 years of age. Accidents are a main cause of blindness.

History of Special Services

The first school for the blind in the United States was founded in 1832 in Boston by Samuel Gridley Howe. Several soon followed in other states. These were residential schools.

Not until 1913 in Boston and Cleveland were "sight saving" classes developed for the partially sighted. Unfortunately, today there are too few programs for the partially sighted associated with regular school systems. It is estimated that at least 50,000 children have need of this service. With the widespread interest in special education, there is no doubt that there will be expansion of the program. Frequent visual tests at school and alertness on the part of teachers will prompt the detection of needy cases.

The trend of the last two decades is to place the visually impaired in regular schools. *This means that every classroom teacher needs to know how to manage and teach the partially sighted and blind.* Occasionally, one will be in attendance.

Education of the Visually Impaired

Programs. There are five types of programs which offer formal schooling for the visually impaired:

1. *Residential School.* This oldest type of program is usually operated on a state level and offers dormitory facilities to a large number of its students. It offers the most concentrated help, but it also offers the most segregation from the sighted public. Most of the states in this country have such a school or cooperate with a school located in an adjoining state.

2. *Special Class.* In this program a blind child attends a regular school, but he has his own segregated classroom, planned specifically for visually impaired students. The students must be transported from many parts of a fairly large community in order to have enough students to form a class.

3. *Cooperative Class.* This differs from the special class in only one basic way. Instead of staying in their own self-contained classroom, the visually impaired are scheduled to attend the regular classes for some of their academic subjects. The subjects, length of time, and grade level may differ for each student; this is determined by the teachers. Such leniency gives a blind child a chance to adjust to the sighted world as slowly or as rapidly as is best for him individually.

4. *Resource Room.* This resembles the two previous programs in that the visually impaired students are all transported to one regular school; but instead of being assigned to a special classroom, they are placed in the regular rooms with the sighted children. Then for an hour or so daily, each visually impaired student goes to a special

teacher who has set up his program in what is called the Resource Room. Here each learns the extra skills needed to compensate for his sight loss. Besides the regularly scheduled visits, visually impaired students may visit the Resource Room for special help or to use the special supplies or equipment anytime they may need it during each school day.

5. *Itinerant Teacher.* This program gives the maximum amount of association with the student's sighted peers. Sometimes in the process little or no association may be had with other visually impaired students. The child attends the same school as the other children in his neighborhood. The special teacher travels from school to school on a regularly scheduled basis to supply the equipment, suggestions, and information needed for the child's good school adjustment. Time, distances, and the size and weight of equipment place some limitations here on the teacher's visits.

The type of program or programs offered in any given area depends upon the need, the density of the population, funds, and trained personnel. Most areas are served, at least, by a residential school. Only the more densely populated regions would have enough handicapped children in a small enough geographical area to make one or more of the other programs possible. The decision as to need and type of program is made by the school district. Decision as to the program best suited for a visually impaired child must be made by a student, his parents, and consultants who judge on an individual basis.

The last three or four programs often give services to both partially sighted and blind children, with the teacher making the adjustments which best fit in with the visual capacities of his various students. Regular classroom teachers must be prepared to work with all degrees of sight loss. The services of the itinerant teacher can be invaluable to teacher and student.

SERVICES OFFERED THE BLIND. Totally blind as well as legally blind students are now found in regular schools. The special teacher will need to help with such skills as braille reading and writing, using tape recorded textbooks, typing, relief maps, models, handwriting, calculating on an abacus, and orientation and mobility.

Services Offered the Partially Sighted. In regular schools these students are encouraged to carry on their schoolwork without fear of damage to their eyes. Eyesight is not conserved by limited use of eyes. The planned program focuses upon certain details: printed matter and typewriters with larger type, sometimes the envy of others in the class; dark-lined writing paper; pencils with large leads to make a clear black line; tape recordings, or other records to which the child listens and learns, again enjoyed by others in the room; various optical aids, including magnifying or telescopic lenses, which are extremely helpful. These students may need to hold reading material close to the eyes. The teacher should not discourage such action. They learn typewriting about the fourth or fifth grade, which increases communication. Their own handwriting tends to be slow, laborious, and difficult to read. Rooms should be kept as quiet as possible so that good use can be made of hearing, as a compensation for visual loss.

HINTS FOR CLASSROOM TEACHER

1. Don't impose limitations. Let him show you what he can do.
2. Accept the student and his special tools.
3. Seat for best view and hearing.
4. Provide good lighting (where needed).
5. Allow student to examine teaching aids individually.
6. Adjust size and due dates of reading assignments.
7. Give face or transcribed copies in place of mimeographed materials.
8. Allow transcribing time to itinerant teacher on handouts, tests, etc.
9. Interpret needs to school personnel.
10. Note areas for itinerant helps.[11]

Orientation and Mobility. This particular area of education is considered the greatest problem the totally blind must master. No matter how much training and experience they have had, getting about gracefully and skillfully is still a great effort which requires the utmost concentration on all tactile clues.

Orientation refers to the person's ability to keep himself accurately "found" or located in his environment in relationship to his surroundings. Where is the street in relationship to his present position? Where are the doorways? Auditory and tactile clues must be used skillfully to answer these questions.

Mobility refers to the blind person's ability to get himself from one place to another skillfully. He may travel without any artificial aid. He might use a long white cane to tappingly feel his way. He may use a seeing-eye dog. However, at some time or another, most use a sighted guide. The blind person should be allowed to hold the arm of the sighted guide (not vice versa) and should be allowed to follow half a step or so behind so that he may use the guide's body movements as clues to approaching steps, doors, and obstacles. When surrounded by crowds in hallways, mobility can become a serious problem to a legally blind student with some vision. To prevent his frustration, he should be permitted to leave each class three to five minutes early so that he can arrive at the next one before the crowd. Or, he may use the help of a sighted guide if both have had some instruction in the techniques which have been most effective.

For those who are in contact with a legally blind individual, the following hints are offered:

If you walk with him:
Let him take *your* arm. Don't push him!
The motion of your body will tell him what to do.

---

[11]Ellen Clint, itinerant teacher of the visually impaired, Granite School District, Salt Lake City, Utah, provided most of the material on education of the visually impaired in this chapter.

If you eat with him:
Read the menu and prices to him. If he wants help, cut his meat, fix his coffee, etc. Tell him the position of the food on his plate.

If he has a dog:
Remember that the dog is a *working* dog, not a pet! Don't divert his attention—his master's life depends on his alertness.

If he is alone:
Always identify yourself when entering a room if a blind person is alone. Don't play any "guess who" games!

If you live or work with him:
Never leave a door ajar! Keep corridors clear of clutter. Tell him if furniture is moved.

If you talk with him:
A blind person can hear as well as you, sometimes better. Always talk directly to him, not through his companion.

If you seat him:
When showing a blind person to a chair, put his hand on the back. He will be able to seat himself easily.

If you direct him:
Give directions as clearly as possible. *Left* or *right* according to the way *he* is facing.[12]

Finally, blind children will be the best ambassadors in the future as they have been in the past. We find over and over again that where people in general education have been permitted to know blind children in regular public schools they have learned to think of them as individuals. We also find blind graduates of residential schools who have moved out into society as efficient adults and have become active citizens in their communities. Perhaps the largest contributions of the present can be found in the parents who, when they are given sufficient help as soon as they need it, are showing that they are capable of accepting and understanding their children. Our final question is: Can we, the professional people, work with resources in behalf of blind children? In so doing, we contribute to a rich educational program which meets each child where he is and thinks of him as a part of a family unit and a participating member of society.[13]

Vocational Guidance

The partially sighted and the blind child have definite need of realistic counseling because they are limited in achieving their potentials. They have social, emotional, and vocational problems which must be anticipated, and they deserve the same educational opportunities as normally seeing children. Those in contact with a visually handicapped child must resist overprotection. He must be disciplined the same as any other child and should not be granted too many privileges. He should not grow up into an adult who blames his

[12] American Foundation for the Blind, Inc.

[13] Georgia Lee Abel: "Education of Blind Children." *Am. J. Pub. Health* 45:905, 1955.

inadequacies on his vision. He travels by bus, plays games and comes into physical contact with his peers.

Vocational guidance in senior high school should stress realistic goals with good counseling which will arouse effective motivation. After the ages of 16 or 17 a visually handicapped person can secure help through the Vocational Rehabilitation Agency. Contact is made through state departments of education or through the Special Education Department of a school system or district. Help is available when vision loss interferes with a person's ability to secure and keep a job and as long as there is reasonable certainty that the individual is capable of becoming a responsible employee.

Basically, State Vocational Rehabilitation agencies will pay tuition, sometimes books and reader's service, for those who have adequate grades and could become employable. The objective is to place a client successfully in gainful employment which suits his personal needs.

School teachers and counselors are not prepared to be vocational rehabilitation counselors. They should offer understanding and encouragement and make sure that the visually impaired student is aware of the services open to him.

Dyslexia (Reading Disorder)

The most important gateway to learning is through the eyes. The eye receives the image; then through an extended path in the brain, a concept develops in the frontal lobe. Letters become words, and words have meaning. Vision is an effective tool in learning.

A significant number of children derive no meaning from letters and words and are unable to read. "In some school districts as many as 15 per cent of the students are two grades or more behind in their reading abilities."[14] The logical and first deduction in the minds of bewildered, distraught parents and worried teachers is that vision must be defective. Usually, the first referral of a dyslexic child is to the eye physician. For this reason a brief discussion of dyslexia is placed in this chapter.

Dyslexia is a complex problem. Only recently has intensive study been devoted to understanding its complexity. No one specialist is involved exclusively.

"Dyslexia is a specific inability to read well or understand printed symbols in an otherwise normal individual."[15] This definition deserves attention because it presents the essence of present-day interpretation for reading disorders, as offered by many authorities. Another definition is: "A difficulty in reading understanding due to a

[14] Harold P. Martin, "Vision and its Role in Reading Disability and Dyslexia." *J. Sch. Health, 41*:9, 469, 1971.

[15] *Op. cit.*, Joint Study Committee of the ASHA and the NSPB, p. 61.

central lesion.[16] By a central lesion we mean a neurological deficit in the area of the brain which perceives an image. The problem is one of immature development in the brain.

Secondary dyslexias ("secondary" meaning the result of or owing to) may occur from such factors as: (1) brain damage, as seen with cerebral palsy or mental retardation; (2) emotional disturbances, anxiety, depression; (3) hyperactivity with its short attention span; (4) environmental conditions: (a) limited social opportunity, cultural and economic deprivations with poor exposure to language, knowledge, and reading, (b) poor motivation, and (c) poor instruction. This outline merely suggests possibilities and is not comprehensive.

Some children are slow readers because of visual or auditory handicaps or poor health.

What is to be done about a dyslexic child? How does a teacher proceed? What counseling is given a bewildered parent?

First, a diagnosis must be established. No one specialist cares to make a decision alone on a diagnosis and management. Skilled teamwork is required. A start must be made. Possibly, an established procedure has been organized in a school system or community. If not, since dyslexia is not an unusual disorder, a plan should be developed. Many disciplines are involved. The specialists on a team to evaluate the dyslexia in a child should include a pediatrician or family physician, a neurologist, a psychologist and, if necessary, a psychiatrist, an eye physician, an otologist, and the teacher. The latter may be the classroom teacher who reports on his observations and the academic performance of the child. Or, he may be from the area of special education. If problems of speech need to be considered, a specialist in this field is consulted. A school social worker or school nurse may be asked to describe the home environment. This team should think and work together and know the contribution that each can bring to the diagnosis and management of the dyslexia. The parents must understand the steps which are being taken and can give invaluable information on health history and behavior.

The steps are these. Eyes are examined. A dyslexic child may suffer from a refractive error or muscle imbalance of the eyes. Rarely would a visual handicap produce dyslexia. Nevertheless, the examination must be made and necessary corrective procedures instituted. Hearing must be evaluated. A complete health examination by a pediatrician or family physician should be followed by a neurological study to determine whether an organic brain lesion exists. A child may not display any gross neurological disturbances, such as spasticity or odd behavior patterns; therefore, a careful study is indicated. Potential academic achievement must be measured. Emotional maturity must be considered.

---

[16] Arthur H. Keeney and Virginia T. Keeney, editors: *Dyslexia Diagnosis and Treatment of Reading Disorders*. St. Louis: The C. V. Mosby Co., 1968, p. 175.

In brief, every facet of the dyslexic child's physical, emotional, mental, and environmental being must be scrutinized. This represents coordinated effort. Once the child is taken by a parent for consultation, one medical specialist, perhaps the pediatrician or eye physician or someone who is interested in dyslexia, should institute investigations and confer with all the specialists involved. He may even gather them all together for a round-table discussion. Hopefully, he finally should formulate a diagnosis.

After a diagnosis is made, a schedule should be planned. All those involved in the management of the youngster at home and at school need to be familiar with the conclusions reached and suggestions for the improvement of the child and his dyslexia. One added observation in this: the team which studied the dyslexic child should continue to function and watch his progress over the years. This is a large order, but if one medical specialist is devoted to this problem, continuing interest is possible, and the results are worthwhile.

To summarize: Once a teacher recognizes a dyslexic child, *early diagnosis* and *early treatment* should be the goals. Responsibility for early detection lies primarily with the elementary teacher. A child is more likely to become a normal reader if careful remedial therapy is started in the second grade rather than a year later. Ninety per cent of these children have learning disabilities to varying degrees in other areas, most commonly spelling and arithmetic. Spelling usually gives the most trouble.

Once the cause of the dyslexia for an individual child is determined and corrective health measures, e.g., glasses or hearing aid, are instituted, the final step is educational. When indicated "a good remedial therapist who is usually a teacher with special education background, learns what is needed as he works with the child and draws out of this knowledge special techniques for that child. There is no one method or one book, because there are no two children quite the same. You have to adapt the approach to what you see and feel in that child, and then move along with him."[17]

SUMMARY

This chapter provides detailed, current information on eye problems of children. As such, it should be a valuable resource. It offers a basic explanation for the various problems and indicates the role of the teacher and school in detection and follow-up. In brief, the following advice is given to all teachers:

> Watch behavior or mannerisms which may suggest visual trouble.
>
> Visual acuity should be checked at regular intervals on all children, beginning at the age of four.

[17] *Ibid.*, p. 119.

Watch for cross-eyes and be persistently persuasive in recommending professional consultation.

Send home every child who has a discharge of pus in an eye. Advise medical consultation.

All injuries of the eye, except such minor ones as a minute foreign body which is readily removed, should be referred promptly through parental cooperation and consent to an ophthalmologist (eye physician and surgeon).

Since visually impaired students are now being placed in regular schools, the classroom teacher needs to be familiar with their management.

Since reading problems (dyslexia) are fairly common, they should be detected early and a routine investigation followed. The elementary teacher bears most responsibility here.

DISCUSSION QUESTIONS AND ACTIVITIES

1. Inquire at two or three schools to discover what types of eye screening programs they provide for their students. Which program did you like the most?
2. Discuss how an eye problem could impair the performance of an otherwise "normal" child in our school system. How is he at a disadvantage?
3. Explain one of the most popular eye screening tests and how it works.
4. Compile a pamphlet of first aid procedures for eye injuries.
5. Make a transparency of the anatomy of the eye, including the details needed for your age-group interest.
6. Blindfold a group and carry on a discussion about eye safety. Then talk about the disadvantages of being blind. Does this exercise make you respect your eyes more? Discuss.
7. Why is color blindness dangerous for some people?
8. Discuss how to handle a situation in which a student is making fun of another student with "coke bottle" lenses.
9. Discuss the importance of direct action for a student with an eye infection.
10. Describe what you could do as a follow-up activity after visual screening has discovered defects in some of your students.

ADDITIONAL SOURCES OF INFORMATION

READINGS

Alonso, L.: "What the Classroom Teacher Can Do for the Child with Impaired Vision." *NEA J.* 56:42–43, 1967.

American Public Health Association and National Association for Prevention of Blindness: "Services for Children with Eye Problems." 1968.
Covers whole process of serving children, including teacher screening, early case finding, and diagnosis.
Campbell, F. W.: "Simple Scanning Devices for Computer Modeling of Visual Processes." *J. Physiol.* (London) 217:18P–19P, August, 1971.
Flax, N. J.: "Problems in Relating Visual Function to Reading Disorders." *J. Am. Optom. Ass.* 47:366–372, May, 1970.
Flax, N. J.: "The Contribution of Visual Problems to Learning Disability." *J. Am. Optom. Ass.* 41:841–845, October, 1970.
Fraser, G. R.: "Genetical Aspects of Severe Visual Impairment in Childhood." *J. Med. Genet.* 7:257–267, September, 1970.
Gibbons, H.: "A Preschool Vision Screening Demonstration Project." *J. Sch. Health* 40:76–77, February, 1970.
Hogan, M.: *Histology of the Human Eye: An Atlas and Textbook.* Philadelphia: W. B. Saunders Co., 1971.
Krippe, S.: "Vision Screening of Preschool Children in Mobile Clinics in Iowa." *Public Health Rep.* 85:41–44, January, 1970.
Lawson, L. J., et al.: "A Technique for Visual Appraisal of Mentally Retarded Children." *Am. J. Ophthal.* 72:622–624, September, 1971.
Lippman, O.: "Vision Screening of Young Children." *J. Public Health* 61:1586–1601, August, 1971.
Moss, H. A., et al.: "The Relation Between the Amount of Time Infants Spend at Various States and the Development of Visual Behavior." *Child Develop.* 41:509–517, June, 1970.
Oliver, M., et al.: "Screening of Preschool Children for Ocular Anomalies." *Brit. J. Ophthal.* 55:462–466, July, 1971.
Potts, A.: *The Assessment of Visual Function.* St. Louis: The C. V. Mosby Co., 1972.
Shaterian, E. T.: "Visual Screening Programs for School-Age Children." *Am. Orthopt. J.* 21:120–126, 1971.

MATERIALS FOR TEACHERS' USE IN SCHOOL

AUDIOVISUAL MATERIALS

Recommended grade levels are designated *pri, int, jh, sh.*

Blindness

29 min. Black and White *sh*, adults
Encyclopaedia Britannica Educ. Corp.*
Shows emotional effect of blindness. Shows how a young man climbs back to normalcy.

Bright Eyes

10 min. Color *pri, int* Avis Films, Inc.
Pupil involvement in a project which teaches facts about care and protection of eyes.

Eyes and Their Care

10 min. Black and White *jh, sh*
Encyclopaedia Britannica Educ. Corp.
Discusses the eyes in terms of structure, function, problems, and care.

Eyes and Vision

10 min. Color *jh, sh*
Encyclopaedia Britannica Educ. Corp.
Animation. Explains structure and physiology of the eye.

*See Appendix A for addresses of film companies.

Eyes: Their Structure and Care

11 min. Color *jh, sh* Coronet Films

Structure, function, common defects.

Our Wonderful Eyes and Their Care

11 min. Black and White *pri* Coronet Films

Explains the structure of the eye, procedures for examining the eye, and wearing glasses.

Protecting Eyes at Work

Filmstrip *jh, sh* McGraw-Hill

See Better: Healthy Eyes

11 min. Color *pri, int* Coronet Films

Explains structure of the eyes, the health and safety practices related to eye care, and the common ways to treat disorders of vision.

You and Your Eyes

11 min. Color *pri, int* Walt Disney Productions

Jiminy Cricket's "adventures" into the realm of eye structure and common rules one should observe for their care and better vision—clever, colorful, amusing.

Your Eyes

11 min. Color *jh, sh* McGraw-Hill

With models and animation, structure of eye is explained. Proper care stressed.

Excellent films are available from the National Society for the Prevention of Blindness, Inc., and its affiliates. The following films are recommended for special eye problems.

"Johnny's New World" (vision problems of children)

"This is the Smartest Kid in Town" (eye safety)

Write for names of recent films.

RESOURCES

American Academy of Pediatrics

American Foundation for the Blind, Inc.

Excellent supply of educational material on the partially seeing.

American Medical Association–Department of Health Education

American Public Health Association

National Society for the Prevention of Blindness, Inc. (State affiliates)

U.S. Department of Health, Education, and Welfare

Chapter 6

HEALTH PROBLEMS OF THE EARS, NOSE, THROAT, MOUTH, AND TONSILS

Such a high percentage of health problems in childhood involves the respiratory system that the teacher's responsibility in their recognition is actually defined by law in some states. Regardless of legislation, every teacher, whether in an elementary grade or in a junior or senior high school, should be sensitive enough to know whether the young person sitting before him is ill. A student may complain of a sore throat or an earache, or suffer from frequent colds which account for many absences. His speech may be indistinct or sound muffled. He may appear inattentive because he cannot hear well.

A teacher may or may not be expected to examine a throat and usually will not know how to check hearing with an audiometer; still, he should be familiar with the various problems of the ears, nose, and throat and be ready to follow through properly with referral. He should appreciate the significance of his observations.

The anatomy and physiology of the ear, nose, and throat regions are interrelated, and infections of one usually involve the others. Disease in one region is not demarcated from the others. The close association of ear, nose, and throat will be quite apparent from the discussion below on causes of impairment of hearing.

EARS

Ears are for good hearing; not only does one need to hear sounds, but one needs to understand them as well. Understanding spoken words is not absolutely necessary for communication of ideas; but with such understanding learning is certainly expedited, and adjustments to living made more readily.

Five out of every 100 children hear so poorly that they may be retarded educationally and lack an acceptable vocabulary. Yet many hearing losses are not detected. Elementary teachers particularly need to be alert; about 85 per cent of hearing problems have appeared by the third grade.

Mechanics of Hearing

The organ of hearing is a complex mechanism (Figure 26), and the hearing process itself is inadequately understood. The accepted explanation is that atmospheric sound waves enter the external canal and cause the tympanic membrane (drum) to vibrate, which in turn sets the three small bones or ossicles of the middle ear (malleus, incus, and stapes) into vibration. These bones are in sequence and interdependent. Their action is like that of a fulcrum in that they increase by about 60 per cent the power which produces sounds. The third small bones, the stapes, inserts into the membrane separating the middle and inner ears and transfers the vibrations through this membrane to the endolymph or liquid in the inner ear. Covering the surface of the cochlea of the inner ear are hair cells (organs of Corti) which react to

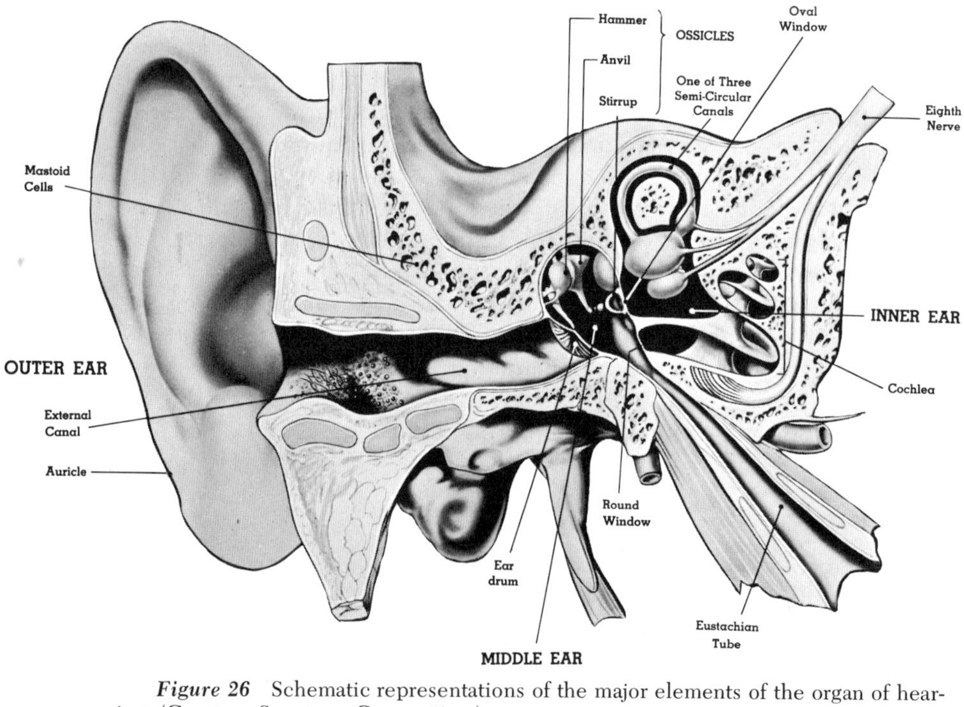

Figure 26 Schematic representations of the major elements of the organ of hearing. (Courtesy Sonotone Corporation.)

the various frequencies of sound transmitted through the endolymph, convert mechanical waves to electrical stimuli, and send these stimuli over nerve fibers which travel through the acoustic nerve to the brain where the sound is finally interpreted. The auditory nerve tract becomes complex as impulses from both ears combine and interact. A great deal still needs to be learned about human hearing.

Deafness. Any impairment along the pathway from the auricle to the cochlea in the inner ear interferes mechanically with the conduction of vibrations; such hearing loss is labeled *conductive deafness*. The term *sensory deafness* is applied when the hair cells of the cochlea are affected. If the nerve elements beyond these cells are involved, the loss of hearing is labeled *neural deafness*. The two terms are usually combined into *sensorineural deafness*.

Conductive deafness may involve only one ear or both and may result in impairment of hearing to varying degrees, but never in a total loss. This form of deafness is more prevalent in children. The reverse is true in older people. Sensorineural deafness usually affects hearing on both sides and may be partial or complete. Mixed or combined deafness involves both types. Conductive deafness is often characterized by hearing loss in the low frequencies; sensorineural deafness results more often in loss of high or middle frequencies (Figures 27 and 28). In conductive deafness there is loss of intensity, and loud speaking helps understanding.

In sensorineural deafness frequencies are dropped, which distorts the reception of sound, and loud speaking will distort sound more. In the latter, a child may respond to loud speech by clapping his hands to his ears with a grimace of pain and protest that he is being hurt.

Two more terms should be explained. A *deaf child has no serviceable hearing; a hard-of-hearing child has a hearing reduction which is still serviceable.* A diagnosis of type, cause, and extent of impairment is necessary because these influence the special education approach to the problem of hearing. About 80 per cent of all cases of impaired hearing are caused by trouble in conduction of sounds. One should think, however, in terms of the amount of hearing present rather than in terms of deafness. Distinction between sensorineural and conductive deafness is essential because the latter may be benefited by a hearing aid and in some instances by surgery. With sensorineural deafness the use of a hearing aid is limited, and surgery is rarely helpful.

Another aspect of this problem of deafness must be understood by the teacher. He needs to understand the complex relationship of auditory problems to learning disabilities, whether these involve spelling, writing, arithmetic, or any subject matter in grade schools. Sounds become words and words must have meaning. Some learning problems may be traced to a developmental disorder in the auditory area of the brain. Such a disturbance in learning requires special management; therefore, every child with a hearing problem must have a

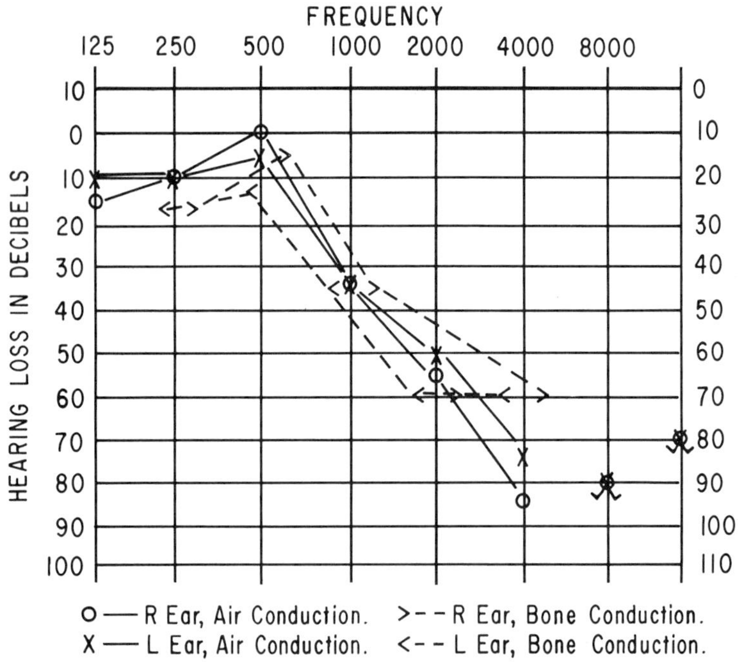

Figure 27 Audiogram showing high frequency loss. The figures along the left border indicate the American Standards Association (ASA) scale. Those on the right represent the international scale (ISO – International Organization for Standardization).

What may be expected from an individual with this type of hearing loss:

1. Typical comment: "The words are loud enough but I can't understand them."
2. There is much greater difficulty with understanding conversation in noisy situations than in quiet ones.
3. When talking with a single individual in a relatively quiet environment, the individual would get along fairly well; but when in a group situation, he would find it difficult to keep up with the conversation.
4. A hearing aid is contraindicated.
5. This person could use lip (speech) reading and auditory training profitably.

(Courtesy W. A. Goates.)

careful analysis of his hearing loss and should be referred to an audiologist.

Outer Ear

Occasionally the auricle or pinna may be absent on one or both sides, either from congenital or accidental causes. When the cause is congenital, frequently other congenital anomalies are also present to account for even more serious hearing loss. The external canal, about one and three-fourths inches long in the adult, is lined by skin which may suffer the usual disorders of such tissue. The skin may be too dry and itch. In many people it may be too oily and produce an excessive secretion. This secretion tends to dry and harden and may become a plug of *wax* which can interfere with the transmission of sound waves.

A surprisingly large number of cases of impaired hearing are cleared when wax is removed from the ears.

Foreign bodies may enter or be placed in the external canal. A curious insect may explore its possibilities. Children tend to poke peanuts, beans, kernels of corn, and other objects into this aperture, or break off the lead points on pencils while scratching or exploring. Under no circumstances should a foreign body in this position by removed by anyone but a physician. Without the proper equipment damage can be done to the skin and cause infection. If a child is frightened and protesting violently, anesthesia may be necessary in order to protect the drum during manipulation.

Infection may follow any attempt to relieve itching in the external canal. Use of instruments to scoop out wax, swabs to clean out the canal, or employment of toothpicks, bobby pins, match sticks, or finger nails can cause breaks in the epithelium and serious complications.

Occasionally, a small localized area of infection (pimple) or pustule may develop in the skin and cause considerable pain. Only a physician can made a diagnosis.

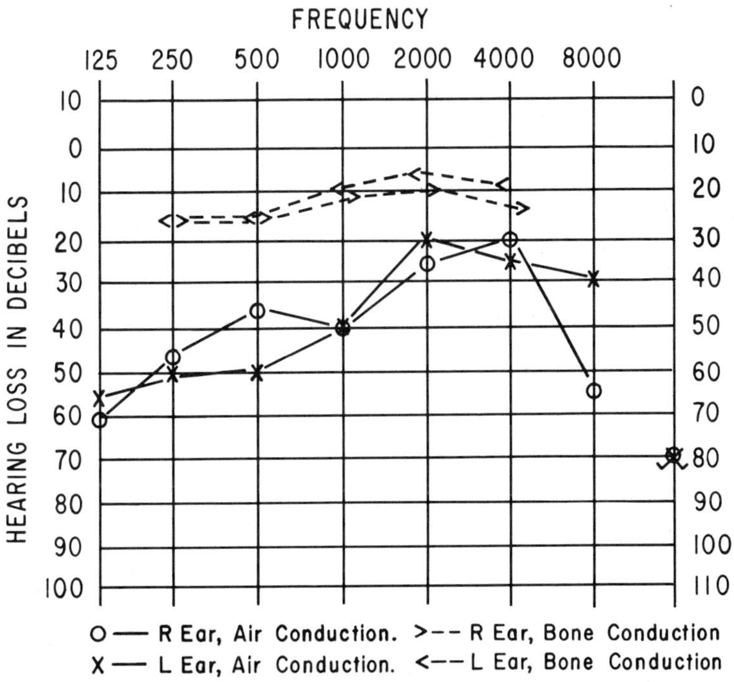

Figure 28 Audiogram showing hearing loss in the low frequencies. Figures on left border—American scale. Figures on right border—International scale.

1. This type of loss usually is overcome successfully with a hearing aid.
2. Owing to the low tone loss, the words heard by this individual would not have the carrying power of the vowel sounds.
3. In any situation, if the speech were loud enough, he would experience little or no difficulty in understanding it. (Courtesy W. A. Goates.)

Middle Ear

This part of the ear contains the indicated air space, the ossicles, the distal openings of the eustachian tubes, and the tympanic membrane (drum). Also, the mastoid air cells drain into the middle ear. A glance at the anatomy of this region will show that the main air space is encased in bone except for its relation to the eustachian tube and external and inner ears. This fact is significant and explains the etiology of pain from infections. The middle ear is lined by mucous membrane which is continuous with that of the eustachian tube and the linings of the contiguous mastoid air cells. Since the lower opening of the eustachian tube lies in the nasopharynx, any infections of the mucous membranes of the nose or throat can sweep up the carpet of mucosa to the middle ear. Since the eustachian tube is relatively short and straight in children, infection can ascend readily.

Otitis media (middle ear infection) practically always results secondarily from infections in the nose and throat. It is the most common disturbance of the ear in childhood and consequently the most common cause of earaches. Infections of mucous membranes produce mucus and pus. If the cavity of the middle ear is filled with this material, impairment of hearing and a sensation of fullness result. The mucous membrane of the eustachian tube is probably swollen at the same time and closes off air from the nose so that air pressure cannot be equalized on both sides of the drum. Acute discomfort develops. If the infection is untreated, mucus and pus continue to be produced, and, since bone is not resilient, these products not only can be pushed back into the mastoid air cells causing mastoiditis, but can also develop pressure against the drum. This pressure will cause the drum to bulge outward. The earache is produced by inflammation and swelling of the mucous membrane lining the middle ear and drum. A throbbing earache is the response to arterial fluctuations in pressure. As a rule, in young people, a throbbing earache indicates otitis media. If infection progresses, pressure causes the drum to rupture, usually in its central portion; discharge of pus and mucus is released into the external canal, pain is relieved, and the child has a "running ear." Except in a few instances, a "running ear" means otitis media with a perforated ear drum. Such a condition demands immediate medical care. As long as there is discharge in the external ear, infection is present, and perforation exists. One or both ears may be affected. Often, hearing is impaired. The discharge may have a foul odor. *The presence of cotton in the canals should make a teacher suspect trouble.* If the discharge clears up quickly, usually after treatment, new tissue is regenerated in the drum with or without its scarring or retraction. With persistent discharge, the perforation may become permanent. Its size, its position in the drum, and the thickness of its edges determine the amount of impairment of hearing. Scarring may result in some reduction of response; some children with a permanent perforation may have a normal audiogram, while others show total conduction loss.

Perforations of the tympanic membrane may also result from explosions. A direct blow on or near the ear (as with an open hand) may rupture the membrane, dislocate ossicles, and even damage the inner ear. Deep diving, landing on an ear in diving, or a fall from water skis may produce a perforation of the drum. With any blow on the head or ear, if a child is knocked unconscious, even temporarily, he should be seen by a physician. If he shows irritability or changes in personality afterwards, he should be referred for medical consultation. And, of course, any fluid or blood coming from an ear after a blow to the head or ear demands prompt medical attention. There is a possibility of a fractured skull.

A child with a *chronic "running ear"* not only suffers from some hearing loss and its consequent learning problems at school, but actually is a sick child. He has a focus of infection where bacteria are growing continuously; he probably has a lowered resistance, and he needs a thorough medical checkup as well as care for the underlying cause of his ear trouble. He may have latent mastoiditis or irreparable damage to the middle ear and partial deafness. A draining or "running ear" resembles a time bomb which may explode into mastoiditis, meningitis, or a brain abscess.

Causes of otitis media:

1. The common cold.
2. Other respiratory infections, such as scarlet fever, mumps, chickenpox, whooping cough, streptococcal sore throat, influenza.
3. Diseased tonsils.
4. Diseased adenoids.
5. Obstructions or infections in the nose, resulting in accumulation of catarrhal material in the nasopharynx.

Every case of an earache lasting longer than a few hours should be watched by a physician. An acute earache is an emergency. The infection can progress so rapidly that it becomes serious in a matter of hours. Underlying causes should be ascertained and corrected. With modern drugs the incidence of otitis media and possible impaired hearing is decreased. Some parents regard an earache as a necessary evil of childhood, and each winter their children report to school daily with cotton in their ears. There is no excuse for such negligence. Ears are for hearing, and this hearing must be preserved.

Inner Ear and Nerve Pathways to Higher Centers

Sensorineural deafness may involve the cochlea, one or both acoustic nerves, or the extended pathways to the brain. A fracture through the organ of hearing may injure the cochlea or a nerve. Infections account for most involvement of the acoustic nerves, and usually affect both at the same time. Any severe systemic infection can produce serious complications. Epidemic meningitis and scarlet fever have been common offenders, but here again, early diagnosis and treatment with antibiotics have worked wonders. This is particularly true in meningitis.

Hereditary deafness is a possibility. The defect is carried in the genes. A child may even be born with an underdeveloped organ of hearing and be totally deaf in the defective ear. Research has revealed that rubella (German measles) contracted by an expectant mother in the early weeks of her pregnancy may cause sensorineural deafness in the child. An aftermath of the 1964 epidemic of rubella in Massachusetts resulted in the birth of some 3500 infants with congenital deafness. Hearing aids will not be of value in these instances. The preventive is immunization for every female child to prevent congenital anomalies.

Congenital brain damage, as found with mental retardation, may be associated with a hearing loss.

It is essential that a differentiation be made between the types of deafness. An otologist or audiologist makes this differentiation. Once a sensory nerve is destroyed, it does not regenerate, and the pathway to the brain is lost. The method of handling a case, including any possible use of a hearing aid, depends upon the amount of hearing present and the type of impairment.

SCHOOL HEALTH PROGRAM FOR HEARING PROBLEMS

Detection

Mannerisms or Behavior

Deafness usually goes undetected until hearing loss becomes critical. The loss may be so gradual that some children become skilled at lip (speech) reading and have such good inflections of the voice that partial deafness may be unsuspected. However, the actions of the child himself frequently suggest a hearing defect. In many instances the classroom teacher is the first person to be aware of this difficulty. Common patterns which are noticed may be:

Abnormal position of the head, forward or turned to one side.
Apparent inattentiveness.
Failure to comprehend spoken words.
Requests for repetition of words.
Inappropriate or irrelevant responses.
Cotton or discharge in the ear.
Complaints of earache.
Complaints of head noises or ringing in the ears.
Complaints of stuffiness or a full feeling in the ear.
Written work better than oral.
Intentness of child's eye upon speaker's lips.
Poor articulation.
Quality of the voice – low or monotonous, or high, or denasalized. (Listen to the speech.)

Erratic, inconsistent responses in which spoken directions are understood one time and missed the next.

Inability to localize sound. If the hearing loss involves only one ear, a child will have difficulty locating sound, particularly without visual clues. Interestingly enough, a child's safety may be threatened as a result. He may not hear warnings or traffic sounds on the deaf side. When hearing response is normal or near normal in the other ear, his hearing impairment may not be detected except by formal testing. Nevertheless, he is handicapped in the classroom.

Emotional disturbances. The continual failure to understand may breed frustrations and withdrawal, "giving up," and no response to speech.

Tests

Rough tests can be given by a teacher. He may simply walk towards the back of an unsuspecting student, pause at varying distances, address him in conversational tones and wait for a response. He can compare this response to the reaction of others.

Watch, Whisper, and Voice Tests. These tests have been used in the past, under very limited conditions. School nurses, physicians, and teachers may use them expeditiously until more accurate screening can be done.

A loud-ticking watch is preferable. The examiner stands behind the child and moves the hand holding the watch at varying distances from the ear to be examined, asking the child to nod when he hears the tick. A tablet or card should be held next to the head on the examining side, obscuring the motion of the hand. Otherwise, the child can see the hand from the corner of his eye and give an incorrect response. He plugs the other ear with a finger during the test. Since the tick of the watch represents only one area of frequency of sound (usually 4000 to 5000) and is not standardized, and since the intensity may be of a wide, unknown variation, this test is only of value to confirm a suspicion. In this test the teacher checks his own hearing by the watch and then compares the child's hearing with his.

The whisper or voice test is evaluated in much the same way as the watch test. The examiner stands 15 feet behind the child. The latter places his finger in one ear, and repeats either the spoken or whispered words of the examiner. Each ear is tested. The test is not reliable because it does not have a standard base nor a controlled level. Conductive deafness often results in loss of hearing of the low frequencies and sensorineural deafness, of the high frequencies. This is not always true but holds to a great extent. Whispers are sibilant and can usually be detected by anyone who hears high frequency sounds. A student with nerve involvement is also quite likely to hear them, or guess the words, if they are loud enough. Both tests depend upon the frequency and intensity of the range of sound. More reliable hearing tests should be used before arriving at a definite conclusion about a child's hearing.[1]

Multiple or Group Testing. Group examinations have been made by using multiple earphones (as many as 40 individual phones) which transmit "fading numbers" dictated by a special phonographic record. "Fading numbers" are numbers recited on the record in gradually receding intensity. The children are instructed to record on special forms what they hear. This test has been used in the past but has proved inadequate. Numbers do not contain a proportional representation of speech sounds in the language, and better tests are available. It should be pointed out that group methods, of all types, are felt to be less valid and reliable than individual pure tone tests.[2]

Group Pure Tone Audiometer Tests. These are sometimes used. Earphones are attached to the audiometer and a group of children is examined at one time. Sounds may be sent into either ear. The child listens and writes on a paper when he hears a signal. Intensity is increased until each child has apparently responded. This method of testing is clumsy and expensive in terms of time and offers the same hazard that all multiple testing involves, i.e., a child may be missed. Since the individual audiometer screening test can be performed so quickly, it is the procedure of choice.

Individual Audiometer Tests. There are two types of audiometers—the precision pure tone instrument and the speech audiometer for more specialized testing. Both instruments may be included in the same cabinet.

The *pure tone* audiometer is widely used (Figure 29). Each child is tested individually and quickly by a "sweep check" method. The technique employed here is to set the intensity dial at a minimum level in decibels which will be satisfactory for hearing in the existing environment. Each ear is tested separately. As many as 20 children can be examined in an hour. This procedure serves to screen out those children who need more careful study later. One fine advantage of this test is that permanent records of audiograms can be kept and progress marked.

An intelligent child of five years and an average child of six or seven years can be tested by the audiometer. Below these ages suspected cases of deafness should be examined by an otologist or audiologist. Psychogalvanometric tests have been devised to detect defects in infants and very young children.

Once a teacher has the recording from a pure tone audiometer in hand, he still does not have the true picture of a child's hearing. This recording shows hearing of tones at the threshold, but does not give adequate information concerning the practical ability to hear and understand the complex sounds which make up speech. If the audiogram from a pure tone audiometer shows defective hearing, further

---

[1]Victor Eisner, and Allen Oblesby: "Health Assessment of School Children. III. Hearing." *J. Sch. Health 41*:9:495–496, November, 1971.

[2]*Ibid.*, pp. 495–496.

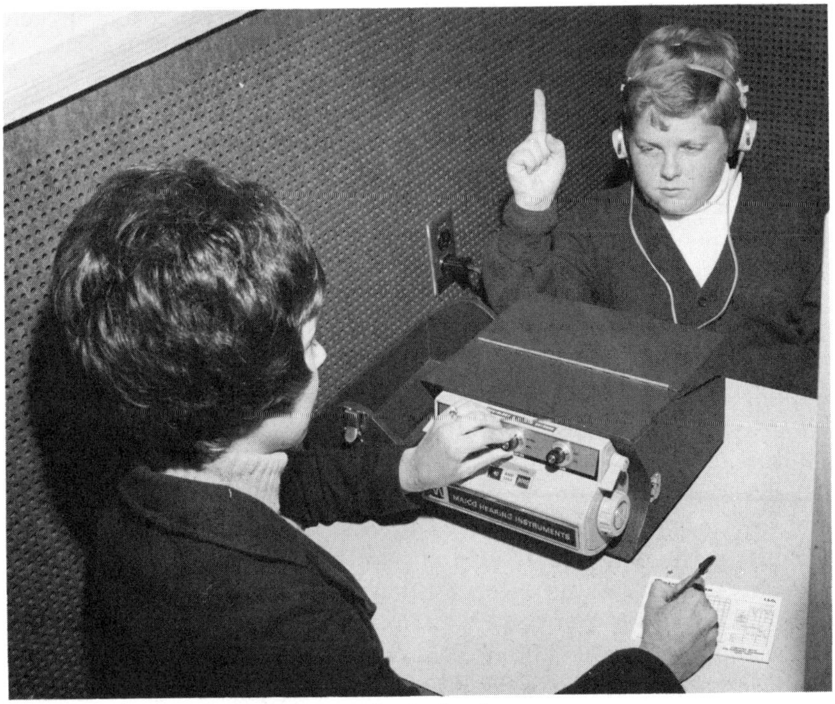

Figure 29 Individual audiometer test.

examination by an audiologist or otologist, using a speech audiometer, is indicated.

It is not difficult to perform pure tone audiometer tests. One instrument is sufficient for a small school system. The tester should be experienced in its use and should know how to handle children. Testing should be routine and done at frequent intervals. An annual examination would be ideal. All children with speech defects should have a hearing check; and arrangements should be made for interim checks if a teacher or school nurse wishes such an examination.

Hearing problems identified by the pure tone audiometer are further investigated by use of the *speech audiometer.* Children may hear pure tones but be unable to correlate them into speech. Evaluations are conducted by specially trained examiners, under controlled conditions with specialized equipment. They are not conducted routinely at a school. Tests consist of presenting to an individual a measured series of carefully selected and valid words which contain all of the sounds in the language in the proportions in which they occur. These words are offered at various controlled intensities and the threshold of hearing of speech in the person being examined is accurately measured. They are also offered at above-threshold levels to determine how this person functions at levels of speech of common occurrence. Such testing measures the degree to which a child hears speech as well as minimum levels of intelligibility.

Measurements derived from use of both the pure tone and speech audiometers will provide a comprehensive understanding of a hearing impairment, aid in diagnosis, and suggest the type of educational program which will meet the needs of a hearing-handicapped child.

Results of surveys show the magnitude of the hearing problem, the importance of examining everyone in a particular group or grade level, and the values in early detection. An example of a mass survey to determine the incidence of hearing defects and the value of various detection methods was a study by the Tennessee Department of Public Health.[3]

Elementary children in 19 counties were examined by three different case-finding methods. These methods were: (1) use of the audiometer in mass survey, with expert testers; (2) referral by teachers using symptom sheets indicating signs and symptoms that might point to a hearing loss; and (3) referral by teachers who were simply asked to refer for testing any children with suspected hearing defect. The results and evaluations in Table 4 are self-explanatory. The most reliable method of detection of hearing defects is mass survey.

This particular study showed that defects were more frequently found in boys (17.6 per cent) than in girls (11.1 per cent). Also, it was interesting to note that both total and major hearing defects tended to increase with the age of the youngsters.

Preschool screening permits early detection of hearing defects, usually leads to an explanation of basic causes, may make it possible for a hearing loss to be cured or arrested by adequate medical care, and encourages early speech training.

A routine study on a grand scale, using audiometrists and supplementary Federal funds, was conducted in the Los Angeles School Districts. These findings in Table 5 give us information on the prevalence of hearing problems in general and upon their distribution by grade level.

[3]Robert M. Foote: "Public Health Aspects of a Speech and Hearing Program." *J.A.M.A. 150*:1390–1392, 1952.

TABLE 4 Defects Among Elementary School Children, According to Method of Case Findings in 19 Counties in Tennessee*

METHOD OF CASE FINDING	ELEMENTARY SCHOOL ENROLLMENT	CHILDREN WITH HEARING DEFECTS		CHILDREN WITH MAJOR HEARING DEFECTS	
		No.	%	*No.*	%
Mass survey	13,010	1790	13.8	430	3.3
Referral by teachers using symptom sheets	46,188	980	2.1	494	1.1
Referral by teachers with preparation	4,505	79	1.8	41	0.9

*Courtesy Tennessee Department of Public Health.

TABLE 5 Significant Statistics, Hearing Conservation Unit, 1966–67 Hearing Tests Performed by Audiometrists in Schools and Clinics

	TOTAL TESTS	REFERRED TO OTOLOGISTS
Preschool (ages 2½–4)	2,420	96 (3.55%)
Elementary	172,036	7821 (4.54%)
Junior high	15,428	1098 (7.12%)
Senior high	8,889	629 (7.07%)

The North Carolina study clearly stablishes the need for periodic audiometer calibration tests.[4] A check of all instruments in use revealed that all were out of calibration, and thus, any testing results had to be suspect. It is recommended that calibration tests be made every six months.

Classification of Hearing Problems

Statistics vary as to the number of children with hearing defects, depending upon the screening methods and standards used. Some type of classification helps in guidance. Table 6 should offer guidance in evaluating learning abilities and in determining need for follow-up.

[4]W. G. Thomas, et al., "Calibration and Working Condition of 100 Audiometers." *Public Health Rep.* *84*:311–327, 1969.

TABLE 6 Difficulty Experienced by School Children With Flat Hearing Losses*

AVERAGE HEARING LOSS (500, 1000, 2000 hz) ASA-1951	ISO-1964	DEGREE OF DIFFICULTY
Up to 10 db	Up to 21 db	No difficulty. Hearing sensitivity within normal limits.
10-15	21-26	Virtually no difficulty. Normally undetectable by patient and others.
15-25	26-36	Slight problem limited to failure to understand faint speech or speech heard in difficult listening situations.
25-35	36-46	Loss begins to produce significant handicap in most children. Child has difficulty with spelling and arithmetic in particular. Child frequently does not recognize loss, and others think child is slow or inattentive, or both. Hearing aid may be indicated.
35-45	46-56	Child has considerable difficulty with most schoolwork. He still may be mistaken for a slow inattentive child. Hearing aid is usually indicated.
45-55	56-66	Most serious loss. Child is usually recognized to have a hearing loss but occasionally the problem goes unnoticed. Hearing aid and therapeutic help are essential.

*Reproduced by permission from Gerald A. Studebaker: "Hearing Problems in School Children." *Postgrad. Med.* *43*:192, 1968.

Follow-up

Importance of Early Detection

A child may be labeled as having normal hearing, when actually he may have unsuspected hearing difficulties which interfere with his progress in school. An individual can lose 20 per cent of his hearing before he becomes aware of the loss. Early detection of such difficulties can affect educational plans for him; expensive and needless repetition of classes can be avoided as well as development of unfavorable emotional and behavior patterns in the individual who fears that he is inferior. A deafened child tends to withdraw into himself and suspect others of talking about him. Since some speech difficulties are attributed wholly or partially to hearing handicaps, early detection of the latter, while speech habits are being developed, can prevent deterioration of the voice and slow and incorrect speech formation.

Management of the Child with Defective Hearing

One specialist should be the coordinator. He works with a team of specialists to secure a diagnosis, establish treatment, and see that the proper educational approach is maintained. He consults with administrators, teachers, parents, and child. Perhaps he is the otologist or the audiologist.

Parents of children with defective hearing should be requested to secure medical advice as soon as possible. The child may be seen first by his family physician who will check his health in general and refer him to an otologist. Medical treatment may not only correct troubles and prevent further hearing loss, but in many instances may improve existing hearing. It goes without saying that a personal contact with a parent by teacher, school nurse, social worker, or principal is always more effective than written notes. Oftentimes more than one reminder is necessary. Prolonged explanation is usually necessary; every assistance should be offered a bewildered parent. Information about a child's hearing should always be placed upon the Cumulative Health Record for use by all of his teachers.

One must remember that hearing aids alone do not solve problems. Special instruction in their use is necessary. The hearing aid is used with a molded ear piece fitted to the ear with better hearing. If one is needed, the aid should be fitted as early as possible in order to use the hearing which is present.

Most youngsters need to know lip reading and have auditory and speech training as well. Auditory training enables a child to use the hearing he has and teaches him to interpret what he hears. He is taught to listen carefully to sounds. Some schools or communities provide such training. More facilities are needed. The child must be encouraged to use his hearing aid, and society must accept this device for improving hearing as being in the same category as glasses.

It is good for a hard-of-hearing child to remain with his peers, if at all possible. If he can maintain progress in his usual environment, he should be kept there. How much better it is to keep him in his own home with his normal social patterns—playing, studying, and developing his speech with children who hear normally. It must be emphasized that many will still require lip reading, auditory training, and speech training, with or without hearing aids.

A clinical psychologist can evaluate the child's intelligence, personality, adjustments, and vocational aptitudes. Parents need counseling and reassurance. A social worker can be useful in establishing home and school relationships. The otologist and audiologist, working together, and working with the special education teacher, can probably offer the most complete guidance for children with problems of hearing.

In regular classrooms, a hard-of-hearing child should select the seat which affords him the best hearing advantage. Each room has its own particular acoustic properties. Let the child experiment and try a number of positions. A child's good ear should never be near such noises as ventilator fans, heavy traffic, or noisy playgrounds. If possible, his back should be to the light.

For teachers who are in contact with hard-of-hearing children, the following suggestions are also offered. Some of them utilize any lip (speech) reading ability the child may have.

1. A teacher should face the pupil as much as possible.
2. A teacher should stand so that the light shines upon his face.
3. A teacher should move around the room as little as possible while carrying on a discussion. He should stand in the child's line of vision.
4. A teacher must secure a child's attention before addressing him. If the child does not watch the teacher's face, there is no communcation.
5. Lip movement should not be exaggerated and speech should be at normal speed.
6. A teacher should check to see if the youngster understands the discussion. Frequently he states that he does when actually he does not. A new idea can be presented in several ways.
7. A hard-of-hearing child should read in advance on the subject to be discussed in class. In this way he will be familiar with the vocabulary and with the ideas involved.
8. A "hearing" student should be appointed to help with assignments.
9. A teacher should remember that the hard-of-hearing child may become fatigued from intent use of eyes and the tension from straining to hear.
10. Other students in the class must understand the problem of their classmate and be helpful and tolerant.
11. The deafened child needs encouragement and self-confidence.

12. He should be included in extra-class activities to that he can feel himself as part of a group.

13. Remember that he is trying to combine faulty hearing with visual clues for the spoken word. The teacher should write clue words on the chalkboard as he talks.

The preceding discussion makes it apparent that a child with some hearing loss can be placed in a regular classroom. Supplementary assistance is usually given. The various programs provided depend upon the size of the school population, the number of handicapped children, and the facilities available in the community. One whole school or one full-time special class may be devoted to these youngsters. There may be a part-time special class, or the child may have access to a resource room with special equipment, or a visiting special teacher may give assistance at regular times.

For those children who cannot benefit from the above program, education is available in schools for the deaf. Since there will be only a few such children in most communities, state boards of education usually provide a residential school. Some parents, where feasible, prefer to live near a school for the deaf and have the child attend during the day. In this way, daily family contact is maintained. Others must send their children away to residential schools. At all times the welfare of the child comes first. He needs to prepare himself for his place in society and must be taught to handle his own socioeconomic problems.

Some educators, physicians, and others interested in the education of a child with an extensive hearing defect are convinced that he should not be placed in a school away from home, especially when quite young. Such a child is believed to experience too much psychic trauma. If he feels unwanted because he is a defective child, then placing him in a special school makes him feel still more insecure because he considers that he is being thrown out of his home. Later he becomes comfortable among his deaf peers, only to be sent back into a hearing world to make his living. Again he will feel insecure. There are those who advocate the education of an intelligent child in his own home, if necessary, rather than placement in a residential school for the deaf. He may secure private tutoring, or be visited by special teachers provided by some branch of the state government. In this way he will be reared in the same environment in which he will eventually expect to live.

The final decision in selection of a school depends upon the following factors: the degree of the child's hearing impairment, his early development in the home, his language and speech skills, and his ability to compensate for his hearing loss in competition with normally hearing children.

One big task in education of the deaf is the development of understanding and expression of language. We first learn language through the ear. Yet, special teachers for the deaf, through ingenious methods, to develop in deaf children a comprehension of words and language and can teach them to speak.

The philosophy of education of children in schools for the deaf has been the subject of controversy, whether to confine communication to the oral speech method (speaking and reading lips) to to the use of oral skills combined with manual skills. Such argument is relegated to the educators. The oral method, however, seems to be replacing the manual.

Hearing Conservation Program

This program involves not only the early detection of hearing loss in children but aims to preserve residual hearing and educate the afflicted child. It should emphasize prevention of hearing problems and should include in its operation the services of classroom teacher, special education personnel, administrators, parents, physicians, otologists, audiologists, and volunteer and welfare organizations in the community. This type of ambitious program looks good on paper and everyone will favor it. It can prove expensive, however, to individual families and to the school system. Financial aspects must be kept in mind. What is needed is a recognition of the problem of hearing loss in children and a desire to do something about it. A hearing conservation program cannot have a haphazard approach. There must be coordination and a center for planning. When a teacher reports a suspected case of hearing loss, the planned program should function smoothly. In addition, mass examinations should be done at intervals (about every three years in schools) to detect new cases and follow-up on old cases.

Health Education

In School. Teaching units on care of the ears are available in curriculum guides provided by local or state boards of education. They not only delineate materials on anatomy and physiology, but stress the significance of earaches and need for prompt medical care. Children and older youth should appreciate their hearing and preventive measures which should be taken to preserve it. The attention paid to the handicapped child serves as a health education experience for his classmates.

In the Community. Education concerning hearing problems involves not only health instruction in the classroom but a more comprehensive program which strives to change the attitudes of the community, utilize its resources, and establish a hearing conservation program.

Aid to Parents. It is difficult for parents to have insight into the problems of their handicapped children without intelligent advice. The parent is the key person in the hearing conservation program. The parent must be responsible for securing medical help and for following educational recommendations. If a parent postpones these, the child suffers. No one in contact with parents should be satisfied simply to acquaint them with the fact that their child has a hearing loss. Their understanding and cooperation is vital. They should not feel that their child is defective. Feelings of guilt should be dispelled; many parents are guilt-ridden. They should be given an opportunity to see a corrective program in action.

Advice to parents may come initially from the teacher, the principal, the social workers, or the school nurse. Further follow-up should be a team approach.

Voluntary clinics have been established to help the deaf child and his parents, for their mutual adjustment, and for the adjustment of the child to society. Private practitioners in audiology are becoming increasingly available. Universities and colleges through their specialists in such departments as Child Development, Speech, Speech and Hearing, Psychology, Social Work, and Special Education can offer invaluable assistance to anxious and bewildered parents. At the same time a fine training program for students interested in this field can be established through the united efforts of these academic areas in holding clinics and workshops. Parents may be invited to attend. There may be special classes for the handicapped children.

The resources listed at the end of this chapter have national headquarters, often with state and local branches. Their trained personnel act as consultants to advise parents, teachers, and hearing-impaired individuals. Some local groups sponsor social programs of various types.

STATEMENTS ON DEAFNESS TODAY*

1. Today, there are 15 million adults and 3 million children in the United States with a hearing loss of some degree, and the number is increasing.

2. Today, between 3½ per cent and 5 per cent of the school age children in the United States and abroad have a hearing loss to some degree.

3. Today, a greater proportion of deaf young people are born deaf or are deafened before language has been acquired than occurred 25 years ago. Due to improvement in obstetric and pediatric care, many thousands of children who would have died are now saved, but at the cost of various kinds of impairments—including hearing impairments.

4. Very few children are *totally* deaf, that is, with no residual hearing whatsoever.

5. The deaf child is triply handicapped—in hearing, in language which comes through hearing, and in speech.

6. A number of deaf children are multiply handicapped due to a brain-centered difficulty.

7. Some hearing impaired children are considered mentally

*Reprinted through the courtesy of the *Alexander Graham Bell Association for the Deaf, Inc. News*, November 1, 1965.

retarded until hearing tests reveal that deafness is their sole problem.

8. The hearing of all children is often not checked early enough. A hearing loss can be discovered long before the child reaches school age.

9. The main types of hearing loss are (a) conductive (middle ear), (b) neurosensory (nerve deafness) and (c) mixture of both types.

10. Less than 50 per cent of the deaf children in the United States, under the age of six, needing specialized preschool instruction, receive it.

11. There is a severe shortage of educational assistance for the hearing impaired in our public schools.

12. The average graduate of a public or private residential school for the deaf has only an eighth grade education. For many this is the end of their formal education.

13. Deaf children who learned speech and lip reading at the elementary school level may be able to attend high schools for hearing persons and a few with better than average skills in communication may obtain degrees from regular colleges.

14. Vocational and professional opportunities for the deaf are very limited.

15. Almost all (five-sixths) of the deaf adults work at ordinary manual jobs, compared with 50 per cent of the hearing adults. Even the so called hard-of-hearing person finds less opportunities and more barriers for promotion than the normally hearing.

16. Past vocational education programs at mechanical and operational levels are now becoming inadequate.

17. Future deaf adults may become victims of the changing occupational outlook unless a more sophisticated occupational education for the deaf is provided to meet the increasingly complex demands of business and professional pursuits.

18. The small percentage of well-educated, successful oral deaf adults in the professions, other than teaching, could be increased if employers realized the potentials of those who speak and lip read.

19. Over 50 per cent of the hearing impaired people in the United States have a family income of less than $4000 per year.

20. The plight of the deaf in the United States—educationally and vocationally—is due to failure to launch an aggressive attack on the basic problems. More research is needed and the findings applied.

21. The deaf must be taught to communicate and communicate well in order to compete in the world of hearing persons.

22. The future of the deaf child is limited unless he has learned to speak and lip read at an early age.

23. All deaf children can be taught to speak and lip read although with varying degrees of proficiency. Just as normal hearing children being taught a foreign language in school have varying degrees of success, so do deaf children have varying degrees of success in learning to speak and lip read. The fact that some children do better than others is not, however, sufficient reason to discontinue teaching a foreign language nor in teaching speech and lip reading to deaf children.

24. Learning to talk and lip read is a difficult task for any deaf child. But the end result, that is, the capability of communicating with family, friends and the man on the street and getting a good education makes it worth the effort.

25. Environment is very important. The child with a severe hearing loss should be kept in an environment of speaking children and adults as much as possible. Without the stimulation of those who use normal speech communication, the deaf child tends to use his voice less and less.

26. Auditory training and speech therapy are vitally important and should be started at the earliest possible age.

27. Infants of less than a year of age can often be fitted with a hearing aid and their entry into the hearing world begun.

28. Residual hearing of deaf children can and must be cultivated and trained by experienced therapists and teachers and enhanced by parent cooperation in the home.

29. Parents must talk to the deaf child.

30. Parents of deaf children need more readily available counsel, guidance and instruction.

31. No surgical cures are known for nerve deafness, which is most common among young deaf children. Parents of such children must be helped to bridge the gap from a search for medical "cures" to acceptance of the fact that this is an educational problem.

32. Speech and hearing centers or clinics provide essential training for the deaf child in preschool years.

*33. For lists of schools and classes for deaf children and preschool classes in the United States and Canada, write The Alexander Graham Bell Association for the Deaf, Inc.

34. "One of the greatest achievements in the world is that of the child born deaf who learns to talk. No deaf child in America should be allowed to grow up mute without earnest and persistent efforts having been made to teach him to speak and read lips."—Dr. Alexander Graham Bell.

NOSE

Anatomy and Physiology
(Figures 30 and 31)

Since health problems of the respiratory tract are most common in childhood, some understanding of the anatomy and physiology is necessary in order to appreciate the initimate relationship of the structures in this region. One should visualize a continuous sheath of mucous membrane which follows the contours of the throat, nose, accessory nasal sinuses, nasopharynx, eustachian or auditory tube, middle ear, and mastoid air sinuses. From the throat this same sheath extends down into the larynx and bronchial tubes. In most areas except the pharynx the epithelial cells forming the superficial layer of this membrane have attached cilia or fine hairs. Over this sheath a carpet of mucus is always present. Through action of cilia in sweeping along this mucus which may be loaded with bacteria and viruses, and also by direct extension of infection in the mucous membrane, disease can

*33 are authors' comments.

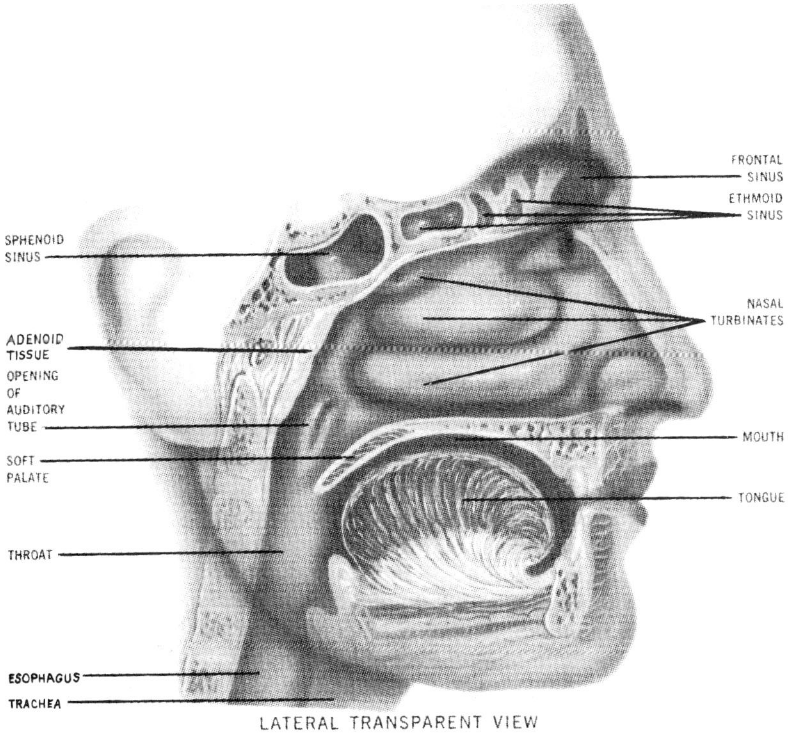

Figure 30 Relations of the eye, ear, nose, throat, and sinuses. (Courtesy Schering Corporation.)

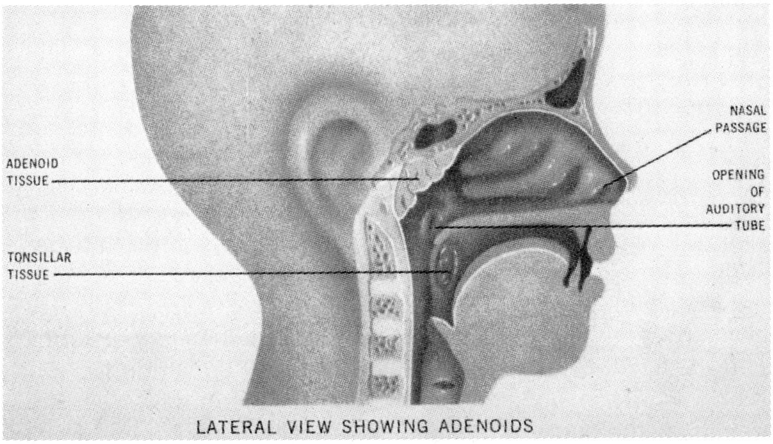

Figure 31 Lateral view showing relationship of adenoidal tissue to opening of auditory (eustachian) tube and tonsils. (Courtesy Schering Corporation.)

spread from one region of the respiratory tract to an adjacent one. Hence, a sore throat or cold in the nose can involve the nasal sinuses, middle ear, and mastoid regions. Or, the sore throat can soon evolve into laryngitis or bronchitis. Thus, infection can extend up or down the mucous membrane.

One rarely sees much discussion of the importance of the nose in the health of the respiratory system. Yet even in early childhood, disturbances in normal air passages are common. It is for this reason that detailed information is being given.

The interior of the nose is divided by a septum or partition into two nostrils; its covering of mucous membrane warms and moistens air during its passage, and the cilia filter foreign material such as bacteria, dirt, and pollen from the air. In order to increase the area of membrane, three wing-like bone structures are present on the lateral walls of the nostrils; these are referred to as the *turbinate bones.* Air hits these bones and spins as if it were in a wind tunnel, thus coming in contact with more mucous membrane for the conditioning mentioned above.

The *accessory nasal sinuses* are air spaces in bone, also lined by mucous membrane, with openings into the nose. Those on the cheeks are the maxillary air sinuses and each has a small opening into the side of the nostril. At the roof of the nose and between the eyes are the sphenoid, ethmoid, and frontal air sinuses, which drain down into the roof of the nose through small outlets (Figure 30). Back of the nostril is the *nasopharynx,* the nasal portion of the throat. Air from the nostrils hits the back wall of the nasopharynx and is deflected down through the pharynx to the respiratory passages below. Attached to its upper and posterior walls is the adenoidal tissue.

An *adenoid* is similar in structure to tonsils and is sometimes referred to as the pharyngeal tonsil. It consists of white blood cells in a fibrous connective tissue network and is soft and spongy in appearance. If it is enlarged, it can occlude the nasopharynx and cause partial to complete obstruction of nasal breathing. If the adenoidal tissue grows towards the nasal sinuses, infection can spread from one area to the other. Although this tissue tends to shrink with age, about 20 per cent of adults still have enlarged adenoids.

The other structures of great importance in the nasopharynx are the *openings of the eustachian (auditory) tubes.* These lie lateral to the mass of the adenoid tissue, which protects the openings and acts as a cushion. The *olfactory center,* in the upper back part of the nasal cavity, transmits responses to smell. Gaseous particles or odorous substances are dissolved into particles which stimulate special olfactory cells in this center. Attached nerve fibers carry the stimuli to the specific brain center. Congestion of the mucous membrane in this region can obstruct the sense of smell. This is noticed when one has a bad cold, or a constant discharge in the back of the nose, or when suffering a siege of sinus infection. The nose protects against dangerous odors and opens up the whole world of fragrance.

Causes of Obstruction of Nasal Breathing

Breathing through the nose should be easy and free. Any obstruction cannot only cause discomfort, but it can alter the physiology of the mucous membrane lining the nose. If air cannot move freely through the nostrils to keep the membrane fairly dry and healthy, mucous discharge, frequently referred to as a catarrhal secretion, accumulates and causes obstruction of breathing. A congested thickening and swelling of the mucous membrane then develops. This in turn causes more obstruction and more secretion, and a vicious cycle is established. This congestion or stuffiness may become chronic; and if the swelling is severe, mouth breathing may develop.

Obstruction of one or both nostrils may be due to:

Enlarged adenoids, most common cause in childhood.

Deviated or crooked septum, congenital or due to injury.

Thickness or congestion of the mucous membrane over turbinate bones.

Polyps (pedunculated overgrowths of mucous membrane).

Acute infections, such as the common cold, whooping cough.

Allergies—hay fever, allergic rhinitis.

Foreign bodies, such as peanuts, beans, beads, kernels of corn, erasers, buttons, marbles, usually placed in right nostril.

Fracture and displacement of nasal bones or cartilage.

Results of Chronic Obstruction of Nasal Breathing

1. Possible middle ear discomfort, infection, and impairment of hearing may result. In the nasopharynx, accumulated mucus, which is usually laden with bacteria, may pass over or extend into the openings of the eustachian tubes and spread infection through the tubes into one or both middle ears.

2. Catarrhal discharge from the mucous membrane of the nose may accumulate in the nasopharynx and pass down into the pharynx as postnasal drip, a common cause of chronic cough.

3. Sinusitis may be a secondary involvement. Swelling and congestion of the mucous membrane in the nose can cause closure of the openings with the resultant accumulation of discharge in the sinuses. Bacteria gain entrance to the sinuses from the nasal cavities by extension along the mucosa. Sinusitis in children can begin between the fourth and ten years of age. It acts frequently the same as in adults.

4. The sense of smell may be impaired or destroyed owing to congestion of the mucous membrane and accumulation of discharge in the roof of the nose where the olfactory buds are located.

5. Mouth breathing may result. In the case of *prolonged* mouth breathing during the early growth period of the child, typical changes in the contour of the face, jaws, and mouth may gradually develop. Most mouth breathing in children is caused by enlarged adenoids.

The "adenoidal" type of face (Figure 42) is characterized by the pinched appearance around the nostrils, the slight swelling below the lower eyelids, the narrow face with protuberant upper front teeth, under-development of the lower jaw, and receding chin. The front teeth do not meet in a bite. The lips do not close. The upper lip may appear shortened; space between the upper jaws is narrowed, forming a V-shaped arch; the palate is high and narrowed laterally. Gradations of these alterations from normal depend upon the severity and duration of the mouth breathing. Malocclusion (poor bite) of the teeth requires the services of a dentist and orthodontic procedures (Figure 43). An open mouth is esthetically unpleasing. It is more socially acceptable to chew with a closed mouth than with an open one.

6. An unhealthy condition in the nose and nasopharynx may predispose to frequent colds. Individual resistance is an important factor.

7. "Bad breath" may be produced from bacterial action in the accumulated catarrhal discharge.

8. Speech is not resonant and clear because of a chronically stuffed-up nose.

Injuries and Nosebleeds

An *injury* to the nose should be examined soon after the accident. There may or may not be associated nosebleed. Blows on the nose from a fist or a thrown ball, or trauma from falling on it usually go unrecorded, but a fracture of the septum or of the nasal bones in the bridge can cause narrowing inside of one or both nostrils, with consequent difficulty in breathing. The bridge of the nose may appear broadened.

Given a child with a blow on the nose, a teacher should recommend to the parent an immediate referral to a physician if (1) the nosebleed is excessive or persistent, (2) the nose is displaced, or (3) the contour of the nose is altered by marked swelling and/or broadening across the bridge. With a fracture the nose is tender. There may be discoloration from bleeding in the soft tissues under the eyes. Occasionally, a fracture of the cheekbone accompanies a blow on the nose. Of course, if the child is unconscious, hospitalization will follow.

With early detection of a fracture, manipulative methods by a physician can be used to restore original contour and preserve air passages. This quick action is particularly important in youngsters, because surgery on the nose is usually not undertaken until late adolescence, owing to the slow growth of the nasal bones and septum. If obstruction is practically total, however, the specialist may occasionally operate sooner.

Nosebleeds are very common in childhood. Examination will usually reveal bleeding from the front part of the septum, in an area just below the bridge, where capillaries are abundant. In this region the breaking of a capillary stretched over an angle of a deviated or crooked septum is a very common cause of nosebleeds. Exercise also may cause dilatation and rupture of a blood vessel, usually at this site. There may be dry crusts or ulcers on the septum which cut the vein and cause bleeding. Injuries may also produce hemorrhage.

One simple procedure in management of a nosebleed is to have the individual lean forward and blow the clot away from the bleeding area. Bleeding will soon stop. Sometimes, simply pinching the nostrils together and keeping them compressed for about five to 15 minutes will be effective. A small cotton or gauze pack may be inserted into the nostril and pressure applied from the outside against the pack. The latter should remain in place for some time and the child should be kept sitting forward rather than lying down. This method should also be effective. Persistent hemorrhage demands more extensive medical care. A child who suffers frequent episodes of nose bleeding should be seen by a physician, particularly while bleeding, so that the physician can locate the affected area and treat it accordingly.

SCHOOL HEALTH PROGRAM

Detection of Mouth Breathing

Mouth breathing can be observed readily. The changes in the contour of the jaw and general facial appearance may be present to varying degrees. Sniffling, chronic nasal discharge, and congestion in the nose are common with nasal obstruction. With pronounced obstruction, both air and food are received through the mouth, and there must be delicate timing of swallowing and breathing. Parents notice the open mouth, the sniffling, the complaints of ear discomfort, and the snoring at night. Teachers notice impairment of hearing, possibly cotton in the ears, and the typical changes from mouth breathing. The child may be inattentive and accomplish little in school because of hearing defects.

Follow-up

All cases of mouth breathing should be examined by a physician; the underlying cause should be diagnosed and corrective measures taken as early as possible before permanent changes occur. Although surgery on the nose itself is not undertaken in other than exceptional cases until late adolescence, other problems may be corrected. The earlier the obstructions are removed, the better, because once the habit of mouth breathing is established, it is difficult to break. Students who have had all obstructions removed and breathe properly may still walk around with their mouths open, offering a pretty stupid appearance. They need to be reminded frequently and must remind themselves to close their lips. This is easier said than done. Appeal in the older group is through vanity and through vigilance on the part of all interested and amused companions. Mothers have tried every trick with the young ones, including trying to keep the lower jaw closed at night with a folded dish towel which is placed under the chin and jaw, then pulled up and tied over the head.

Few people actually appreciate the importance of the nose. Some examples of the worthwhile effects from correction of mouth breathing are indicated:

> A student in senior high school had been advised about two years before that a surgical operation, referred to as a submucous resection, should be done to correct a markedly deviated septum. Finally she became so disgusted with her high incidence of "colds" which seemed almost continuous, that she took time off one weekend in the fall to have the correction made. A checkup late in the spring produced the enthusiastic report that not only had her nose and nasopharynx been clear all winter, but that she had noticed an unusual phenomenon. As she would be walking along with her classmates, she amazed her friends by calling attention to aromas never noticed before. Actually she had never to her knowledge experienced the sense of smell. Constant congestion had prevented stimuli from reaching the olfactory buds.
>
> A school health examination record of an older boy contained the following notation: "Mouth breather. Extensive deviation of the septum." About a year later this student was asked to report to the school physician because of the persistent, offensive bad breath noticed by a counselor who asked for the medical consultation. The student at first refused to discuss his mouth breathing or any possibility of seeking advice from a nose and throat specialist. Naturally, he was embarrassed at the cause of referral. When it was explained to him that the accumulation of postnasal catarrhal discharge, which usually has bacteria in it, was the probable source of foul odor, he decided to discuss the problem with his parents. Soon after, he had an operation. Checkup a year and two years later revealed a correction of the original complaint.
>
> The following incident occurs often: A child seen by the school physician at preschool "roundup" seemed very quiet and somewhat in a monotone. His mother reported frequent earaches and colds. Consultation with an ear-nose-and-throat specialist was recommended. Follow-up later by the school nurse when the child entered the first grade revealed that after his adenoids were removed the incidence of colds and earaches was reduced and hearing seemed improved.

THROAT (PHARYNX)

The part of the throat which is located back of the nostrils is designated as the *nasopharynx*. The anatomy and physiology of this region and its importance have already been discussed. An examination of this part requires medical skill; however, a teacher should be able to examine a child's pharynx. A good light, either a flashlight or light from a window, is satisfactory. It is possible to see the back of the throat in some youngsters without the aid of a tongue blade. If the tongue blade is used, it should be placed on the front part of the tongue and pressure applied gently to prevent gagging. Breathing through the mouth also prevents gagging. When the sound "ah" is produced, the soft palate is elevated, the base of the tongue is lowered, and a better view of the throat is permitted. Children are so accustomed to having their throats examined that this procedure should offer no difficulty.

Ordinarily the mucous membrane of the throat is pink. The teacher should observe color and any unusual appearance. A reddened inflamed color, an appearance of swelling, patches of gray or white membrane, or spotty areas of pus are significant. No attempt should be made by a teacher to make a diagnosis. Diphtheria, streptococcal sore throat, or Vincent's disease may present some of these characteristics. Scarlet fever usually starts with a bright red, swollen throat. In all of these diseases the children are sick and have a fever. The lymph nodes at the angle of the jaw are usually swollen and tender. Any child whose throat presents any of the characteristics described above should be taken home immediately.

In the common sore throat associated with a cold, there may be no fever. The throat may present no unusual appearance or may be slightly inflamed. The lymph nodes in the neck may or may not be enlarged. If there is fever present, the student should be sent home.

It must also be kept in mind that, even in the absence of positive findings in the throat, a record of frequent sore throats is sufficient cause for requesting an examination by a physician.

MOUTH

Inspection (See Figure 32)

Following an inspection of the throat, the teacher's glance naturally proceeds forward into the mouth. The tonsils are inspected and then the tongue blade should be moved within the mouth to expose all of the teeth and gums to careful scrutiny.

Injuries to the Mouth

A fall or a blow on the mouth may catch the tongue between the teeth, and sometimes the tongue is literally almost bitten in two. The gory results usually arouse panic. Immediate suturing by a physician produces excellent results with very little scarring and no loss of function.

Teeth may accidentally gash the lower lip, externally or internally, or as a completely penetrating wound. If the laceration is bleeding profusely, or extends more than superficially, it should be seen by a physician.

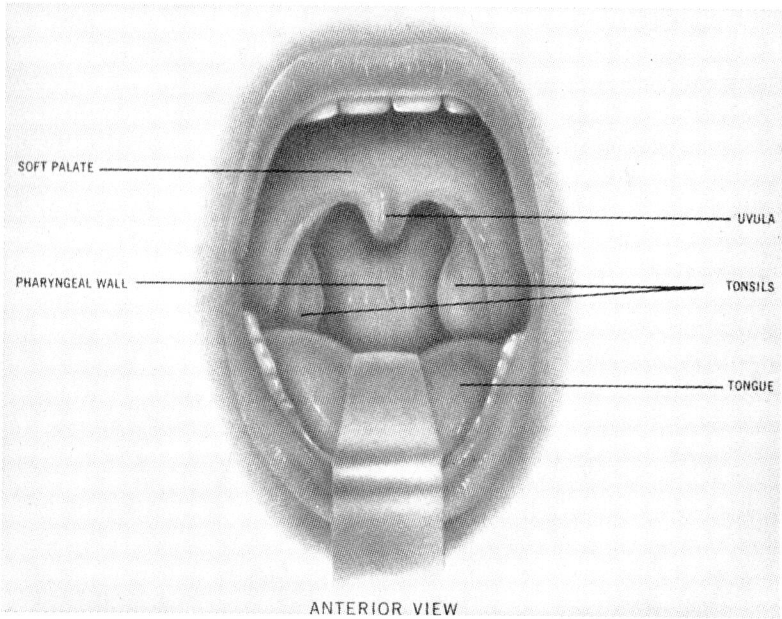

Figure 32 Normal throat. (Courtesy Schering Corporation.)

Canker Sores

Canker sores are blister-like sores which appear in various parts of the mouth—on the inner surface of the cheeks, floor of the mouth, on the edge of the tongue, on the palate, and on the red or mucous surface of the lips. Fever blisters (herpes simplex) (see Skin) are usually found on the outside of a patient's lips at the point where the mucous membrane adjoins the skin. Sometimes both fever blisters and canker sores are present at the same time.

Canker sores start as blisters and become painful when the blisters break; then yellowish ulcers with red margins develop. They may occur singly or in numbers, occasionally, frequently, or almost continuously in crops. Some people seem to be afflicted all of the time with "sore mouths."

> There is some evidence that canker sores "run" in families. Thus a youngster developing these sores may very likely have brothers or sisters, or one or both parents suffering from the same illness.[5]

The exact cause of canker sores has not been determined. Foods, such as nuts and chocolate, have been indicated. An "upset stomach" has been offered as an explanation. Some observations are pertinent:

[5]U.S. Department of Health, Education, and Welfare: Public Health Service. Publication No. 1329. "Canker Sores." 1965, p. 6.

canker sores tend to appear when an individual is under physical or emotional stress. "A slight injury while brushing the teeth, eating harsh foods, and possibly some allergies are also factors which tend to produce canker sores."[6] In some instances a viral infection is suspected.

Canker sores heal spontaneously in ten to 14 days. Various treatments have been advocated. Some cauterizing agents add insult to injury. No cure has yet been found.

Tonsils

Description

The tonsils are almond-shaped, lymphoid bodies, 1 to 1½ inches long, ensconced in lateral niches or pockets in the back of the mouth on a level with the root of the tongue. They form part of a lymphatic ring which includes the adenoids and lingual tonsils, to form Waldeyer's tonsillar ring. Lymphoid tissue consists of a connective tissue network filled with white blood cells, many of which are produced locally in the germinal centers.

There are many theories concerning the function of this lymphoid ring. Since these lymphatic tissues contain and also produce white blood cells, they act as a protective mechanism against organisms; they act as filters or strainers. Both the adenoids and tonsils have crypts or tunnels filled with debris from broken-down tissue and dead bacteria. There is some belief also that the harbored bacteria and viruses tend to stimulate the formation of antibodies. Tonsils and adenoids tend to be enlarged in childhood and shrink somewhat in size after four or five years of age. Theoretically then, the tonsils and adenoids do protect in the first few years, until the body becomes accustomed to its environment, by forming a barrier against bacteria and possibly producing some immunity.

The tonsils continue growth until about the age of four. Since it is now believed that they have a protective value, there is extreme reluctance in the medical profession to remove them before that age. Only if the damage to the body from diseased tonsils outweighs the protective benefits are they removed early.

General Indications for Removal

1. Frequent attacks of tonsillitis. With acute tonsillitis, bacteria in the crypts of the tonsils are forced into the blood stream every time the child chews, and may cause development of a high fever. Since not all of the bacteria are killed by antibiotics, recurrences are not unusual. The usual complaints are acute sore throat and "swollen

---

[6] *Ibid.*, p. 7.

glands." Tonsils are not removed until the infection subsides. With chronic tonsillitis pus is present in the crypts, a foul odor is present, and the lymph nodes in the neck are enlarged and uncomfortable. Blood vessels in the area surrounding the tonsil are enlarged. Occasionally the appearance of a tonsil gives no clue to its diseased condition. The surface may present no unusual changes or be covered with a thick capsular tissue and yet the interior will be filled with pus and bacteria. There probably is a history, however, of chronic tonsillitis and other indications of diseased tonsils.

2. Enlargement of tonsils. Sometimes tonsils are so big that they tend to rub together. The child may gag and be unable to handle food. Only if the large tonsil gives trouble mechanically with swallowing or breathing should it be extirpated. Otherwise, the size alone is not an indication for surgery. There is no correlation between a diseased condition and the size of a tonsil.

3. Repeated earaches and deafness. Bacteria can spread from diseased tonsils to surrounding tissue and may be associated with diseased adenoids. If the tonsils are at all infected, they are removed along with the adenoids for correction of middle ear disease.

4. A diseased tonsil may serve as a focus for infection and disseminate toxins and bacteria to other portions of the body, either through the blood stream or locally through the lymphatic system. In recent years this interpretation of a focus has provided controversy in medical circles and is not acceptable to some physicians. Nevertheless, in selective cases of arthritis, rheumatic fever, asthma, kidney trouble, or markedly "run-down condition," a physician may recommend tonsillectomy. Asthma due to bacterial sensitivity may be improved with elimination of this focus. A child who suffers frequent bouts of enlarged painful lymph nodes in the neck ("enlarged glands") may experience relief after a tonsillectomy.

5. Malocclusion of teeth. Occasionally with greatly enlarged tonsils, the child cannot maintain normal position of the tongue. This may be instrumental sometimes in forward thrusting of the tongue and reverse swallowing. (Malocclusion in Chapter 7.)

Tonsillectomies are no longer considered routine protective surgical procedures. Each child's problem is weighed carefully, with a complete medical history and physical examination taken into consideration. More observation and caution are exercised in making a decision for removal. Complete surgical extirpation of diseased tonsils is often technically difficult; and if incompletely removed, particularly early in life, bits of lymphoid tissue, sometimes almost microscopic in appearance, may be left in place. These may increase in amount and even reach the size of the original tonsil. The same holds true of the adenoids.

Since lymphoid tissue is growing in small children, reappearance of this tissue after surgery explains their "growing in" again. Sometimes the lingual tonsils, which are in the throat and usually not seen, move into more prominent position and give this illusion. Bits of lymphoid tissue in the tonsillar niche are referred to as tonsil "tabs" or "tags." They may become badly diseased and require removal.

Since the adenoids are the chief source of disease in the nose and throat area, if diseased tonsils are removed, the adenoids are usually removed also. Adenoids alone may be the offenders. Surgery is the approved method of extirpation. Sometimes radium or x-ray is used for shrinking bits of adenoidal tissue.

The Lymphatic System

In order to understand the significance of the lymph nodes ("glands") in the neck, a description of the anatomy and physiology of the whole lymphatic system is necessary. This system serves as a major defense mechanism against infection. It consists of an organization of closed vessels, beginning with the small capillary networks which drain the fluid that is continually bathing cells in the various tissues of the body. These vessels unite into a few large ones and finally conduct lymph into veins in the neck.

Lymph consists of tissue fluid in which white blood cells, principally lymphocytes, as well as other elements are present. These cells act as phagocytes or scavengers, and attempt to destroy foreign material in the body. They can engulf and destroy invading organisms; in this way they defend against infection. Sometimes the cells themselves are destroyed in the process.

Interspersed among the collecting lymph vessels at certain strategic areas in the body are nodes, which may occur singly or in clusters. More frequently, they are arranged as a chain, close together, separated by lymph vessels. On their way to join finally the veins in the neck, these vessels enter the lymph nodes where they break up into capillaries. Finally lymph is spread through the lymphoid tissue; much of it is absorbed through the venous system, and the remainder is collected again into closed vessels before leaving the nodes. In the node the lymph is filtered and replenished with lymphocytes.

Lymph nodes consist of lymphoid tissue, similar to that of tonsils and adenoids in morphology and function. They are small, split-pea shaped bodies, consisting of connective tissue filled with white blood cells, principally lymphocytes, and contain germinal centers which produce these cells. Some nodes are superficial and palpable; others are located deep within the body; they drain specific areas.

Within a lymph node, during the process of combating infection, the accumulation of white blood cells, dead bacteria, broken-down cells, and debris results in an inflammatory reaction with resultant enlargement and tenderness. A swollen, sensitive lymph node, regardless of location indicates the presence of infection in the area it drains. If the infection is overwhelming and one discrete node cannot contain it, organisms will be spilled over through the connecting lymph vessel into the next node. As the severity of the bacterial or viral invasion demands it, successive nodes in the chain will be involved. If this defense is still inadequate, lymph nodes at a more distant point will take over. Finally, if not contained and filtered out by these protective barriers, infection may pour over into the blood stream and a generalized septicemia or blood poisoning results. Severe infection spreading up the lymph channel usually is demarcated by redness or streaking. Red streaks leading from an infected area are danger signals.

A common example of this protective phenomenon is an infected area on the foot. Streaks may or may not be present. Tender, swollen nodes may be felt in back of the knees; and if the infection is severe or has been present for a while, the lymph nodes in the groin may be large and painful. Immediate medical treatment is mandatory. Individuals have died of generalized septicemia from an infected blister on the foot. With any infected area, regional lymph nodes are palpated.

The lymphatic system reaches its peak in development of lymphatic tissue during the ages of seven to ten and gradually undergoes regression toward the smaller amounts usually found in adults.

Lymph Nodes (Glands) in the Neck

The chains of lymph nodes, deep and superficial, in the side of the neck, beginning on each side with the angle of the jaw and extending down obliquely to the sternum, drain an extensive area—the throat, tonsil, side of the cheek, skin around the ear, the region of the jaw, chin, and tongue (Figure 33—cervical nodes). Any infection in the tissues mentioned above can ultimately cause enlargement and tenderness of at least the uppermost nodes in the side of the neck. Severe infections can cause successive involvement of the lower nodes until they all can be felt like beads on a chain. Drainage from the adenoids leads to the nodes in the back of the neck.

In making an evaluation of the health of tissues in the nose and throat regions, lymph nodes are always palpated for enlargement. With a mildly diseased tonsil, for instance, only the upper nodes at the angle of the jaw may be felt. With mumps, however, all of the nodes on the side affected are greatly swollen and painful. Enlargement of lymph nodes in the neck, therefore, usually indicates infection somewhere along their drainage area. Investigation must be made for the source.

Some children suffer severely from frequent attacks of "enlarged glands" (adenitis) in the neck. They are quite ill and may have elevated temperatures. Repeated medical investigation sometimes fails to reveal the source of infection. With frequent adenitis it is surprising how many children are relieved after a tonsillectomy.

Persistently enlarged hard lymph nodes should be called to a physician's attention.

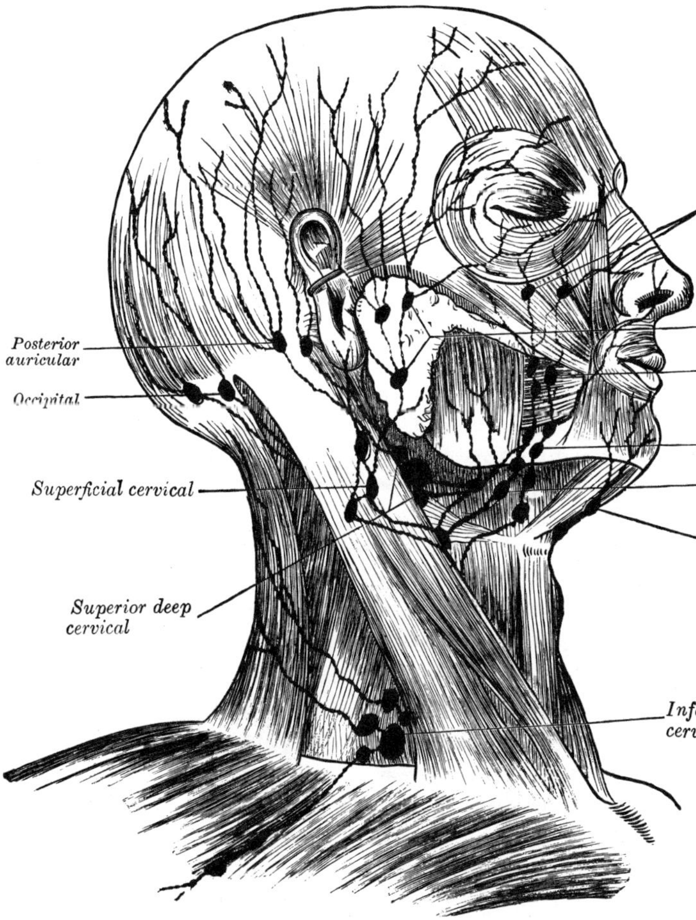

Figure 33 Superficial lymph nodes (dark, split-pea shaped masses) and lymphatic vessels of head and neck. (From C. M. Goss, ed.: *Gray's Anatomy of the Human Body.* Lea & Febiger, 1966.)

SCHOOL HEALTH PROGRAM

Detection

Most teachers will have no need to examine a student's throat or mouth. There are some, however, who are expected to make routine inspections and are competent to do so. Nursery school and, in some instances, kindergarten teachers, have this responsibility. Oftentimes it is difficult to identify tonsils or to evaluate their health. Instruction and repeated examination can provide necessary experience. Criteria used are size, appearance, color, the presence of membrane or localized pockets of pus, and enlargement of the upper lymph nodes in the neck. Frequently the appearance of the tonsil gives no clue to the diseased condition within. As has been stated, many factors must be weighed. The student's complaint of sore throat, and the presence or absence of fever are some factors to be considered.

Teachers can secure an evaluation during the school health examination, when they may refer suspected cases to the school physician. A request for examination by the family physician is always in order.

Follow-up

Parents should be urged to seek medical advice for their children, who may be suffering from any of the indications for tonsillectomy mentioned above. Most parents make provision for private financing of such care. For indigents, however, various channels are readily available, mostly through welfare departments, but occasionally through boards of education or through funds provided by PTA groups or civic organizations.

DISORDERS OF SPEECH

Speech is the most common avenue of communication between a teacher and those in his classroom. An elementary school teacher, particularly, needs to realize that it is one of his responsibilities to help the child communicate effectively. When a voice draws attention to itself, there is a problem. The voice may be unusual in quality, pitch, intensity, or its monotony. Words which are spoken too rapidly or too slowly make listening difficult. If a teacher's ears are attuned to the child's speech, he will be surprised and pleased with his ability to become aware of defects in delivery of words. With experience one notices if the speech is inadequate, if the sounds are indistinct, and if the words are rapid, jumbled, and confused. He will also be able to discern whether there is defective production of specific consonant sounds. He will notice whether speech is interrupted, associated with blinking of eyes, facial distortions, and other evidences of stress. Teachers are cautioned to watch the child on the playgrounds who yells and screams instead of talks, who may develop a hoarse, breathy voice.

Speed disorders are not remote problems; on the contrary, they are commonly observed in the classroom. Between five and ten of every 100 school children have a disorder of such severity that educational, social, and emotional adjustments are affected. The most frequent difficulties are defective articulation, delayed speech, voice abnormalities, and stuttering. These account for 70 to 75 per cent of speech defects in elementary schools. No attempt is made here to present a classification of speech disorders or detailed explanation of their causes.

Defective articulation accounts for about 70 per cent of speech problems in school-age children. Variations occur from a slight lisp to severely impaired speech. *Speech is entirely learned.* Contributing factors to speech disorders may be faulty training or learning, example of poor speech in members of the family, poor motivation to use good speech, and emotional stresses. Physical defects in the mouth and poor alignment of teeth may offer an explanation. A marked protuberance of the upper incisors, for example, may produce an articulation problem.

Delayed speech in the lower grades is quite common. It ranks second to articulation disorders. A number of explanations are possible. Lack of sufficient stimulation to talk and inadequate rewards for early speech attempts are frequent factors leading to delayed speech. If a child has defective hearing, his attempts at speech may be absent or delayed. Prolonged illness, emotional adjustments, and needs to communicate are also factors. Mental retardation is commonly associated with retarded speech.

Sometimes articulation disorders and delayed speech may correct themselves before the age of eight. But since most children talk before the age of three, it is not fair to a child to wait and wait, hoping that later, by intermediate grades, his speech will correct itself. By then serious social and psychological problems may have developed. While waiting for improvement, parents should have taken the child to a speech pathologist to determine what course of action to follow.

Stuttering usually begins in pre-school years. It is not common and accounts for only about one tenth of all speech disorders. Theories on its mechanism are complex and inconclusive. An over-simplified version observes that small children tend to repeat words or part of words and are not aware of doing so. Worried, correcting parents and teachers can create awareness and tension in a child, thereby fixating this speech pattern and producing increased stuttering. Other indications of emotional disturbances often accompany the speech problem. Whether they are a cause or an effect is not always clear. Stuttering seems to appear more often in boys than in girls. Handled wisely and early, incipient stuttering will disappear in about 25 per cent of affected children. Severe or persistent manifestations should receive speech therapy without delay.

What does a teacher do about a child who stutters? He recommends that the youngster be seen by a speech pathologist. Do not try home remedies. Stuttering is not amenable to drills. "Do it slowly. Say it over again. Take deep breaths." A child cannot go through life taking deep breaths.

Other speech problems may be explained by various organic anomalies, including cleft palate and cerebral palsy.

Watch for persistent, long-time or recurrent hoarseness. Such a condition should be referred to a physician, and possibly to a speech pathologist.

The preceding discussion touches only the most important points. Emphasis here is upon teacher responsibilities. A teacher's primary concern is with detection of speech disorders and with procedures to secure help for them. The teacher refers a child through the avenues available in the community. The school system may employ a speech correctionist or clinician, referred to occasionally as a speech therapist. This individual is usually familiar with the facilities provided for evaluation and rehabilitation of less complicated cases. Referral may be directed to a speech pathologist. This specialist, usually with the degree of Doctor of Philosophy, acts as a consultant, diagnostician, and therapist for disorders of speech. Speech training classes and auditory training classes should be available in school systems of any size. Parents, physicians, specialists in speech disorders, health agencies, welfare organizations, and others unite with the schools to furnish guidance. This means cooperative effort of school and community, with a designated coordinator. Provision of facilities and specialists by the school system may not necessarily be the economical way. Engagement of services on a private basis may at times be more feasible.

Not only must a teacher be alert to discover speech defects and refer them for early diagnosis and therapy, but he must cooperate in the classroom with the recommendations made by those in charge of the child's speech training. With proper assistance a teacher can improve a child's specific problem; with a little extra effort he can improve the general speech effectiveness of all the pupils in his classroom.

SUMMARY

Problems of the ear, nose, and throat regions are discussed together because of anatomical continuity and the close physiological relationships. Diseased conditions in one area may affect another. Problems can arise from the time the child is born. Hearing should be checked as early as possible, by the physician in his office, in preschool surveys, and at regular intervals throughout the school years.

Descriptions of health problems given in this chapter should serve not only as background information for all teachers, but should make them alert to complaints and to signs and symptoms of significance. For those teachers who are immediately responsible for detection of defects in the ear, nose, and throat areas, the material presented is invaluable. Methods of follow-up and health education implications are indicated. The philosophy and techniques of education of the hard of hearing or deaf are discussed briefly.

A closely related topic, disorders of speech, is discussed here.

DISCUSSION QUESTIONS AND ACTIVITIES

1. Explain the effects of the attitude of a partially deaf student on his own learning process.

2. Discuss the importance of early detection of hearing defects. Include physical, social, and emotional aspects.
3. Obtain an audiometer and perform the test on another individual in the class.
4. Obtain the latest methods of stopping a nosebleed and teach these to your classmates.
5. Make a list of all the infections possible with a sore throat.
6. Explain how a cold can affect not only the nose but can also affect hearing, speech, and taste.
7. Organize a panel discussion on the value of introducing a unit on ear, nose, throat into the school system. At what ages should these programs and tests be administered?
8. Find out what screening programs in hearing exist in the local school system. Do you think these are adequate?
9. Find out what a speech and hearing specialist's duties are in a school system.
10. Discuss the function of the lymphatic system in problems of ear, nose, and throat.

ADDITIONAL SOURCES OF INFORMATION

READINGS

Allen, E. Y.: "What the Classroom Teacher Can Do for the Child with Speech Defects." *NEA J.* 56:35–37, 1967.

Alpiner, J.: *Speech and Hearing Disorders in Children.* New York: Houghton-Mifflin, 1970.

Bothwell, H.: "What the Classroom Teacher Can Do for the Child with Impaired Hearing." *NEA J.* 56:44–46, 1967.

Byrd, O. E.: *Medical Readings on Vision, Speech, and Hearing.* San Francisco: Boyd and Fraser, 1971.

Davis, H., and Silverman, S.: *Hearing and Deafness.* Revised edition. New York: Holt, Rinehart and Winston, Inc., 1964.

Drumheller, G. H.: "Nasal Fractures in Children." *Postgrad. Med.* 48:123–127, August, 1970.

Egland, G.: *Speech and Language Problems: A Guide for the Classroom Teacher.* Englewood Cliffs, N.J.: Prentice-Hall, 1970.

Fiedler, M. F., et al.: "A Speech-screening Procedure with Three-year-old Children." *Pediatrics* 48:268–276, August, 1971.

Gifford, G. H.: "The Management of Electrical Mouth Burns in Children." *Pediatrics* 47:113–119, January, 1971.

McConnell, F., and Ward, P. H. (eds.): *Deafness in Childhood.* Nashville: Vanderbilt University Press, 1967.

Perkins, W. H.: *Speech Pathology: An Applied Behavioral Science.* St. Louis: The C. V. Mosby Co., 1971.

Rose, F. C.: "Speech Disorders in Children." *London Clin. Med. J.* 11:39–46, July, 1970.

Wells, C. G.: *Cleft Palate and Its Associated Speech Disorders.* New York: McGraw-Hill, 1971.

MATERIALS FOR TEACHERS' USE IN SCHOOL

AUDIOVISUAL MATERIALS

Recommended grade levels are designated *pri, int, jh, sh.*

Good Health Practices

10 min. Color *pri, int* Avis Films, Inc.*

Portrays good health practices in regard to teeth, eyes, ears, and nose in the course of a day on vacation spent at the beach.

NOSE

Learning About Your Nose

10 min. Color *int, jh* Encyclopaedia Britannica Educ. Corp.

The Nose, Structure and Function

11 min. Black and White *int, jh, sh* Encyclopaedia Britannica Educ. Corp.

Nose, Throat, and Ears

11 min. Black and White *sh* McGraw-Hill

Animated drawings—structure and function of these organs. Shows spread of infection.

EARS

Ears and Hearing

11 min. Black and White *jh* Encyclopaedia Britannica Educ. Corp.

Discusses physiology, impaired hearing, and hearing aids.

Function of the Ear in Health and Disease

30 min. Color *jh, sh,* teachers Do-Ho Chemical Company (Usually available from local film libraries)

Presents five case histories of ear defects and new methods of treatment. Shows accomplishments of leading otologists.

Hear, Now

10 min. Color *pri, int* Avis Films, Inc.

You and Your Ears

11 min. Color *pri, int* Walt Disney Productions

Jiminy Cricket "adventures" into the realm of ear structure and some do's and don't's about the care of ears.

RESOURCES

American Hearing Society
American Public Health Association
American Speech and Hearing Association
National Society for Crippled Children and Adults (state and local affiliates—Easter Seal societies). Publishes the *News.*
The Alexander Graham Bell Association for the Deaf, Inc.
The John Tracy Clinic (for preschool deaf and hard-of-hearing children and their parents)
The New York League for the Hard of Hearing
The Volta Bureau. Publishes *Volta Review.*
U.S. Department of Health, Education, and Welfare

*See Appendix A for addresses of film companies.

Chapter 7

PROBLEMS OF DENTAL HEALTH

ANATOMY AND PHYSIOLOGY OF TEETH

Teeth are constructed to provide the hard chewing surfaces so necessary in breaking food into small particles for swallowing and easier digestion. Teeth are necessary for good speech, and they also govern the contour of the lower part of the face. If a tooth is infected, it can not only cause pain, but can become a health and economic liability. Neglected or uncontrollable infection can descend through the tooth to the root where it may produce an apical abscess.

A tooth has three parts (Figure 34): the *crown* above the gum line, the *root* or roots below, and the *neck* where crown and root meet. The crown is covered with *enamel,* a hard substance, alkaline in chemical reaction; the root is covered with a thin layer of bone-like material, the *cementum.* A softer, less dense calcified substance, the *dentin,* lies inside these outer coverings. Within the dentin is a hollow space called the *pulp chamber,* containing a spongy pulp which holds the nerves and blood vessels that maintain the life of the tooth. These nerves and vessels enter the root and travel up a narrow canal to the pulp chamber. The blood brings food and oxygen and takes away waste products. The nerve supply maintains viability of the tooth and responds to pain, thereby giving warning of infection or injury. The teeth are held in the jaws by a layer of elastic tissue, the *periodontal membrane,* which connects the cementum to the bony sockets. The bone is referred to as *alveolar bone.*

GROWTH AND DEVELOPMENT OF TEETH

For the formation of dentin and enamel, the following are particularly essential: calcium, magnesium, fluorine, protein, and vitamins A, C, D and E.[1] With the earliest development of teeth in

[1]Samuel Dreizen: "The Importance of Nutrition in Tooth Development." *J. Sch. Health* Volume 43:2:114, February, 1973.

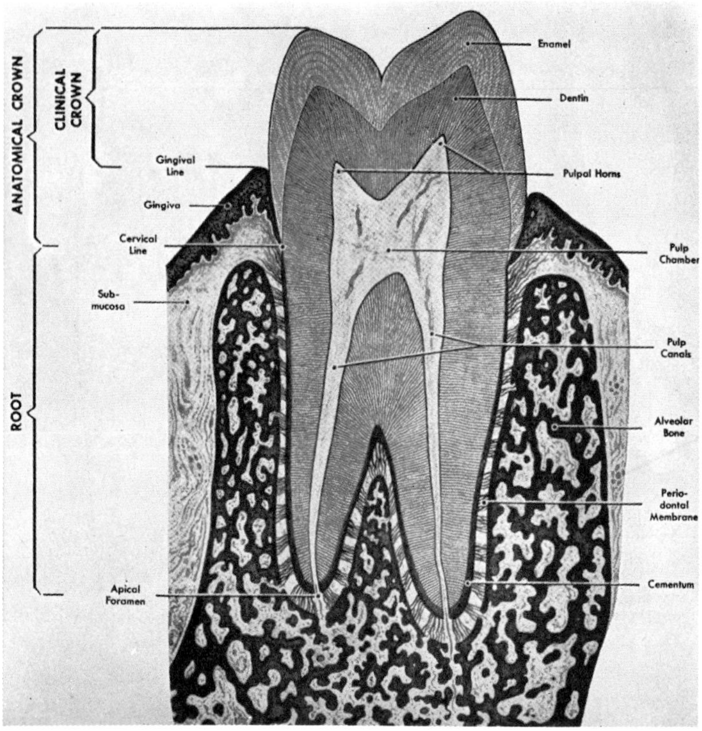

Figure 34 Longitudinal section of a tooth. (Zeisz and Nuckolls: *Dental Anatomy*. The C. V. Mosby Co.)

prenatal life, the diet of the mother provides these substances. They may be taken in addition to her regular diet. Later the child's diet should supply them in ample amounts until such time as the permanent set is developed, a span from birth until ten or 12 years of age. It is understood, of course, that a well-balanced diet is essential at all times for good health of the teeth, gums, periodontal membrane, and supporting bone.

During the growing stages of teeth the cells which form enamel and dentin are very sensitive to metabolic changes in the body, such as those produced by birth injury, nutritional deficiencies, endocrine insufficiencies, and severe illnesses. Defective calcification may be observed as opaque or chalky areas or as pits and lines or rings in the enamel at the level where enamel was being formed during the time of illness. Thus, appearance and durability of teeth are affected.

Since the jaw of a child is too small to contain a full quota of adult-sized teeth, nature has provided two sets (Figures 35 and 36). The primary ones (deciduous, "baby teeth") begin to form early in prenatal life, and at the time of birth the crowns are partially developed. They are located below the gums but gradually erupt at varying times

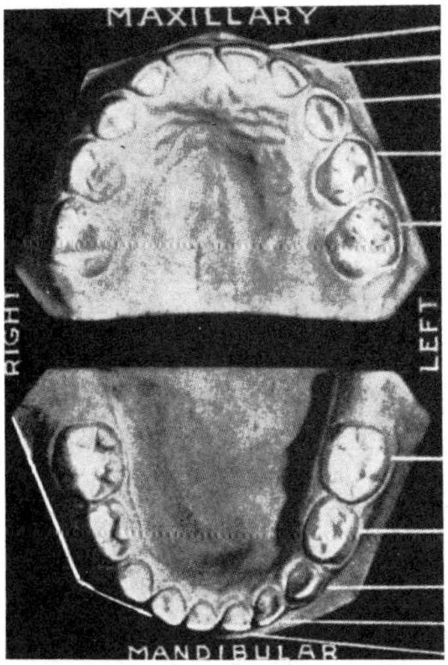

UPPER	ERUPTION	SHEDDING
Central incisor	$7\frac{1}{2}$ mo.	$7\frac{1}{2}$ yr.
Lateral incisor	9 mo.	8 yr.
Cuspid	18 mo.	$11\frac{1}{2}$ yr.
First molar	14 mo.	$10\frac{1}{2}$ yr.
Second molar	24 mo.	$10\frac{1}{2}$ yr.
LOWER		
Second molar	20 mo.	11 yr.
First molar	12 mo.	10 yr.
Cuspid	16 mo.	$9\frac{1}{2}$ yr.
Lateral incisor	7 mo.	7 yr.
Central incisor	6 mo.	6 yr.

Figure 35 Plaster casts of primary or deciduous dentition. (Modified from Wheeler: *Dental Anatomy and Physiology.* Fourth edition.)

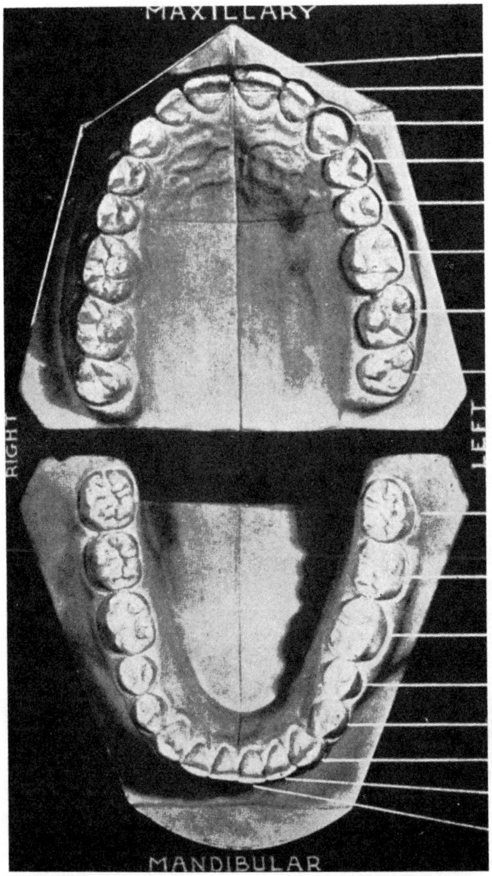

UPPER	
Central incisor	7–8 yr.
Lateral incisor	8–9 yr.
Cuspid	11–12 yr.
First bicuspid	10–11 yr.
Second bicuspid	10–12 yr.
First molar	6–7 yr.
Second molar	12–13 yr.
Third molar	17–21 yr.
LOWER	
Third molar	17–21 yr.
Second molar	11–13 yr.
First molar	6–7 yr.
Second bicuspid	11–12 yr.
First bicuspid	10–12 yr.
Cuspid	9–10 yr.
Lateral incisor	7–8 yr.
Central incisor	6–7 yr.

Figure 36 Casts of permanent dentition. (Modified from Wheeler: *Dental Anatomy and Physiology.* Fourth edition.)

until all 20 have made their appearance by two years of age or so. These "baby" teeth suffer the wear and tear of mastication until replaced by their permanent successors. They are important for clear speech and for development of the face. In addition, they maintain space and serve as guides for the permanent teeth which will gradually replace them.

During childhood the primary front teeth gradually become widely spaced as the jaw grows to make room for the permanent ones. The latter are developing underneath. As a permanent tooth forms and begins to erupt, it exerts pressure on the root of the primary tooth above. The root is gradually resorbed; when only the crown remains, it is shed; then the permanent tooth moves into place. The crown of this tooth is full-grown and does not become larger. A child begins to lose his primary teeth about age six (Figure 37). The incisors are usually the first to loosen and fall out. The gape-toothed smile at the age of six or seven is familiar. At about the same time four permanent teeth make their appearance, one back of each of the primary second molars. These are the six-year molars; they started to develop in the jaw before one year of age; they are the keys to the arches of the upper and lower jaws. Other permanent teeth align themselves in relation to these molars (Figure 38). They also carry the burden of chewing during the years when the primary teeth are being shed and have not as yet been replaced. The six-year molars are subject to a good deal of trauma; their surfaces are liable to decay; they should be watched closely. When the child reaches about the age of 12, all the permanent teeth except the third molars (wisdom teeth) should have erupted.

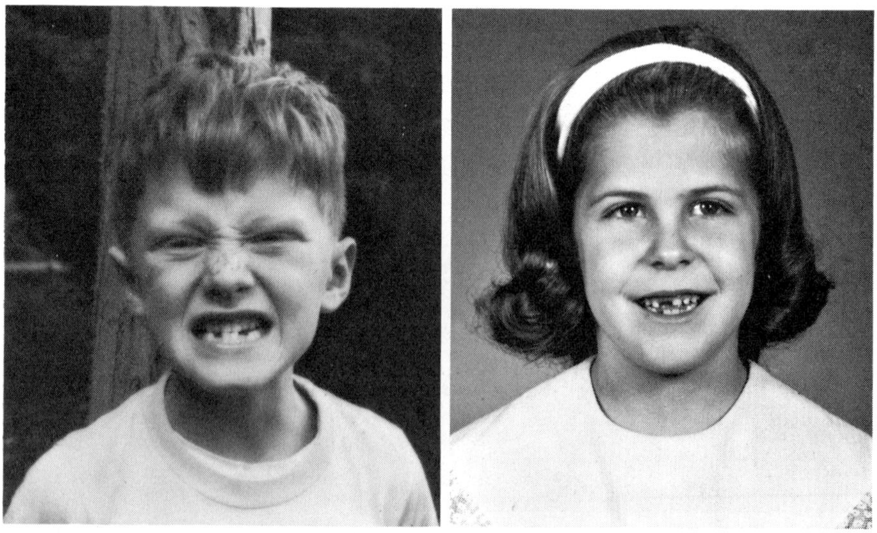

Figure 37 Six years old.

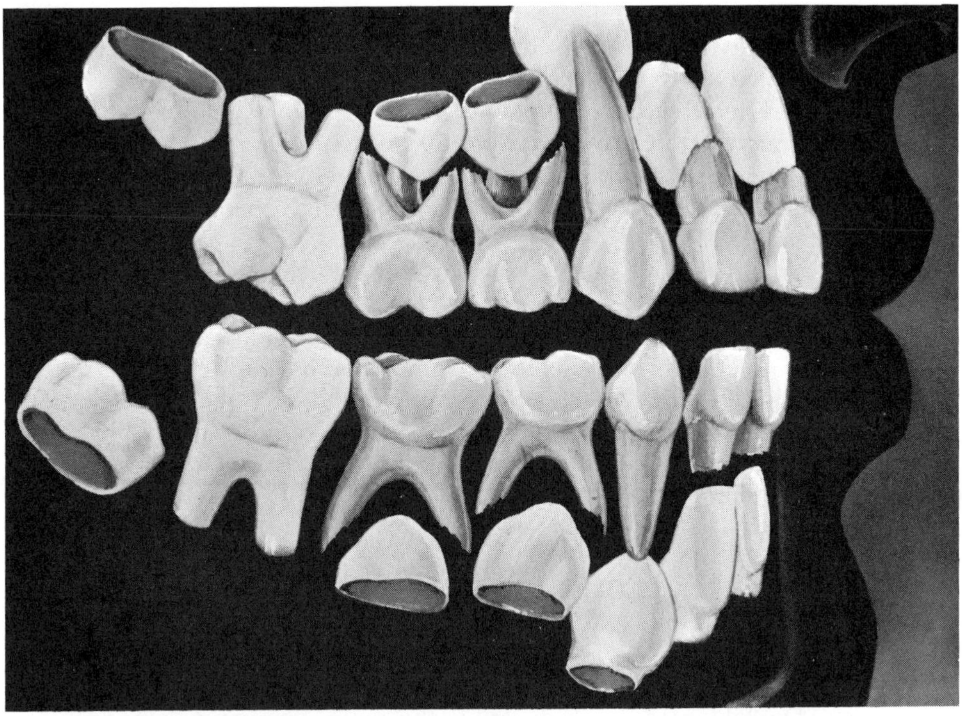

Figure 38 Dentition of six-year-old child. Note the buds of permanent teeth in the jaws below the primary teeth. The six-year permanent molars have erupted (the last fully developed teeth in back).

INCIDENCE OF DENTAL DEFECTS

About 95 to 99 per cent of children and youth suffer from dental problems, the first ranking physical defects in our school population.

A nation which prided itself on its standards of dentistry was shocked to learn during World War II that the most common cause of rejection for physical reasons from the armed services was poor dentition. Among the first two million men examined in 1941, almost 10 per cent did not have six sound front teeth and six in the back of the jaw, a total of 12 teeth, which met in a good bite.[2] By 1943, in order to secure sufficient manpower, men were accepted who had no teeth (almost 5 per cent) – men who should have been in the prime of their physical vigor and who had been exposed for years to routine dental health education in their schools and communities. Then there followed a program of rehabilitation in the armed services unprecedented in the history of either dentistry or military science.

What are the statistics today concerning incidence of dental defects?

In preschool years approximately one half of three-year-olds

[2]L. G. Rowntree: "Health of Selective Service Registrants." *J.A.M.A.* *118*:1223, 1942.

average one or more decayed teeth. This number increases to three or more decayed teeth within the next two years. In senior high school by the age of 16, the average is seven teeth which are decayed, missing, or filled. In young adults of 15 to 24 years one out of 100 has lost all of his teeth. Currently about 20 million men and women (18 in 100) have lost all of their natural teeth. Another 90 million have an average of 18 teeth, which, if not missing, have been filled or need filling.

Nevertheless, successive surveys by the American Dental Association do reveal some improvement in dental health. Observe Tables 7 and 8. The last survey of 1965 shows a noticeable decline in dental needs. "This can be accounted for by multiple factors: increasing fluoridation, steadily improving dental technics, greater utilization of dental services by an increasingly aware public, the relatively improved economic situation, and other socio-economic causal phenomena."[3]

COMMON DENTAL PROBLEMS

Dental Caries

Dental caries (tooth decay) is the most common defect of teeth. The disease involves the calcified tissues—enamel, dentin, or cemen-

[3]American Dental Association: "Survey of Needs for Dental Care, 1965." p. 38.

TABLE 7 Average Number of Fillings Required According to 1940, 1952, and 1965 Surveys of Dental Needs, by Age and Sex*

AGE	MALES			FEMALES		
	1940†	*1952†*	*1965†*	*1940†*	*1952†*	*1965†*
–4	‡	3.1	2.9	‡	3.4	2.3
5–9	‡	2.6	3.0	‡	3.7	2.9
10–14	‡	4.2	2.9	‡	4.6	3.0
15–19	7.0	6.0	4.2	6.5	5.4	4.0
20–24	6.5	4.4	4.2	6.5	4.6	4.2
25–29	5.7	3.8	3.8	5.4	4.0	4.0
30–34	5.4	3.3	3.1	4.4	3.3	3.1
35–39	3.7	2.6	2.5	4.0	2.7	2.9
40–44	3.6	2.2	2.6	3.2	2.3	1.8
45–49	2.7	1.7	2.0	2.8	1.9	1.8
50–54	2.1	1.4	1.8	2.3	1.7	1.8
55–59	1.8	1.0	1.4	1.9	1.2	1.4
60–64	1.1	0.8	1.4	1.1	1.1	1.1
65–	1.6	0.7	0.9	1.1	0.9	0.8
Total	§	2.9	2.9	§	3.1	2.9

*Copyright by the American Dental Association. Reprinted by permission.
†Not strictly comparable, because of exclusion of return-visit patients in 1965 survey.
‡Not included in survey.
§Total omitted because of exclusion of first three age groups.

TABLE 8 Average Number of Extractions Required According to 1940, 1952, and 1965 Surveys of Dental Needs, by Age and Sex*

AGE	MALES			FEMALES		
	1940†	*1952*†	*1965*†	*1940*†	*1952*†	*1965*†
–4	‡	0.3	0.1	‡	0.3	0.2
5–9	‡	0.9	0.3	‡	0.9	0.5
10–14	‡	0.6	0.4	‡	0.6	0.5
15–19	1.0	1.1	0.6	0.8	0.9	0.5
20–24	1.3	1.4	0.9	1.3	1.3	1.2
25–29	2.6	1.5	1.1	1.4	1.4	1.2
30–34	1.9	1.6	1.0	1.9	1.5	1.2
35–39	2.6	2.0	1.0	2.1	1.6	1.0
40–44	3.2	2.3	1.1	2.5	1.6	0.9
45–49	4.8	2.4	1.9	3.1	2.2	0.8
50–54	4.2	2.5	1.9	2.9	1.8	1.1
55–59	4.7	3.0	1.4	3.1	2.1	1.4
60–64	4.1	3.2	1.6	3.2	2.1	1.1
65–	3.5	2.7	0.7	2.9	2.0	0.8
Total	§	2.0	1.0	§	1.6	0.8

†Not strictly comparable, because of exclusion of return-visit patients in 1965 survey.
‡Not included in survey.
§Total omitted because of exclusion of first three age groups.

tum—and is characterized by destruction of the tooth as a result of bacterial action. Hence, dental caries is defined as a bacterial disease; it is not a hole in a tooth. Although it occurs at all ages, it is primarily a disease of childhood and adolescence. The times of greatest carious activity are at ages five to eight in the primary teeth and 12 to 18 in the permanent set. The teens represent an age of great susceptibility when 90 per cent of rampant caries occurs.

Factors Influencing Dental Caries

This most prevalent health problem is the subject of extensive research. The whole process is not wholly understood; complex systemic, chemical, and bacterial factors are involved.

Systemic Factors. Systemic factors which produce an inherent individual caries resistance are *heredity* and *nutrition* during the development of teeth. Systemic implies that the body as a whole is affected, and the teeth as an individual organ are involved incidentally. "In all probability each tooth and each person have an inherent caries-susceptibility that is determined by both genetic and nutritional factors. . . . If the tooth and its host environment are caries-resistant, all oral environmental requirements for a high caries-attack rate may be present with little or no caries activity."[4]

[4] James H. Shaw: *"Factors Controlling the Incidence of Dental Caries." J.A.M.A. 177*:304–305, 1961. Introductory article to an excellent symposium on tooth formation and dental caries.

Perhaps the preceding statement explains why a situation can exist in identical twins; in such a case, although reared in the same environment with the same foods, one child will have perfect teeth and the other will have teeth riddled with cavities.

Heredity. Those who have occasion to examine children's mouths are sometimes confronted with a baffling observation. Occasionally a child is seen who has never visited a dentist in his entire life and has never possessed a toothbrush; yet he will present a beautiful set of well-aligned teeth. Another child who has had every care from prenatal life on and has enjoyed an excellent diet will need to spend hours in a dental chair. The latter's mother will protest that the child has "soft" teeth and always has a cavity to be filled. Undoubtedly, inherent differences in the ability to resist caries accounts to some extent for variations in susceptibility. In addition, the anatomy of teeth, their size and shape, is determined largely by heredity. There may be some relationship of anatomy to caries-susceptibility in the pits and fissures of teeth.

Nutrition. Alterations also result from such factors as nutrition, both in the diet of the expectant mother while primary teeth are developing as well as later in the diet of the child, endocrine metabolism, illness, and intake of fluorides during the years that teeth are being calcified.

Oral Environment. The environmental offenders are bacteria, food debris, especially carbohydrates, and saliva. A working hypothesis which is generally accepted is that saliva and food debris are deposited in plaques on teeth, in areas where there is little traffic, such as gum margins, fissures, and crevices in enamel, or on surfaces in contact with adjacent teeth.

Plaque is a soft, tenacious, colorless adherent bacterial deposit which forms on the surface of teeth and gingiva when inadequate oral hygiene exists. It is the pathogenic factor that causes dental caries and periodontal disease, which is a disease that destroys the tissues surrounding the teeth, the gingiva, the bone, and the periodontal fibers. The bacteria in plaque yield products of bacterial action including acids, toxins, and dextrans. The acids cause tooth decay by decomposing the enamel of the teeth. The toxins, or poisons, help to cause periodontal disease by weakening and eventually destroying the periodontal fibers which hold the teeth in place. The dextrans, which are gooey, sticky substances, hold the bacteria, acids, and toxins next to the teeth and gingiva creating a "mushrooming effect." Calculus (tartar) is formed when plaque is not removed every 24 hours. These hard deposits must be removed by dental instruments. If the calculus is not removed, it will irritate the gingiva and increase the disease process.[5]

---

[5]Dr. Darwin Dennison, Associate Professor of Physiology and Health Science at Ball State University, provided much of the material on plaque, nutrition, and flossing.

Figure 39, which shows a ground section of a carious tooth, deserves study.

A graphic and simple explanation is:

Oral *bacteria* + *food,* especially fermentable carbohydrates, → *acids.*

Acids in *dental plaques* on a *susceptible tooth surface* initiate and continue *process of dental decay* (dissolve and erode enamel).

Bacteria. Bacteria in the mouth, therefore, are important agents in the production of caries. The majority of these are streptococci, although several strains of lactobacilli are also known to produce caries. Bacteria concentrate in the dental plaques.

Nutritional Aspects. The national per capital average of sugar ingested daily is approximately 30 teaspoonfuls. This results in 600 calories per day. In this situation, an individual who eats 2400 calories per day would have 25 per cent of his caloric intake in sugar.[6] This is excessive when one considers that there is no need for sugar in our diet, and that its only effects are taste and calories. In fact, there would be no ill effects on our health if all sugar was eliminated from our diets. This high usage of sugar has deleterious effects upon our health. It contributes to the high incidence of dental disease and body overweight. Also, foods high in sugar content reduce the appetite for nutritious foods if they are eaten between meals as a snack.

Research has indicated that there is a direct relationship between the ingestion of sugar products and the incidence of dental decay.[7] The most significant factor related to increased caries was the between-meal eating of foods high in sugar content. Popular snack foods (candy, soft drinks, gum, donuts, etc.) are high in sugar content. A popular candy bar had 12 teaspoonfuls of sugar which generate 240 calories; a sweet carbonated soft drink, 4⅓ teaspoonfuls; a piece of apple pie, 10 teaspoonfuls. These foods create intense bacterial activity for about 20 minutes after eating. This activity produces acids which literally bathe the teeth in a substance which can break down the enamel of the teeth, causing decay. The destructive action continues even after the sugar products are swallowed. Generally, individuals who frequently snack have significantly greater dental decay than those who confine their eating to three meals per day.

Other nutritional factors that contribute to the high incidence of dental disease include the use of white refined flour and soft impacting foods. Individuals using large quantities of white refined wheat flour in their diet were found to have considerably more tooth decay than those using moderate to small amounts.[8] Impacting foods are those that are soft and require little chewing. There is a tendency for these foods to become impacted between the teeth and gingiva,

---

[6]"Interpreting Dietronics," Dietronics Division of Hanson Research Corporation, Northridge, California, p. 6.

[7]American Dental Association, "Diet and Dental Health," Chicago, 1967, p. 3.

[8]*Ibid.*, p. 6.

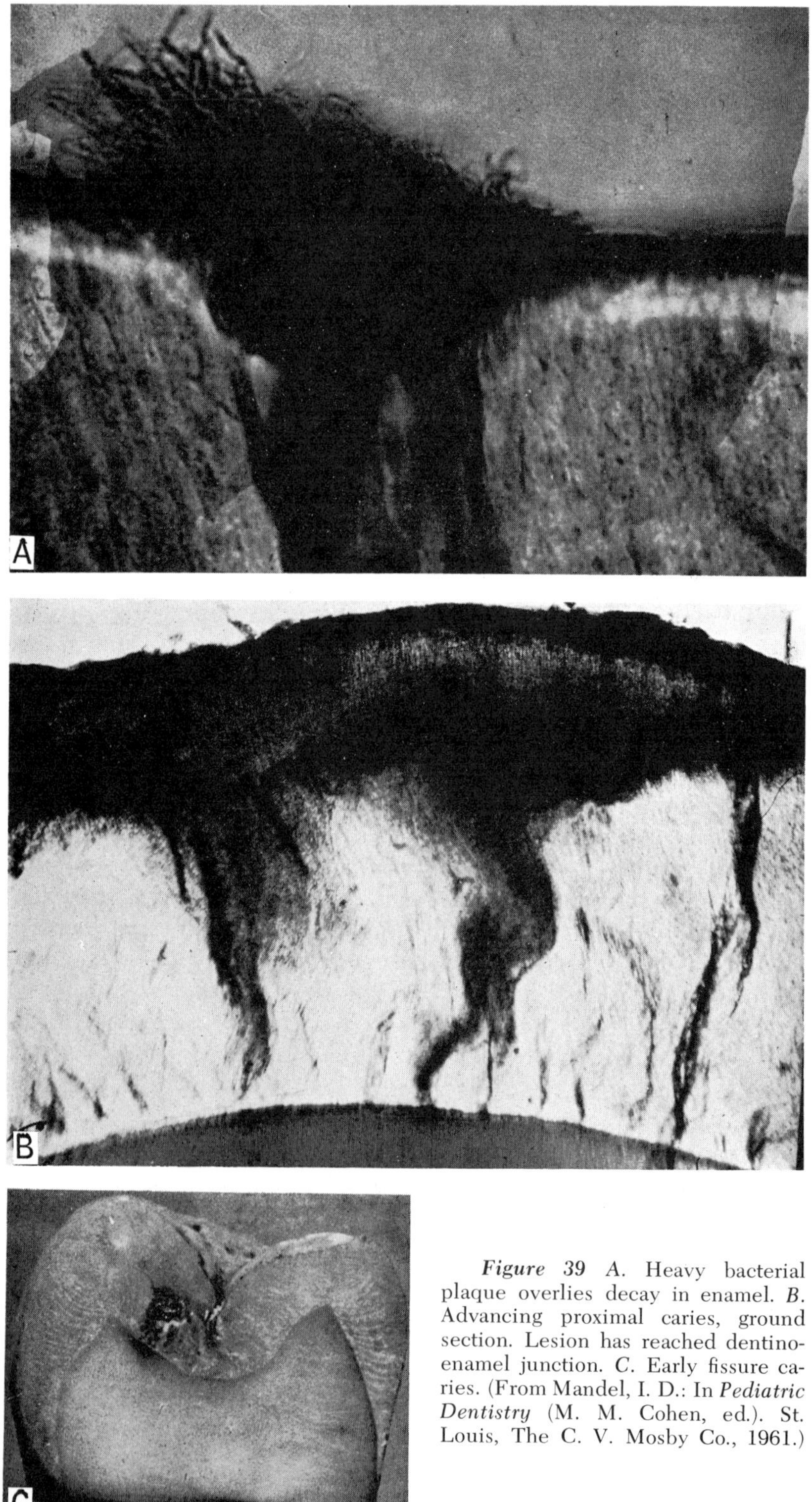

Figure 39 *A.* Heavy bacterial plaque overlies decay in enamel. *B.* Advancing proximal caries, ground section. Lesion has reached dentino-enamel junction. *C.* Early fissure caries. (From Mandel, I. D.: In *Pediatric Dentistry* (M. M. Cohen, ed.). St. Louis, The C. V. Mosby Co., 1961.)

and in fissures and grooves on the teeth. White refined flour products and impacting foods tend to nourish bacteria on the teeth and gingiva. The products of this bacterial action increase the probability of dental caries and periodontal disease.

Nutritionally, there are certain basic safeguards an individual can take to lower the risk of dental disease. A few of these safeguards include: (1) reducing the intake of sugar products in the diet, (2) eliminating snack foods that are high in sugar content and have impacting qualities, and (3) replacing white refined flour products with whole wheat products or crackers whenever possible. Also the use of lozenges, cough drops, hard candies, and lollipops should be discontinued. They are particularly harmful to the teeth because of the continuous bacterial action occurring in the mouth during their use. One individual who was a habitual user of candied cough drops "developed 21 cavities in a period of six months."[9]

If white refined products and/or impacting foods are consumed, it would be best to do so at a time when the teeth and mouth could be thoroughly cleaned afterwards. Sugar products and sweets should be eaten all at one time—preferably as a dessert—rather than eaten periodically throughout the day.

The following list includes snack foods that do *not* have impacting qualities and high concentrations of sugar. Substitute these foods for between-meal snacks whenever possible.

- Potato chips, corn chips
- Raw vegetables: carrots, celery sticks, turnips
- Fresh fruit: apples, grapes
- Diet soda
- Cold meat
- Orange juice, unsweetened fruit juices, whole milk
- Sugarless gum
- Whole wheat bread and crackers
- Peanuts
- Popcorn

Saliva. In children with extensive caries the composition of the saliva differs from that of children with little or no caries. Saliva is slightly alkaline in action, but under some conditions of poor health, poor appetite, soft non-cleansing diets, and poor oral hygiene, the quality and quantity of the saliva may be altered so that its buffering capacity is lost. More acid will be present. The beneficial action of saliva is also related to its mechanical washing and cleansing ability.

PROGRESS OF CARIES IN A TOOTH

The progress of decay presents a typical picture (Figure 39). The action of bacteria upon various foods, particularly fermentable carbohydrates, was described above. Acids produced from fermentation cause a local erosion of enamel and start the process of cavitation. As food and bacteria become impacted in the cavity, more

[9] "Effects of Acids on Teeth," *Consumer Bulletin*, February, 1972, pp. 22–24.

fermentation, more acid formation, and more destruction of calcified tissue occur.

In the *acute* process decay extends rapidly. There can be quite an undermining of enamel with a small opening on the surface. If the decay is not detected and checked by professional care, it can spread down into the dentin and pulp. The final results may be a "dead tooth" (devitalized pulp) with a root abscess, possible destruction of bone and formation of a gum boil.

When the decay is limited to enamel and dentin, the tooth is sensitive to heat, cold, and sweets. When the pulp is involved, a toothache develops. When the nerve is destroyed, pain ceases.

In *chronic* caries, destruction progresses slowly towards the dentin over a period of months and occurs more on the smooth surfaces of teeth. Cavities have a relatively large opening on the surface. Usually the decay does not penetrate far into the dentin. Such a process will be observed in primary teeth or with moderate caries susceptibility in the ages from 11 to 19.

Control and Prevention of Dental Caries

Early Detection. In the control of dental caries early detection is essential. This can be accomplished successfully in frequent examinations by a dentist. Parents, teachers, and physicians can detect gross caries. A definite cavity will be visible. Experience has shown, however, that a high proportion of caries will be missed unless all children receive a dental examination with mirror and explorer, supplemented by x-rays. A dentist or dental hygienist as a part of the health-appraisal team can make an invaluable contribution. Their services may be available either at school, a clinic, or a private office.

Restorative Dentistry. In operative or restorative dentistry the removal of decay and placement of a filling will prevent further spread of caries within the tooth and preserve the tooth for mastication and good appearance—all at minimal expense.

Preventive Dentistry. Following are the approaches of preventive dentistry in caries prevention:

1. Promote optimum development of teeth through proper nutrition of the expectant mother and the growing child (discussed earlier in this chapter).
2. Increase the resistance of enamel to acids.
3. Reduce bacterial activity.
4. Reduce the amount of carbohydrates in the mouth.
5. Use of sealants.

Increased Resistance of Enamel by Fluoridation. If fluorine is ingested in drinking water while the teeth are still developing, the teeth become decay-resistant. The precise chemical mechanism which produces this resistance has not yet clearly been determined.

The effects of fluorine on teeth were first observed in children from communities where the drinking water naturally contains a relatively high fluorine content (above four parts per million). If the ionizable fluorine in the water is excessively concentrated during the development of the tooth, a varying degree of brownish staining occurs, referred to as "dental fluorosis," or mottled enamel. These teeth may be considered unsightly but have been observed to be relatively free from dental caries and are more resistant to the process of decay. Mottling occurred only from an excessive intake of fluoride during the growth of teeth.

As a result of observations on caries resistance and after many years of careful research, many communities have introduced fluorine into the drinking water in low concentrations (one part per million in the northern United States and 0.7 per million in the warm southern areas where more water is consumed). In these concentrations mottling of enamel does not occur. Fluoridation of water is gradually revolutionizing the dental health program. The city of Newburgh, New York, one of the first to undertake a controlled fluoridation project, celebrated its tenth anniversary in 1955 and commended the beneficial results. Extensive physical examinations of its children who consumed fluoridated water for ten years were made by pediatricians. No ill effects were observed. A number of states have adopted mandatory laws on statewide fluoridation of water supplies.

Currently, more than 6100 communities with an estimated population of over 82 million are drinking adequately fluoridated water. Some fluoridation occurs naturally; but more than 3800 cities and towns add fluoride to the water supply as a public health measure. In Canada more than six million people are drinking fluoridated water. The cost is low. Scientific studies all indicate the possibility of reducing dental caries by as much as 65 per cent in those who receive fluoridated water from birth through the developmental period of their teeth. In other words, dental caries is still found in the teeth of most children who live in areas where the public drinking water supply is fluoridated, but the size and number of cavities are smaller than in comparable groups in fluoride-deficient regions.

Such scientific organizations as the American Dental and Medical Associations and the United States Public Health Service approve the addition of fluorides to community water supplies. A high per cent of reduction in caries represents a corresponding reduction in the cost of dental care; also, there will remain the beauty, comfort, and service of good teeth.

In communities which have no fluorine in the drinking water, fluorides may be applied directly to the enamel by the dentist or dental hygienist. Reduction in decay with this procedure has been estimated to be 30 to 40 per cent on the average. Referred to as a topical application, a solution of fluoride compound is applied to the surfaces of thoroughly cleaned and dried teeth at the ages of three, seven, 11, and 13. The enamel of teeth, presumably, is more permeable immediately after eruption. Annual treatments and other schedules are also used by dentists. Results vary with individuals, of course; it must be emphasized that the fluorides are only partially protective. They help prevent tooth decay.

In rural areas or where the public water supply is not fluoridated, suggested means for taking fluorides are fluoridation of the drinking water in the individual home by means of an automatic dispensing unit or by adding a measured amount of fluorides to a container of water kept in the refrigerator. Such methods will provide only a partial supply of fluorides, since water is also consumed away from home. Besides, a consistent, persistent motivation is demanded.

Physicians may prescribe supplementary fluorides for children. Some preparations are combined with vitamins. The casual or indiscriminate use of fluoride products for children is to be condemned; they should only be given under professional supervision.

Combinations of some of the preceding methods on use of fluorides may be advised by the dentist or physician. Dietary supplements and later topical applications could be a desirable combination.

Research has shown that fluoridated toothpaste is an effective aid in decay prevention.

Reduction of Bacterial Activity. Bacterial activity can be reduced by good hygienic practices which include proper brushing of teeth and flossing.

All bacteria cannot be eliminated from the mouth. No attempt is made to kill them. So-called antiseptic mouth washes have little practical value as bactericidal agents.

Limitation of Fermentable Carbohydrates. Another approach to prevention of dental caries is by limiting fermentable carbohydrates, particularly between meals. This definitely arrests decay. The objection is not primarily to consumption of sweets, but to the presence of sugars in the mouth where they may be fermented to form acids. Even so, consumption of sugar is high in our country. It has been recommended in general that sweets—syrups, jams, jellies, candies, sweetened beverages, and pastries—be kept at a minimum. Popcorn, vegetables, cheese, milk, and fruits can replace cookies and candies as snacks. Such a control program would lead to better eating habits, which alone will reduce markedly the incidence of caries.

Home Care. Care in prevention and control of caries involves brushing and flossing every 24 hours and eating a well-balanced diet with control of sweets as discussed above.

Flossing Procedure

1. Cut off a piece of floss approximately three (3) feet long.
2. Wrap the floss lightly around the middle fingers at the lower joint.
3. Use thumbs for upper teeth and forefingers for lower teeth. (Thumb and forefinger for front interproximal areas.)

4. The area of floss to be used should be approximately 1/2 inch and not more than 3/4 inch.

5. Start with distal areas at the end of each arch.

6. Gently slide the floss between the teeth with a sawing motion. (Caution: Do not "pop" the floss from the contact point into the open space.)

7. Contour the floss around each tooth and move the floss up and down on each tooth until it is "squeaky" clean. (Notice the floss disappearing under the gingival margin.)

8. Move to clean sections of floss by turning from one middle finger to the other.

9. Rinse mouth with water.

The physical character of foods is important. Children should eat chewy foods, crusts of bread, and fairly large pieces of fibrous foods, such as apples, celery, and carrots. Firm chewing promotes good bony development of the jaw.

Regular visits to the dentist from early childhood will assure skilled supervision.

Periodontal Diseases

Periodontal diseases involves the tissues surrounding the teeth—the gums, and frequently the periodontal membrane and alveolar bone. The gingivae (gum tissue) cover the necks of the teeth and extend over the alveolar bone. Gums are normally pink and firm and hug the teeth closely. Unhealthy gums appear red to purple in color, puffy or swollen, and may bleed easily. The area around one tooth or group of teeth only may be involved, or the inflammation may involve all of the gum tissue.

Our concern has been focused principally upon the health of children's teeth. Surprisingly, about 50 per cent of elementary children have diseased gums; even more adolescents present red, puffy gum tissue.

Gingivitis

Gingivitis refers to inflammation of gum tissue. The gums appear red, swollen, possibly tender (more frequently not), and tend to bleed if pressure is used. The latter occurrence has prompted the term "pink toothbrush," which, of course, is merely a descriptive term and not a diagnosis. Anything which lowers the resistance of gums may result in an unhealthy condition.

Causes of gingivitis may be:

1. Local irritation caused by malocclusion, faulty restorations or overhanging fillings, accumulation of tartar (salts from saliva which have precipitated on teeth and hardened with age), impacted food, bacteria, poor oral hygiene, abnormal tooth contour, improper use of toothbrush, mouth breathing, soft diet, or trauma (as produced by

faulty use of toothpicks, sharp or hard food, or digging into the gums with a thumbnail or pencil).

2. Systemic disorders—those associated with such nutritional deficiencies as lack of the vitamin B-complex and vitamin C, acute or chronic illness, and some drugs used in the treatment of epilepsy, blood diseases, and allergies.

3. A transient gingivitis accompanying the normal hormonal disturbances of adolescence.

Gingival disease is quite noticeable whenever oral hygiene and dental care are neglected. We find it more in children of the lower socioeconomic level and in the handicapped and mentally retarded group. Gingivitis, common with both primary and secondary dentition, is caused mostly by local factors in the mouth. In the prepuberty and adolescent years, there may be, in addition, some association with hormonal changes. If gums are not kept healthy during the intermediate years and junior and senior high school, serious periodontal disease may develop.

Neglected gingival disease may result in advanced periodontal disease or periodontitis, commonly called pyorrhea.

Periodontitis (Pyorrhea)

Pyorrhea is not uncommon in teenage students. A teacher may notice it particularly in the gum tissue around the lower incisors. Secondary to lowered resistance from gingivitis, bacteria invade the gum tissue; with the inflammatory process, the gum recedes from the tooth, forming a pocket in which bacteria, pus, and food debris accumulate. Tartar is deposited, which adds to the gum irritation, and promotes more recession and a deeper pocket. Infection spreads to the periodontal membrane and gradually invades the alveolar bone. After extensive bone loss with pocket formation, the tooth becomes loose. Pyorrhea may be localized around one tooth or one surface of a tooth or may involve all of the teeth. Bad breath accompanies the process. An individual with the disease should be under the care of a dentist for treatment and control. A teacher does not need to make a positive diagnosis of pyorrhea. His observation of unhealthy gums is sufficient for referral to a dentist. Pyorrhea is not a communicable disease.

Ulcerative Necrotizing Gingivitis ("Trench Mouth")

Sometimes, but not too frequently in childhood, gingivitis occurs in an acute form with the typical picture referred to as necrotizing ulcerative gingivitis (Vincent's disease, "trench mouth"). Onset is sudden. It is characterized by red, puffy, tender gums which bleed easily. Tenderness or soreness is a prominent complaint. Chewing foods and brushing teeth become painful. Ulcerations may appear along the gum margin. Only a small area of gum tissue may be involved, or the disease may be present in both upper and lower mucous membranes. The involved gums usually appear grayish. The breath is malodorous. Sometimes the infection extends to the throat (Vincent's angina). An individual may become quite ill, suffer from swollen lymph nodes in the neck, poor appetite, and a fever. Diagnosis is based upon the clinical picture and the presence of the typical organisms in a bacteriological examination.

Interestingly enough, this disease is the object of a great deal of controversy. The following observations are pertinent. It occurs more in winter, more when resistance is low, sometimes in those recovering from a cold or influenza, at times of emotional stress or crises as in college students during final examinations, and under adverse living conditions. It occurs in what appear to be epidemics, or in conditions which may be attributable to intimate oral contact. It tends to recur. Older adolescents, beginning about the age of 15, are commonly afflicted.

The exact, conclusive, scientific explanation of the cause and method of transmission of "trench mouth" has not been reached. Most authorities do not consider it contagious. Of course, a person suffering from this acute disease needs dental and symptomatic relief.

Malocclusion

Occlusion is a term used to designate the relation of the upper and lower teeth to each other when the jaws are closed (Figure 40). In other words, it is used to describe the bite. If this relation is ab-

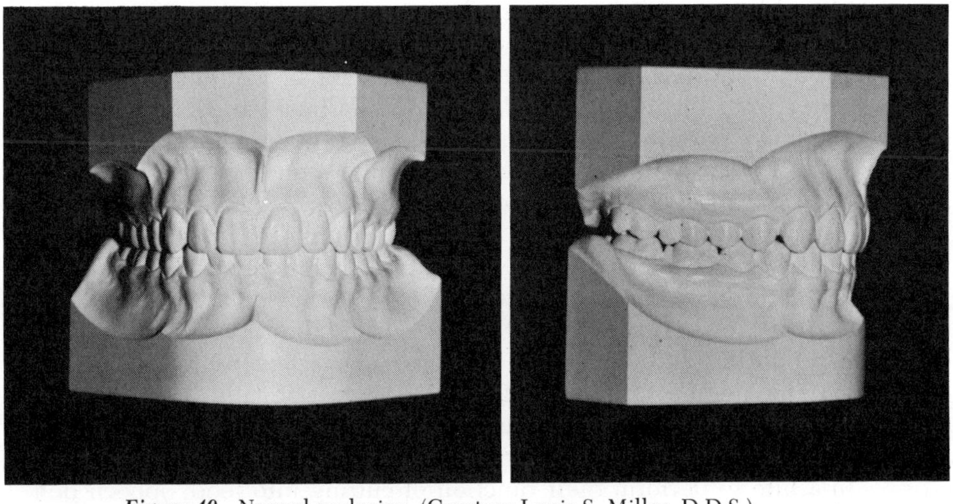

Figure 40 Normal occlusion. (Courtesy Louis S. Miller, D.D.S.)

normal, the teeth are considered to be in malocclusion ("crooked" or irregular). Not only the alignment of teeth but the actual contour of the face may be affected, producing dentofacial abnormalities. Teeth are seldom completely fixed in one position and are interdependent for proper alignment. When it is realized that the position of teeth can actually be altered in growing jaws, then a good occlusion should be a planned objective for children.

Causes

Malocclusion may occur occasionally in the primary teeth, the cause of which is uncertain. Usual causes of malocclusion in permanent teeth are:

Heredity. This may be quite a factor in determining both the form and size of alveolar bones, and the size, contour, and position of the teeth. One has seen families where facial contours of many of its members will show a narrowing of the jaws and face laterally with prominence of the upper incisors and possible recession of the chin. Occasionally, the lower jaw is abnormally prominent.

Premature Loss of a Primary Tooth. This results in a drifting of the adjoining teeth towards the empty space with a subsequent crowding of the permanent successor. Moreover, when a primary tooth is lost too soon, there is poor development of the bone in the area which held the tooth, again producing an inadequate space for eruption of the permanent one. From necessity it breaks through on the side or rotates to fill the narrow space. If an upper cuspid protrudes in front, it is sometimes referred to as a "tusk." Preservation of the primary teeth until the proper time for shedding is vital to normal growth and development of the jawbones. If a tooth must be extracted prematurely, a dentist can attach a space maintainer so that the space for the permanent successor can be held.

Loss of a permanent tooth before eruption of all teeth is completed can also cause a severe disturbance of alignment.

Reduction in dental caries reduces incidence of loss of primary teeth. Children who have had the benefit of drinking fluoridated water from birth are less likely to lose primary teeth prematurely. Evidence indicates that less malocclusion occurs in fluoridated areas.

Mouth Breathing. Mouth breathing is another major cause of malocclusion. (See discussion under nose.) With chronic or persistent longstanding mouth breathing in children, the mandible is held slack and does not grow well, the palate is high, the upper jaw is narrowed on the sides and develops a V-shaped arch with protrusion of the incisors ("buck teeth"). The underdeveloped lower jaw in apposition to the protruding one above results in overbite of varying degrees (Figures 42 and 43). Occasionally, the condition may be crippling when the lower teeth impinge upon the hard palate above, causing bruises and bleeding. The incisors may not meet in a bite to perform their function of cutting into food; speech defi-

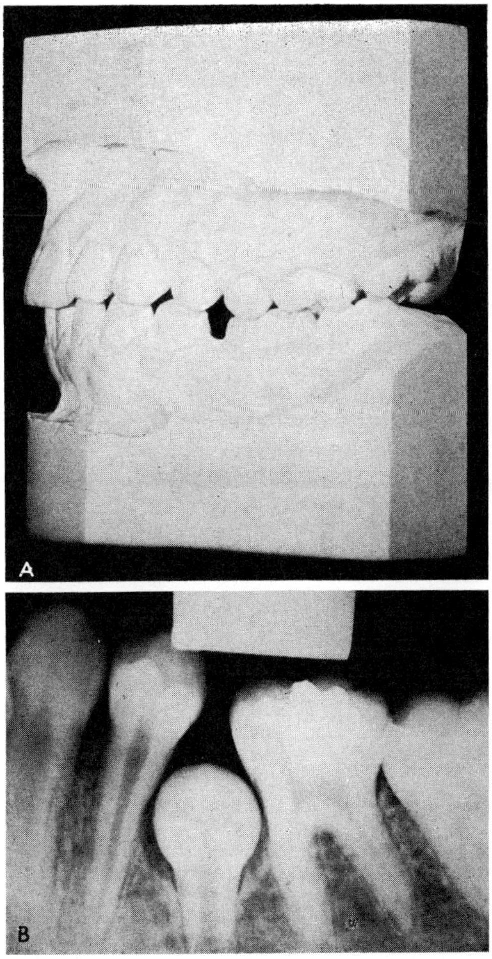

Figure 41 *A*, Casts showing the end result of the early loss of a mandibular second deciduous molar. *B*, A radiograph of an impacted second bicuspid. Space needed for the eruption of this tooth has been almost completely lost. (From McDonald, R. E.: *Pedodontics.* The C. V. Mosby Co., 1963.)

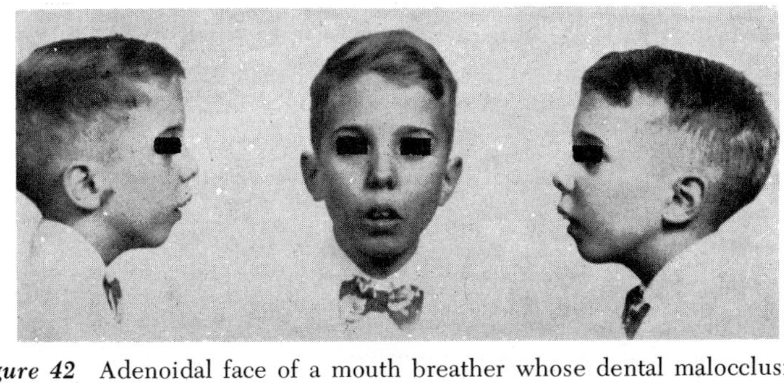

Figure 42 Adenoidal face of a mouth breather whose dental malocclusion prevents him from closing his lips properly. The extreme picture is seen occasionally. (From Graber, T. M.: *Orthodontics.* Third edition, 1972, W. B. Saunders Co.)

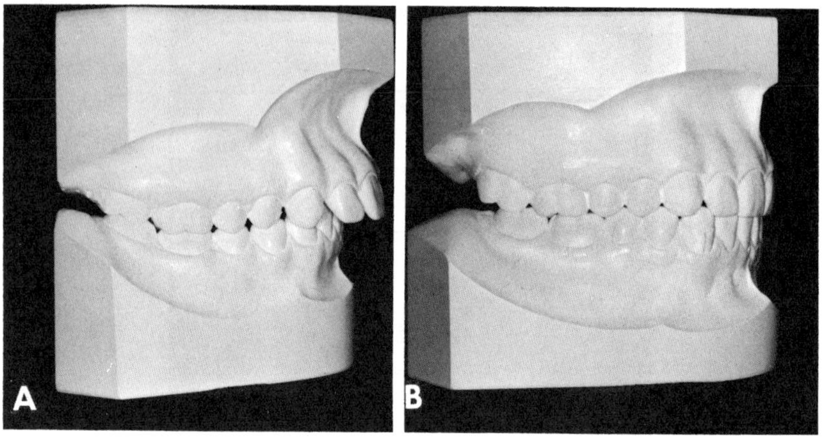

Figure 43 *A*, Model of teeth of a 13-year-old girl, showing upper protrusion, a result of mouth breathing and detrimental swallowing habit (tongue thrust). *B*, Same teeth 18 months after orthodontic treatment. (Courtesy Louis S. Miller, D.D.S.)

nitely is affected; and the receding chin can be an affront to vanity. Many a youth who reaches the late teens without any treatment of this overbite has wept in bitterness. In many cases early orthodontic care makes lip closure possible and encourages nasal breathing.

Habitual Pressures. Habitual pressures on various portions of the jaw or teeth, while the jaws are growing can produce an improper bite. Some of these are:

Oral Habits. For example, frequent thumb or finger sucking with intense activity of muscles around mouth, prolonged beyond early childhood, sucking in the cheeks, lip biting, lip sucking, tongue biting, tongue sucking, tongue thrust against either lower or upper incisors for prolonged periods, and nail biting or cuticle biting.

Postural Habits. Some examples—resting the jaw in the same position against a fist or hand for long periods of time, as children frequently do in school, habitual sleeping with the arm under the cheek in one position (pillowing), resting the head on a thumb which is pressed against one tooth, and habitual sleeping on abdomen, with face always to the same side.

Prolonged Retention of a Primary Tooth. This can cause the deflection or impaction of its successor. The tooth will probably need to be extracted, once the dentist is assured that a permanent one is present below the gum.

Enlarged Tonsils. Enlarged tonsils may cause protrusion of the lower teeth and narrowing of the arch. The child is unable to maintain a normal tongue posture and swallowing habit.

Enlarged Frenum. This may separate the two upper central incisors. The frenum is a muscle which extends from the upper lip to the hard palate, passing between these two teeth. If the muscle band is greatly thickened, it prevents approximation of the incisors and may need to be removed. The usual age for this minor surgical procedure is 11 or 12 years of age.

Endocrine Glands. The endocrine glands, through their influences on the growth of bony structures and on calcium metabolism, are involved in the development of malocclusion.

Impacted Teeth. Failure of impacted teeth to erupt because surface space is encroached upon by adjacent teeth may cause malocclusion.

Congenital Problems. Cleft palate, cleft lip, and cerebral palsy also affect alignment of teeth.

Indeed, an orthodontist pioneered the establishment of a cleft palate clinic for research and treatment.[10] Cleft palate occurs once in 700 live births, which is a rather high incidence.

Children with cerebral palsy are difficult to manage in the dental chair. They have difficulty brushing their teeth because of uncontrolled movements of hand and mouth. Orthodontic problems develop from uneven pressures of the muscles of the cheeks and jaws.

RESULTS

Malocclusion renders adequate home cleansing of teeth difficult and thus may favor inception of dental caries, gingivitis, and periodontal disease. It also disturbs the balance of stress in mastication, resulting in painful occlusion, painful chewing, and possible loss of supporting bone around the teeth. It may change the dental arch itself. Malocclusion also increases likelihood of injury to protruding, unprotected front teeth, may influence speech and articulation, and even alter facial contours, producing unfortunate psychological and social effects. The child may be referred to as "Bucky Beaver" and other nicknames of derision. His poor appearance can set him aside from his classmates.

PREVENTION AND TREATMENT

In orthodontics, which is the science of correction of malpositioned teeth, the underlying causes must be corrected first. Enlarged tonsils and adenoids should be removed; poor postural habits must be discontinued; normal oral muscle balance should be achieved in children with detrimental swallowing habits; endocrine studies may be considered. All caries should be removed and restorations placed. Good operative dentistry is important, also, in preventing malocclusion.

The orthodontist studies each case carefully—the facial lines, the alignment of teeth—to determine the course of treatment. Orthodontic procedures secure the best results during the growth period of the

[10]Jean Carper: "Normal Lives for Crippled Mouth Victims." *Today's Health* *46*:55–57, 1968.

jaws when the position of the teeth can actually be changed. Such a change requires a great deal of time—from months to years in the hands of an orthodontist. The results are worthwhile (Figure 43).

In the prevention and treatment of malocclusion the dentist is the final authority. In the school health program, however, inspections of the mouth are usually made by teachers, school nurses, dental hygienists, and physicians. These individuals must be alert to notice more than caries. Detection of early malocclusion with recommendations for referral is an important part of the dental program.

As far as the school is concerned, several problems arise with these recommendations for orthodontic referral. In many communities there may not be an orthodontist. Since orthodontic correction requires close supervision and frequent visits over a long period of time, such a referral may not be feasible if the orthodontist lives at a distance. Some parents will consult one in a nearby city and transport the child to his appointments, or will even send a child to live in a community where such a specialist is available. Orthodontic care is not only time-consuming but it involves considerable expense. To recommend such treatment to an impoverished family is futile. In cases, however, where the malocclusion is crippling, special welfare care is usually available.

Injuries to Teeth

Except in the case of a fractured jaw, injuries usually involve the incisors, especially the upper ones. A child may fall and crack or chip his tooth against a sidewalk or step, be hit in the mouth with a ball or fist, or not uncommonly be hit on the head as he leans over a drinking fountain. Falls from stairs and bicycles take a toll. Protruding incisors are particularly vulnerable. Certain careless practices encourage injury or fracture of teeth—biting on hard objects, cracking nuts, chewing ice, jerking a thread to break it, chewing pencils, opening bobby pins with the teeth, shoving, pushing, and tripping in hallways, playground, and bus. Properly fitted mouthguards should be used in athletics.

If one or more primary incisors are lost completely too early, the bone usually does not develop sufficiently to permit good alignment of the succeeding permanent teeth. Orthodontic correction will be more difficult.

Injured teeth should have *immediate* treatment by a dentist. His management of the case depends upon the extent of injury. A tooth that is broken off near the gum will require different treatment from one which is only partially severed or chipped. There is always the possibility that a nerve may die in an injured tooth. Sometimes it may be only lightly tapped and the nerve dies without any outward manifestation until later when it assumes the grayish discoloration of a devitalized tooth. An injured tooth may give pain and even become abscessed. Since a "dead tooth" may not give pain, it should be x-rayed at regular intervals to permit early detection of a possible periapical abscess.

If a tooth has been knocked out completely, it should be found and reinserted in the socket promptly. Speed is important, even if the youngster has to push it in himself. Then, he should be seen by his dentist as soon as possible. Such a tooth can often be reimplanted successfully. The pulp and periodontal membrane may remain vital and, if so, the root will continue to develop.

DENTAL HEALTH PROGRAM

Objectives

These are:

1. To teach the facts of dental health;
2. To operationalize a plaque control program;
3. To promote proper attitudes and desirable dental health practices, including good food habits, oral hygiene, and professional care; and
4. To graduate finally youth with healthy teeth in good alignment, motivated to maintain the good health of their teeth.

Detection

Inspection of a mouth is a simple procedure. A teacher should be able to examine the teeth and gums of a child, either in a good light from a window or with a flashlight. A tongue depressor does help in exposing the structures of the mouth. It is manipulated inside the cheeks to expose teeth and gums. The glance observes occlusion, the amount and quality of dental repair, the presence of cavities, the number of missing teeth, the appearance of gums, and the condition of oral hygiene. The odor of the breath is noted. This type of inspection is done by teacher, school nurse, dental hygienist, or physician.

If all children visited their dentists regularly, there would be no need for the inspection at school. Unfortunately, comparatively few do. Teachers should remember that if an examination reveals no gross cavities, caries is still not ruled out. If, on the basis of such an inspection, a parent or child is notified that no diseased condition exists in the teeth, a false sense of security will be instilled. A dentist or dental hygienist will make a more thorough examination. Sometimes caries is revealed only by x-ray.

The services of a dental hygienist are invaluable in the detection of dental defects and in the whole dental health program. For example, in 1955 the Clay County, Missouri Health Department engaged the services of a school hygienist to survey the dental health of students from kindergarten through high school. Referral cards were sent to parents. This specialist also was a resource person in dental health education to students, teachers, PTA groups, and public health nurses. A well-planned program which has involved between 8000 and 10,000 students annually has shown an improvement over 13 years in the incidence of visual dental defects from a beginning level of 70 per cent to as low as 39 per cent.[11]

The dentist is part of a school health-appraisal team. Some dentists like to participate in screening procedures at school and do so on a voluntary basis. They are better prepared, however, to do a more thorough and leisurely examination in a clinic or private office, with the x-ray machine handy. Under no circumstances should the purpose of the inspection at school be interpreted as a substitute for the thorough examination by the family dentist. If the dentist should be present at school during health examinations, his most valuable contribution is in dental health education. It is assumed that over 90 per cent of the children in most schools have dental defects. The dentist's findings will merely confirm this observation. Nevertheless, his presence will provide an excellent teaching situation, by creating an appreciation of the role of the dentist in a complete health examination and motivating the children to care for their teeth.

It has been shown that in instances when a dentist visits a school for teeth inspections, there follows a noticeable increase in visits to private dental offices for care. The same is true when a dentist speaks on dental health at a PTA meeting. The tendency officially is to preclude the dentist from the health examination at school and utilize his services instead as a health educator. In local situations, however, the attitude of the dental society and of the dentists themselves will determine their contribution to a school health examination. The school health committee of a local dental society is an excellent resource for assistance and advice.

The preschool round-up offers an opportunity to start the little ones on a regimen which will educate parents and the children themselves, encourage early dental care, and save teeth.

Teacher observation need not involve a formal inspection. One can listen to the child's complaint of a toothache, can observe the swollen jaw, the caries, and unhealthy gums that are revealed during a smile, note the poor position of teeth and missing teeth, and detect readily some types of malocclusion. It is not difficult to decide that a child rarely, if ever, brushes his teeth.

A few school systems have the services of dental hygienists who work under the supervision of a dentist, assisting with the whole dental health education program.

Follow-up

No program for inspection should be undertaken at school unless routine provisions are made for follow-up. Parents should

[11]*J. Sch. Health* 38:230–232, 1968.

receive notices of the dental findings. At times a series of notices or oral reminders may be necessary. Regardless of whether dental inspections are conducted at school, all children and youth are urged to have dental care at the intervals prescribed by their dentists. Excuses for dental appointments during school hours are permitted. All arrangements for a follow-up program should be made in consultation with the local dental society or local dentists. The dentist is the key to the dental health program. A teacher usually asks for a note from him upon completion of his work. (See forms on dental health in Appendix B.)

Even though the burden for follow-up falls upon the elementary classroom teacher, or in secondary schools upon the health or physical educator, all teachers should be interested in this most common health problem. If there is rapport between a student and his teacher, a casual word with encouragement in seeking professional care and adopting good dental practices will reap everlasting benefits.

One big problem is care of indigent children. Since dental defects are so common, neglected mouths will in most instances require extensive attention. Who is to pay for it? Communities have various plans for care of these children. Some offer minimum provisions, such as extractions and fillings, made possible by a municipal or county welfare department with local or state funds. Some expenses are paid from funds raised by PTA or other civic groups. The local dental society may accept some responsibilities.

Federal funds have been available in the last few years. Amendments to the social security act and other legislation will provide comprehensive dental services for some children. Educators and school nurses can secure necessary information on funding from their state board of education.

In some instances a state board of health provides personnel with a mobile dental trailer or portable dental unit to visit periodically areas where no dentist or a limited number of dentists is available. Such a project will have as its primary objective the promotion of a dental health education program for school and community. There may be provisions for correction of dental defects in individual children at full, partial, or no cost, according to the recommendations of local school officials or welfare workers. This latter function is gradually being abandoned because easier transportation facilities reduce the difficulty of miles; also departments of health are interested primarily in preventive dentistry and health education. The field dentist may make surveys of the incidence of caries in a school and apply fluoride solution to teeth as a preventive measure. He teaches constantly the importance of good nutrition and care of teeth.

Health Education

Nowhere in health education is there a finer opportunity for school-community cooperation than in the dental health education field. Education of the child, the parents, and of larger groups in the community is essential in planning any organized school dental program. Each year National Children's Dental Health Week is proclaimed far and wide. The school administration, school health council or committee, teacher, public health nurse, the school nurse, dental hygienist, dentist, local dental society, local board of health, physician, social worker, responsible civic worker, parents, and child serve as a team in accepting responsibility for comprehensive organized planning of a dental health education program. The decision to install a fluorine-treated water supply concerns a whole community, where discussion should be held under able and scientific leadership.

The attitude of the child and his family towards care of teeth forms the basis of success or failure in a dental program. Lack of interest or understanding must be combated. Parents need to be taught current concepts.

Health instruction in the classroom should provide information on teeth—their development, preservation, and care—and should strive to promote receptive, constructive attitudes. For example, the new Bass method of brushing teeth might be taught at school.

BASS METHOD OF BRUSHING

1. Do *not* use this method of brushing with a hard bristle brush.

2. For the outside surfaces of all teeth and the inside surfaces of the back teeth hold the brush horizontally with the bristles at the junction between the teeth and gums.

3. The brush should be on a 45° angle toward the gum line.

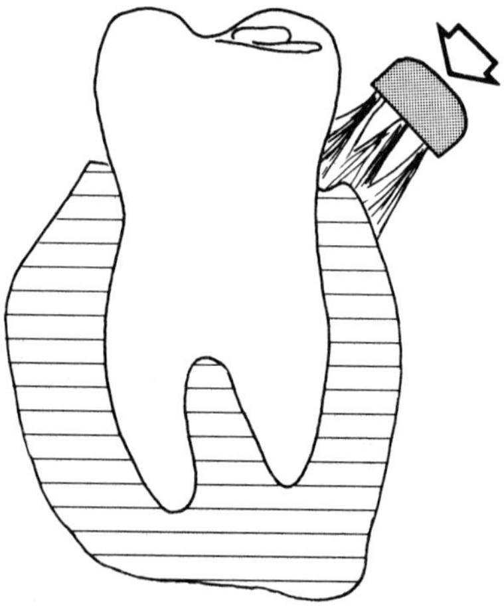

4. Brush no more than two teeth at one placement.

5. Brush gently with a short "back and forth" vibratory motion; hold the brush with tips of fingers.

6. For the inside surfaces of the upper and lower front teeth, hold the brush vertically and make several gentle "back and forth" strokes over the gum tissue and teeth.

7. Brush "back and forth" on biting surfaces.
8. Rinse with water.

The findings of the dentist, the services he performs, as well as the advice he gives on diet and home care offer a springboard for effective instruction on dental health practices.

The slight but significant decline in needs for fillings and extractions, as shown in the 1965 dental survey of the American Dental Association, indicates some progress from health education.

SUMMARY

Since dental problems affect more than 90 per cent of our school population, every teacher will have to assume some responsibility if the incidence is to be decreased. Attention should be focused upon a comprehensive dental health program from kindergarten through high school.

The most common defect is dental decay. Causes and methods of control and prevention are discussed. Part of the program of prevention is the public health aspect; fluoridation of drinking water supply is recommended.

Another problem is malocclusion (poor alignment of teeth). Causes and results are discussed in detail because the psychosocial effects of malocclusion may be serious. The best time for correction is in the school years.

Detection of gross dental defects is a simple procedure. Any teacher can observe many of them while talking to students. Teachers can be influential in persuading children and youth and their parents to seek professional advice and care.

A good dental health program involves prevention, treatment, and education. Such a program includes children, families, schools, medical and dental personnel and their organizations, social workers, and the community, with all participating in the planning. Fluoridation is a community-wide effort to reduce the prevalence of tooth decay.

DISCUSSION QUESTIONS AND ACTIVITIES

1. Explain the advantages of preventive dental health, rather than restorative dental care. Include physiological, financial, and social aspects.
2. What factors make the development of dental caries probable?
3. Develop a skit or puppet show, showing in an amusing way the fundamentals of preventive dental care.
4. Take a poll in the class to see how many students visit the dentist

annually. Then try to correlate the number of dental caries to this number.

5. Research the influence of diet on positive dental health.
6. Develop two activities that would promote proper attitudes toward dental health practices. Positive reinforcement is desirable.
7. Find out what dental health programs exist in the local schools. Do you agree with their approach?
8. Explore the possibilities of jobs in the dental health area. Besides the dentist, what other occupations are open in this area of dental health? What are the duties involved in each?
9. Examine activities that are unwise for good dental health. Then try to put these ideas into a positive presentation.
10. Discuss why it is important to start positive dental habits as early as possible.

ADDITIONAL SOURCES OF INFORMATION

READINGS

American Dental Association: Catalog. current issue. A comprehensive list of publications and teaching aids—charts, posters, films, and exhibits. "Dental Health Facts for Teachers." A pamphlet. *J. Am. Dent. Assoc.* 74, (January) 1967. Special issue devoted to fluorine and dental caries.

American School Health Association: *J. Sch. Health* Many articles on dental health education.

Barr, G.: *Young Scientist and the Dentist.* New York: McGraw-Hill, 1970, juvenile literature.

Boffa, J., et al.: "Development and Testing of a Junior High School Oral Hygiene Education Program." *J. Sch. Health* 40:557–560, December, 1970.

Dreizden, S.: "The Importance of Nutrition in Tooth Development." *J. Sch. Health* 43:114–115, February, 1973.

Dunning, J. M., et al.: "Influence of Cocoa and Sugar in Milk on Dental Caries Incidence." *J. Dent. Res.* 50:854–859, July–August, 1971.

Dunning, J. M.: *Principles of Dental Public Health.* Cambridge, Mass.: Harvard University Press, 1970.

Jelliffe, D. B., et al.: "Linear Hypoplasia of Deciduous Incisor Teeth in Malnourished Children." *Am. J. Clin. Nutr.* 24:893, August, 1971.

National Dairy Council: Catalog. Articles on nutrition and teeth.

Sicher, H.: *Oral Anatomy.* St. Louis: The C. V. Mosby Co., 1970.

AUDIOVISUAL MATERIALS

Basic Dental Health Education

2 × 2, 29 slides Color Parents and teachers

American Dental Association

Good for in-service education on dental health.

Set the Stage for Dentistry

28 min. Color Parents and teachers

American Dental Association

"A resourceful dentist with an imagination presents an evening program of basic dental health facts to parents and teachers. To enliven his presentation, this dentist developed portable 'props' and models and incorporated nearly every type of audiovisual device in his program. The facts are important to all adults who are interested in preserving the dental health of their children, as well as their own, and to teachers who are responsible for any phase of a dental health education program in a school."[12]

MATERIALS FOR TEACHERS' USE IN SCHOOL

AUDIOVISUAL MATERIALS

Recommended grade levels are designated *pri, int, jh, sh.*

The following films and film strips are available from the Bureau of Audiovisual Service, American Dental Association, as a purchase or for a slight rental fee. Some of them may be secured from local film sources.

The Beaver's Tale

4½ min. Color *pri*

Animated. Bobby Rabbit is going for his first visit to a dentist. He talks to Mr. Beaver, who explains what will happen.

A Dentist in the Classroom

14½ min. Color Grades 4 and 5

Fourth grade class seeks further information on dental problem. Dentist invited; he uses teaching aids to explain dental caries, malocclusion, and dental injuries.

Donald Visits the Dentist

Filmstrip, 23 frames Color *pri*

This filmstrip introduces the child to the dental office and what to expect during his visit.

Healthy Teeth, Happy Smile

20 min. Color *jh, sh*

"Designed to teach good oral hygiene, regular dental care, and proper eating habits, this film stars a prominent Negro dentist and a young patient who—in real life—won the Smile Championship of a large city school system. Sally, a high school student, is motivated as a result of a school dental examination to practice good grooming habits as related to oral hygiene and proper dietary rules. This film will help to teach youngsters and their parents about the value of preventive dental care."[13]

Project Teeth: Dental Health and Classroom Science

14½ min. Color *int*

Fifth grade classroom. Following an experiment in nutrition, using white rats, children want to learn more about oral health. One groups discovers why cavities develop in teeth; another group with the help of an orthodontist learns about tooth growth and importance of straight teeth.

Teeth Are For Life

15 min. Color *int*

Three children, two ten-year-old girls and a little brother, are the main characters in this interracial film, which teaches young children preventive oral care, and creates favorable attitudes towards dentistry. The girls and their dentist discuss the functions of the various teeth. The relation between food and dental health is discussed as well as how the dentist helps us maintain healthy teeth. Animation and models. Includes the proper way to brush teeth.

---

[12]American Dental Association: "Audiovisual Materials in Dentistry," (1967) p. 69.
[13]*Ibid.*, p. 74.

The Things That Really Count

4½ min. Color *jh, sh*

Teenagers can change or improve quite easily such things as clothing and hair styles. But an attractive smile can be had only by routine and conscientious care of the teeth. An attractive smile is an asset to appearance and to general health.

What Do We Know About Teeth

14½ min. Color Second grade

Filmed in second grade classroom. Pupils, teacher, and school nurse learn about teeth and oral health. Useful ideas in teaching dental health.

Why Fluoridation

14½ min. Color *jh, sh* Free loan

Filmed in cooperation with United States Public Health Service, this film provides basic information on the safety, effectiveness, and feasibility of fluoridation of the community water supply.

Recommended films from other sources:

Dental Health: How and Why

10 min. Color Grades 4–6 Coronet Films*

Excellent review on structure of teeth, good diet, progress of tooth decay, proper brushing, and fluoride applications.

How and Why

11 min. Black and White or Color *int, jh* Coronet Films

Current thinking on diet, dental decay, fluorides, and oral hygiene.

Judy's Smile

10 min. Color *pri, int* Avis Films, Inc.

Take Time for Your Teeth

14 mins. Color *jh, sh* Johnson and Johnson, Film Department *New Brunswick, New Jersey*

Approved by the American Dental Association.

Teen-Age Teeth

11 min. Filmstrip *sh* National Film Board of Canada

Good dental habits are reflected in positive attitude on studies, social activities, and appearance.

Teeth Are to Keep

11 min. Color Grades 1–5 Encyclopaedia Britannica Educ. Corp.

Roger learns the uses and importance of teeth when his baby brother cuts his first tooth. His dentist teaches him the four rules for healthy teeth.

Teeth: Their Structure and Care

11 min. Color *jh, sh* Coronet Films

Your Children's Teeth

24 min. Parents and teachers New York University Film Library

Structure and growth of two sets of teeth. Diet of children. Emphasizes importance of care of dental decay.

Many films on teeth are available from the libraries of schools, universities, departments of health and education, and from professional organizations.

---

*See Appendix A for addresses of film companies.

Chapter 8

COMMUNICABLE DISEASES

DEFINITION

A communicable disease is "an illness due to a specific infectious agent or its toxic products, which arises through transmission of that agent or its products from reservoir to susceptible host, either directly as from an infected person or animal, or indirectly through the agency of an intermediate plant or animal host, a vector, or the inanimate environment."[1]

The usual childhood diseases are caused by *bacteria* or *viruses*. Just as a reminder on the bacteria, the general types are designated by their shape and arrangement. A coccus (cocci, plural) tends to be rounded, may occur in clusters (staphylococci), or in chains (streptococci). A bacillus (bacilli, plural) tends to be rod-shaped.

Other infectious agents which may cause disease (examples in parentheses) are: *protozoa* (malaria), *rickettsiae* (Rocky Mountain spotted fever), *fungi* (ringworm infections), *insects* (lice), and *worms* (hookworm, tapeworm).

METHODS OF SPREAD AND ENTRY INTO THE BODY

These various organisms enter the human body and produce damage to tissue and to health. The methods of their transmission from one human being to another and their methods of entry into the body vary. They are spread from a sick person or carrier to a well person by direct or indirect contact. A *carrier* is an individual who harbors the infectious agent without apparent symptoms of the disease, e.g., typhoid, diphtheria. An infection by *direct contact* is one

[1]American Public Health Association: *Control of Communicable Diseases in Man.* Eleventh edition, 1970, p. 288.

in which the organisms are transferred directly, as by inhalation or sex contact, e.g., tuberculosis, venereal diseases. *Indirect contact* implies that the organisms are acquired through a contaminated medium, such as floor dust, bed clothes, wash rags, towels, handkerchiefs, pencils, door knobs, utensils, milk and other foods, water, and other mutually contacted materials. Flies may transfer organisms mechanically on their bodies.

The most common group of communicable diseases is the *respiratory* type in which bacteria or viruses are transmitted by contaminated nose and throat discharges from an infected individual. They enter the body of another person through inhalation. In talking, laughing, sneezing, or coughing, a spray is ejected for quite a distance in front of an individual. If the spray contains organisms in the droplets of moisture, the individual nearby may breathe them in. Such an infection is called a *droplet infection.* Droplets of moisture can be carried through the air for several minutes and are referred to as "droplet nuclei." It has been proved that bacteria can be ejected as far as 10 feet in front of a child during a forceful cough; hence it is obvious that avoidance of respiratory diseases is difficult. They are also spread indirectly by the avenues mentioned above; sometimes milk and other foods are polluted by the nose and throat discharges of food handlers. A child coughs into his hands, then plays games and handles objects which are used by others.

The *gastrointestinal* group of communicable diseases involves this system; organisms are passed from one individual to another through infected bowel contents. Failure to wash hands thoroughly after toileting or to dispose of excreta under strict sanitary conditions can result in contamination of food, water, and milk; so one may state that the infection is swallowed. Flies are often intermediaries, spreading disease from excreta to food. Water in our watersheds may be crystal clear in appearance and yet be polluted with typhoid or dysentery organisms. Salmonella infections are transmitted through food contaminated by a food handler or an infected animal, e.g., eggs from infected chickens.

Another source of entry into the body is by way of *skin* or *mucous membrane.* We are all familiar with the possibility of development of tetanus (lockjaw) in the puncture wound from a dirty nail or of the dreaded appearance of rabies from the bite of a rabid animal. Bacterial conjunctivitis, commonly referred to as "pink eye," can spread quickly through a schoolroom by indirect contact from handling doorknobs, books, pencils and such, tainted with the infected pus from the eye of a suffering classmate. A child rubs his eye because it is uncomfortable, gets pus on his fist and fingers, and then handles objects; if these are handled soon after by another child, who in turn touches his own eyes, the infection is on its way. The venereal diseases are transmitted principally through skin and mucous membranes of the genital tract. Communicable diseases of skin, such as impetigo and scabies, are discussed under Health Problems of Skin.

Infection may also occur by way of *insects,* through inoculation of organisms during the insect bite, e.g., malaria from the *Anopheles* mosquito and Rocky Mountain spotted fever from the tick.

PROGRESS OF A DISEASE

Incubation Period

Once the disease-producing organism has entered the body, it begins to multiply; when sufficient numbers are present, the first symptoms and signs of the sickness occur. This period, between entry of organisms and appearance of the disease, is referred to as the incubation period. It varies with the disease and also varies with the amount of organisms introduced in the initial dose. If only a few viruses were inhaled with exposure to chickenpox or mumps, for instance, illness may not appear for about three weeks. It is good to know in general how long this period may be, because, once a child is known to have an infection, the teacher, principal, and nurse must be constantly on the alert for new cases. A teacher does not always have readily available a handbook on communicable diseases, but he can rely fairly well upon the following rule of thumb: Most childhood diseases have an incubation period of two to three weeks except scarlet fever and streptococcal infections, which usually show up within three to five days.

Prodrome

The stage in which the early signs and symptoms of the infection appear is referred to as the prodrome. This is the stage before the typical picture of the disease is full-blown. It may last from a few hours to a few days. The discomforts of the prodrome are similar in all of the respiratory diseases. Here the complaints are usually those of the early "cold"—general malaise and aching, lassitude, possibly a headache and nausea and vomiting, a congested sniffling nose, with or without an associated sore throat and swollen lymph nodes in the neck. Sometimes the neck is a little stiff. A mild fever may be present. This prodrome may presage one of many communicable diseases—the common cold, influenza, whooping cough, measles, German measles, poliomyelitis, chickenpox, infectious hepatitis, infectious mononucleosis, scarlet fever, or streptococcal throat.

How is one to decide from the early symptoms of a cold which disease will develop? Only time can tell. The truly stiff neck which cannot be bent forward should be called immediately to a doctor's attention. There are those who feel that a child presenting the prodrome of a cold, regardless of whether fever is present or not, should be sent home; one cannot predict future developments. Some children are sent home only if fever is present. Keep in mind that headaches in a young child are not to be disregarded and may be an early warning of an on-coming infection. One kindergarten teacher who has a keen appreciation of the spread of the communicable diseases greets each of her pupils every morning just as he enters the door, asks about his health, and observes him closely. With any complaint of an upset stomach or headache or general malaise or appearance of any respiratory disorder, she does not permit him to join his classmates. He is isolated until a member of the family can call for him.

Acute Stage

During the acute stage of the illness, fever and other signs and symptoms of the disease are manifest; the child should be in bed; rash, if any, begins to appear with onset of fever; infectious discharges as well as excreta (if indicated) should be handled in sanitary fashion; contacts with others should be disrupted in order to prevent spread of the infection. The length of time the child stays home varies with the disease and its severity; today this period is often shortened. The use of antibiotics and immune bodies has hastened convalescence and even modified the course of many diseases.

Convalescence

The child gradually recovers and usually returns to school during convalescence. This is the period during which he should be watched closely by both parents and the teacher. Physical exertion should be avoided for a week or more after infections. Resistance is usually low after any disease and a convalescent may "catch" another ailment. Children sometimes have one communicable disease after another "in a row." Rest during the day, good nutritious food, and plenty of sleep are required. Every school should have a quiet room with comfortable beds where children rest. Avoidance of contact with active cases of other diseases is mandatory. School personnel must also keep in mind that sometimes a youngster returns to school with undetected and unsuspected complications which may be noticed only by an alert teacher. A child may return to school after a siege of a common cold or scarlet fever with impaired hearing. Physical activities should be watched after any absences for illness; the endurance of the child should be evaluated. Convalescence may be slow and endurance poor. The child who continues under par should be called to the attention of the parents.

SCHOOL HEALTH PROGRAM IN HANDLING COMMUNICABLE DISEASES

General Measures

The measures taken in a school for handling communicable diseases are exactly the same as those adopted in a community public health program. The objective is to prevent infections and control organisms by blocking their spread and destroying them. To accomplish this objective, the following procedures are basic:

1. Sick children must be discovered, isolated, and taken home with request for referral to the family physician.

2. The routes of spread at school must be blocked. Control of spread by milk, food, water, and insects has been quite effective in our country but still demands constant vigilance. The school plant must provide adequate classroom space with wide separation of seats, good ventilation, sanitary water supply and sewage disposal, sufficient toilet and hand washing facilities, clean lunchrooms which conform to regulations for eating establishments—in general, a healthful environment. Every food handler, even if part-time, should have a permit from the local board of health and should be familiar with hygienic regulations in handling food. Infections and food poisoning can occur in a lunchroom of any size. (See discussions in chapters on Nutrition, Problems of the Digestive System, and Healthful School Living.)

The respiratory route, which involves respiratory discharges conveyed through the air, is more difficult to control. Health education must be the weapon. Education in personal hygiene blocks spread of infected respiratory and intestinal discharges. The following practices must be emphasized:

a. The body should be kept clean by soap and water baths.
b. The hands should be washed with soap and water after toileting and before eating.
c. Keep hands and unclean articles away from the eyes, ears, nose, mouth, genital areas, scratches, and sores.
d. Do not use common or unclean eating, drinking, or toilet articles, cups, glasses, or toothbrushes, combs, head covers, or towels.
e. The mouth and nose should be covered during a cough.

3. Immunizations should be given to confer resistance to disease.

4. Health education gives information which will promote cooperation among school personnel and students for the development of an effective preventive program.

Communicable diseases are gradually occupying less prominence as a major health problem. Pneumonia and the respiratory diseases once were the leading causes of death in this country. With the advent of the sulfa drugs in the 1930's their incidence dropped. Use of the antibiotics has reduced the serious bacterial complications of the viral diseases, complications such as pneumonia, ear infections, and meningitis. Poliomyelitis vaccine has proved effective against that dread disease. Venereal diseases can be controlled by antibiotics. Effective vaccines against more diseases are being produced. The viral infections generally still constitute a large group of uncontrolled illnesses. As drugs are discovered which will combat this group, communicable diseases will become a lesser problem for the health authorities.

Since a high percentage of communicable diseases occur in childhood, and since a child must attend school, a responsibility lies upon the board of health, board of education, principal, teacher, parent, child, custodian, food handler, bus driver, and everyone in association with a school. This responsibility calls for a well-organized program which will prevent and control communicable diseases.

Detection

A teacher should be alert constantly for early indications of illness. He is familiar with a child's usual appearance and behavior, notes any deviations, and *listens to complaints*. He is responsible for protecting the health of pupils and excluding those who are ill. He serves a primary role in the school's communicable disease program. He inspects each child who walks into the room, may ask questions concerning health, and continues his observations throughout the school day. This should be true, regardless of grade level.

About 46 per cent of the common childhood diseases fall into the respiratory group. Parents and teachers are warned to watch for:

unusual pallor or unusual flush of the face,
sniffles, excessive nasal discharge,
complaints of headaches,
complaints of sore throat,
enlarged lymph nodes in the neck,
complaints of stiff neck,
complaints of generalized aching,
diarrhea,
persistent coughs,
complaints of earaches,
jaundice,
itching,
excessive irritability,
unusual quietness,
unusual listlessness,
red or "watering" eyes,
rash,
fever,
nausea and vomiting,

or other deviations from normal. Most rashes first appear at the base of the neck. A shirt or blouse can be pulled back to expose this area. As a rule teachers become quite shrewd in their observations and are conscientious in their desire to protect the health of children. A wise teacher will never voice his opinion about a suspected infection in the presence of the sick child or in the hearing of his curious classmates. He could be in error; actually *it is not the diagnosis of the disease which is important, but rather knowing enough to send a child home and prevent further contacts.*

As for the gastrointestinal group, common complaints are nausea, vomiting, diarrhea, and abdominal pain. Jaundice may be observed.

In order to sharpen a teacher's observations a more detailed description of each of the common communicable diseases in children and youth is given at the end of this chapter. *The intent is not to make the teacher a diagnostician, but to give pertinent descriptive information for practical application at school.*

Aside from his knowledge of the clinical picture of a disease, certain additional information enables a teacher to form an impression concerning an illness. Newspaper accounts of health department data may indicate that a certain type of epidemic is impending or is in progress. If the teacher knows that mumps is sweeping the pupil population and that several from his room have already been afflicted, he is more confident in his observations. If a child is home ill with a communicable disease, it is the duty of a parent to notify the school. This responsibility should be impressed upon parents at PTA meetings.

Follow-up

Once he suspects that a child has a communicable disease, the teacher follows the policies and procedures set up for his particular school. In some areas the teacher accepts all responsibility and arranges for the ailing child to be taken home. If one is fortunate enough to have a school nurse, further confirmation is helpful. The teacher may confer with the principal first. Actually, he should be self-reliant and make his own decisions. Excluding a child is sometimes an unpopular procedure because parents are prone to minimize the whole respiratory disease problem with, "It's only a cold." The presence of a fever is a convincing argument. To explain that the "cold" may develop into a more serious infection is sometimes futile for parents who find it inconvenient for many reasons to have children at home during school hours. One can understand the feelings of a teacher who, having heard for days a sticky cough from one of her fourth-grade pupils, was informed one morning that his father was going to pick him up at noon and take him to the doctor to "find out whether he had whooping cough."

On the other hand an administration may be reluctant to send a child home because of illness. When funds are allocated from the state to the school on the basis of average daily attendance (A.D.A.), an absence represents a loss of money. One policy has been to hold a child for a short while in the morning until attendance has been taken, then arrange to take him home for sickness. One state adopted the ruling that children who were absent because of illness were counted as present as far as A.D.A. funds were concerned. Students who were absent more than three days were requested to bring a note from a physician. The latter is a good plan also because it assures medical supervision.

If a child is ill, he should not be permitted to go home alone. Someone who has had the disease should accompany him, or a parent may come for him. There must be a responsible individual at home to receive him.

Teachers are sometimes punitive in their attitude towards the absent child—not mindfully so, but nevertheless they can discourage an ailing child. The following incident has many implications:

> A tenth-grade boy of fine intelligence suffered a severe streptococcal sore throat. Because of the specter of possible rheumatic fever complications, his physician requested that he remain home for two weeks, then attend school with no extra activity there and immediate bed rest upon returning home. Gradually his activity was increased. While he was home in bed, his buddies brought him homework and he was able to keep up fairly well with his classmates. It was decided not to request a visiting teacher because of the short duration of the absence and the heavy loads these instructors were already carrying. When time for giving grades arrived, his teachers decided to award him B's and C's in his courses. The health teacher, of all people, protested that because of his absence he should receive D's. Her opinion prevailed. The child was discouraged; the mother was outraged and remonstrated so vigorously that the grades were altered.

Consider the reaction of a class when a teacher makes the following statement: "This flu epidemic cost us $500 because so many children were absent. We need the money for equipment." Incidentally, she did not know that in her state the A.D.A. is calculated on the three-year average in case of epidemics. Regulations on A.D.A. allotments are gradually being changed. The whole structure for financing education may have to be changed by legislation in some states.

Children who have been absent from school with a communicable disease should be interviewed before re-entering a classroom. The routine varies with the school. In many instances, the teacher questions and inspects a child before permitting him to join his mates; a school nurse may perform this function. Has his doctor given him permission to return to school? Have there been complications? Is he tired? Whenever it is indicated, particularly for highly communicable infections which have been under a physician's care, a note of clearance may be requested. Frequently such notes accompany the child, sometimes with instructions as to precautions on rest and activity.

Isolation of the Individual

With our newer knowledge and treatments of communicable disease, the isolation period tends to be shorter. In general, as soon as the symptoms and signs of the disease have disappeared, the child is released from isolation.

Handling of Contacts

What about the classmates who are contacts? Health authorities are not as concerned as formerly with the contacts of a sick child. Changes have occurred gradually from the rigid quarantining and placarding of whole families to simple isolation of the child and disposition of his infectious discharges. Isolation of a few contacts in the family will not control the spread of a disease. During an epidemic of scarlet fever, for instance, as many as 10 to 15 per cent of the population may carry in their throats the particular streptococcus causing the disease. It is estimated that from ten to 15 times as many normal individuals carry the organisms of a disease as there are people who develop the disease. How is one to identify each carrier? There is no practical way to determine these carriers and the numbers would be too great to isolate.

The handling of siblings and exposed children varies with the disease and with local regulations of the board of health, but the tendency is to liberalize procedures. In general, those who have had the disease are permitted to attend school and are kept under close supervision. In many diseases one attack of a disease usually confers a lifetime immunity, but occasionally a second attack may occur. Children exposed to serious diseases, such as streptococcal sore throat, may remain home, especially when the incubation period tends to be short. In diseases such as mumps or chickenpox, pupils are sometimes permitted to attend school for the first few days after exposure, then to remain home for the latter part of the incubation period. In rural areas, or where it is difficult to maintain close supervision at school, it is probably better for susceptible exposed children to remain home. Common sense and observation of local health regulations will dictate procedures. Teachers must remember that they also are contacts and watch for development of infection in themselves. Since a teacher is expected to serve as an example, he should exclude himself if suffering from a cold.

Detection of contacts for pulmonary tuberculosis presents a different problem. The spread from person to person is insidious, for the presence of the infection may not be suspected in an individual until serious damage to health has occurred. The interval between the first exposure until the disease has been diagnosed may be so prolonged that all infected contacts cannot be found. Hence a follow-up program is complex, involving not only the school but the family and the community. The social worker, school or public health nurse, physician, health authorities, and even police may be called into action. All teaching and administrative personnel should cooperate in any medical investigation.

These same observations apply to the detection of individuals who have been exposed to one of the venereal diseases. In such instances, because of the stigma attached to these diseases, an infected person hesitates to divulge information concerning contacts. Follow-up will require the assistance of health authorities.

Procedure During Epidemics

An *epidemic* is an unusual increase in the occurrence of a disease for a limited time. During epidemic periods schools should be kept open unless advised to close by the city or state health officials. Since many children, not only in a classroom but also in the entire school have been exposed to a given disease agent during an epidemic period, closing the doors will not prevent disease spread. The youngsters simply have more play time and opportunity for direct contact. Under close observation of teaching personnel, new cases are more likely to be detected. A good example of an epidemic outbreak is the spread of influenza.

A great deal of pressure from public opinion may force administrators and public health officials to close schools, but the gesture serves to allay apprehension only. Children will wander through neighborhood stores, theaters and recreation grounds; infections can spread just as readily through these channels. Where school administrators are faced with pressure based upon fear and misinformation, an agreement may be reached to discontinue classes if the children are barred from all public gatherings and kept strictly at home. Usually parents come to realize that close observation at school may result in the safest situation possible with the exception of the home; and if parents fail to be observant, earlier detection is more likely in the classroom.

If a sudden outbreak of a disease should occur, peculiar to one class or to one school only, the source of such a disease agent will probably be local. The help of the school nurse and public health officials will be needed to find it. The source of infection may be milk or other foods, water supply, sewage contamination, a member of the teaching staff, a food handler, the custodian, or even one or more pupils.

Epidemics of the common childhood diseases frequently occur in waves or cycles every few years. These diseases are considered *endemic,* which means that they exist in the community, with a few children constantly being infected. From time to time the diseases flare up into epidemic proportions. Chickenpox is one of these diseases. Several thousand cases may appear in one year and only a few hundred within the next three or four years. During the epidemic period, many seats in the elementary grades will be vacant from one to two weeks. Gradually absenteeism decreases and in general remains at a low level until a new group of susceptible children enters school.

IMMUNIZATION

Immunization procedures constitute another phase of follow-up. *Immunity* is defined as resistance to infection. Resistance occurs because of antibodies, protein substances in the human tissues and blood, which combat or neutralize the action of the infecting organism or the toxin produced by it. Antibodies are specific. An antibody which combats poliomyelitis will not protect against smallpox.

Active Immunity. Active immunity develops when a person creates his own specific antibodies by:

1. Having the active disease, as in measles, whooping cough, and other common childhood diseases;

2. Vaccination, in which a suspension of viruses or bacteria is introduced into the body orally or by injection for such diseases as smallpox, poliomyelitis, measles, and typhoid fever; and

3. Inoculation with harmless toxins (called toxoids), to protect against tetanus and diphtheria.

Immunity may last for a number of years and can be intensified or redeveloped by "booster shots" at recommended intervals. Several weeks are required before the body has manufactured an adequate supply of antibodies.

Passive Immunity. To create a passive immunity, antibodies are taken from either an immune person or from a specifically immunized animal and injected into the person to be protected. This *immediate* "borrowed immunity" lasts only a few weeks at most; but for certain diseases the temporary protection will prevent the individual from developing the disease process. This defense mechanism is utilized to combat diphtheria, tetanus, and rabies. One source of antibodies is out-dated blood from blood banks. Gamma globulin, the globulin fraction derived from the pooled blood of several hundred adult human donors, has a good chance of containing antibodies against a number of diseases. It is used to prevent or modify the progress of such diseases as measles and infectious hepatitis, and possibly prevent the development of German measles in a nonimmune woman who has been exposed to German measles in the early weeks of her pregnancy.

Tetanus Immunization. Since everyone should be protected against tetanus and since there is confusion concerning the uses of tetanus antitoxin and tetanus toxoid, clarification is necessary. Tetanus toxoid is used to create active immunity. It is prepared in a laboratory from a culture of tetanus bacilli and is harmless. Toxoid is injected into an individual to stimulate the formation of antibodies against tetanus toxin. These antibodies are called specifically tetanus antitoxin (against toxin), and since the individual produced his own antibodies, the process is active immunity. Immunity will last for quite a number of years. To keep up immunity, booster doses of tetanus toxoid are given at intervals of ten years. Also, if a person suffers an injury where there is a possibility that tetanus may occur, and if he has been previously immunized, he is given a booster injection of toxoid to boost the antibody titer in the body to assure protection. This procedure is the best method of preventing tetanus. In World War II only 12 cases of tetanus developed among 2,785,819 hospital admissions for wounds and injuries. Of the 12 cases, six did not complete the immunization series and two had not received booster doses at the time of injury.

On the other hand, there are some people who have never been actively immunized against tetanus. Or, possibly one has had the toxoid so many years before that the physician is afraid to rely upon its protection in an emergency where immediate coverage is necessary. Then, tetanus antitoxin will be injected into the patient. This tetanus antitoxin has already been produced in a laboratory animal or in a human being (preferably the latter) and is measured in standardized units. It confers immediate passive immunity. Any person who has had tetanus antitoxin injections is usually given injections of toxoid concurrently in order to produce his own active immunity. In the United States in 1967 there were 263 cases reported. Essentially all infections were in persons who had had no previous tetanus immunization. The mortality rate is 60 per cent.

Immunization Schedule. The usual timetable recommends primary immunizations during infancy for whooping cough, diphtheria, tetanus, poliomyelitis, possibly influenza, and, in some areas, typhoid fever. Measles vaccine is given after one year of age. Mumps vaccine should be given to children over one year of age.

German measles vaccine is recommended for boys and girls between the ages of one year and puberty. "Children in kindergarten and the early grades of elementary school deserve initial priority because they are commonly the major source of virus dissemination in the community. A history of rubella illness is usually not reliable enough to exclude children from immunization. . . .

"*Routine* immunization of adolescent girls and adult women should *not* be undertaken because of the danger of inadvertently administering vaccine before pregnancy becomes evident.

"Women of child-bearing age may be considered for vaccination only when the possibility of pregnancy in the following two months is essentially nil; each case must be considered individually."[2]

One program, which received its impetus under the Vaccination Act of 1963, is now being adopted in state after state. Procedures are implemented through joint efforts of the U.S. Public Health Service, the state boards of health, and the state medical associations. The mother of every newborn receives through the mail a copy of an immunization record with the urgent recommendation that the baby be protected against the mentioned diseases. When the basic series of immunizations are completed (between ages one and two), the parent sends the record to the local board of health. In exchange an embossed

[2]Public Health Service Committee on Immunization Practices: "Morbidity and Mortality Weekly Report." April 12, 1969, p. 125.

plastic copy is returned, with the suggested schedule for further boosters and revaccinations imprinted. When a youngster enters kindergarten, he will probably have such a record and is ready for boosters. Observations show that response has been good. Continuation of the recommended schedule is urged.

As time goes on, more and more vaccines will be tested, adjudged safe and effective for human use, and be made available to the public.

Our biggest public health concern in regard to the immunization problem is the apathy or ignorance of the public. Immunization drives against poliomyelitis and measles were successful. Nevertheless, there remain small pockets of non-immunized, susceptible children in our population. Flare-ups of these and other immunizable diseases may occur among them. Another threat results from relaxation of vigilance so that new infants are not vaccinated and provide a reservoir for possible infections. Also, an occasional small outbreak may appear when a virus is introduced to this country.

School officials should offer continued protection. The immunization program should be a well-planned, continuing one which anticipates and prevents a threatening epidemic, rather than one which is quickly mapped out in a feverish attempt to take care of an immediate emergency. Not only should immunization procedures be readily available to parents and children, but there should be an educational program, promoted by administrators, teachers, school nurses, social workers, physicians, PTA groups, private health agencies, and public health officials, to acquaint the population with the needs and benefits of such procedures. This type of school-community and even national effort has been effective in the campaigns for poliomyelitis and measles vaccinations.

Parents are encouraged to preserve immunization records on their children and to keep up their immunity by having them receive the recommended booster doses at regular intervals (Figure 44).

Methods of control at school for each communicable disease likely to be found in the classroom are presented below under Descriptions of Individual Diseases. Children should never be awarded prizes for perfect attendance. A sick child should stay home for his own sake and to prevent exposure of his classmates to a disease.

Health Education

No one aspect of the school health program is exclusively concerned with the control of communicable diseases. Knowledge of the cause of disease, its spread, its prevention, and its control forms the basis for practical application in providing a healthful environment, adequate health services, and meaningful health instruction. The cohesive agent throughout the control program is education.

To promote an immunization program among children and their parents, medical and teaching authorities have a selling job to do.

Tuberculin Test (P.P.D.)	Date Result	Date Result	Date Result

IMMUNIZATION RECORD

Smallpox Vaccination	Date Result			Due every 5 years		
	Date Started	Second Dosage	Third Dosage	Date Booster	Date Booster	Date Booster
Diph. – Tet. A.P. Toxoid				Due every 10 years		
Tetanus Toxoid				Due every 10 years		
Poliomyelitis Vaccine (Oral)	Type I	Type II	Type III			
Triple Typhoid Vaccine						
Others						

Front

I am allergic to:

Penicillin Yes _ No _

Other ____________________

I am a diabetic Yes _ No _

Please notice:

I suffer from____________________

Name and address to be contacted in case of emergency.

____

____

PHONE

PERSONAL HEALTH RECORD

Name____________________

Keep this record up to date. Present this card each time you have a skin test or immunization.

Always carry this card with you

Back

Figure 44 Sample immunization record. Record is folded in half and may be carried in a wallet. Reminder for older students. Blood type may be included.

Needless to say, the attitude of the teacher is important. The teacher who makes an announcement of the impending visit of a medical team to carry out immunization procedures and then hands out the permits to be signed by the parents with an off-hand comment, "I don't believe in vaccinations myself; I've never been vaccinated," is sure to have a poor response to this important health procedure. Most of the permits will never be taken home for signature.

Administrators, teachers, parents, pupils, and all employees must be given accurate medical information so that they may understand their responsibilities in the prevention and control of communicable diseases. Since the school is only one agency which cares for the health of the child, there must be intermeshing relationships with other groups in the community.

DESCRIPTIONS OF INDIVIDUAL DISEASES

The following diseases[3] may be encountered in children and youth. Some are very common. Some occur more in the preschool years. Others may occur infrequently; but since they are communicable, personnel in schools should have information concerning them. Some are discussed in detail under other topics and will be so indicated. The methods of control of all these diseases are the same: (1) isolation of the sick child when necessary, (2) close observation of contacts and early detection of new cases, and (3) immunizations where effective.

Botulism

Cause. Bacillus.

How Spread. "By ingestion of contaminated food from jars or cans inadequately processed during canning and eaten without subsequent adequate cooking. Most poisonings in U.S.A. are due to home-canned vegetables and fruits or to fish; meats are infrequent vehicles. In Europe, most cases are due to sausages and to smoked or preserved meats or fish."[4]

Incubation Period. Usually within 12 to 36 hours after eating contaminated food. In general, the shorter the period, the more severe the infection and the greater the fatality.

Description of the Disease. Principally central nervous system involvement with such manifestations as hoarseness, slurred speech, and double vision. Headaches, dizziness, weakness, vomiting, and diarrhea occasionally initiate the attack. About two thirds die of respiratory or heart failure within a week.

---

[3]Outline in general for each disease based on "Control of Communicable Diseases in Man." Eleventh edition. An official report of the American Public Health Association, 1970.

[4]*Ibid.*, p. 93.

Control at School. If infection occurs among a number of school children, search for contaminated food. This disease should be considered along with salmonella and staphylococcus infections as possible causes of a food poisoning or gastroenteritis outbreak. (See discussion in Problems of the Digestive System.)

Chickenpox (Varicella)
(Figure 45)

Cause. Specific virus.

How Spread. Direct and indirect contact. From pox and from respiratory discharges. Spreads readily.

Incubation Period. Two to three weeks; average 13 to 17 days.

Period of Communicability. Probably not more than one day before appearance of rash and six days after first crop of blisters. Highly contagious.

Description of Disease. Prodrome of a cold. Rash starts as red bumps (papules) which soon develop into blisters (vesicles). This vesicle has been vividly described as a "dewdrop on a rosy base." Gradually the vesicle dries to form a scab which drops off and occasionally leaves a scar. Vesicles come in crops, and all stages of the

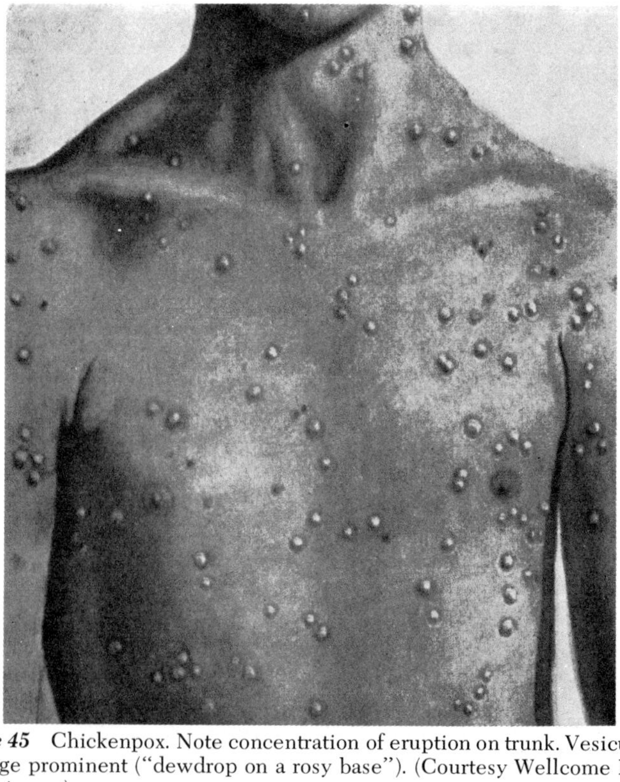

Figure 45 Chickenpox. Note concentration of eruption on trunk. Vesicular (water-blister) stage prominent ("dewdrop on a rosy base"). (Courtesy Wellcome Museum of Medical Science.)

pox may be present at the same time (papule to scab). Span of one lesion is two to four days. Rash occurs more on trunk, scalp, and mucous membranes. Itching evokes scratching and possible secondary infection of a lesion, with pus formation and a deeper pit upon healing.

School Control. Take child home.

Common Cold

Most prevalent communicable disease at all ages.

Cause. One or more viruses.

How Spread. Direct and indirect contact. Respiratory discharges.

Incubation Period. Twelve to 72 hours.

Period of Communicability. Just before and for several days after signs and symptoms develop.

Description of Disease. Upper respiratory infection with nose and/or throat discomfort. General malaise. Possible mild fever. Lymph nodes in neck may be enlarged.

Control at School. Difficult because so common. Close observation to make sure infection is common cold and not prodrome of another disease.

Immunization. Indeterminate results.

Conjunctivitis

Bacterial, commonly labeled "pink eye." See discussion of Health Problems of Eyes.

Diphtheria

Cause. Diphtheria bacillus.

How Spread. Direct and indirect contact. Respiratory discharges.

Incubation Period. Usually two to five days.

Period of Communicability. Variable. Until organisms have disappeared from throat, usually about two weeks.

Description of Disease. Prodrome of a cold, especially sore throat. Usually becomes an acute illness, with high fever and prostration. White or gray membrane in patches on tonsils and/or throat. Dangerous disease. Highly toxic. Severe manifestations may be asphyxia, neuritis, cardiac damage, or combinations of these. Attack rate in the United States ranges from 200 to 300 cases a year in recent years, highest in children under ten years of age, mostly early school age. Most patients had not been immunized or were inadequately protected by immunization.

Control at School. Once the diagnosis is made, the school authorities will be notified. Procedure will be dictated by health officials, working with principal and teacher for investigation of contacts, detection of new cases, and planning immunizations.

Immunization. Passive (antitoxin) for patient and very close contacts. Active with use of toxoid inoculations for whole population. All children should be immunized against diphtheria in infancy. Booster dose should be given before entrance to school.

Food Poisoning

See Problems of the Digestive System, Botulism, and Salmonellosis.

Fungus Infection (Ringworm)

See Health Problems of Skin.

Gastroenteritis

See Problems of the Digestive System, Botulism, and Salmonellosis.

German Measles (Rubella, "Three-day Measles")

Cause. Specific virus.

How Spread. Direct and indirect contact. Respiratory disease.

Incubation Period. Fourteen to 21 days; usually 17 to 18 days.

Period of Communicability. For about one week before and at least four days after appearance of rash. Highly contagious.

Description of Disease. Prodrome of a cold. Lymph nodes back of ears and/or neck are large and tender. Mild disease. May be very little in way of respiratory complaints. Rash may be transitory and missed. Forty per cent may not have a rash. Rash consists of red dots, each a separate one, more on exposed parts of body, arms, legs, face, spreads to body. Serious disease to contact during first third of pregnancy and perhaps even longer, since it has caused development of many congenital abnormalities (defects in hearing, vision, etc.). More prevalent in winter and spring.

Control at School. Take home. Watch for other cases.

Immunization. Passive—gamma globulin to prevent or modify disease (moderately effective). Vaccine for active immunity.

Impetigo

See Chapter on Skin.

Infectious Hepatitis (Infectious Jaundice, Catarrhal Jaundice)

Cause. Suspected virus.

How Spread. Water-borne route of infection has been demonstrated from fecal contamination. Cases traced to raw shellfish from water contaminated by sewage, to uncooked vegetables, and to milk. Tendency to household contacts. Exact mode of spread not certain. Considered a "hand-to-mouth" infection from intestinal discharges.

Incubation Period. Fifteen to 50 days or longer; average 25 days.

Period of Communicability. Several days before to usually not more than one week after onset of obvious disease.

Description of Disease. Mild fever, nausea with or without vomiting, general malaise and weakness, loss of appetite, headache, aching, abdominal pain, especially under ribs on right side. As acuteness subsides, in a few days jaundice appears, noticed in "whites" of eyes and skin. Disappears after seven to ten days. Disease may be mild and unrecognized. Disease is more prevalent in fall and winter and is mostly a disease of childhood and adolescence. Increasing incidence. Almost 39,000 cases were reported in 1967.

A similar clinical picture, called serum hepatitis, is produced by introduction of a viral infection directly into the blood stream through transfusions and from dirty, unsterilized needles and syringes. This type of hepatitis is seen in drug addicts.

Control at School. Take home. Isolation is about one week. Watch for others with same illness. If more occur, public health authorities should be notified.

Immunizations. Passive—gamma globulin to active case and household contacts.

INFECTIOUS MONONUCLEOSIS (GLANDULAR FEVER)

Cause. Herpes-like virus.

How Spread. Respiratory discharges.

Incubation Period. Two or more weeks.

Period of Communicability. Probably in prodrome and until fever and throat involvement clear.

Description of Disease. Prodrome of a cold. Sore throat may be dominant complaint. Fever. Lymph nodes in neck, under the arms, and in the groin enlarged. Student feels a persistent weakness and lack of ambition. Convalescence slow. Occurs more in children and young adults, anytime of the year, as isolated cases and in epidemics, the latter noticeable in schools and institutions for children.

Control at School. None. Sick child should remain home, but if disease is mild he attends school later in disease.

Immunization. None.

INFLUENZA

Cause. Several types of viruses.

How Spread. Direct and indirect contact. Respiratory discharges.

Incubation Period. Twenty-four to 72 hours.

Period of Communicability. Possibly during prodrome as well as in acute phase.

Description of Disease. Prodrome of a cold, gradually intensified with generalized aching, low back pain, fever, chills, and excessive weakness. Onset may be sudden. Recovery in two to seven days. Sometimes complicated by secondary bacterial infection which may affect ears or lungs and produce severe illness and high mortality. Virus not affected by present-day antibiotics. These are used for bacterial complications. May occur in epidemic proportions which sweep over large areas of population and even over many nations of the world. When the latter occurs, the outbreak is referred to as *pandemic.*

Control at School. Take home. Watch for other cases. During epidemics closing of schools not an effective control measure. With excessive absenteeism of pupils or teachers or because of community pressure, may need to close.

Immunization. Since mutations are common, it is necessary to isolate specific types of viruses. Vaccine is useful if it contains specific viruses which are current invaders.

MEASLES (RUBEOLA, "RED MEASLES")

Cause. Specific virus.

How Spread. Respiratory discharges. Direct and indirect contact.

Incubation Period. Eight to 12 days; about 14 days until rash appears.

Period of Communicability. Several days before and after appearance of rash. Highly communicable.

Description of Disease. Typical rash (Figure 46). More in ages two to six. Prodrome: a cold. Eyes and nose watering. Fever. Rash develops between second and fourth day of prodrome. Rash looks similar to that of German measles but remains much longer. First seen in mouth (Koplik spots). Discrete red spots scattered more on exposed parts, especially the face, then spread to body. These last four to six days. Itching, peeling of skin present with convalescence. Complications may involve ears and/or lungs; occasionally encephalitis occurs. Serious disease among malnourished children.

Control at School. Take home. Watch for other cases.

Immunization. Active. Vaccine introduced in 1963. Millions of children have been immunized. Some states require compulsory vaccination before entering school. Final goal is total eradication. Must continue to immunize children. (See Figure 44.)

MUMPS (INFECTIOUS PAROTITIS)

Cause. Specific virus.

How Spread. Respiratory discharges. Direct and indirect contact.

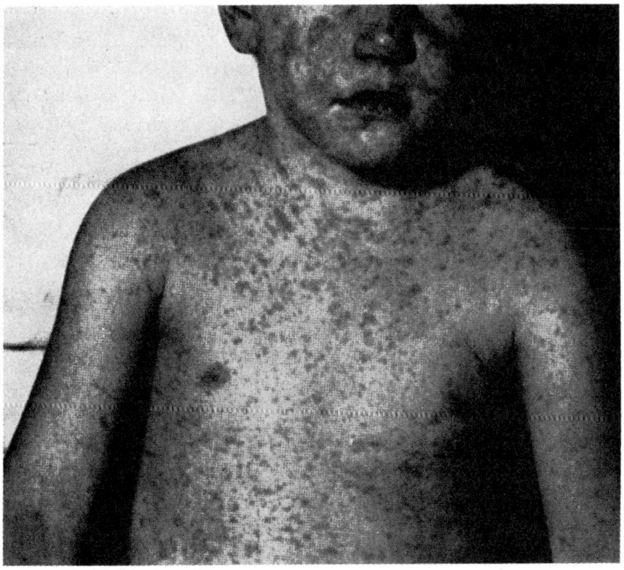

Figure 46 Measles. Eruption noticed first on either neck or face, then spreads rapidly over trunk and extremities. (Ormsby and Montgomery: *Diseases of the Skin.* Lea & Febiger.)

Incubation Period. Twelve to 26 days, usually 18 days.

Period of Communicability. Several days before swelling of salivary glands until swelling has subsided, mostly about time swelling begins.

Description of Disease. Fever. An acute swelling of one or more of the salivary glands, occasionally involves only those under the chin, more often affects one or both parotid glands (Figure 47).

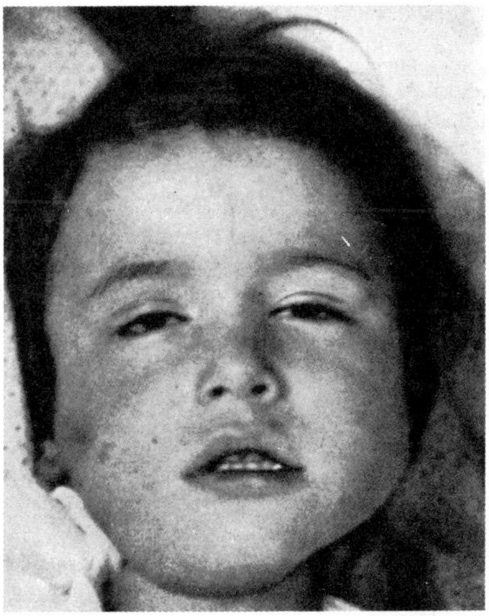

Figure 47 Parotid mumps. (Grulee and Eley: *The Child in Health and Disease.* Second edition. The Williams and Wilkins Co.)

These lie on the sides of the cheeks, just in front of the ears. The outline of an infected, swollen parotid gland can be mapped out by the fingers, and the tissue is tender to pressure. The lymph nodes in the neck on the involved side become tender and greatly enlarged until the individual looks almost "square" on that side. If lymph nodes in the neck are enlarged, and there is *no* tenderness with pressure over any of the salivary glands, a diagnosis of mumps cannot be made.

Control at School. Take home. Watch for other cases.

Immunization. Active. Given after one year of age.

PEDICULOSIS (LOUSINESS)

See Health Problems of Skin.

POLIOMYELITIS (INFANTILE PARALYSIS)

Cause. Three types of viruses.

How Spread. Respiratory discharges—direct and droplet infection. Virus also found in feces. Portal of entry—the mouth.

Incubation Period. Three to 21 days, average seven to 12 days.

Period of Communicability. Prabably from latter part of incubation period through first week of disease.

Description of Disease. Prodrome of a cold. Many cases are never diagnosed, but have been considered as a cold or influenza. There may be generalized aching, sore muscles, and a stiff neck. Sometimes the infection is not suspected until later when muscular weakness develops. If the paralytic involvement is extensive, diagnosis can be made easily.

Control at School. Difficult to recognize cases. Watch for complaint of stiff neck and be particularly alert if some cases have occurred.

Immunizations. Active immunity, protects over 70 per cent against the paralytic form with dead virus vaccine (Salk) and over 90 per cent with oral live virus vaccine (Sabin). With the vaccine the incidence has remarkably decreased. Boosters are recommended upon entrance to school. With adequate immunization, the anticipation is life-time protection. A few cases do occur, scattered over the country, and a cluster of cases could occur in the slums or other areas where children are not too well immunized. A total of 48 cases were reported in the United States in 1968. Five of them died, and these deaths were in non-immunized persons. Some states and some school systems have a compulsory vaccination requirement.

RABIES

Animal injuries, including dog bite. Since rabies is almost 100 per cent fatal,[5] and since a common source for human infection is

[5]Charles L. Barrett: "If Dog Bites Man That's News Today." *Monthly Bulletin*, Indiana State Board of Health, March, 1973, p. 1.

dogs, *a dog bite must be considered suspect in every instance.* Occasionally, a case of rabies develops in a human being; then great excitement and almost panic results. Police power is evoked; all dogs in the neighborhood are inoculated, and anyone else bitten by the infected dog must undergo the Pasteur active immunization treatment.

Any animal bite is suspect.

Cause. Virus of rabies. Found in saliva of infected animal.

How Spread. Bite of rabid animal usually. Reservoirs of infection are infected animals. Found in livestock (cattle, horses); cats; bats; wild predatory animals, such as fox (reservoir in eastern and southern U.S.), coyote, skunk (reservoir in west-central and northern Mississippi basin and central California), squirrel, beaver, muskrat, weasel, wolf, and woodchuck. Dogs and coyotes are reservoirs in southern Arizona and southern California. Unconfirmed diagnoses have been made in gophers, mice, rabbits, and rats. It has been shown that man can contract rabies by walking into a cave populated by infected bats. Viruses can be airborne in caves.

Incubation Period. Usually four to six weeks; may be longer.

Handling the dog bite which occurs at school.

I. The Dog

First, identify the dog. Know where it is. *Notify public health authorities.* Most laws concerning rabies include the statement that it is unlawful for any individual having knowledge that a person has been bitten by a dog to refuse to report such to local health authorities.

The rabid dog. Earliest signs may not be noticed. Dog may bark at everyone who passes and then become unusually quiet. Gradually he becomes extremely nervous, paces back and forth, starts wandering, and becomes glassy-eyed. As the disease progresses, he starts chewing and biting at everything in his path. These dogs placed in wire cages have bitten so hard at the wire that they have pulled their teeth out. Finally, the swallowing muscles are paralyzed, saliva accumulates in the mouth and becomes frothy in appearance. This latter sign is commonly associated with the "mad dog."

If the dog lives in the neighborhood and is in good health, he should be confined within an authorized place for ten days. If the dog continues well, there is no danger of disease. If a strange dog, he should be impounded by proper authorities, placed in a sturdy cage that he cannot chew out of, and watched for ten days. If the dog has been killed or dies, the head should be removed, packed in dry ice and sent to the nearest diagnostic laboratory. Cooperation between school authorities, private physician, public health personnel, and often the police, is necessary to handle this problem. If the dog was rabid, as established by examination of the brain, public health authorities will take over. Family and physician will be notified immediately. Owners of dogs in the area will be requested to have their pets inoculated. Police power may be necessary. There must be strict control of all dogs in a known area of rabies. Owners should have their dogs protected against rabies as a routine procedure. Any quarantines against dogs should be obeyed.

II. The Child

A. Teacher should scrub wound thoroughly to its depths with a handbrush and detergent or soap and warm water as a first aid measure to remove virus transferred in saliva. This is effective only within two hours of bite. The child should be seen immediately by his physician. *No medication should be applied at school.*

Identifying the dog is a *must.* Care of the wound or the child usually is secondary unless the injury is extensive. More than one teacher or individual can give aid at school.

B. Call parent immediately and recommend prompt attention of physician.

C. Take child home or to physician's office if the latter is directed. *The dog bite is an urgent medical problem.*

Immunization. Active for suspected individual and animals. For passive immunity, hyperimmune antirabies serum may be administered early (within 72 hours of exposure), especially with bites around the face, even before diagnosis is made. There should be a law requiring immunization of all dogs and cats against rabies. Control of wildlife is a difficult problem.

SALMONELLOSIS (SALMONELLA FOOD POISONING)

Cause. Salmonella bacillus.

How Spread. "Epidemics are usually traced to foods such as meat pies, poultry products, raw sausages, lightly cooked foods containing eggs or egg products; unpasteurized milk or dairy products; foods contaminated with rodent feces or by an infected food handler; or to utensils, working surfaces or tables previously used for contaminated foods such as egg products."[6]

Incubation Period. Six to 48 hours, usually less than 24 hours.

Period of Communicability. Throughout infection. May be in a carrier for months.

Description of Disease. Sudden onset, usually 12 to 14 hours after a meal, of stomach cramps, nausea, vomiting, and diarrhea. Fever.

Control at School. Methods employed for investigation of all food poisoning outbreaks. Intensive search for source and means of contamination. Prevention consists of following all public health regulations for eating establishments and food handlers.

Immunization. None.

---

[6]*Op. Cit.*: "Control of Communicable Diseases in Man." pp. 101–102.

SCABIES (THE "ITCH," "SEVEN-YEAR ITCH")

See Health Problems of Skin.

SMALLPOX (VARIOLA)

Cause. Specific virus.

How Spread. Direct and indirect contact. From respiratory discharges and from pox itself.

Incubation Period. Seven to 16 days. Average nine to 12 days.

Period of Communicability. From first symptoms until all scabs have dropped off, about two to three weeks.

Description of Disease. Prodrome of a cold—gradually increasing in intensity. Rash starts four to five days after fever appears. Cycle of a pox consists first of a red spot (macule), which becomes raised (papule), develops into a blister (vesicle) whose contents gradually accumulate pus (pustule). The center of the pustule becomes withdrawn or umbilicated, gradually dries to form a scab that eventually drops off. A scar indicates the site of one pox.

In the active disease, pox are present over the whole body, more so on the exposed parts, noticeably on the palms and soles. In contrast to chickenpox, which rarely develops pustules and in which all stages of the pox may be present at one time, smallpox shows only one stage at a time and the pox progresses through the whole cycle. Smallpox can be fatal and in the past accounted for high mortality rates throughout the world.

Immunization. The United States Public Health Service has been opposed to immunizations for smallpox since 1972. Further, they are opposed to mandatory school entrance vaccination laws. The reason cited for their position is the low incidence of the disease and the resulting low risk of coming down with the disease.

However, the American Medical Association suggests to physicians that they use their own judgment on this matter, citing outbreaks of this disease in various parts of the world.

STREPTOCOCCAL INFECTIONS

Respiratory. Scarlet fever and streptococcal sore throat.

Cause. Group A streptococcus.

How Spread. Respiratory discharges. Direct or indirect contact.

Incubation Period. Usually one to three days.

Period of Communicability. In mild cases during incubation period until a few days after clinical recovery. Cases with sinus and lung complications may be infectious from discharges for a longer period.

Description of Disease. Severity of infection varies. May be mild or may become serious with ear, lung, sinus, kidney, heart, and other complications. (See chapters on Ear, Nose, and Throat and Heart Problems in the School Child.)

Scarlet fever is actually streptococcal sore throat with toxic manifestations of a skin rash. Prodrome of a cold. Complaint of sore throat is dominant, with lymph nodes in neck enlarged and tender. Throat is red and swollen. Tongue appears a strawberry red color. The rash is bright red, fine, tends to "run together," appears more on the trunk and more often in the folds of the body—neck, under arms, groin, folds of elbows and knees. After the infection subsides the skin peels over the whole body, beginning at the tips of fingers and toes (desquamation).

Streptococcal sore throat is considered to be scarlet fever without the rash. The patient is sick, has a high fever, flushed face, and a severely infected throat with enlarged lymph nodes in the neck.

Control at School. Take child home with any complaint of sore throat accompanied by fever. Readmission on physician's clearance. Watch closely for other cases in classrooms. Incubation period is short.

Immunization. Vaccine under study.

TUBERCULOSIS

Cause. Tubercle bacillus.

How Spread. (1) Respiratory (human strain of bacilli)—transmitted from one person to another by air in minute droplets of sputum or moisture, produced during coughing, sneezing, or laughing. These droplets evaporate, leaving "droplet nuclei" which remain suspended in air indefinitely. Tubercle bacilli in nuclei will be inhaled directly into depths of bronchial tree and implanted on lung tissues, where they will start to multiply. (2) Bovine strain of bacilli—swallowed in unpasteurized milk or dairy products from infected cow. May be airborne infection in barns; also transmitted from contaminated animal products.

Incubation Period. At least 30 days from infection to progressive disease. May take years.

The development of a positive tuberculin test after infection requires three to eight weeks.

Period of Communicability. As long as patient is discharging bacilli.

Description of Disease. Early tuberculosis is hard to detect. Active disease may involve lungs, lymph nodes, bone, and other tissues. Children under the age of five are most susceptible and vulnerable—susceptible because of intimate and perhaps repeated contact, vulnerable as seen by the high mortality at this age. Those aged five to 14 years are less susceptible and vulnerable. Mortality is high among young adults, 15 to 30 years of age. It is a disease of the teens. The time required for treatment has been greatly reduced, and recovery has been expedited by modern drugs, which may be given while the patient is ambulatory. The pulmonary type is accompanied by loss of weight, fatigue, persistent coughing, and low-grade fever. Coughing of blood from tuberculosis is rare in childhood.

Control at School.

1. Children with active tuberculosis located anywhere in the body should be excluded until cleared by physician.
2. Detection of unrecognized cases of tuberculosis.
   a. There must be a follow-up on all contacts (associates) with known cases. This is done with the aid of the teacher, school social worker, school or public health nurse, private physician, or health authorities. Several of these will probably work together. Active cases should be identified as quickly as possible in order to prevent spread.
   b. All administrators, teachers, members of the counseling staff, secretaries, bus drivers, and food service personnel should have an x-ray of the chest once a year.
   c. All athletes should have an annual x-ray of the chest.
   d. Mass tuberculin testing of children and adult personnel must be carried out regularly. Positive reactors, those showing a positive skin test, must follow through with complete health examination and chest x-ray. Mass testing should not be undertaken until there has been extensive education preparation in the classrooms and among the parents. The meaning of a positive tuberculin test must be interpreted so that there will be no fear if the child should be a positive reactor.

A teaching unit on tuberculosis, preceding the testing, will help the school children understand the program.

A tuberculin test is a tissue-sensitivity skin test. *A positive test does not necessarily indicate active disease.* All it indicates is that the individual has been exposed at some time to tubercle bacilli and the body has reacted. The tuberculous process may be either active or "arrested" (nonactive); hence the need for physical examinations and chest x-rays of all positive reactors. Provisions must be made in advance to make this follow-up available for indigents.

If a child who has had a consistently negative tuberculin reaction converts to a positive, it is assumed that active infection has developed. Recent converters should be evaluated by a physician for possible therapy. Once a positive reaction occurs, no further skin tests are done unless there has been a long lapse of time, but chest x-rays are taken at intervals. Occasionally, a positive reactor will revert to negative.

With all positive reactors there must not only be a medical follow-up, but their close contacts should be studied by tuberculin tests followed by x-rays on all positive reactors. It is essential to find the active case or cases which are disseminating bacilli and thus protect uninfected people.

Severe outbreaks in schools are sometimes reported. One of the most tragic,[7] resulted from relaxation of vigilance with the hiring in the midyear (January 1962) of a young teacher for the sixth grade, who "was not required to furnish evidence of freedom of tuberculosis." All other teachers had had x-rays of the chest the previous fall. Late in April an ailing child from the classroom was diagnosed as having tuberculosis. The case was reported to the County Health Commissioner and immediately every person in the school was given a tuberculin test. The newly hired teacher had advanced pulmonary tuberculosis. All 44 students in the sixth grade room had a positive reaction. As for the remainder of the school, there were 22 positive reactors out of 590 for a rate of 3.7 per cent in contrast to 100 per cent for the sick teacher's classroom. Public health nurses visited the homes of the positive reactors, explained the problem to parents, and checked all siblings by tuberculin test or x-ray. Checking contacts revealed that the teacher's sister, age 20, and brother, age 15, needed to be hospitalized.

The final score: July 20, 1962–
- 1 teacher with active primary tuberculosis
- 1 teacher hospitalized with active pulmonary tuberculosis
- 16 students diagnosed as having active, primary tuberculosis and placed under medication for at least one year
- 66 students to be checked every year of their lives
- 6 adults to be checked every year of their lives.

Another recent tragedy was revealed in May, 1967 in a second-grade room where a teacher was found to have an active pulmonary tuberculosis with bacilli in her sputum. Previous x-rays of the chest over a period of years had shown no pathology. The last previous x-ray was August, 1965. Her attendance during the school year had been perfect. After her active disease was diagnosed, tuberculin tests administered to her class of 25 pupils uncovered four positive reactions. These pupils had negative reactions the year before. The teacher's son also had a positive test. All the children were started on antituberculous chemotherapy. Repeat testing in June, 1967 of the remaining 21 negative children (five weeks after the contact was broken) showed two additional converters making a total of six tuberculin conversions among 25 pupils. Beginning in the fall of 1967, all teachers in the public and parochial school system were required to have annual tuberculin tests.[8]

The American Student Health Association, in order to promote an effective tuberculosis detection and control program, issues a certificate to a school or school system, kindergarten through twelfth grade, if 95 per cent of children and 100 per cent of employees and teachers have had a tuberculin test and follow-up on positive reactors.

---

[7]L. L. Taylor: "100% Is Not Always Good." *J. Sch. Health* 32:385–386, 1962.

[8]Weekly Report on Morbidity and Mortality: National Communicable Disease Center. June 17, 1967.

This certification program is a case-finding program. In schools with this certification the problem of detection of contacts is much less difficult. Such a program prevents spread of tubercle bacilli and prevents outbreaks in schools.

Eradication is the objective. This will be a stupendous project, screening every school child in the United States, screening not just once but at intervals over a period of time. A joint committee of the Section on Diseases of the Chest of the American Academy of Pediatrics and the American College of Chest Physicians makes the following recommendation:

> Infection with tuberculosis in children is still a problem. Since early treatment has been found valuable for tuberculin converters, particularly in the very young, it is mandatory that tuberculin testing be carried out early in life. This Committee strongly suggests that routine tuberculin testing be initiated between six and 12 months of age, preferably before measles or smallpox vaccination, and be repeated annually up to four years of age and thereafter every two years, depending on the risk of exposure of the child and the prevalence of tuberculosis in the population group.

3. Education for personal and community health.
   a. Children and older students still need to be reminded of the hygienic principles to be observed in care of respiratory diseases. They must understand the importance of pasteurized milk. They must appreciate the importance of general good hygienic principles of rest, nutrition, and maintenance of good health.
   b. The cooperation of individual parents and of the PTA is necessary in a tuberculosis-detection survey.

      The usual routine in communication with parents is to send a form which notifies them that the program is to be conducted, explains the significance of the tuberculin test and the need for a chest x-ray on a positive reactor. The parent or guardian then signs a request for the test on his child and gives permission for periodic follow-up x-rays, if necessary. After the test is read, the parent receives the report with appropriate recommendation for follow-up. All parents should receive notifications as to whether results indicate positive or negative reactions, again with interpretations and indicated follow-ups.
   c. School-community relationships are particularly important in this area. Mobile x-ray units are often provided by state boards of health, who also provide the costs, technical assistance, and medical interpretation of films. The local branches of the National Tuberculosis and Health Association assist with this program. Every state board of health has a division of tuberculosis control and should be ready to carry out a screening program covering the state.

Local health authorities and medical societies must be included in all plans.

The final goal is a uniform, practical, and effective program to eradicate tuberculosis throughout the country. Regardless of our information and new methods of attack, this disease still demands close attention. In 1967 case-findings in the United States were:

Ages	New Active Tuberculosis Cases
0–4 years	2,247
5–14 years	2,794
15–24 years	4,315
all ages – total	45,647

If we still have a tuberculosis problem in the United States, imagine what confronts the poverty-stricken populations of the world! In some countries tuberculosis is the leading disease.

Immunization. Live vaccine, the most widely used being the BCG vaccine, first introduced in France in 1923. Can produce variable amounts of resistance to tuberculosis, but not complete protection. Used on nonreactors only. Used by World Health Organization in many countries. Where prevalence of disease is low, as in U.S., public health authorities do not promote use except occasionally for selected population groups. Rather, chemical therapy on positive reactors is usually preferred.

Typhoid Fever

Cause. Bacillus.

How Spread. Swallowing contaminated food or water.

Incubation Period. Seven to 14 days, may be longer.

Period of Communicability. During infection and variable time during convalescence, organisms are present in excreta. Infection may persist indefinitely in about 3 per cent as carriers.

Control at School. Public health precautions for eating places and food handlers. Screens on windows and doors to keep out flies. See Healthful School Living for discussion of lunchroom personnel.

Immunization. Active.

The description of *paratyphoid fever* is similar in all respects except that the disease is usually milder and is caused by another bacillus of the same basic group of organisms.

Venereal Diseases

The incidence of the most common venereal diseases, *gonorrhea* and *syphilis*, in school populations including the college level, is low. The incidence rate has been approximately one per thousand for syphilis and possibly two per thousand for gonorrhea. With the excellent response to antibiotics, their incidence throughout the country has been decreased. Nevertheless, because individuals have become too reliant upon the cure and have become careless, or because moral standards are relaxed, or because health officials have relaxed their vigilance in tracing down contacts and keeping the public educated, the venereal disease rate has been climbing again. *The incidence in teen-agers is definitely increasing.* A summary of the reported cases in the United States between 1957 and 1972 reveals the dramatic increases in the incidence of these diseases over a fifteen year period. Reported cases of venereal diseases represent only a fraction of the cases treated. The remainder may have been treated but are not reported. Indiana has devised a recommended procedure to be followed when a case of venereal disease is reported in schools.

INDIANA STATE BOARD OF HEALTH DIVISION OF COMMUNICABLE DISEASE CONTROL*

A Suggested Procedure to be Followed by School Administrators When it is Reported That One or More of Their Students Has a Venereal Disease

Once in a while an alleged case of venereal disease among the students of a junior or senior high school is reported to the school nurse or administrator. In many cases this information is handled judiciously by those on the school staff and the matter is processed without anyone knowing about it except the persons directly involved. In other cases mistakes in reporting procedure have been made, allowing the information to become common knowledge among the students of the school. Infinite harm is thereby done to the infected person, and unnecessary excitement is created among both students and parents. It is for this reason that the following suggestions are made.

1. If it comes to the attention of any teacher, nurse, or other school official that one of their students is purported to have a venereal disease, it should be reported at once to the principal. *It is confidential information and should not be discussed with any other person in the school or member of the staff.*
2. Principals should call the health officer of the county or city in which the school is located—or the Director, Division of Communicable Disease Control, Indiana State Board of Health, 1330 West Michigan Street, Indianapolis, Indiana 46206. Phone (317) 633–6310.
3. The local or state health officer will assign the case to an investigator who will pursue the case in the following manner:
   a. The investigator will visit the school administrator and gather all available information on the case.
   b. He will then visit the person or persons involved and advise them to report to their private physician or to an appropriate local agency for diagnosis, if they have not already done so. Private physicians or local clinics may legally examine and

*Courtesy of Indiana State Board of Health, Division of Communicable Disease Control.

treat minors for venereal disease without consent of parents or guardian.

c. If the person involved is infected, he will be interviewed for sexual contacts. If individual is under care of a private physician, the investigator will obtain permission from the physician to interview the patient.

d. The named contacts will be traced and any student contacts will be approached outside the school and after school hours, if possible. Each contact will be impressed with the confidential nature of venereal disease information and the legal consequences which can follow any breech of this confidence.

e. All contacts will be referred to their private physician or to an appropriate local agency for diagnosis and treatment if necessary.

f. If the investigator finds venereal disease to be of epidemic proportions in a given school, he will consult with the local health officer who will, in turn, consult with the school administrator relative to the procedure to be followed.

g. At the end of his investigation, the venereal disease investigator will report the results of his work to the school administrator. He may advise the administrator of the number of students involved in that school, and provide other useful information, but the names of those involved will not be divulged.

There are three reasons for the above procedure.

1. The health departments have trained personnel to handle such situations. Venereal disease control is their responsibility and so defined by law.
2. The confidential nature of venereal disease information is clearly defined by regulation. If such information becomes common knowledge and injures the reputation of an individual, even though this information is true, the person responsible may be subject to legal action.
3. This procedure will relieve the teacher and other school staff members from involvement in a situation which could be embarassing to them legally, and for which they can be severely criticized by students, parents, and the general public.

Each case which is not identified, reported, and investigated as to contacts contributes to the spread of the disease, increases the reservoirs for infection, and hinders or prevents effective control.

Gonorrhea

Cause. Gonococcus.

How Spread. Mainly by sexual contact. Possibly in a newborn an eye infection during passage through the birth canal in delivery.

Incubation Period. Usually three to four days, may be longer.

Period of Communicability. Indefinite. For months unless individual is treated. Response to antibiotics usually prompt and satisfactory.

Description of Disease. Primarily an infection of the mucous membranes of the genital tracts, producing in the acute phase discomfort and heavy discharge of pus from male urethra or from female vagina. Infection may extend into the epididymis in the male or into the fallopian tubes in the female and produce sterility. Further progress can extend beyond the reproductive system into other tissues of the body. Arthritis and heart damage are possible complications. In the chronic stage signs and symptoms may simulate other mild infections of the male urethra and of the vagina.

Since the description of gonorrhea is the description of an infection of mucous membranes, and since there are various causes of local infections, acute or chronic, no attempt should be made at self-diagnosis or self-treatment. Medical consultation and bacteriological investigation are always indicated.

Control at School. An infected individual must be treated. Cases have been traced back to students. If health authorities request cooperation from the principal, social worker, school nurse, or guidance personnel at school, such help is given, and the information imparted should be kept confidential.

One stumbling block to early detection and treatment of venereal diseases in teen-agers has been the reluctance of a minor to seek medical help. Under the laws of most states he has to be sent home for written consent of parents before he can receive treatment. Recently, several states have passed laws providing for a confidential communication between a physician and his patient, making it permissible for a minor to give his own consent to treatment against syphilis and gonorrhea. The attending physician is not required to report the treatment to parents or a legal guardian unless this is considered essential.

An informative and motivating sex education program should be a part of health instruction in a school.

Syphilis

Cause. *Treponema pallidum*—a corkscrew shaped organism called a spirochete.

How Spread. Almost always by direct sexual contact. Indirect contact—relatively little occurrence. Prenatal infection through placenta after fourth month of pregnancy.

Incubation Period. Ten to 60 days, average three weeks.

Period of Communicability. Indefinite. Certain infection with local primary lesion. Possible with any subsequent skin eruptions. Response within 24 hours to adequate treatment.

Description of Disease. Primary lesion appears as a sore (chancre) on skin or mucous membrane of the penis or in the vagina about three weeks after sex contact. Highly contagious. Heals spontaneously in 30 to 40 days. Organisms invade blood stream, may appear in mucous membranes or skin as an infective eruption weeks to months later in what has been termed the secondary stage, and then remain dormant in various tissues of the body for years, in the blood vessels, brain and other vital organs, causing an assortment of disabilities. The last stage is called tertiary syphilis. When the organisms are in the blood stream, they can be transferred to the fetus through the placenta. If the mother is untreated, the baby will be born with congenital syphilis. Blood tests used in diagnosis of syphilis are expected to be positive about three weeks after appearance of the chancre.

Control at School. Same as for gonorrhea.

Immunization. Research being done on vaccine for active immunity.

WHOOPING COUGH (PERTUSSIS)

Very common. More in preschool.

Cause. Pertussis bacillus.

How Spread. Respiratory discharges. Direct or indirect contact.

Incubation Period. Seven to ten days, may be to 21 days.

Period of Communicability. Early stages until about three weeks after onset of characteristic cough.

Description of Disease. Prodrome of a cold followed by appearance of a "sticky" cough which develops a paroxysmal pattern. Experienced teachers have ears attuned to this cough. An attack consists of a series of rapid coughs which end in a crooning inspiration (the whoop). The child may even turn blue as breathing is suspended during the attack, and after the whoop he often vomits. Frequent paroxysms followed by vomiting can cause dehydration and starvation. Whooping cough accounts for a high mortality rate in children under two years of age. Cough starts one to two weeks after onset of disease and may last one to two months.

Control at School. Exclusion of sick child until released by physician. Watch for other suspected cases. During epidemics nonimmune children checked each day on arrival at school by a physician or nurse.

Immunization. Active—in infancy. Repeated as boosters.

SUMMARY

A general discussion introduces the subject of communicable diseases—causative agents, their methods of spread and entry into the body, the progress of a disease, and general measures to be followed in prevention and control at school. A specific school health program is outlined, which describes the role of the teacher. Immunization is discussed in detail, since this principle is a key to prevention, control, and possibly to eradication in some instances.

A description of individual communicable diseases (presented in alphabetical order) which are likely to be encountered at any age level in school affords background knowledge. The intent is not to promote diagnoses but to give teachers enough information so that they may suspect the presence of a communicable disease and take proper steps for handling it. The information also affords a basis for health instruction. In effect, teachers serve an important role as personnel in the public health program.

DISCUSSION QUESTIONS AND ACTIVITIES

1. Discuss the effectiveness of treatment for the common cold.
2. Discuss past and present measures effective in reducing incidence of and death from tuberculosis.
3. Explain why the classroom can be a good medium for the spread of a communicable disease.
4. Discuss at what point a teacher should send home a student who believes he is sick. Why should the teacher take action at that particular point?
5. Does the school you attend have an immunization requirement? Was this a local or state requirement?
6. Find out if the degree of physical fitness can be correlated with susceptibility to a communicable disease.
7. Find a U.S. morbidity report and discuss which communicable diseases are more prevalent for school-aged children. Can this information help you in making up a curriculum?
8. Discuss the difference between bacterial diseases and viral diseases—the organisms' mode of eating, make-up, and other differences.
9. Discuss how measles or mumps can affect a prenatal child.
10. Discuss the possibilities of a communicable disease's seriously invading a vital organ. How can it do this?

ADDITIONAL SOURCES OF INFORMATION

READINGS

American Association for Health, Physical Education and Recreation: "Facts about Syphilis and Gonorrhea." (1965). "Teacher's Handbook on Venereal Disease Education." (1965).

American Medical Association: "Venereal Disease." The Association, 1972.

American Public Health Association: "The Control of Communicable Diseases in Man." New edition published at intervals. Similar outlines on diseases are published by state departments of health.

Khanduja P. C., et al.: "Some Experiences During School Health Surveys." *Indian Journal of Pediat.* 37:612–614, December, 1970.

Lamb, G. A.: "The Natural History of Infectious Diseases as Manifested at Different Ages." *J. Periodont.* 42:453–459, August, 1971.

Smith, P. E.: "Infectious Diseases in Schools." *Lancet* 1:1293–1294, June, 1970.

MATERIALS FOR TEACHERS' USE IN SCHOOLS

AUDIOVISUAL MATERIALS

Recommended grade levels are designated *pri, int, jh, sh.*

Body Fights Bacteria

15 min. Black and White *sh* McGraw-Hill*

Story of the never-ending battle between disease-producing organisms and the human body. Active and passive immunizations are discussed.

Common Enemy . . . the Common Cold

26 min. Color *sh* Association Films, Inc. (Free)

A clever combination of fun, fact and fantasy starring the common cold. Historical and modern day sequences.

Community Health and You

10 min. Black and White *jh, sh* McGraw-Hill

Dance Little Children

25 min. Color Adults, parents, teachers Available from all boards of health

The story of teen-agers and the pressures they are under today, such as lewd publications, sex magazines, provocative dancing. The VD investigator on a case shows what must be done, how to uncover early cases of syphilis, and stresses that all cases must be located, contacted, and treated in order to break the chain of syphilis.

Health In Our Community

13 min. Color *int, jh, sh* Encyclopaedia Britannica Educ. Corp.

Dramatizes the work of public health departments. Stresses teamwork among health personnel, medical workers, and citizens.

How Our Body Fights Disease

8 min. Black and White *int, jh* Encyclopaedia Britannica Educ. Corp.

How to Catch a Cold

11 min. Color *pri, int, jh* Walt Disney Productions

Animated Jiminy Cricket film.

Louis Pasteur (Man of Science)

30 min. Black and White *jh, sh* Sterling Films, Inc.

Portrays discoveries of this great scientist from 1856 to 1895.

Magic Bullets

30 min. Black and White *sh* Available from boards of health

The life of Paul Ehrlich who discovered the first scientific cure for syphilis.

Quarter Million Teen-Agers

16 min. Color *jh, sh* Churchill Films Available from boards of health

Animated. Explains physiological aspects of syphilis and gonorrhea. Shows progress of disease. Stresses treatment.

Sneezes and Sniffles

10 min. Black and White *jh, sh* McGraw-Hill

Soapy the Germ Fighter

10 min. Color *pri, int* Avis Films, Inc.

The Common Cold

11 min. Black and White *int, jh* Encyclopaedia Britannica Educ. Corp.

Gives rules for care. Discusses complications.

---

*See Appendix A for addresses of film companies.

The Elusive Enemy

22 min. Color *jh, sh* Local chapters American Tuberculosis and Health Assn.

Current information on nature, cause, detection, diagnosis, treatment, and prevention of tuberculosis. Interviews teen-agers who have had disease. Produced 1967.

The Innocent Party

17 min. Color Grades 9–12 Available from boards of health

Shows how one young man in a moment of indiscretion contracts venereal disease from a pick-up and what happens to him and his "steady girl." A simple, sincere document of the nature, recognition, cure, and control of syphilis.

The Magic Touch

9 min. Color *pri, int* Avis Films, Inc.

A nurse explains immunization to young school children. Shows children receiving immunization fearlessly.

Your Health: Disease and Its Control

10 min. Black and White *int, jh* Coronet Films

Causes, spread, and control of diseases.

Your Health in the Community

10 min. Black and White *int, jh* Coronet Films

Important services of a health department and individual's contribution to community program.

RESOURCES

American Association for Health, Physical Education, and Recreation
American Medical Association – Department of Health Education
American Public Health Association
American Social Health Association
National Foundation. Write for current catalog.
National Tuberculosis and Health Association (and local chapters). Write for current catalog.
State and local boards of health
U.S. Department of Health, Education, and Welfare

Chapter 9

ALLERGIES IN CHILDREN AND YOUTH

INTRODUCTION

A teacher passes by a boy's desk in a history class and leaves a wake of perfume. The student grabs for absorbent tissue paper to hold over dripping nose and eyes. All is serene in the fourth grade until someone brings a pot of flowering chrysanthemums, and one of the youngsters starts to wheeze. An elementary teacher has her teaching plans all laid for a unit on reproduction. Birds, hamsters, and rabbits are brought to the classroom for care and observation by the youngsters. The teacher herself is very fond of animals. In the afternoon of the day the animals are introduced, one little boy finds difficulty breathing and has such a stuffed-up nose that he has to go home. Repeated attempts to stay in school are futile. Since he is allergic to animal dander, his school days are miserable. A boy in senior high school refuses to participate in physical education activities and shower because of a severe skin rash. Self-conscious about the appearance of his skin and following his physician's instructions which forbade showers, he finally secures a medical excuse from "gym."

These are not isolated instances, but are very common. (See Figure 48.) These are allergic manifestations. Allergic disease in the United States reaches phenomenal proportions. It is the leading chronic disease in the pediatric group, about one third of the total, and accounts for 33 million days of school absences annually. In the spring when trees are shedding pollen, on windy days when dust and pollen are in the air, and in the fall when the grasses are drying up allergy becomes a critical problem.

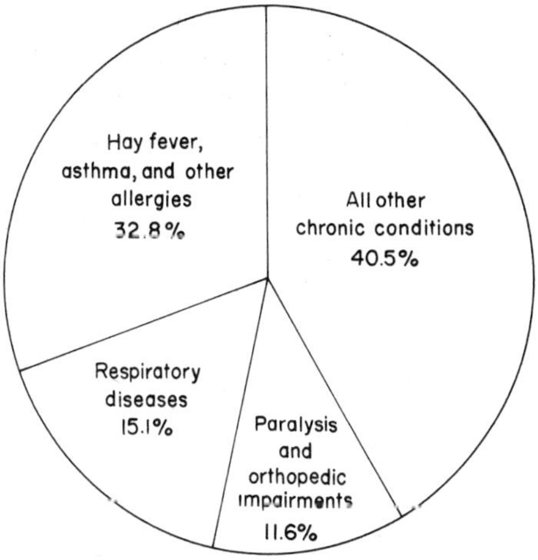

Figure 48 Hay fever, asthma and other allergies account for one-third of all chronic conditions reported for children under 17 years old. (Courtesy of Dr. John P. McGovern, McGovern Allergy Clinic, Houston, Texas.)

BASIC EXPLANATION

An *allergy* is an oversensitive state or hypersensitivity to some particular substance that is referred to as an *allergen*. (See Figure 49.) The tendency towards an allergy may be inherited, or allergy may be induced. If one or both parents have allergies, a child is likely to have them as well; but he does not necessarily have the same type of allergy as his parents. If a tissue or more than one tissue in the body is overly sensitive to an allergen, then exposure again to the allergen precipitates a chain of symptoms and signs characteristic of the disease. The nature of this response is not too clearly defined. It is believed that when an allergen comes in contact with a sensitized cell, a severe reaction occurs, destroying the cell and releasing histamine in the process. Histamine causes irritation of tissue and produces characteristic changes, such as dilatation of

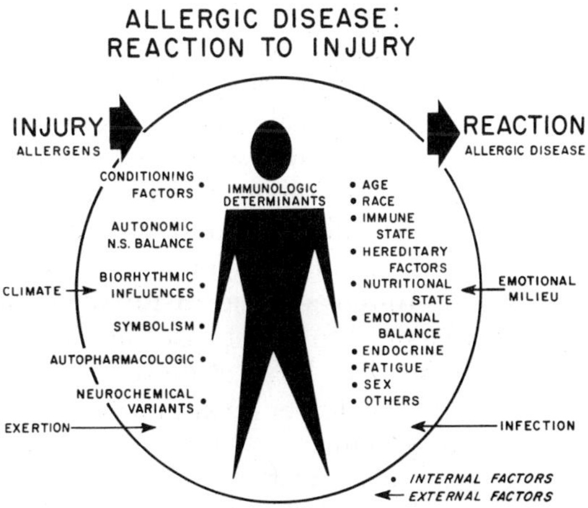

Figure 49 A holistic approach to allergic disease shows disease as being a process of "reaction to injury" with many factors both within the body and in the external milieu modifying its expressions. (Courtesy of Dr. John P. McGovern, McGovern Allergy Clinic, Houston, Texas.)

blood vessels, swelling of mucous membranes, and spasm of muscles. Several tissues may be irritated at the same time, so that several diseases or manifestations of allergy are present.

The psychosomatic aspects of allergies should be appreciated. Psychosomatic factors may result from and contribute to allergic responses.[1] Allergic children tend to be perfectionists, which can produce stress. Or, a combination of psychological stress plus allergen may trigger a response. In other words the child who is unhappy in his various relationships, particularly in the home, is more likely to have trouble, given a predisposition to allergies. Moreover, a child plagued by chronic allergic manifestations tends toward fatigue and irritability.

CHANNELS OF ENTRY OF ALLERGENS

Allergens are introduced into the body by:

Mouth. They may be swallowed, e.g., various drugs and foods. Predominant offenders among foods are wheat, eggs, milk and milk products, cocoa, and chocolate.

Inhalation. Seasonal substances which may be inhaled (particularly in spring and fall) are pollens and mold spores which are present on plants and grasses. Substances which may be inhaled at any time (nonseasonal) are dust, feathers, bacteria, viruses, animal dander (skin or hair shed by animals), perfume, chalk dust, smoke, smog, insecticide sprays, and many others.

External Contact. Allergens may touch a sensitized skin, e.g., wools, silks, synthetic textile fibers, dyes, poison oak, poison ivy, drugs, plastics, rubbers, chemicals, and cosmetics. Physical factors, such as heat, cold, and light, produce effects on some individuals.

Injection. Offenders may be biological products, particularly antibiotics or horse serum containing antitoxin. They may be toxins injected by an insect bite, as from a bee, wasp, or mosquito. Venom from snakes is injected.

Autosensitivity. Sensitization can occur to substances within a person's own body. These may be bacteria or viruses residing in diseased tonsils and adenoids or toxins produced by streptococci.

The tissues which are sensitized most readily are the skin and the mucous membranes of the respiratory and gastrointestinal tracts. Some headaches are definitely attributed to allergies. A combination of tissues may respond.

Initial allergic disturbances appear more often in the first 15 years of life. Most cases of asthma appear before the tenth year, and about two thirds of these occur before the age of five. Some babies will develop eczema immediately after birth when placed on a feeding formula.

---

[1]John P. McGovern, Kenneth E. Pierce, and Rufus E. Lee: "The Allergic Child and His Challenge to the School." *Clin. Pediat. 10*:11:640, November, 1971.

TYPES OF ALLERGY

Nasal Allergy

Nasal allergy is characterized by swelling of the mucous membranes of the nose, watery secretions resulting in a "runny" or stuffed-up nose, and red and itchy conjunctiva (see Eyes) with tearing. Sneezing and paroxysms of sneezes in succession are a dominant sign. Two mannerisms are noticeable—nose rubbing, pushing the tip of the nose upward and outward, ("the allergic salute") and nose wrinkling. The throat feels itchy. The individual is unable to sleep because of difficult breathing.

Hay Fever

Hay fever is seasonal nasal allergy. Pollens from trees, weeds, and grasses, and the mold spores present on them are inhaled. The seasons are spring and fall, with hay fever reaching a peak in late summer and early fall. Hay fever is worse on dry, sunny, windy days when pollens are in the air. Pollens are increased in the morning, less at dusk. Some people feel worse on damp, cool days, however. Hay fever usually starts in childhood. The disease causes misery but is not dangerous.

Allergic Rhinitis

Allergic rhinitis (year-round hay fever) is nonseasonal. It persists throughout the year, with periods of increasing discomfort when exposed to greater quantities of allergens. When exposure is minimal, a child will be fairly comfortable. Common allergens are the inhalants previously enumerated.

Results of nasal allergies may be development of sinusitis, difficulties in hearing, and polyps in the nose. (See chapter on Ear, Nose, Throat, and Mouth.) One third of these children develop asthma.

Asthma

Asthma is the most serious of the allergies; it may be handicapping. "In the United States an estimated 1,600,000 children through 16 years of age have asthma."[2] In the prepuberty years twice as many boys as girls suffer from it. Asthma may occur seasonally or at any time

[2]John P. McGovern: "Allergy Problems in School-Aged Children." *J. Sch. Health,* *44*:5:260, May, 1974.

of the year. The same allergens which precipitate nasal allergies may produce this disease. Foods often cause trouble—wheat, milk, fish, eggs, beans, nuts, and many others. Severe air pollution increases the prevalence of asthma. Fumes and smoke may act as irritants.

Psychic stress may trigger an asthmatic reaction. Emotional disturbances, particularly in the child-parent relationship, are important.

"It is most important to prevent the child from using his allergies for primary or secondary gain. Teachers as well as parents will frequently ask physicians to recommend that an asthmatic child be excused from participating in physical education or other school activities, usually because of an unwarranted degree of anxiety. Often one finds a rather continuously projected apprehension: 'Should we let him do something because this might precipitate an attack.' Needless to say, much of this anxiety spills over to the child."[3]

Asthma is characterized by swollen mucous membranes of the bronchial tubes in the lungs, the presence of a sticky mucus in the tubes, and a spasm of the muscle surrounding the tube. The result is a narrowed air passage obstructed by mucus. Expiration is difficult.

Description of Acute Attack

During an acute asthmatic attack the child sits or leans forward to breathe better. He brings into play the muscles of his chest, shoulders, neck, and abdomen. He is straining to breathe and get rid of the mucus accumulated in the bronchial tubes. Expiration is prolonged. The individual feels that he is choking. The attack usually ends when a considerable amount of thick mucus is expelled. Wheezing is quite loud and can be heard nearby. If paroxysmal coughing is prolonged, the child is exhausted. An attack may last from 30 minutes to several hours.

Handling Acute Attack at School

If a child should have an attack of asthma at school, it can be a frightening experience for a teacher. Do not try to lay the victim flat. He breathes better sitting up. He probably carries his own medicine, usually tablets or some type of inhaler. If the teacher or principal is worried—particularly when the attack is severe—he can call the parent or the child's physician. The parent may come to take the child home, especially on a windy day. If a child has frequent attacks and is under no medical supervision, the principal can insist on medical care in order to avoid too much distraction at school.

Effects

The effects of asthma on young people are readily observed. A chronic mild asthmatic suffers from shortness of breath and wheezing.

[3] *Op cit.*, McGovern, Pierce, and Lee, p. 641.

When he is resting and at peace with the world, this may not be noticeable; but coughing and loud wheezing may begin, following exposure to various irritating factors: chalk dust or dog hair, a sudden change in temperature, unusual exertion, a respiratory infection, a stress situation, unusual excitement, or sometimes a long laugh. This reaction can become quite embarrassing to the victim. The asthmatic limits his physical activities. He knows when to quit. Cold showers may be forbidden because of change in temperature. The type of adjustment he makes to his limitations is important. Many children with asthma have emotional and behavior problems as a result of physical illness. A child may feel frustrated and inadequate, restless, nervous, fearful, insecure; he may suffer from poor appetite and insomnia; may be self-conscious and quiet and not want to talk (which worries the teacher) or may compensate by becoming hostile and aggressive (which again worries the teacher).

Asthma accounts for the highest percentage of days lost from school and is offered commonly as an excuse for restriction of activities in physical education classes.

Skin Allergies

Skin allergies produce a large variety of lesions which can confuse the teacher. Since the reactions here are due to foreign materials, the diseases are not contagious, and the child need not be sent home. Probably the best criterion in making a decision is the child's history of recurrent attacks over the years. Many times the child himself can name the irritating source. The skin manifestations of allergy vary in appearance. There may be round dry areas which are scaling and itch, the type one sees when the child returns to school in the fall after gorging on such fruits and vegetables of late summer as cucumbers, peaches, and tomatoes. This reaction has been called a *food rash.* The lesions on the skin may resemble those of measles—punctate, red dots, distributed mainly on the trunk. They may be in the form of welts—raised white patches with red borders—which itch intensely, commonly referred to as *hives* (urticaria). A child with chronic hives may have trouble breathing because of swelling in the mouth and throat. This is a medical emergency, and a physician should be called.

Allergies to cold, heat, and light produce rashes, hives, and other skin changes.

Eczema usually has a long-standing history of chronicity from infancy or early childhood, disappears at times, then recurs. The child himself usually knows the diagnosis. The lesions are circumscribed scaling areas, dry or weeping (oozing), with prominent skin markings. They are commonly found in the folds of the skin, namely the neck, the bend of the elbow or knee, the front of the wrist, back of the hand or front of the ankle. These eczematous patches may be in any location, however. They should not be confused with ringworm or fungal infection, since the ringlike formations are absent. Strictly speaking, the word eczema is not a diagnosis, but refers to that group of skin conditions due to allergy. *Allergic dermatitis* is a preferred term.

Eczema frequently persists into the teens and, because of its appearance, may create deep-seated emotional problems which will affect a student's athletic activities as well as his social and occupational goals.

Since the skin lesions of allergy may not be so simple to identify, a word of warning is indicated. A teacher should never hesitate to contact the family concerning the diagnosis; he may request a physician's statement in regard to communicability.

Other Allergic Responses

Some individuals develop *gastrointestinal disturbances* after eating certain foods, or coming in contact in other ways with allergens. There may be nausea, vomiting, and abdominal pain. Since it is not the province of a teacher to attempt an explanation of such disturbances, the parent should be notified of the problem and the child taken home.

Some *headaches* may be explained on an allergic basis and are relieved by proper medication.

Any tissue of the body may become sensitized and cause health problems.

EFFECTS OF ALLERGIES ON CHILDREN AND YOUTH

Since asthma is quite serious, most of the effects of allergy have been discussed under this disease. All of these children with chronic allergies can suffer from lack of sleep because of itching or difficulty in breathing. Since stress, fatigue, overexertion, and upper respiratory infections may precipitate an attack, many absences are scattered through the school year. A child stays home after a windy day, or a cold, or after overindulgence in some food. It may be difficult for him to keep up with his school work in view of so many absences. This can be discouraging. He must learn to study during the times when he is free of illness. Hence, his progress will be uneven. He may be quite hyperactive in his behavior until he quiets down under treatment.

MANAGEMENT OF THE INDIVIDUAL WITH ALLERGY

In general, close cooperation should exist between the physician and the home. The physician's diagnosis is based on history, clinical picture, skin tests, and response to medication. Treatment consists of:

1. Avoidance of allergens as much as possible. This means elimination of guilty foods from the diet and alteration of environment as much as possible with attention to chalk dust, feather pillows, pets, flowers, etc. Airborne allergens are difficult to avoid.

2. Medication.

3. Immunization (so-called desensitization) with injections of specific allergens in increasing doses to build up tolerance of the allergic individual to his allergens.

4. Investigation of stress in the child's relationships.

At school a teacher, particularly in elementary grades, should confer with the mother of an asthmatic at the beginning of the year. The latter may need reassurance that she will be notified when an attack occurs. A teacher can cooperate intelligently, if he is made aware of the problem by either the youngster or the parent. Once he appreciates the basic difficulties and precipitating factors, he can understand the absences from school, the wheezing on a windy day, the apparent self-coddling, the personality problems. The history teacher smiled when told about the perfume and discontinued its use. The elementary teacher was reluctant to give up the unit on reproduction, when the child's physician called to explain the allergic difficulties; but after the whole class discussed the situation, the decision was made to forego the presence of pets. One child's health problem became an educational experience.

Stress at school should be avoided as much as possible. A teacher can encourage a student to continue his immunizing injections. Prognosis under the regimen outlined above is good. There should be no overprotection. He conforms to the same scholastic requirements as his classmates. If the teacher suspects that a child is using his asthma as a weapon to control others or is being overcome by anxiety, efforts are directed toward group activities and working with others.

As far as physical education activities are concerned, the asthmatic limits himself because of difficulty in breathing. "In our experience, tennis provides the best of all forms of competitive exercise for the respiratory allergic child."[4] This activity is suggested because it is an outdoor activity that is generally played on cement or asphalt with built-in rest periods. The instructor should appreciate the absences from school, and should work under the supervision of the student's physician.

In the long-term management of allergies, especially asthma, the teacher should watch for behavioral disorders. If emotional elements are prominent, an understanding, non-critical, tactful interview with the parents should initiate some adjustments. They should be encouraged to promote the independence of their child. In some instances psychiatric referral may be indicated.

---

[4]*Op cit.*, McGovern, Pierce, and Lee, p. 640.

SUMMARY

An allergy is an oversensitivity to foreign substances (allergens) which may enter the body through the mouth, be inhaled, be contacted externally on the skin, or be injected. The common diseases which result are nasal allergies, asthma, and eczema and other skin rashes. Some headaches and gastrointestinal disturbances may be explained on an allergic basis. Severe or prolonged manifestations of these diseases, especially asthma, produce marked effects on a growing child—physically, emotionally, and socially. A teacher must understand the basic explanation of allergy and its effects in order to cooperate with the child or adolescent, with his parents, and with his physician.

DISCUSSION QUESTIONS AND ACTIVITIES

1. Discuss the first aid procedure for handling an asthmatic child.
2. Explain the basic principle involved in hay fever. What type of medication is associated with this ailment? How would this medication affect a child in your class?
3. Describe the physical and emotional ramifications of eczema for a child.
4. Describe the relationship of the parent, teacher, and student in dealing with the problems of severe allergies.
5. Discuss how stress can play an important role in managing a child with allergies.
6. Investigate the procedure for finding specific allergic reactions.

ADDITIONAL SOURCES OF INFORMATION

Aas, K.: *The Allergic Child.* Springfield, Ill.: Charles C Thomas, 1971.

Barkin, G. D., and McGovern, J. P.: "What the Classroom Teacher Can Do for the Asthmatic Child." *NEA J.* 56:40–41, 1967.

Carson, R.: *Asthma—How to Live with It.* Public Affairs Committee, 1969.

McGovern, J. P., and Knight, J. A.: *Allergy and Human Emotions.* Springfield, Ill.: Charles C Thomas, 1967.

Normon, A. P.: "Asthma in Children." *Nurs. Mirror* 123:355–357, 1967.

Rapaport, H. G.: "Emotional Factors in Eczema and Asthma in Childhood." *Ann. Allerg.* 24:496–498, 1966.

Salvin, R. G.: "Pediatrician's Attitude toward Allergy." *J. Allerg. Clin. Immun.* 47: 80–83, February, 1971.

Speer, F.: "Allergic Children and Parental Attitudes. Understanding the Parents Helps the Child." *Clin. Pediat.* (Philadelphia) 9:642–647, November, 1970.

Chapter 10

HEALTH PROBLEMS OF SKIN

INTRODUCTION

Nothing in the field of health problems is more baffling to a teacher than rashes or lesions on the skin. He is confronted frequently with the necessity of making disposition of a skin problem, particularly if there is possibility of contagion. To the untrained eye many lesions appear the same, yet present different diagnoses. Rashes occur as part of the clinical picture in the common communicable diseases, such as chickenpox, German measles, and scarlet fever; they also occur with allergies; sometimes they may be insect bites. At all times a decision must be reached as to whether a child should be sent home and whether his referral to a physician is recommended. Is it a cold sore (fever blister) or is it impetigo? Is it a wart on the sole of the foot, or is it a callus, or is it both? A child states that he has eczema. Is eczema contagious?

In addition to these perplexing conditions, teachers in junior and senior high schools are presented with a special skin problem. Adolescents are beginning to develop acne at a time when they are becoming interested in their own appearances and in the opposite sex. Grooming, charm, and personality development are being emphasized in class and literature; so the student watches every blemish on the face with a magnifying mirror. If the acne is severe, he feels that his whole life is ruined, and he may even suffer severe personality difficulties.

The discussions and descriptions below are intended only to give a teacher or principal sufficient information for intelligent handling at school of the more prevalent skin problems of childhood. There is no question of medical treatment. Nor is the aim to make him a diagnostician. As a matter of fact, it is not wise for a teacher to make a diagnosis, either oral or written. In his own mind he may have a distinct impression, but prudence dictates that his references should be in general terms. In this way he protects himself should he be in error. He may also avoid causing needless anxiety. Even doctors are at a loss to diagnose a skin lesion sometimes and must await developments. Nurses are always cautioned against making a direct verbal diagnosis, even though they may make the final decision as to disposal of the case. It must be kept in mind at all times, however, that when a skin condition is considered as probably communicable, the welfare of the affected child is important. Since other children also must be protected, the teacher, nurse, or principal has discretionary powers in asking for a note from a physician concerning contagiousness before permitting a child to remain in school.

Functions of Skin

The skin is one of the most important organs of the body, particularly because it contributes immeasurably to the regulation of the temperature of the body. Fairly uniform temperature is maintained through the circulatory system and sweat glands of the skin. It serves as a protective organ, owing to the response of its nerves to heat, cold, pressure, and pain, and its almost total impenetrability. Bacteria and other organisms, cosmetics, and soaps do not penetrate to the structures below, if the surface is intact. Breaks in the skin do permit infections; hence the need to use sterile coverings for protection of any cut. The skin also molds the surface of the body and gives form to its underlying structures.

The physiology of the skin is similar to that of other organs of the body. Oxygen and food products are conveyed to the cells of the skin through the blood stream and the waste products removed by the same means. There is no other way of "nourishing" skin, nor does the skin or its pores "breathe." Good health of skin in general results from good health of body.

Skin and Cleanliness

Cleanliness of skin is desirable, not only for appearance's sake, but because dirt and bacteria can cause irritation and local infection in a hair follicle. Simple hygienic rules dictate frequent washing of the hands, particularly before meals and after toileting. Courtesy and consideration for others demand a clean skin, free from body odors. Adequate washing facilities should be available in every school. Unfortunately, they are not always present, even in schools in large cities. Soap, water, and towels are essential in washrooms; the children, especially the younger ones, should be taught to use them. Even when these facilities are available, time is usually not sufficient to permit all to wash their hands before eating. Thus, we defeat in practice our own educational program. Children with dirty skins should be encouraged to shower at school; despite the dirt, some resist, and any appeal to their pride is futile. Lastly, the environment in washrooms and showers should be kept clean, to guard children who are barefoot.

COMMON BACTERIAL INFECTIONS

Boils and Carbuncles

Boils are infections of single hair follicles; carbuncles involve more than one hair follicle. They are usually painful; they are potentially dangerous because of the possibility of spread of bacteria (frequently staphylococci, occasionally streptococci) through the lymph or blood stream, resulting in systemic infection (blood poisoning). If the inflammatory barrier around the localized infection is broken, either by nature or by squeezing, disseminated infection is possible. Hence the dictum, "Never squeeze a pimple." The occurrence of many or frequent boils or carbuncles deserves medical investigation. Under no circumstances should a teacher advise hot compresses or soaks and undertake treatment; in many instances cure is effected only by the use of antibiotics, and delay can be serious.

Impetigo Contagiosa

The contagious bacterial disease that causes the most concern is impetigo (Figure 50). The bacteria grow in the epidermis and form superficial vesicles (small blisters), followed by ulcers covered with yellow or straw-colored crusts or scabs. When the crust is removed, a smooth, oozing surface is exposed. The area involved in impetigo

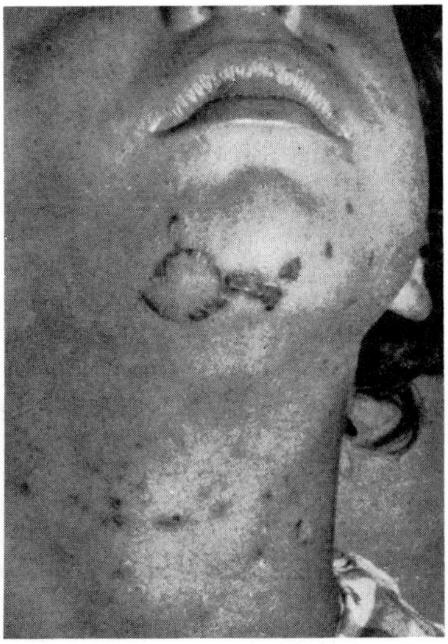

Figure 50 Impetigo contagiosa. (Pillsbury, Shelley, and Kligman: *Dermatology.* 1956, W. B. Saunders Co.)

not only grows larger, but the infection can spread to other parts of the face or body. The initial infection is usually on the lower part of the face, a commonly fingered area, particularly around the chin or lower lip. In the latter position it can be confused with a cold sore, which is also characterized by vesicles (blisters). A cold sore, although there may be an increase in the number of vesicles, usually does not increase much in size, does not spread to other parts, and lacks typical honey-colored crusts.

Impetigo can spread rapidly at school among children through indirect contact, by means of contaminated articles—toys, pencils, books, and door knobs. The infected child fingers the uncomfortable area, then touches these objects. Another child handles them also, touches his own face, and transfers the infection.

The best method for handling impetigo at school is simply to *bar the student from all classes.* He should be sent home and not permitted to return until he brings a note from his physician stating that he is free of infection. Under treatment he should not be absent longer than a few days.

COMMON VIRAL INFECTIONS

Verruca (Wart)

The disease in this group which provides a frequent school health problem is the wart (verruca). Many authorities consider warts as only mildly infectious. An immunity can be developed against them. As the body develops resistance or immunity, a skin which was "covered with warts" gradually clears. This latter phenomenon can explain the efficacy of "charms" of all types which apparently cause the spontaneous disappearance of these skin lesions. Children often have their own pet charms or cures. Huckleberry Finn recommended that a dead cat be taken to the cemetery at midnight where certain ceremonies should be performed that would "fetch any wart." In fact, those warts would have disappeared anyway. Sometimes they seem to occur in epidemics among school children. A high percentage of youngsters will have them for a while; then immunity apparently develops, so the warts become scarce. Some people do not develop an immunity, however, and must have their warts treated.

The formation of warts is the same regardless of their positions on the body. They appear as hard, dry, grayish projections of skin, usually with distinct roundish borders, sometimes flat, sometimes conical in shape (Figure 51A); they often contain darkish flecks in the center. They can occur anywhere on the body. There may be only a few isolated lesions, or they may grow luxuriantly with absence of individual delineation to form a mosaic pattern. On the knuckles of the fingers, they may not only be disfiguring but disabling. Those

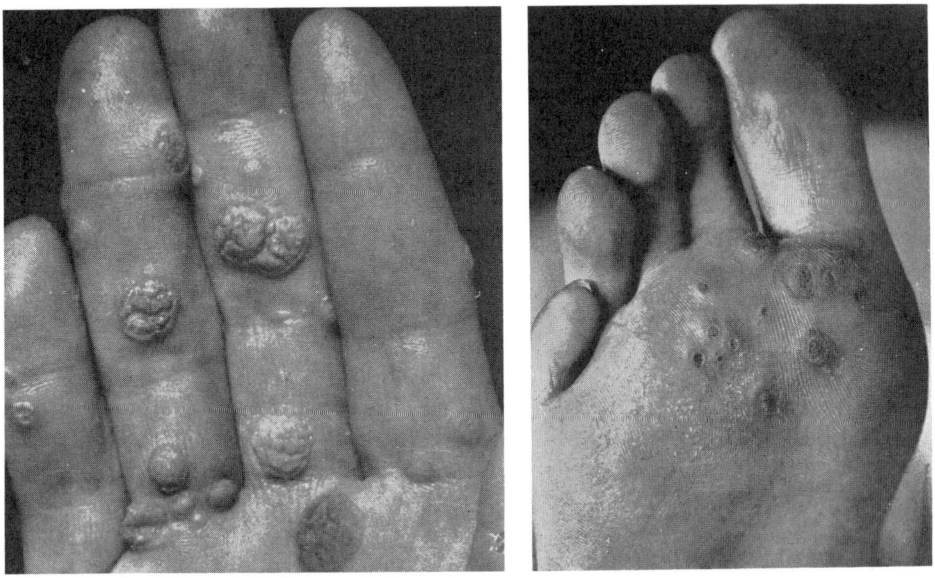

Figure 51 A. Warts. *B.* Warts on sole of foot (plantar warts). (From Andrews and Domonkos: *Diseases of the Skin.* Fifth edition, 1963, W. B. Saunders Co.)

located on the soles of the feet are designated as *plantar warts* (Figure 54B). In this site the conical part presses in and can become quite painful. A plantar wart is often located in a callus, which sometimes masks the wart. To add to the confusion, plantar warts have been referred to by some sources as "tumors" or "papillomas," thereby lending a fearful impressiveness to a simple infection.

Warts may not only become larger but can increase in number on the body. Home remedies should never be used. In susceptible individuals, they are sometimes hard to eradicate and may recur several times, even though all of the area of infection seems to have been removed. Nevertheless, there should be a persistent effort to treat recurring warts as soon as they appear.

The school program for warts is to encourage medical management. In the prevention of plantar warts, students should not be permitted to walk barefoot around dance floors, dressing rooms, showers, or decks of swimming pools. The rigid attitude of barring students with plantar warts from participation in all physical education classes has been relaxed. Because a high percentage of their classmates are immune, those infected may participate provided they wear foot covering.

Herpes Simplex (Cold Sore, Fever Sore, Fever Blister)

Herpes simplex is a viral infection. The lesions appear first as small vesicles (blisters), either singly or in a cluster, sometimes with swelling of the surrounding tissue, and are usually found around the lips. Gradually, the vesicles dry, scab, and disappear. Despite attempts to do so, healing cannot be particularly rushed. They are associated with the common cold, with such irritants as sunburn, ultraviolet light, or exposure to the elements, and at times with emotional upsets. These factors apparently activate a dormant virus; hence, fever sores tend to recur at the same site, the site of a former primary infection.

FUNGAL INFECTIONS

This type of infection is so prevalent that a good deal of discussion is being devoted to it. A fungus is a plant, grows actively in the skin by spreading projections (mycelia), yet can develop a spore stage in which it lies dormant and resists medication. This phenomenon in the growth of fungi explains how the disease apparently disappears after active treatment, only to flare up later if medication is discontinued too soon. Spores form during the treatment and await their chance to grow again. Therefore, treatment needs to be continuous and persistent for quite a while after the skin is apparently normal.

A fungal infection is a *communicable disease,* regardless of its location on the body. It has been variously labeled: "ringworm," because the growth on the skin sometimes is ringlike in appearance and not because it is due to a worm; "jockstrap itch" or "dhobie itch," if it occurs in the groin; "athlete's foot," if it occurs between the toes; and "jungle rot," if it occurs anywhere and even suggests a fungal infestation. The infection is more scientifically termed *dermatophytosis* or *tinea.*

Fungal Infection on the Trunk, Legs, and Arms

This does not occur often. It presents a ringlike formation. The lesion is dry, scaling, has sharply demarcated edges, and sometimes has vesicles in the outer border. Infection spreads from the outer portion while the center appears healed. These cases should be under medical care.

Fungal Infection of the Scalp (Tinea Capitis)

Tinea capitis or ringworm of the scalp is probably the most contagious and most difficult variety of fungal infection to manage (see Figure 52). It is endemic in various regions of the United States and can become a serious health problem to a whole school or community. This infection of the scalp occurs chiefly in childhood and *is rarely*

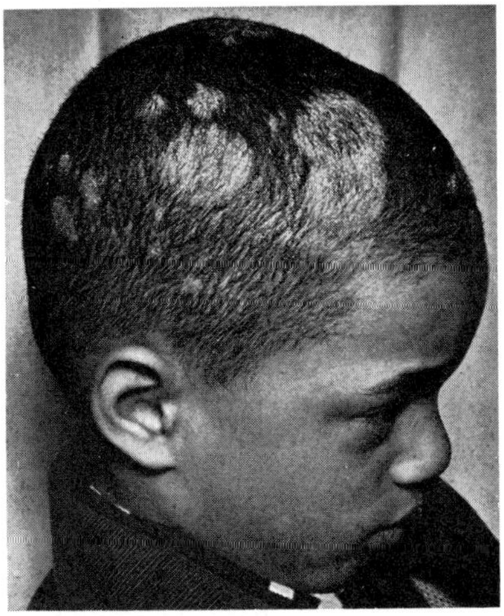

Figure 52 Fungal infection (ringworm) of the scalp. (Pillsbury, Shelley, and Kligman: *Dermatology.* 1956, W. B. Saunders Co.)

seen beyond the age of puberty. It is a problem of the elementary schools.

One type of fungal infection of the scalp, contracted from cats, dogs, and pet animals, involves the hair shafts and results in spotty baldness. Another common variety is transferred directly from child to child in contact activities, as in scuffling. Indirect transfer may occur from the interchange of articles, such as hats, combs, scarfs, towels, and pillows; from scissors and clippers; or from rubbing the head against the contaminated upholstery on a theater or bus seat. The onset is insidious, but the growth gradually produces areas of partial baldness. The infection may involve at first only one hair shaft and may continue to spread for six months before it is detected.

Fungal infection of the scalp will present coin-sized patches in which the hair appears "nibbled off"; the scalp is covered with fine whitish, grayish, or dirty yellowish scales. The skin may appear reddened and may itch mildly. These patches may increase in number to involve the whole scalp.

If one child is found diseased, all of his classmates in the room are screened with a filtered ultraviolet lamp (Wood's light, black light), a device which causes infected hairs to show a green fluorescence. Children in other classrooms may need to be examined also. Nurses are trained to perform these screening tests. Other methods of diagnosis are by examining a suspected hair under the microscope and by culture.

Once a teacher or nurse suspects the presence of ringworm of the scalp, the child should be placed immediately under the care of a physician. Drugs seem to be effective, but require a number of weeks to cure the infection. All children under treatment are permitted to attend school. The victims and their parents must follow the prescribed regimen strictly.

Teachers have a vital role to play in the health education program for handling ringworm of the scalp. One major problem involves the education of children and their parents. The disease is contagious. There must be close cooperation between parents, teachers, and medical staff. Daily observation of all the youngsters is necessary; children need to be encouraged to continue treatment.

Fungal Infection of the Groin (Tinea Cruris)

Tinea cruris or "jockstrap itch" presents a picture similar to fungal infection elsewhere on the body. The groin should be kept dry and cool. Each student should use his own personal undergarments. These should be boiled, washed thoroughly, or cleaned at frequent intervals.

Fungal Infection of the Feet (Tinea Pedis)

Description. (See Figure 53). Since fungi like to grow in heat, perspiration, and moisture, the feet, especially the region between the toes, easily fulfill requirements for optimum growth. Wet benches and floors in dressing rooms, shower rooms, and surfaces around swimming pools offer ideal environments for maintenance of the organisms. Indeed, those who frequented gymnasiums were so commonly infected that the disease was nicknamed "athlete's foot." Summer is a time for flare-ups, when the feet perspire a great deal.

Between the toes the infection may be either acute or chronic. In the *acute* condition, the skin is peeling, red, itching, tender, and may show blisters. Infection with secondary organisms may occur, which will be manifested by pain and the presence of pus. If this latter complication is neglected, there can be invasion of the lymph stream, enlargement of lymph nodes in the groin, threatening blood stream invasion, and possible critical generalized illness.

Of more usual occurrence is the *chronic* infection between the toes. If not extensive, it is usually found between the fourth and fifth toes, when the little toe is pressed close to the fourth and moisture accumulates. The manifestations may be only slight scaling with some alteration of the sheen of normal skin; there may be more inflammation with more extensive scaling and itching, accompanied by "cracking" of the skin in the webs between the toes ("cracking" in itself is not diagnostic of fungal infection); it can spread between other toes and towards the soles of the feet; it may spread to the tops of the toes and involve the nails; small vesicles may be present. Lesions on top of the toes which show pus formation are usually due to bacterial infection and not to fungus.

Prevention of Infections. Administrators, physical education teachers, and custodians are confronted with a perennial problem in this area. Fungi are everywhere in the school environment, and

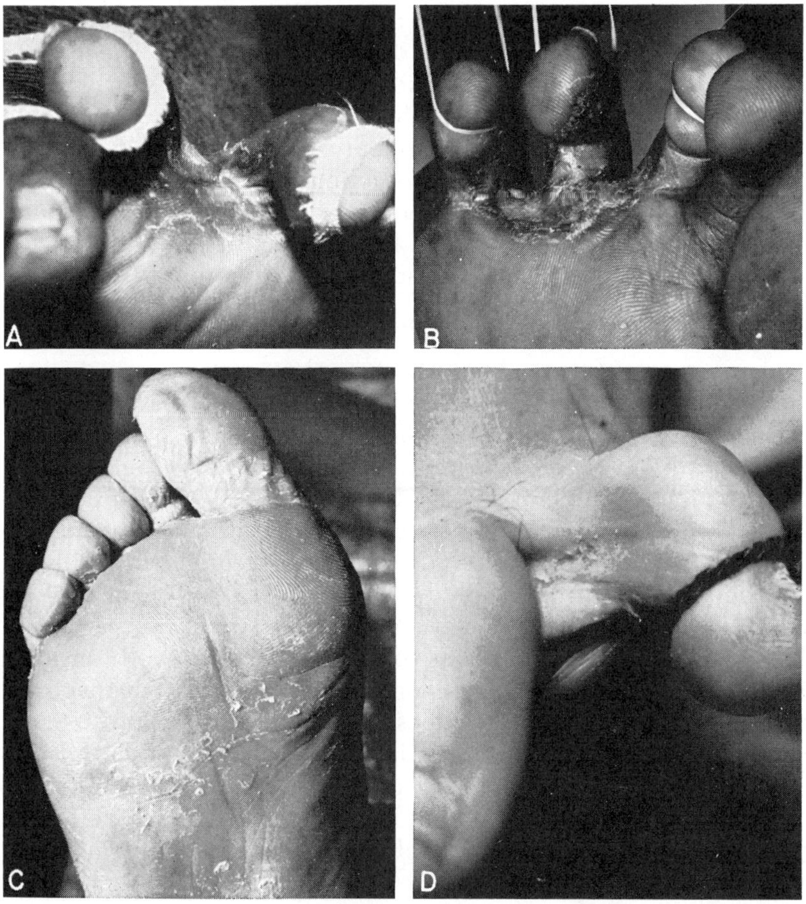

Figure 53 Various clinical manifestations of fungal infections of feet. Scaling is a constant feature of subacute or chronic lesions. (Pillsbury, Shelley, and Kligman: *Dermatology.* 1956, W. B. Saunders Co.)

extensive preventive measures are apparently futile. The school health program should have two objectives: (1) maintenance of an environment which is antagonistic to growth of fungi; (2) detection of existing cases.

An attempt should be made to prevent the spread of organisms, or at least keep them at a minimum by keeping all gymnasium facilities dry and cool. Everything should be well-aired in dressing and shower rooms and around swimming pools. Wet floors should be mopped and permitted to dry. The usual hypochlorite foot baths are of no value and only serve to give the individual a false sense of security. Feet should always be covered; some type of foot wear should be mandatory around facilities where there is moisture.

Some facts concerning the spread of fungus infections of the feet must be kept in mind. The harsh and rigid regulations of the past are not realistic. The experience of the armed services in World War II demonstrated that the ever-present fungi cannot be eradicated; so the requirement of foot baths was discontinued in 1944. The infection is not highly contagious; an individual may build up his own immunity. Those who are not susceptible do not acquire the disease. One often observes that only one member of a family may be infected despite negligence and lack of precautions.

If the environment is antagonistic to luxuriant growth of fungi, and if contamination of floors and benches can be minimized by foot covering, then the susceptible individual can be protected to some extent.

Handling Existing Cases of "Athlete's Foot." Students with frank, severe infections should be barred from the gymnasium and showers and advised to have treatment by a physician. No two cases of tinea are necessarily treated alike, particularly if acute; thus, *it is assumed no specific medication will be recommended by a teacher.* Mildly infected students should be kept under observation of the physical education teacher; treatment by a physician is recommended, and some type of shower slippers should be used. Persons with mild infection or normal feet should keep the feet cool, clean, and dry; avoid hot or tight shoes which make the feet perspire, particularly those with rubber or nonporous soles; wash the feet well, rinse, and dry thoroughly, especially between the toes; use plain talcum powder (not medicated) between the toes; change hose frequently. Such a cool, dry environment is not conducive to growth of fungi; infection can usually be prevented; mild cases may be cured or controlled by these simple measures. Stressing hygienic environment, both of the gymnasium and of the individual's feet, offers the best method of prevention and treatment.

INFECTIONS CAUSED BY ANIMAL PARASITES

Scabies

Scabies (itch, seven-year itch) is produced by an itch mite which travels in the skin, forming burrows about one-eighth inch long. Where the burrows occur, minute grayish vesicles may be seen, sometimes in a row ("runs"). In the process of burrowing, an itching occurs which is intensified at night and after physical exercise, when the body is warm and the insects are more active. The common scabetic areas are the webs of the fingers, fronts of the wrists, the armpits, on the breasts, around the umbilicus, over the buttocks and external genitalia.

Diagnosis is usually based upon three factors: (1) itching; (2) the fact that more than one member of the family usually has the same complaint; and (3) scratch marks, sores, and scabs caused by infection from scratching.

A child with scabies should be sent home; he can infect an entire classroom through close contact. The simple treatment involves only about 24 to 48 hours, but usually a social problem is involved. All members of the family, regardless of whether they think they are infected or not, should receive treatment at the same time. Otherwise, one keeps giving it to another. Clothing, bedclothes, furniture, and rugs should be washed or boiled or shampooed or cleaned. Unless complete cooperation is followed, there will be no eradication of the infection from a home. It has been said "It is no disgrace to have scabies, but it is a disgrace to keep it. The Itch is no respecter of society."

Interestingly enough, the disease seems to occur in cycles. For as long as a number of years no cases will be seen; then the infection makes its appearance, especially in underprivileged areas. There is some immunity to scabies.

Pediculosis (Lousiness)

Pediculosis is a disease caused by infestations of an insect, the louse, which may have preference for the hair, the body, or the pubic region. Again, it is not a disgrace to have this infection. The incidence is low, except in deprived areas.

Head Lice. These are diagnosed in the presence of the following: (1) itching; (2) the presence of the active louse itself, a grayish insect about one-eighth inch long; (3) the presence of nits or eggs, minute whitish objects which resemble flakes of dandruff but are actually cemented on the hair shaft close to the scalp; and (4) secondary infection from scratching, with the presence of sores containing pus. Diagnosis is not difficult (Figure 54).

Body Lice (Cooties, "vagabond's disease," "seam squirrels"). Lice live in the clothing, not on the body, are found in the seams, and are associated with filth. They crawl on the human body to feed. The site where the proboscis penetrates the skin can become infected and form a pustule. Scratch marks, scabs, and pigmented scars form the common picture. Diagnosis is made by examining the clothes for nits and insects. Since the parasites can live in clothing for a long time, all garments should be washed or cleaned.

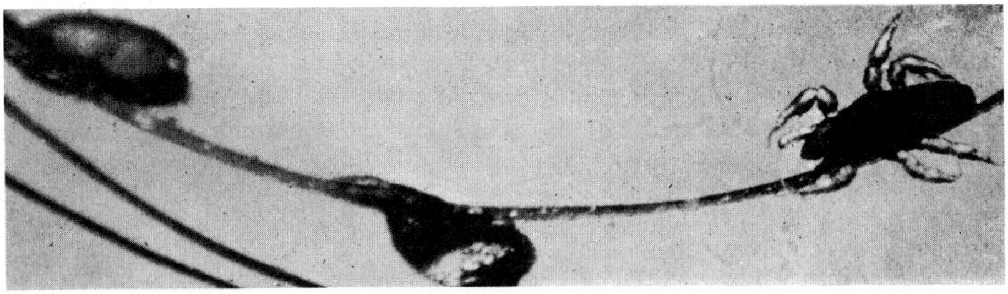

Figure 54 Head louse and nits on hair. (Courtesy Dr. O. G. Costa. From Sutton, R. L.: *Diseases of the Skin.* Eleventh edition. 1956, The C. V. Mosby Co.)

Crab Lice. These are easily acquired, usually from toilet seats or from contact with an infected person. The louse lives on the skin, bores into the hair follicle in the pubic region near the base of the hair, and is hard to find. Diagnosis is based on the presence of itching, nits, and lice. Infestation may spread to other hairy portions of the body except the scalp. It may be at the edge of the scalp hair and in the eyebrows and eyelashes. Secondary infection can result in a good deal of discomfort.

Management of Pediculosis at School. The school program in handling pediculosis also involves socioeconomic factors. Every member of a family or group may be infested. In some parts of the country, practically all the children at school and their families are troubled with the insect. In such instances, school and public health nurses, welfare workers, teachers, physicians, and the public health officials are all concerned. The school cannot handle the problem alone. Effective treatment requires only 24 to 48 hours. Cleanliness is essential. Isolation from school and immediate treatment of active cases are indicated. The school is also interested in prevention effected by detection of active cases and isolating them. Toilet seats should be washed daily with hot soap suds containing an antiseptic. The seats should be rinsed after application of the antiseptic. The benches in the dressing room where students sit should be washed with the same mixture, and then rinsed.

ALLERGIES

The allergic rashes include eczema and hives. These are discussed in Chapter 9 (Allergies in Children and Youth).

RASHES IN COMMUNICABLE DISEASES

Rashes in communicable diseases may be toxic manifestations, as in scarlet fever, or may actually contain the organisms, as in chickenpox or smallpox. Descriptions have been discussed in Chapter 8 (Communicable Diseases).

ACNE VULGARIS

A discussion of acne deserves special consideration, since this skin disease is probably the most common, the most irksome, and the most frustrating health problem of adolescents. Sulzberger states, "The usual age for acne starts at thirteen, and, if fortunate ends for good before the age of about twenty-three."[1] If a teacher appreciates

[1] Marion B. Sulzberger: "Acne and Skin Eruptions from Plants and other Allergens." *J. Sch. Health 43*:6:381, June, 1973.

the physiological explanation of acne, more understanding counseling will make an adolescent a happier or at least a more reconciled individual.

Basic Explanation or Cause

Acne (Figure 55) is a chronic inflammatory disease of the skin, involving chiefly the sebaceous or fat gland structure, characterized by blackheads (comedones), papules, pustules, scars, and pits, located on the face, chest, shoulders, and back. It is associated with sexual development during adolescence and is linked with the appearance of the gonadal hormones. The male hormone, androgen,

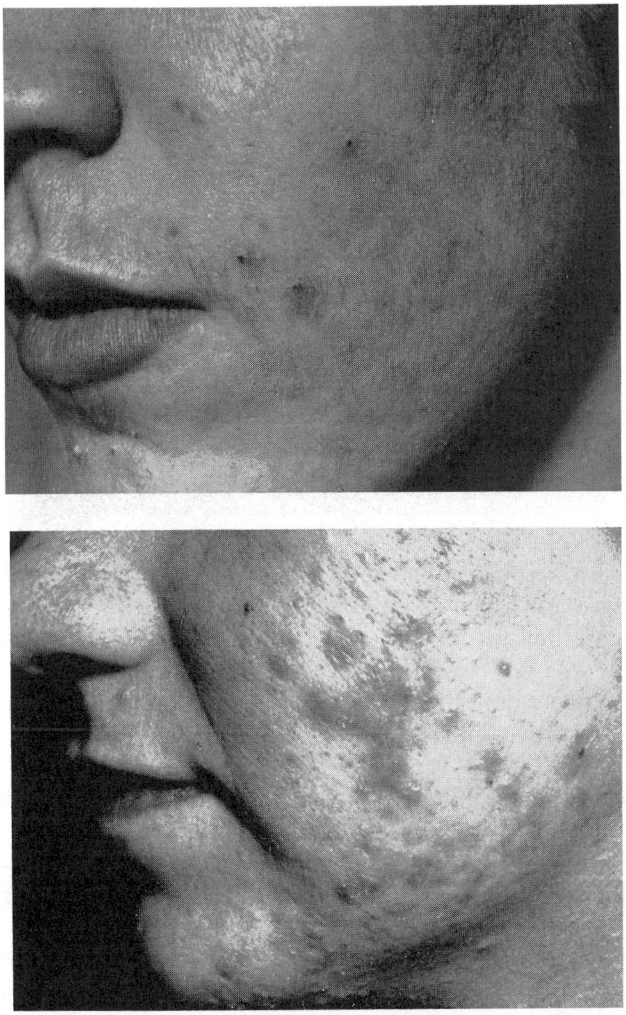

Figure 55 A. Acne Grade I. Each small papule arises around a comedo (blackhead). *B.* Acne Grade II. More severe inflammatory lesions, all arising around comedones. (Pillsbury, Shelley, and Kligman: *Dermatology.* 1956, W. B. Saunders Co.)

and the female hormone, estrogen, influence the activity of the sebaceous or fat glands in the skin. Both sexes possess both hormones; androgens increase the activity of the sebaceous glands with overproduction of sebum or oil; estrogens decrease their activity. Usually the hormones are balanced; a disproportion between the two hormones may create an excessive secretion of sebum, a typical condition in adolescence, resulting in the production of acne.

Increased oil on the surface of the skin encourages plugging of the pores with oils, cosmetics, dirt, and bacteria. The plugged pore is called a *blackhead* or *comedo*; reaction of the surrounding tissue to this irritating plug produces a raised, indurated lesion, a *papule*, sometimes referred to as a pimple. The invasion of bacteria, which are always present on skin, stimulates the formulation of pus in the papule, producing a *pustule*. With healing, scarring or pitting of the skin may be the end result. At first the scar or pit may be an angry red color, but with time it fades and smooths over so that after adolescence a badly pitted skin does not necessarily present a marred appearance.

A quick explanation of acne in outline form can be given as follows:

SEX HORMONES		ACTIVITY OF SEBACEOUS GLANDS	ACNE
male——	androgen——→	increased——→	blackheads
female——	estrogen——→	decreased	papules (pimples)
			pustules
			scars

In brief, the remote or underlying cause of acne vulgaris is hormonal or endocrine; the immediate cause is abnormal fat-gland activity. Acne in some form is practically universal at adolescence.

Factors Influencing Acne

Diet. A well-balanced diet is necessary, with plenty of calories, proteins, vitamins, and minerals for the growing adolescent. Restrictions on diet are the subject of controversy. Some dermatologists propose a low-fat regimen with the explanation that there is an association between high-fat intake and sebaceous gland activity. Usually, an individual becomes aware of the foods that seem to stimulate a flare-up of acne lesions. Those to which one is allergic should be avoided. Whatver dietary restrictions may be observed, a well-balanced diet is essential.

Cleanliness. Washing the skin reduces excessive oils and decreases the number of bacteria. Repeated rough scrubbing can irritate skin; gentle washing is worthwhile.

General Health. Illness and infections which lower resistance can encourage the development of acne. Poor hygiene health practices—inadequate rest and sleep, constipation, lack of exercise, and low intake of liquids—may be contributory factors.

Nervousness. Nervous tension and emotional disturbances contribute to the production of acne. Acnes are definitely aggravated during periods of tension. Moreover, nervous youngsters tend to pick and squeeze the lesions. Unusual concern, by the patient, and particularly by a doting mother, makes acne worse. The concern over the acne frequently approaches a mania and definitely requires corrective management for the patient and for the mother.

Counseling the Adolescent with Acne

With the preceding explanation in mind, a teacher should be able to reassure the student who is worried about his complexion. Almost all of his peers have the same skin problem. The average case of acne improves gradually with time and needs no special care. A few severe cases need intensive investigations and treatment by a physician. Most acne conditions disappear in the early twenties; a few linger on. One can be reassured that the severest pitting usually smooths over with normal skin after the active period of acne regresses. Even though, at the time of greatest vanity, charm and complexion seem utterly hopeless, a student can look forward to ultimate improvement in appearance of his skin.

SEBORRHEIC DERMATITIS (DANDRUFF)

Scaling, mild to severe, affects practically every scalp. When mild, it is called dandruff. Severe scaling is referred to as seborrheic dermatitis. It is frequently associated with increased activity of the sebaceous glands, producing excessive oiliness, and with increased vulnerability of the skin to secondary bacterial infection. The infectious element is mildly communicable and can be transferred by the common interchange of combs, brushes, caps, pillows, and similar articles. There is no "cure" for seborrheic dermatitis, but it usually can be controlled. Seborrheic dermatitis and acne vulgaris frequently occur together, and both should be treated simultaneously.

OTHER HEALTH PROBLEMS

Lacerations

Lacerations or cuts need to be clean in order to heal well. The immediate first aid procedure is to remove all foreign material, dirt, cinders or gravel, with plentiful use of soap and running water. If the skin edges are gaping, the child should be seen by a physician. Sutures (stitches) are probably indicated in order to expedite healing and prevent unsightly scars. Moreover, deep, gaping wounds which are soil-contaminated or deep puncture wounds, such as those produced by nails or glass, may need not only surgical first aid but also prophylaxis against tetanus. Most physicians will probably agree that, aside from soap and water, antiseptics should not be applied at school to lacerations. The use of pretty salmon-pink tinted mercury antiseptics is of dubious value and lends a false sense of security. If indicated, dry sterile gauze may be placed over the wound as a first aid measure.

Floor Burns

Floor burns and denuded areas of skin from slipping on floors or on dirt and gravel, if superficial, need only to be washed with soap and water. Usually they are left exposed to the air. If gravel or dirt is embedded and cannot be removed by gentle washing, the child should be seen by a physician. Children who fall on the black-asphalt substitute for grass may rub some of the dark mixture into the skin. Unless all of this foreign material washes off with soap and water, the child needs a physician's care in order to prevent a tattoo. One physician relates an incident in which his own daughter had asphalt deeply embedded in her chin. After trying tweezers, he finally resorted to rubbing the epidermis with a stiff brush in order to remove all of the foreign body. Sometimes a student must be taken to surgery and have gravel and other extraneous material removed under anesthesia. With the plentiful abrasions on knees, palms of hands, and all exposed areas of skin on a child, teachers are called upon frequently to administer first aid.

SUMMARY

A discussion of common skin diseases which are encountered at school is presented in enough detail so that a nurse, teacher, or principal will have sufficient information to form a decision in the handling of a problem at school. The intent is neither diagnosis nor treatment, but provision of background knowledge. Skin lesions can occur at any age in school. Material presented on fungal infections will be of interest to physical education teachers. All teachers and counselors in secondary schools will benefit from the discussion of acne.

DISCUSSION QUESTIONS AND ACTIVITIES

1. Devise a list of the important functions of the skin.
2. Make a check of the locker rooms in a school to see if athlete's foot is being discouraged from growing. What recommendations can you make?
3. What physical, social, and emotional factors may be affected by acne?

4. Discuss the importance of having hot water and soap available in the school. What part does washing with soap and water play in the prevention of skin diseases?
5. Discuss your opinion about the correlation between lousiness and socioeconomic factors.
6. Discuss which should be emphasized more in school health—detection or prevention of skin problems.
7. Make a list of the factors that can influence acne growth. Can any of these be eliminated through education?
8. Explain your position on letting a student with impetigo in your classroom.
9. Report on new research dealing with the causes of warts.
10. Discuss the influence of diet on the condition of the skin.

ADDITIONAL SOURCES OF INFORMATION

READINGS

American Medical Association: Department of Health Education. Write for articles on skin problems. *Today's Health.* Each issue usually has a column devoted to skin problems.

Andrews, G.: *Andrews' Diseases of the Skin: Clinical Dermatology.* Philadelphia: W. B. Saunders Co., 1971.

Bauer, M.: "Skin Diseases and the Adolescent." *J. Sch. Health* 40:236–238, May, 1970.

Behrent, H. J.: *Patterns of Skin pH from Birth through Adolescence with a Synopsis of Skin Growth.* Springfield, Illinois: Charles C Thomas, 1971.

Bryan, D.: "Skin Problems of School-Age Children—A Nursing Responsibility?" *J. Sch. Health* 40:437–439, October, 1970.

Kerns, D. L., et al.: "Ampicillin Rash in Children." *Am. J. Dis. Child.* 125:187–193, February, 1973.

Robin, M.: "How Emotions Affect Skin Problems in School Children." *J. Sch. Health* 18:6:370–373, June, 1973.

Ruppe, J. P.: "Skin Infections: Their Role in Health Today." *J. Sch. Health* 18:6:373–380, June, 1973.

Zeller, W.: "Adolescent Attitudes and Cutaneous Health." *J. Sch. Health* 40:115–120, March, 1970.

MATERIALS FOR TEACHERS' USE IN SCHOOLS

AUDIOVISUAL MATERIALS

Recommended grade levels are designated *pri, int, jh, sh.*

And Everything Nice

23 min.	Color	*int, jh*	Discovery Teaching Films 1275 Lincoln Avenue San Jose, California 95725

For girls. Shows how diet, exercise, and care with make-up can make a girl more attractive.

Body Care and Grooming

17 min. Black and White *sh*
Encyclopaedia Britannica Educ. Corp.*

Develops the theme that good grooming starts with personal care. Demonstrates good habits of skin care, hair care, and manicure of nails. Emphasizes that clothing deserves care.

Care of Hair and Nails

11 min. Black and White *int, jh*
Encyclopaedia Britannica Educ. Corp.

A fairy tale character teaches children good habits for care of hair and nails.

Care of the Skin

11 min. Black and White *int, jh*
Encyclopaedia Britannica Educ. Corp.

Three attractive children prepare for bed, show proper way to wash hands and face and bathe. Common skin ailments illustrated. Animated drawings of structure of skin.

Cleanliness and Health

11 min. Color *int* Coronet Films

David's visit to a doctor teaches him about cleanliness.

Good Health Practices

10 min. Color *pri* Avis Films, Inc.

Compares human body to an engine burning fuel. Stresses food habits, elimination, and cleanliness.

Healthy Skin

11 min. Color *sh* Coronet Films

Structure and functions of skin. Maintaining a healthy skin.

How to Be Well-Groomed

11 min. Color *jh, sh* Coronet Films

Demonstrates the four fundamentals of appearance: good health, good posture, cleanliness, and neatness.

How Billy Keeps Clean

11 min. Color *pri* Coronet Films

"How can Billy play hard yet keep himself clean and healthy?" Film shows how to wash skin, when to wash, and how keeping clean helps make a person more attractive and healthy.

Personal Hygiene for Boys

11 min. Black and White *jh, sh* Coronet Films

Explains to boys the proper way to shower, shave, guard against athlete's foot, and care for the complexion. Emphasizes the value of a balanced diet.

Your Hair and Scalp

13 min. Color *jh, sh* Film Associates

Describes structure of hair and follicles. Best way to care for hair.

Your Skin

15 min. Color *jh, sh* Film Associates

Some basic facts on structure and functions of skin.

---

*For addresses of film companies see Appendix A.

Chapter 11

PROBLEMS OF THE DIGESTIVE SYSTEM

SIGNIFICANCE OF AN "UPSET STOMACH"

A very common complaint is a "stomach ache," "upset stomach," or abdominal pain. Complaint of pain, nausea, or vomiting must not be taken lightly. The quick recovery which youngsters make from suspected digestive disturbances is often amazing. A little girl may have a high fever, appear prostrate, and frighten the family; a few hours later she is alert, afebrile, and demands her dolls. Nevertheless, these disturbances demand serious consideration.

Sometimes it is not easy to differentiate between a minor gastrointestinal disturbance and an illness which demands surgical intervention. The latter may also start with nausea and vomiting. Negligence may be fatal in this instance; therefore, *every child complaining of abdominal pain should be under medical supervision.* A few general facts on abdominal pain are pertinent: (1) Pain is a protective mechanism. (2) Pain is not necessarily located over the diseased area inside the abdomen. (3) The severity of the pain is not necessarily correlated with amount of disturbance, i.e., severe pain may be associated with a minor problem. The converse may be true. (4) Pain should be considered as reflecting a major disease disturbance until proved otherwise.

An "upset stomach" may be characterized by nausea, vomiting, abdominal pain, diarrhea, constipation, or any combination of these discomforts. A sudden attack may be:

1. A precursor of a communicable disease. (See Communicable Diseases.)
2. An indication of an emotional upset.
3. Due to injudicious eating.
4. Associated with gastroenteritis.
5. An early indication of appendicitis.

6. A manifestation of allergy.

7. An early indication of a more complex or progressive disturbance which will require medical or surgical treatment.

8. The onset of a migraine headache, associated with nausea and vomiting.

9. Urinary tract infection.

This outline is presented so that a teacher can appreciate the difficulties in determining the cause of abdominal pain and also appreciate the fact that in an individual case the diagnosis should only be made by a physician. No one else should accept the responsibility of making a diagnosis.

A child may suffer from a chronic or recurrent abdominal pain. This may occur over any area of the abdomen and recur at intervals. There is a tendency to ignore the complaint because no serious consequences occurred in the past. Even so, as far as a teacher is concerned, whenever the complaint of pain is made, management is the same as for an acute attack. The parent should be notified.

EMOTIONAL DISTURBANCES

Emotional disturbances are frequently reflected in gastrointestinal disturbances. A new baby in the family, a visit from relatives, quarrels or tensions between mother and father, nonacceptance by peers, poor grades at school, dread of reporting to a classroom or to a special recitation (frequently mathematics)—any one of many excitements, fears, or frustrations can upset a youngster.

Feigned gastrointestinal upsets are also a part of school life. A child voices an urgent need to go to the toilet room as a dreaded class period approaches, or when soon to be confronted by a certain teacher. He may remain away from his classroom an hour or more. The comment has been frequently repeated, "It's a poor teacher who cannot compete with a lavatory."

Every teacher is familiar with the complaints the morning following a holiday, either due to excitement or dietary indiscretions, such as eating the conglomeration gathered on "trick or treat" Halloween visits the night before. Older students have similar disturbances, but usually do not complain as readily. An abdominal pain may not even be mentioned until it becomes severe.

APPENDICITIS

Appendicitis can be quite sudden in onset, and the infection can progress very rapidly in a few hours to the acute surgical stage. A teacher cannot rely upon any one typical clinical picture to guide him in a decision to send a pupil home. All that can be accurately stated about appendicitis is that there is abdominal pain. There may or may not be nausea or vomiting; abdominal distress may be more a diffuse colicky pain which may later localize in the lower right side; or localization to the region of the appendix may be immediate; or the complaint of pain may be minimized. The child may or may not appear acutely ill. Abdominal examination and diagnosis by school personnel is definitely contraindicated. He should not be sent to the rest room to lie down on a cot for a while.

INJURIES

A *penetrating wound* into the abdominal wall, caused by a stick, a piece of glass or wire, or any other instrument, *should be seen immediately by a physician*, even though there is no complaint of pain, and even though the wound appears to be superficial. The following case explains the possible significance of a wound:

> A little boy of ten, in a hurry to get outside, pushed into the glass panel of a door and broke it. A small laceration in the upper mid-abdomen was sutured. Deep pressure in the region of the wound elicited no discomfort. The mother called the physician about three o'clock in the morning to state that the boy was whimpering with pain. The child was taken to the hospital; x-ray showed a vague shadow which might be considered that of a piece of glass. Surgery revealed perforations of the larger curvature of the stomach; a piece of glass was lying on the pancreas.

A blow to the abdomen followed by pain, either immediate or delayed, or a sudden, severe, persistent abdominal pain without history of an injury demands immediate medical attention. Children sometimes forget injuries. Again, a note of caution. Only a physician should feel the abdomen. An organ, such as a liver or spleen, may be bruised or perforated. Sudden hemorrhage may have occurred. *Consider every blow to the abdomen as serious.*

Do not send or take a child with abdominal injury to his home. A parent should come to the school and pick up the injured one. Play it safe.

ULCERS

Ulcers of the stomach or duodenum are not unusual in children. The children bring their medicines to school and take them at regular intervals.

> A principal in one school was confronted with a nine-year-old boy who had been under treatment for an ulcer since the age of six. He presented a severe personality problem—bullying, hostile, resentful of authority, hovered over by a smotheringly protective mother and rejected by his stepfather.

One college student reports that he suffered his first hemorrhage from an ulcer at the age of 12. Another recalls lying upon the grass, as a small boy, writhing in pain. This pain which recurred intermittently over many years was later explained by the presence of a stomach ulcer. He was an only child. During psychotherapy at college he came to appreciate the strain imposed on him by parental demands for perfection and excellent grades.

A physician hospitalized a boy of ten who had been complaining of vague abdominal pains for several years. X-rays demonstrated a duodenal ulcer. In probing for sources of stress, it was revealed that the boy was constantly being picked on by his classmates because of his small stature. Nevertheless, this was not sufficient explanation of his stress. The physician noted that the child never asked when he might go home. His mother, a self-centered, socially ambitious woman, visited him once at the hospital and showed no anxiety. Finally, after the diet had been regulated and the boy was comfortable, the physician called the mother, only to have her protest the inconvenience of having her son home for the next few days. Later visits to the home confirmed the suspicion of neglect and disinterest in the boy's welfare.

Sometimes a child with an ulcer of the stomach or duodenum needs psychological evaluation as well as medical treatment. Ulcers can heal. A regimen of medication and relief of tensions must be outlined and followed. The whole family situation must be taken into account, and the cooperation of the physician, school nurse, social worker, psychologist, and teaching personnel will be needed.

GASTROENTERITIS

Gastroenteritis is frequently the diagnosis used in referring to an attack of nausea, vomiting, diarrhea, abdominal pains, and general malaise. It may not be recognized as a disease entity, but outbreaks do occur. Many individuals will be afflicted at the same time. It is sometimes referred to as "intestinal flu." The cause is probably respiratory and viral in origin, although there may not be respiratory complaints. Similar symptoms and signs may be produced by organisms mentioned under Food Poisoning. Under no circumstances should medication to allay abdominal pain be given at school. The child should be *taken* home with a recommendation for medical consultation.

Food Poisoning

Food poisoning occurs occasionally at school. It usually afflicts a group at one time: a classroom, a bus load of children on a picnic, or a great number of students in a school who use a common eating place. Food poisoning has been inaccurately referred to as "ptomaine poisoning." The term applies to illnesses caused by contaminated foods. The symptoms and signs are those of gastroenteritis. Onset is sudden, characterized by severe nausea, vomiting, colicky pains, prostration, and usually diarrhea. Onset occurs within 30 minutes to four hours and even up to 24 hours after intake of food, depending upon the infectious agent.

It is not incumbent upon school personnel to determine the cause, source, or means of an outbreak of suspected food poisoning. Health authorities are called in, and all cooperation is extended. However, the following explanation is offered concerning possible diseases. Detailed description of them will be found in the chapter on communicable diseases.

One possibility is a *botulinus* infection. Actually, this is not likely unless home-canned vegetables or meats are used without the precaution of being boiled for about five minutes after removal from their containers.

Another possibility is a *salmonella* infection. The disease is quite prevalent. Occasionally, an epidemic occurs. The description of this infection and the foods which are usually contaminated can be found in Chapter 8. Sometimes this infection is referred to as gastroenteritis.

Other diseases which have been spread by contaminated food or water are in the *typhoid-dysentery* group. A food handler who is a carrier may be the offender. If water is the source of infection, the whole community will suffer, not just the school.

The most likely explanation of an outbreak of food poisoning at school is the growth of certain strains of bacteria, called *staphylococci.* A toxin produced by these organisms acts rapidly and causes severe illness and prostration. Onset of symptoms occurs from one to six hours after ingestion of food, usually two or four hours. Recovery should be in one to two days, but the time may be longer. Staphylococci may be transferred from food-service personnel to foods, where the organisms multiply and produce toxins. Foods which are left in a warm environment for several hours encourage growth of bacteria. Outbreaks have been traced to pastries and puddings with a custard or cream content, and to such a variety of foods as "ham, tongue, and other processed meats, cheese, ice cream, potato salad, hollandaise sauce, chicken salad. . . ."[1] Some cases have developed from milk of infected cows.

"Preventive measures:

1. Prompt refrigeration of sliced and chopped meats and of custards and cream fillings to avoid multiplication of staphylococci accidentally introduced; fill pastries with custard just prior to sale, or subject finished product to adequate heat treatment. Immediate disposal or proper refrigeration of leftover foods.

---

[1]Paul B. Beeson and Walsh McDermott, editors: *Cecil-Loeb Textbook of Medicine.* Twelfth edition. Philadelphia: W. B. Saunders Company, 1967, p. 1699.

2. Temporary exclusion from food handling of persons suffering from pyogenic (containing pus) skin infections, especially of the hands.

3. Education of food handlers in strict attention to sanitation and cleanliness of kitchens, including refrigeration, handwashing, attention to the fingernails, and the danger of working while having skin infections."[2]

MANAGEMENT AT SCHOOL OF A CHILD WITH ABDOMINAL PAIN

If a child is suffering from a digestive upset, abdominal pain, or an injury to the abdomen, the teacher should notify a parent directly. In the meantime, *keep the child lying down. Give no medicine and no water. Do not feel the abdomen. Accept no responsibility.* A mother or father may call for the sufferer and take him home, to a physician's office, or to the hospital.

If a child is to be taken home by someone from school, good judgment dictates that he be accompanied by a responsible individual. *Make sure that someone in authority is there to receive him.* With acute pain or abdominal injury he should not walk home.

SUMMARY

Young children suffer frequently from an "upset stomach." The cause may be transient or may be serious; each case should have a medical evaluation.

No pupil or student with an abdominal injury or a complaint of abdominal pain should be kept at school. Some responsible member of the family should be notified.

Outbreaks of food poisoning are public health problems.

DISCUSSION QUESTIONS AND ACTIVITIES

1. Explain your procedure as a teacher when a students complains of a stomachache.
2. Discuss how emotions can play an important part in the digestive system.
3. Compile a list of the few drugs popularly used to relieve "upset stomach" and explain the significance of each.
4. Explain the role of the food service in schools in preventing digestive system disturbances.

[2]American Public Health Association: *Communicable Diseases in Man.* New York: The Association, 1970, p. 91.

5. Discuss the procedure for and the rationale behind the first aid treatment for a blow to the abdomen.

ADDITIONAL SOURCES OF INFORMATION

RESOURCE

American Medical Association
Department of Health Education.
Reprints on gastrointestinal problems.
Today's Health. Occasional pertinent article.

READINGS

Davenport, H. W.: *Physiology of the Digestive Tract: An Introductory Text.* Chicago: Year Book Medical Publications, 1971.

Go, V. L.: "Digestion, Maldigestion and the Gastrointestinal Hormones." *Am. J. Clin. Nutr.* 24:160–167, January, 1971.

AUDIOVISUAL MATERIALS

Recommended grade levels are designated *pri, int, jh, sh.*

Alimentary Tract
11 min. Color *jh, sh* Encyclopaedia Britannica Educ. Corp.*
Shows movements involved in digestive process.

Digestion of Foods
11 min. Black and White *jh, sh* Encyclopaedia Britannica Educ. Corp.
Explains processes of digestion.

Digestive System
17 min. Color *jh, sh* Encyclopaedia Britannica Educ. Corp.
Shows by x-ray the entire process of digestion.

*For addresses of film companies see Appendix A.

Chapter 12

HEART PROBLEMS OF CHILDREN AND YOUTH

GROWTH OF THE HEART

The heart in a growing child must fullfill the demands made upon it to maintain basic metabolic processes, permit normal growth, and care for physical activity. The organ grows steadily towards adult size, not proportionate to skeletal and muscular growth at all times, with an acceleration during adolescence. The average heart size is observed as follows: newborn – 24 grams; one year – 45 grams; six years – 95 grams; puberty (12 to 13 years for girls, 14 to 15 years for boys) – 150 grams; and adults – 300 grams.[1]

The heart rate is rapid at birth (about 140 beats per minute), remains rapid in the early years, decreases to about 95 times per minute in the six-to ten-year-old, and slows gradually towards the adult rate of 70 to 80.

Note the slow growth of a rapidly beating heart over quite a span of time. The heart grows fast and doubles its weight *after* the growth spurt. During the years of growth to adult size, the heart must maintain the good circulation and blood pressure necessary for normal metabolic functions. Excessive physical activity produces additional demands upon the circulatory system. For this reason, in the early growing years, *sustained effort for any period of time is not desirable.* The heart will suffer no damage; but a young person is simply not capable physically of the same performance as an older student. Practical application of this knowledge of the physiology of the heart is shown in the planning of athletic programs for the preteenager and early adolescent. "High pressure" programs are to be avoided.

HEART FUNCTION IN HEALTH AND DISEASE

Normal Function

When the heart is healthy, its valves and muscle function well. The physiology of the heart is described in the legend of Figure 56.

[1]Ernest H. Watson and George H. Lowery: *Growth and Development of Children.* Fourth edition. Chicago, Illinois: Year Book Medical Publishers Inc., 1962, p. 232.

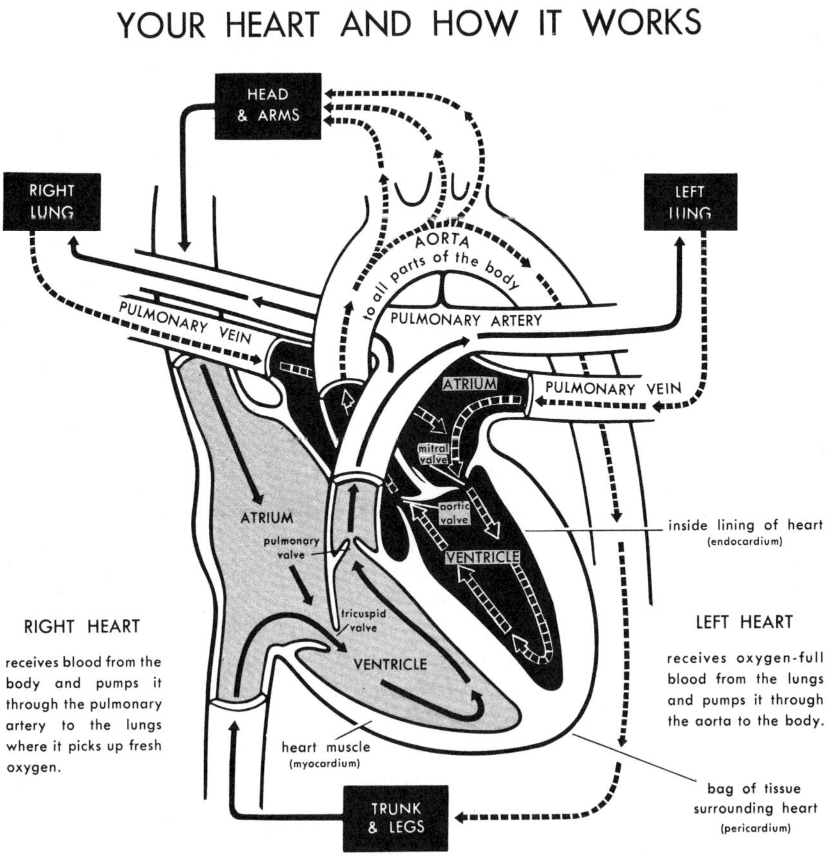

Figure 56 Your heart weighs well under a pound and is only a little larger than your fist, but it is a powerful, long working, hard working organ. Its job is to pump blood to the lungs and to all the body tissues.

The heart is a hollow organ. Its tough, muscular wall (myocardium) is surrounded by a fiber-like bag (pericardium) and is lined by a thin, strong membrane (endocardium). A wall (septum) divides the heart cavity down the middle into a "right heart" and a "left heart." Each side of the heart is divided again into an upper chamber (called an atrium or auricle) and a lower chamber (ventricle). Valves regulate the flow of blood through the heart and to the pulmonary artery and the aorta.

The heart is really a double pump. One pump (the right heart) receives blood which has just come from the body after delivering nutrients and oxygen to the body tissues. It pumps this dark, bluish red blood to the lungs where the blood gets rid of a waste gas (carbon dioxide) and picks up a fresh supply of oxygen which turns it a bright red again. The second pump (the left heart) receives this "reconditioned" blood from the lungs and pumps it out through the great trunk-artery (aorta) to be distributed by smaller arteries to all parts of the body. (Courtesy American Heart Association.)

Effects of Heart Damage

Any disturbance of valvular or muscular action alters efficiency and influences general health. Disease may affect the inner lining of the heart, the valves, the muscle, or the outer covering. Various diseases have predilections for certain of these tissues. For instance, rheumatic fever involves muscle or valves or both. Usually the valves in the left side of the heart are attacked.

When valves are injured by toxins or bacteria, their thin tissue margins become inflamed. As healing occurs, the latter frequently become thickened and lack delicacy of motion for perfect opening and closure. With much involvement the margins may become scarred and deformed. The end result may be a narrowed, rigid valvular ring, a *stenosis.* With such a condition the valves meet in closure, but do not retract enough to permit full flow between the chambers. Another condition may exist. If the valves do not close perfectly, then with contraction of the heart muscle to send the stream of blood forward, some will leak back into the chamber from which it has just been expelled. Such a process is referred to as a *leakage* or *insufficiency.* Both a stenosis and an insufficiency may be present. Difficulty in forcing blood into the next chamber through scarred, stiff valves affects the adequacy of blood supply to the body.

If the heart muscle, however, is healthy, it can to a great extent overcome the handicap of damaged valves and provide satisfactory circulation. The child will then be able to maintain normal nutrition, growth, and activity, and show no signs of decompensation or heart failure. Disturbances of muscular function can result from disease, from poor nutrition of the heart itself, or from the action of toxins produced by some infections. It also goes without saying that good health in general is essential for good heart function. Anemia, high blood pressure, kidney disease, malnutrition (especially group B-complex deficiency), and metabolic disturbances in thyroid or glucose metabolism can affect heart function. If heart damage is slight, no particular warning signs will be noticed by a teacher.

If circulation is impaired to any great degree, the *manifestations of decompensation* can be observed by the teachers, particularly those who supervise physical activity. Comparatively few children fall into this category. The prominence of the signs naturally depends upon the degree of decompensation. If insufficient oxygenation of the blood occurs, mucous membranes may appear a bluish red color (cyanotic), noticeable particularly in the lips. The cheeks may carry a purplish flush and the nail beds, a similar appearance. The child appears tired, limits his activity because of fatigue, and becomes short of breath easily with exercise. Growth can definitely be affected. The teacher who observes any of these abnormal signs should notify parents and request an examination by a physician.

The Meaning of a Murmur

A *murmur* is defined as an abnormal heart sound. Its presence does not necessarily mean that a diseased heart exists. As a matter of fact, most murmurs in childhood are what we term *innocent.* An innocent murmur is sometimes referred to as functional, physiological, or accidental. In contradistinction, a small percentage are *organic*, actually due to heart damage or abnormality. The presence of the murmur serves as a clue to the possibility of organic heart disease; differentiation between an innocent and an organic heart murmur must be made by the physician. Sometimes the diagnosis is made readily; in other cases definite conclusions can be made only after thorough medical histories, electrocardiograms, x-rays, and repeated examinations.

A survey to determine the incidence of heart disease was made in Grand Junction, Colorado, on a young age group[2]—6311 pupils between the ages of six and 11 (95.6 per cent of the population at this age level). Innocent murmurs were heard in 2068 children (33 per cent); 33 cases of congenital heart disease and seven of rheumatic heart disease were found. Of these 40 cases, 29 were previously unknown. This finding is important. Only by mass surveys can a high percentage of organic heart disease be detected early. At least 15 children had been diagnosed falsely as having heart disease. This finding is also important. A child should not be labeled unjustifiably as having heart damage.

Innocent murmurs occur frequently in the early years, sometimes involving as many as 50 per cent or more of children, with a peak of incidence between five and nine years. Innocent murmurs appear to be unrelated to any cardiac or anatomical abnormality. Little is known about their cause. They may be transitory or may occasionally persist through the years. Sometimes they disappear completely. They often develop during an acute illness, fever, or severe anemia and disappear during convalescence. Since murmurs are not consistently present, conflicting findings will be reported. One physician may hear the sound; another may not. There may also be a history of an organic murmur which is no longer present. The intensity of a murmur may vary. Its loudness gives no clue to the amount of organic impairment or improvement. Hence there is no such thing as a murmur being "better" or "worse," and a doctor does not treat a murmur. It is important to recognize that a heart murmur is not, in itself, a heart disease. Further, parents should not employ excessive caution with their child, because they may cause unnecessary invalidism in a healthy child.

COMMON CAUSES OF HEART DISEASES IN CHILDHOOD

The two most common causes of heart disease in childhood are congenital anomalies and rheumatic fever. About 30 to 40 thousand children are born each year with heart defects. These account for the

[2]William Martin, Margaret E. N. Beaver, and Richard C. Arnold: "Heart Disease Screening in Elementary School Children." *J.A.M.A.* *169*:1163–1168, 1959.

most predominant heart problem today in elementary schools. One mass field study to detect heart disease, using tape recordings of heart sounds on more than 8000 pupils in elementary and junior high schools, showed an overall prevalence of 3.4 cases per thousand; 2.4 cases were congenital heart defects; 0.7 cases represented rheumatic fever.[3]

Congenital Heart Disease (Malformations)

This type of heart disease is due to developmental anomalies in embryonic life. If the faulty anatomical structure is in a site which is incompatible with living, the infant is either stillborn or dies soon after. Otherwise, the prognosis is dependent upon the adequacy of circulation which can be maintained despite the handicap. If the defect permits fairly good circulatory function—as with small openings between the ventricles or auricles (atria) of the heart, or with a patent ductus arteriosus—the child may have a normal life expectancy and be comfortable. The ductus is a residual vessel from embryonic life which joins the aorta and pulmonary artery. Diagnosis of the abnormality is important these days because developments in surgery permit correction in about three out of four cases of heart defects.

A detailed investigation of 182 cases of suspected congenital heart disease referred over a period of eight years to the Idaho Crippled Children's Service revealed 50 cases of openings between the ventricles and 30 between the auricles. Thirty children had no heart disease. Surgery was performed on the favorable cases.[4] The increased incidence of persons with congenital heart disease is explained by the greater survival rate of premature babies and the benefits of surgery.

Rheumatic Fever

The major manifestations of rheumatic fever are: migrating polyarthritis (many joints involved), chorea (St. Vitus' dance), and carditis (heart infection).

Rheumatic fever occurs more frequently between the ages of five and 18 years, with the first attack usually suffered between five and ten. It occurs more frequently in our migrant populations, in slum areas, and generally in the lower economic stratum of society where crowding in homes and unsanitary conditions prevail among children who suffer from poor nutrition, poor health, and lowered resistance.

---

[3]Robert A. Miller et al.: "The Detection of Heart Disease in Children. Results of Mass Field Trials with Use of Tape-recorded Heart Sounds. II. Michigan City Study." *Circulation* *32*:956–965, December, 1965.

[4]F. L. Fletcher and R. H. Wilson: "Screening for Suspected Congenital Heart Disease." *J.A.M.A.* *179*:9–13, 1962.

It tends to "run in families." Fatal first attacks have struck young adult Negroes and Puerto Ricans who have recently migrated to northern cities in the United States.

The preceding observation does not rule out the fact that children from all strata of society and from homes that stress medical care may also suffer from rheumatic fever.

Rheumatic fever has definitely been associated with the presence of streptococci; some speculate that it is a sensitivity reaction to the toxins produced by the organisms. It is not a communicable disease. The exact mechanism which produces symptoms is not known. Observations are definite, however, that the disease may develop in 1 to 3 per cent of untreated cases[5] of scarlet fever or streptococcal sore throat or other streptococcal infection, usually after a lapse of one to four weeks. A "bad" year for scarlet fever or "strep throat" is a "bad" year for rheumatic fever. The disease has been associated with the temperate zone at a time when upper respiratory infections are present—winter and spring; still, it is probably quite prevalent in the tropical and subtropical climates, where the manifestations are less severe and may go unobserved. About 30 to 40 per cent of streptococcal infections are silent, so that the presence of rheumatic fever may not be suspected until complications appear.

The clinical picture of rheumatic fever varies and is not necessarily easy to diagnose. It may be acute and pronounced, or it may be insidious. The initial injury, particularly in the nonarthritic form, may not be detected; and not infrequently the first indication of a damaged heart is found in the routine examination by a physician. In such children there may be no history of sickness, or more likely only a vague complaints of "growing pains," fatigue, or frequent sore throats. Incidentally, growing is not painful. Recurrent attacks of arthritis, chorea, or carditis are typical of the disease. Frequently a second attack returns a year or two after the first episode. For instance, a child who has had arthritis one year may have chorea or carditis the year following. Occasionally, no further illness is suffered. If a child has apparently been well for five years or more, the prognosis is good. The tendency to recurrent attacks decreases after puberty. The greatest incidence of recurrence is in the first few years after an acute attack.

POLYARTHRITIS (RHEUMATISM, ARTHRITIS, JUVENILE RHEUMATISM, INFLAMMATORY RHEUMATISM)

With this manifestation of rheumatic fever, varying degrees of discomfort in the joints may occur. Usually the larger joints are involved—ankles, knees, hips, wrists, elbows, shoulders. The discomfort may migrate from one joint to another and may last only a day

[5] Ralph Bugg: "Rheumatic Fever." *Today's Health* 46:36–39, March, 1968.

or two in each one, or may last longer. Commonly, the joint is swollen, tender to touch, and painful to move; it may or may not be red and hot. The child may cry with pain. If there has been much involvement, he has a lasting impression and can usually remember when and how long he had to stay at home. Absences from school may be for as long as a year. Recurrent attacks tend to be more severe. No deformity of the joints remains after rheumatic fever.

Chorea (St. Vitus' dance)

Chorea is the initial manifestation of rheumatic fever in about 20 per cent of cases. Sometimes a child will give a history of a "nervous breakdown" and describe something of the typical picture of this disease. Chorea involves the central nervous system; it is characterized by emotional instability, bizarre, purposeless movements, and muscular weakness. The onset is insidious yet is frequently noticed first by the teacher. This child, who heretofore has been quiet, becomes fidgety, nervous, and restless. He shows quick irritability, rapid changes of moods, and sometimes maniacal excitement. He becomes inattentive and forgetful, and is unable to remember recent events. Gradually the muscles become weaker: the child endeavors to stand and the knees may buckle under; the arms and hands shake; the handgrasp becomes weak; the child cannot hold a pencil or a glass. The arms are more involved than the legs. Script becomes illegible. The gait may become clumsy and staggering. At this stage, involuntary motions are noticed; gestures occur which follow no stereotyped pattern; parts of the body jerk unexpectedly; grimaces startle onlooking persons. These involuntary, purposeless movements are accelerated by excitement or emotion. Because the muscles around the eyes are weak, tearing occurs; the weak muscles around the mouth allow drooling and protrusion of the tongue. Speech is rapid and indistinct. All of these changes appear over several days and are soon detected. The child is sick, and bed rest is mandatory. The disease is self-limiting and lasts four to six weeks. Recovery may leave no complications. Chorea occurs mostly between seven and 14 years, with a high incidence at the age of eight. It occurs more in girls than boys. It is rarely seen after puberty and never after 20 years of age.

Carditis

This is the most severe manifestation of rheumatic fever. Either the muscles or valves of the heart, or both, may be affected. There may have been no known preceding occurrence of chorea or arthritis. One must also bear clearly in mind that a child who has had chorea or arthritis is not doomed to have heart damage. Only about 20 per cent will develop heart disease after a first attack of rheumatic fever. However, having had one attack, a child is more susceptible to a recurrence of rheumatic fever and also to heart damage (as much as 50 per cent). Those who already suffer from carditis tend to develop increasing heart damage. Hence, the need for continuous prophylactic antibiotics to prevent a recurrent streptococcal infection.

In rheumatic carditis the course of the disease varies and appears to be self-limited. If detected and treated early, heart damage may be minimal. The prognosis depends naturally upon the severity of heart involvement. Damage can be extensive and permanent and can cause marked disability. An occasional child may become bedridden indefinitely. Sometimes the valves become badly scarred and rigid. Surgery today is performing miracles on valvular defects. Children who have mild cases of heart damage live comfortably and suffer few ill effects. Some children apparently recover. Repeated examinations and observation of performance in physical activities are necessary in evaluation of a child's physical status.

In the past, rheumatic fever has accounted for more deaths in the five to 19 age group than all of the infectious diseases of childhood combined. This is no longer true. The incidence of the disease is definitely declining, a decline estimated at as much as 90 per cent or greater. Such a change is credited to health education, to alertness of parents and medical personnel in the detection and prompt treatment of streptococcal infections and early rheumatic fever, to the marvelous boon of antibiotics, to prophylaxis in cases of heart disease, to the progress of heart surgery, and to improved living conditions. Nevertheless, constant vigilance is necessary. The disease is by no means eradicated.

In the states where rheumatic fever occurs infrequently, it is still important for a teacher to have knowledge of the disease. Teachers often notice the first indications and need to be intelligent about the difficulties involved in caring for the afflicted youngsters at school. With migrations of our population, any school is likely to have some children with a rheumatic history and possibly with rheumatic heart disease. Because of this possibility and the seriousness of the problem, especially with the threat of recurrences, quite a bit of space has been devoted here to this subject.

SCHOOL HEALTH PROGRAM

Detection of Heart Disease

Avenues of detection may be: (1) the presence of the acute phase of rheumatic fever—arthritis or chorea; (2) the history of rheumatic fever, a congenital heart problem, or a murmur; (3) actions and appearance of the child; (4) performance in physical education activities; and (5) the health examination.

The *acute phases of rheumatic fever* may be detected during a school health examination if the doctor is so fortunate as to be examining a child at that opportune time. This seldom happens. It is usually the teacher or a member of the family who observes early symptoms and signs of arthritis or chorea. Any pertinent information should be placed upon the child's cumulative school health record, because a rheumatic history or knowledge of organic heart disease may be important in making decisions for future guidance.

History

A history of rheumatic fever, a congenital heart problem, or a murmur is a valuable clue. The child himself may discuss his past rheumatic complaints, in terms of a rheumatism which kept him out of school for a definite period of time, or in terms of a "nervous breakdown." The latter term deserves close questioning, however. It may be a term applied to chorea, or to a period when a child may have been very nervous and emotionally disturbed or reacting to a grave crisis in his home. Questioning the parent should produce more definite information about a heart problem. The family physician may provide a diagnosis. Usually this precise information is not necessary unless there is a question of heart damage and adjustment to school activity. Some children know whether they have heart murmurs or heart trouble or have been restricted. Other children have intentionally not been told about their heart damage by parents or physician, yet have been watched closely. Some parents worry about making heart invalids of their children and resent information's being given or discussed before a child. An older student, as a rule, knows about any abnormalities of his heart and can discuss the problem calmly and intelligently with those interested. He often knows whether he was a "blue baby," which would suggest a congenital defect.

Teacher Observation

Most cases of heart disease will be difficult to detect. The school relies upon the recommendation of the physician. However, teacher observation is important. The *actions* or *appearance* of a child at school may lead a teacher to suspect cardiac trouble, or at least the need for a thorough health examination. The child who restricts his own activity, who appears breathless after short exertion, or who shows pallor or a tired expression or faints after mild exercise is suspect. These signs should be kept in mind. The behavior is not diagnostic of heart trouble. A child with influenza might act the same. Nevertheless, a checkup is indicated.

Major signs of decompensation are occasionally observed, such as breathlessness, flushed cheeks, and bluish lips. No diagnosis should be made by a teacher, but his alertness leads him to suggest further investigation by a physician.

Health Examination

Another method of detection of heart disease is provided by the health examination conducted by a private or school physician. The Colorado survey mentioned above revealed a high per cent of unsuspected cases. If a child does not know that he has cardiac damage, the condition of his heart should not be discussed in his presence. For example, a little girl was told at school that she had a heart murmur and ran all the way home, crying, to tell her mother. The parents and physician in this particular instance did not want the child to have such information nor any fears instilled in her. Nor should the findings on one child be mentioned before another.

A current development in the detection of heart disease in children and youth by mass surveys has been the use of tape recordings of heart sounds. These are recorded by prescribed techniques in school and listened to leisurely by a panel of specialists at a later date. Follow-up on suspected cases is then done by recall stethoscope examination of each child.

Another recent technique in mass screening of heart sounds uses a portable computer. In one experiment the heart sounds of 3797 school children were analyzed. A small microphone and bipolar electrocardiographic timing leads were the inputs from the child. Heart sounds were studied on a beat-to-beat basis, and an immediate analysis was possible. Sixteen cases of heart disease and two cases of conduction disturbances were found. Eight of the cases of heart diseases were unknown. No known cases were missed.[6] Dennison and Fenimore found similar results in their Indiana study.[7] Eisner and Oglesby[8] conclude that this new technique makes it possible to eliminate routine physical examinations. This technique shows great promise.

Follow-up

Medical

When the family physician conducts the health examination in his office – this is the procedure of choice – communication with the school on a heart problem should follow a mutually designed pattern, similar to channels suggested below.

If the examination takes place at school, *follow-up on a heart murmur* is indicated unless the examining physician is satisfied in his own mind and labels it as innocent. Even in these cases it would

---

[6]Robert E. Durnin et al.: "Heart-Sound Screening in Children. Use of a Portable Analog-Digital Computer." (Field Study-Los Angeles 1966). *J.A.M.A. 203*:111–116, 1968.

[7]Darwin Dennison and Joy Ann Fennimore: "A Heart-Sound Screening Program for Elementary Children." *J. Sch. Health 41*:7:349–351, September, 1971.

[8]Victor Eisner and Allan Oglesby: "Health Assessment of School Children." *J. Sch. Health 42*:5:270–271, May, 1972.

not be amiss for a teacher to observe physical performance. Since the school examiner has no facilities for thorough examination of a heart, all children designated by him should be referred to family physicians or to specialized clinics for further check-ups. The *method of referral* in itself is important. Printed forms may be sent home with the pupil. They usually request an additional physical examination with a return communication from the family physician. At no time should the heart be mentioned specifically on these forms because of the anxiety which may be aroused in some parents. In serious cases the school examiner himself may bar all physical activity until further study is made and may suggest that a nurse make direct contact with the parent.

Channels for handling suspected heart cases vary with school systems. Some children are taken directly by their parents to heart clinics maintained by the board of health. Others are seen by the family physician. Procedures vary also for referral to the school of the needed information for guidance. Sometimes the student brings a note directly to the teacher or principal indicating the amount of activity permissible, and possibly the diagnosis. The channels may be from a clinic or family physician to the school physician. In this instance, usually the diagnosis is included; the school physician in turn sends a memorandum to the school. The main question is, "How much activity is safe for this child?" Forms should be provided by the school which enumerate the usual physical education activities done at a grade level, and the physician is asked to check off the type of activities permitted. Some children should have rest periods. (See forms in Appendix B.) And despite all notes, *the teacher still watches physical endurance.*

SUPERVISION AT SCHOOL

A child who has had successful heart surgery is usually not restricted in his activities. Similarly, if a child recovers completely from rheumatic fever without evidence of heart damage, he is not restricted. With known heart involvement, most children can tolerate quite a bit of activity. They should be observed closely and permitted to set their own pace.

The attitude adopted toward organic heart disease is very important for the mental health of the youngster. Instructions to the school on the care of a pupil should come from the physician and not the parent. Overcautious parents who are continually admonishing a child to be careful may have either a rebellious, defiant offspring or a heart invalid on their hands. Parents who use a child's heart murmur as a disciplinary weapon (and there are such) can produce bizarre results.

> One school physician recalls a sophisticated blonde from the seventh grade, with mascara on her eyelashes, who immediately upon sitting down for her health examination announced that she

had a heart murmur. Nothing unusual was heard with the girl in the sitting position. Finally, in the supine position, a suggestion of an abnormal heart sound was detected. Since the girl persisted in questioning the presence of a murmur, the physician reluctantly but honestly reported a very slight abnormality and reassured the girl that it was of no significance whatsoever. She immediately dissolved into tears and kept repeating, "Mother said my heart murmur would come back if I stayed out late last night." When the physical education teacher reported later that the girl was in the locker room, sobbing and moaning and frightening her classmates with her exhibition, she was brought back into the examining room. An attempt was made to reason with her, but the general impression was gathered that she was having a wonderful time with all the attention aroused. Anyone with insight recognizes the presence here of deep-seated problems. The physician and teacher were greatly disturbed, and a school nurse, acquainted with the significance of this episode, was immediately dispatched to the home.

The elementary teacher not only teaches but has a supervisory responsibility for the activities of his youngsters. If one needs to attend part time, or needs to rest instead of play when he has a cold, sore throat, or infection, allowances are made. An understanding should be secured from the attending physician; the child is handled as much like his classmates as possible. He is entitled to a happy school life.

As for students in secondary schools who have heart problems, vocational guidance and general counseling are important. Every effort should be made to be realistic and neither minimize nor exaggerate the handicap. Those who experience difficulty in climbing steps should have their classes scheduled in such a way as to save effort. There is evidence to support the observation that students who experience no symptoms of heart damage need not be restricted in gymnastics or sports, industrial work, or stair-climbing; nor do they need elevator passes.

Cardiologists today feel that even the child with organic heart disease needs some activity in order to maintain good tone of the heart muscle. The amount of this activity, of course, is determined by the physician and by the actual performance of the child. If the heart muscle is in good condition, he is comfortable with quite a bit of exercise. Otherwise, he will limit himself. The older student, particularly, may feel inferior to his peers because of these restrictions, withdraw into himself, feel that he cannot plan vocational goals, feel that he cannot plan marriage and a family, may use his heart disease as an escape mechanism, or otherwise isolate himself from living. Close cooperation between the teaching personnel and the physician, with reports by the teacher on quality of performance, will avoid making a heart invalid of a child, enable him to feel that he is part of a group, and help him to a well-adjusted life.

Since those with organic heart disease tolerate varying amounts of exertion, a physical education teacher can often provide an adapted program in activities and sports, which will offer needed exercise and social adjustments. Nor should a note from a physician one year suffice for that child's whole school career. A checkup should be done each year, at least, and a note be placed upon the cumulative health record. These precautions are necessary to protect the child and the administration, and one may need to explain this regulation to parents. Besides, youths frequently improve or "outgrow" their handicaps; and a well-worn doctor's note may no longer apply. Children usually enjoy play and resent being placed in a different category from their peers.

> One junior high school student who was restricted because of a patent ductus arteriosus finally went to her physician and pleaded for some activity. A phone conversation with the physical education teacher resulted in a program whereby the girl could "suit-up," keep the roll and inventory on equipment, and take a shower with the other girls. She was happy with this arrangement. Incidentally, this girl had an operation for her congenital heart defect seven years later, noticed more comfort immediately, has since married, and had several children.

Competitive activities may or may not be barred, depending upon the individual medical evaluation. "Cardiac" students have played on golf teams. They may serve as team managers or participate in football as punters or field goal specialists. Some well-known athletes have compensated heart conditions. Good supervision in high school activities and a close working relationship between a coach and physician may enable a boy to satify his ambitions in athletics.

Children who are convalescing from acute illnesses or who are barred from all strenuous physical activities may need to rest a part of each day at school. Cots or beds and blankets should always be available at each school, placed in a quiet, pleasant room. The best time to rest is in the middle of the day, dividing the day's activities and exertions into two parts. A child should not be kept in at recess unless he does not feel well or the weather is forbidding. He needs the companionship of his friends and should not be isolated. He must identify with his group.

No discussion on heart disease in children would be complete without mentioning the program for the bed-ridden child. He may be in bed for months or years. Some are extremely ill and may not survive. It is difficult for a child to remain quietly in bed. Indeed, the bedridden one has been described as often having *one foot* in bed. The teacher of the home-bound is a welcome person to a harassed mother and a bored victim. An attempt is made to keep him abreast of his classwork and to occupy his many hours with some interests. Psychological responses to illness and possible invalidism are described in Chapter 15.

Most convalescents from rheumatic fever eventually return to school. They must be watched for fatigue; their activities are directed; they should not be "heart cripples."

Public Health Aspects

Heart disease in children and youth is a public health problem. A good current estimate is that four children per thousand suffer from heart disease.[9] Many of them are unrecognized in our schools.

One approach to the problem is *early detection of existing cases.* Then there can be wise supervision at school. Heart surgery may be a possibility.

A second approach is *early detection of streptococcal infections.* Serious consequences, including heart damage, may be prevented by proper treatment. Every child with a severe cold or sore throat should be sent home with a recommendation for medical referral.

Lastly, those who have a history of rheumatic fever are urged to take *antibiotics for prophylaxis* according to the individual physician's advice. Teachers can encourage this procedure. Many boards of health provide the drugs at the physician's request.

Any suggestion of a "strep throat" epidemic at school should be called to the attention of health authorities. Also, a teacher should notify a parent of each child with a history of rheumatic fever that an epidemic exists or that one or more cases of streptococcal sore throat have occurred in the classroom.

Vigilance involves the knowledge and the cooperative efforts of the young person himself, parents, teacher, family physician, school physician, school nurse, social worker, and public health official. Vigilance and education on management of respiratory infections are powerful weapons.

SUMMARY

Heart disease in children and youth may be congenital or caused by rheumatic fever. Every school and every teacher will have an occasional pupil or student who is handicapped to some extent by heart damage. The role of every teacher is to encourage as normal a pattern of activity as possible, with the minimum amount of restrictions as prescribed by the family physician. There must be understanding and skill in building the morale of those who feel inferior physically to prevent social and psychological handicaps.

The teacher and school have an important role to play in the public health program for prevention and control of heart disease.

DISCUSSION QUESTIONS AND ACTIVITIES

1. Discuss how heart problems can affect the social, emotional, and physical aspects of a child's life.

---

[9]Leland M. Corliss, Mildred E. Doster, and Gertrude E. Cromwell: "Summary Analysis of Recorded Incidence, Amount of Medical Care, and Follow-through on Organic Heart Disease in 95,000 Pupils." *J. Sch. Health 34*:181–184, 1964. Excellent bibliography.

2. Make a transparency, showing the heart in detail, that corresponds to the age level interest of the class. Then, demonstrate to the class how the heart works.
3. Discuss the significance of a heart murmur.
4. Discuss how rheumatic fever could develop in association with a sore throat.
5. Discuss the cooperation needed between the teaching personnel and the physician in the case of heart problems.
6. Discuss the importance of referral for the teacher.
7. Discuss the provision that can be made with the physical education teacher regarding a student with heart problems. Is total abstinence from physical activity necessary in all cases?
8. Discuss the progressive differences between heartbeat of a newborn and heartbeat of a high school senior.
9. Discuss how you would handle a class that mocked a student who had heart disease and was restricted in physical activity.
10. Learn the proper way of taking blood pressure and heartbeat. Try it on two or three people.

ADDITIONAL SOURCES OF INFORMATION

READINGS

Alpert, N. R. (ed.): *Cardiac Hypertrophy.* New York: Academic Press, 1971.
American Heart Association (National, state, or local affiliates): Excellent educational materials on murmurs, rheumatic fever, heart disease. American Medical Association: Department of Health Education.
Gaylor, G. G.: "Benefits From Mass Evaluation of Schoolchildren for Heart Disease." *Chest* 58:349–351, October, 1970.
Heintze, C.: *The Priceless Pump: The Human Heart.* New York: T. Nelson, 1972.
Longmore, D.: *The Heart.* New York: McGraw-Hill, 1971.
Morse, R. L.: *Exercise and the Heart: Guidelines for Exercise Programs.* Springfield, Ill.: Charles C Thomas, 1972.
Phibbs, B.: *The Human Heart: A Guide to Heart Disease.* St. Louis: The C. V. Mosby Co., 1971.
U.S. Department of Health, Education, and Welfare: Publications on various heart problems.

MATERIALS FOR TEACHERS' USE IN SCHOOLS

AUDIOVISUAL MATERIALS

Recommended grade levels are designated *pri, int, jh, sh.*

		Circulation	
17 min.	Color	*jh, sh*	Universal Education and Visual Arts*

*For addresses of film companies see Appendix A.

Circulation and the Human Body

11 min. Color *jh, sh* Churchill Films

Shows the processes of circulation, supplying the body cells from capillaries to the heart.

The following films are often available from boards of health and are usually in the library of the local affiliate of the American Heart Association:

Better Odds for Longer Life

19½ min. Color *jh,sh*

Functions of heart and circulatory system, diseases of heart. What you can do to reduce risk of heart attack. Animated. Excellent.

Circulation

16 min. Black and White *sh* Universal Education and Visual Arts

Animated.

Circulation of the Blood

8½ min. Color *jh, sh* Churchill Films

Animated film. Popular use.

Common Heart Disorders and Their Causes

17 min. Black and White *jh, sh*

Congenital Heart Defects

9 min. Color *jh, sh*, teachers

Excellent presentation of normal heart action and explanation of common congenital defects.

Rheumatic Heart Disease

8 min. Color *sh*, teachers Churchill Films

Scientifically accurate description of disease. Discussion of prophylaxis.

Smoking and Heart Disease

9½ min. Color *jh, sh*

Animated. Discusses relation of smoking to circulation.

Chapter 13

JUVENILE DIABETES MELLITUS

Every teacher at some time will have a diabetic in his classroom. It is estimated that one child in 2500 under the age of 15 suffers from this metabolic disturbance. National surveys suggest that there are more than 2,500,000 diabetics in the United States today. About 5 to 8 per cent of these are children.

Teachers and administrators should be acquainted with known diabetics in the school; indeed, it is a parent's responsibility to discuss the management of his child with someone in authority. Teachers can watch for unusual behavior patterns; they can assist a youngster with his adjustments to restrictions; they will cooperate with the family.

PHYSIOLOGY

Basic Explanation

Diabetes mellitus, frequently referred to as "sugar diabetes," is a disease in which there is a disturbance of carbohydrate metabolism because of insulin deficiency or inability to utilize insulin, characterized by an increase of glucose in the blood and urine. Predisposition to diabetes is inherited as a recessive mendelian trait. The biochemical aspects are actually quite complicated and to some extent unknown. It is a metabolic disease in which the glucose produced from the digestive action on carbohydrates cannot be utilized effectively. Insulin, a hormone secreted by specialized cells in the pancreas, found in the islands of Langerhans, is necessary for the transformation of glucose to glycogen. This is stored in tissues as a reserve and can be changed back to glucose when needed, in the presence of insulin. Ordinarily, with ample amounts of insulin, glucose is readily oxidized into carbon dioxide and water, producing energy in the process. Glucose can be used directly without insulin but is utilized more efficiently if the hormone is present. Without insulin the processes of carbohydrate metabolism, although not ceasing entirely, proceed very slowly. Glucose then accumulates in the body. Glucose is often referred to as sugar. In diabetes, secretion of insulin is diminished.

Insulin was discovered in 1921.

There is no known cure for diabetes mellitus. It is a lifetime disease. Injections of insulin merely supplement insulin produced in the pancreas and do not stimulate it to increased activity. There is no substitute as yet for insulin. Scientists are investigating the use of an oral medication as a substitute for injected insulin; but results so far are inconclusive. This disease has become the butt of quackery, and occasionally parents and children or adult diabetics, tired of the daily schedule of injections and dietary restrictions, succumb to the persuasion of cultists. If the diabetes is severe, the results can be fatal.

Diabetes in childhood can be quite severe. Once diagnosed by the physician, the child is placed upon a fairly strict regimen which involves dietary regulations, frequent examination of urine for glucose, and, most likely, injections of insulin. If the diabetes is mild, a balanced carbohydrate diet may be sufficient. There are occasional cases in which a diabetic is given a free selection of food, but care must be taken to cover it with insulin. Under such circumstances, very close supervision is mandatory. In all instances extensive education of parents and of the patient himself, if old enough, is undertaken by the physician, the nurse, and possibly by the dietitian. The whole family needs to understand the physiological and psychological problems involved. It is surprising how the parents and the child concerned become authorities and are self-confident about diet, insulin dosage, and warning signs. One can learn a great deal about nutrition and treatment from an intelligent mother of a diabetic. It must be kept in mind, however, that some parents experience a sense of shame; there may be overprotection or rejection.

Acidosis

With the diminution in amount of insulin and accumulation of glucose in the body, fat and protein are utilized in more than usual amounts as sources of energy. Intermediate products of fat metabolism, diacetic acid and acetone, may be produced in excess and accumulate in the blood stream; if excessive, they are likely to produce a condition called acidosis.

Acidosis develops slowly and gradually, producing significant changes in behavior. It would be a rare mishap for a serious complication, such as coma, to occur at school. An observing, suspicious mother will keep her child at home for the day. At school every teacher who is in contact with a diabetic child needs to remain alert and never give him the benefit of a doubt. *The warning signals of impending diabetic coma* develop slowly, may be confusing at first, but finally are striking. These signs may be flushed cheeks, deep, sighing respirations, possible nausea and vomiting, dry mouth and skin, apathy and inattention, and, above all, increasing drowsiness. If asked to walk, the child may not only appear stuporous, but may stagger, be disoriented and incoherent, and resemble a drunken individual. If his condition has developed thus far, coma and eventually death may be the end results.

Insulin Reaction

Another type of comatose condition is also possible. If too much insulin is present in the blood stream and there is an insufficient amount of glucose to be oxidized, the blood sugar level becomes too low and an insulin reaction, sometimes referred to as insulin shock, may develop. Among other causes, this condition commonly occurs when an insulin injection has been taken, and the meal which it was to cover, often breakfast, has been skipped or has been inadequate. An older diabetic is usually familiar with the early signs and symptoms of excessive insulin and can correct it himself with the sweets he carries—candy, lump sugar, raisins, an orange. With an *insulin reaction* the child notices sudden weakness; he looks sick, is strikingly pale, nervous, acutely hungry, breaks out in a profuse sweat, or feels that he is in a cold sweat, may be drowsy and inattentive, may even tremble and have mild convulsive seizures; he may be dizzy, feel lightheaded, and lack coordination in walking; he may only show irritability and belligerence; he may finally drop into a coma. An insulin reaction can develop quickly, particularly after excessive exercise.

The preceding descriptions of comatose conditions may breed undue anxiety, but there is reassurance in the fact that there is still time for action early in a coma, and panic should be avoided. Most diabetic children know the common early signs of an insulin reaction.

DETECTION

The onset of diabetes mellitus in children and young adults is relatively sudden. Detection may be incidental during the periodic health examination if a parent is accustomed to taking the children to a physician at regular intervals. A urinalysis, including a test for sugar, is part of that examination. Or, a youngster may be ill and undernourished and present some or all of the usual warning signs of diabetes. These are: frequent and copious urination, abnormal thirst, rapid loss of weight, hunger, weakness, fatigue, and drowsiness.

School surveys may reveal an occasional unknown diabetic. A simple glucose test is done on a urine specimen voided preferably two hours after a high caloric, high carbohydrate meal. All positive glucose tests are followed up by a physician. A positive test is only a clue and is not diagnostic of diabetes. Positive test which are not due to diabetes are common in children, but subsequent tests of various types are conducted under medical consultation. Although hundreds of the urine tests will show no sugar, a single case of diabetes detected early is worth all the efforts of the survey.

A rapid, simple blood glucose test is also used in both individual and mass screening. However, since blood must be taken from the child, parental consent for the procedure is necessary. The blood test is more accurate and predictive. Failing a permit from the parent, a urine test may be done.

MANAGEMENT OF THE JUVENILE DIABETIC AT SCHOOL

The parents should notify the school directly that their child has diabetes. If he is relied upon to tell the teacher, this may not be done. Some diabetics wear special metal tags to indicate a diagnosis.

A teacher or principal may find it helpful, especially with a younger diabetic, to confer with the child's parents at the beginning of each school year. In some instances, a conference among parents, school nurse, physician, and teacher will be advisable.

The alert teacher quietly watches a diabetic child and talks to him frankly about his problems, if he wishes it. A teacher observes any deviations of behavior which make him suspect drowsiness. A teacher *should never attempt under any circumstances to determine the basic cause of a comatose condition. There is no need to assume any responsibility for diagnosis or treatment. His first duty is to call the parent; and failing this contact, he should call the physician,* whose name should *always* be available for reference in every case, describe the clinical picture, and receive instructions as to procedure. A child should never be given any sugar or other sweet food upon a parent's request. A coma or impending coma is definitely a medical emergency and demands prompt attention. Untreated coma can result in death.

With the preceding physiological explanation of diabetes, it follows that any demand for increased energy may upset the glucose-insulin balance. For instance, growth itself, infections, such as the common cold, exercise, and emotional disturbances and tensions can create needs for more energy. Diabetics react differently to these demands. Whereas one student may strive unsuccessfully to keep up regular physical education activities, another with the same handicap may be unrestricted. Some students have too much insulin immediately after exercise because of depletion of supplies of glucose and glycogen and will usually eat food at an earlier time. For this reason, it is recommended that physical education classes be scheduled *after lunch*. Infections are threats, but some diabetics take them in their stride. Each case is handled on its merits; there is no generalization; the attending physician is the advisor.

If his diabetes is controlled adequately, the youngster should require no allowances. A teacher should not be unnecessarily solicitous, nor focus the attention of the class upon this child. He does need help, however, in order to become a well-adjusted individual. Normal play and associations should be permitted and encouraged. It is sometimes pathetic to watch the eagerness and joy of a child who is being given the special treat of a piece of birthday cake; nevertheless, he should be treated in matter-of-fact fashion. He should maintain a feeling of adequacy at all times. The best results are achieved in a well-adjusted family where good control of living habits is exercised.

The uncontrolled diabetic can become a source of worry, even at school. He does not adhere to a restricted regimen, lapses from his diet, fails to take insulin, or may be the victim of indifferent parents. He may not understand the nature of his disease, or he may be exposed to severe tensions or unhappiness at home. It is estimated that one third of the children with frequent acidosis come from broken homes where the parents are either divorced or separated, or from families where the mother works.

The diabetic child tends to be introspective. With the constant care necessary, restrictions on diet, frequent urine examinations at home, blood sugar determinations by the laboratory, daily injections of insulin, and occasional hospitalization, it is remarkable that he is an otherwise normal individual.

The diabetic may show irritability when he is hungry and has to wait until mealtime. He may express anger and hostility and complain about the monotony of his diet. He may flare out in self-pity and frustration because the future holds no promise of cure, and because he feels different from others.

Summer camps for diabetics are scattered around the country. They offer an opportunity for supervised recreation and at the same time give parents a well-deserved rest. They teach the diabetic that he has plenty of company and that with a controlled regimen, he can live a normal life.

Counseling the Diabetic. The preadolescent diabetic child is usually amenable to medical control and adjusts well to his living conditions. His mother selects his food and gives him his injections. The adolescent has personally assumed more dietary responsibility and usually administers his own injections. With his natural rebellions he frequently offers a problem to himself, his parents, his physician, and the school. He wants to eat what the gang eats and will not accept his handicap. He may have been excessively regimented and is defiant and resentful of advice. Encouragement and understanding on the part of school personnel may tide him over this crucial time of activity, growth, and expanding social relations. In all instances, however, the young diabetic should be considered a normal, growing, healthy individual.

Adolescent diabetics need to be assured repeatedly concerning their growth and development and normal functions, possibilities of parenthood, and any restrictions in the selection of a career. They need to be reassured that they face the same problems as their peer group, and self-dramatization will only exaggerate groundless fears. Except for jobs which might create a hazard to a diabetic or to the public as a result of possible insulin reaction, the whole vocational field of business or industry can be surveyed with his qualifications in mind. "With modern-day management of diabetes, there is every reason for the diabetic boy or girl to approach the possibility of marriage secure in the knowledge that he or she will be every bit as good a partner as the non-diabetic, physically, emotionally, socially, and intellectually."[1]

Health knowledge surveys reveal that some juvenile diabetics, many parents, and many apprehensive teachers are not acquainted with diabetes mellitus. Compliance and cooperation on the part of the child or young adult as well as understanding observation and guidance by parents and teachers can be promoted by the educational efforts of physician and school nurse.

SUMMARY

One or more diabetics may be present in a school. A teacher must understand the basic problem of juvenile diabetes in order to relieve his own apprehension and to cooperate with parent, child, and physician. A sympathetic understanding of the social and psychological problems of the diabetic enables a teacher to contribute to the welfare of a student.

DISCUSSION QUESTIONS AND ACTIVITIES

1. Make a chart comparing the symptoms and manifestations of diabetic coma and insulin shock.
2. Contact the American Diabetes Association to see what literature is available to prospective teachers.
3. Explain the need for close contact among parents, school nurse, and teacher in the case of a diabetic student.
4. Discuss the first aid treatment for diabetic coma.

---

[1]Henry Dolger and Bernard Seeman: *How to Live with Diabetes.* Revised edition. New York: Pyramid Books, 1966, p. 147.

5. Discuss the problems of adjustment for an adolescent recently discovered to be a diabetic. What habits must be established or broken?

ADDITIONAL SOURCES OF INFORMATION

READINGS

American Diabetes Association, Inc.: "Facts About Diabetes." 1966.
Bashell, B. R.: *The Diabetic at Work and Play.* Springfield, Ill.: Charles C Thomas, 1971.
Cole, H. S., and Camenini-Davalas, R.: *International Symposium on Early Diabetics.* New York: Academic Press, 1970.
Jackson, W. P.: "Racial and Geographical Factors in Diabetes." *Lancet* 1:601–602, March 20, 1971.
McEvedy, M. B.: "Inheritance of Diabetes." *Brit. Med. J.* 1:458–459, February 20, 1971.
Orzeck, E. A.: "Diabetes Detection with a Comparison of Screening Methods." *Diabetes* 20:109–116, February, 1971.
Today's Health:
"Are You a Hidden Diabetic?" 44:86, 1966.
Kaye, L.: "Camping for Diabetic Youngsters." 43:50–53, 1965.
"Taking the Danger Out of Diabetes." 43:56–57, 1965.

MATERIALS FOR TEACHERS' USE IN SCHOOLS

AUDIOVISUAL MATERIALS

Diabetes and You, Too

21 min. Color *sh* Int. Film Bureau*

Early identification of diabetes. Story of a 15-year-old diabetic.

Diabetics Unknown

29 min. Black and White *jh, sh,* adults Public Affairs Film Library
State Boards of Health

Goals: detect unknown cases, teach people early signs of diabetes, overcome apprehension, persuade them to have tests. Describes early signs and treatment.

RESOURCES

American Diabetes Association
Health education materials. Publishes *Forecast*, a bimonthly publication for diabetics and their families.

American Dietetic Association
Diets, printed materials.

American Medical Association
Department of Health Education

U. S. Department of Health, Education, and Welfare
Public Health Service. Publications on Diabetes mellitus.

---

*For addresses of film companies see Appendix A.

Chapter 14

EMOTIONAL PROBLEMS

INTRODUCTION

"Mental health is that emotional adjustment in which a person can live with reasonable comfort, functioning acceptably in the community in which he lives. The mentally healthy person is for the most part able to handle his emotions and cope acceptably with situations in his environment. The pupil who shows unacceptable behavior may be showing signs of emotional stress and may need specialized help."[1]

An emotionally healthy individual is one who appreciates his own worth and has a strong sense of responsibility toward others. In considering the whole child, emotional as well as physical health problems must be detected and handled. An emotionally disturbed youngster, or one who is poorly adjusted in his social relationships, may be more severely handicapped than if he had a known physical ailment.

How does the individual, as a personality, reach optimum health and strength? The keynote to a good emotional adjustment is a feeling of security. The time to start is the moment the child is born. His basic tissue needs, shown by hunger, thirst, and rest are fundamental, but beyond these he also needs *love, acceptance, security, protection, independence, faith, guidance,* and *control.*[2] Every child needs to be loved, to be wanted, and to feel secure during his early dependent years. He needs to feel worthy, confident of himself, and have confidence in others. Within this warm framework he also needs to be guided and controlled and yet be able to grow towards independence. He needs to acquire a set of values which will enable him to accept his relationships in society.

---

[1]Report of the Committee on Mental Health in the Classroom, American School Health Association: *J. Sch. Health* 38(No. 5a), May, 1968.

[2]The National Association for Mental Health, Inc.: "What Every Child Needs for Good Mental Health." Pamphlet.

"The major source of personality growth for the child resides in the maturity and harmony of his parents; hence parents inevitably provide the model which the child consciously and unconsciously emulates. In short, the effect of training on personality is a matter of the continuous, persistent influences with which the child comes in daily contact."[3]

A child's emotional development is measured to a great extent by his behavior.

DEVELOPMENTAL PATTERNS AT VARIOUS LEVELS OF GROWTH

Tables 1 and 2, pp. 32–35

Infancy

A feeling of closeness is important. If the infant can develop in a world relatively free of the pangs of fear, if he can find trust and security from the people with whom he is in contact, and similarly find comfort in his environment, then he can relax and be at peace. He can devote his energies to growing. When he cries, he can be held and reassured. The feeling tones in the home are warm, and he feels loved, wanted, and secure. Any jarring note, either in quarreling, worry or tension, is sensed by a baby even when he has no comprehension of the spoken word or of adult environment. Infants thrive not only on food but on loving care. Both are necessary. Babies in institutions who are given scientific formulas but no individual attention grow up very poorly. It has been demonstrated that loving attention, reassurance, and snuggling from a nurse, an attendant, or a constant visitor produce surprising improvement in a lonesome waif. The infant who is happy, peaceful, and loved is ready for the next stage of growth.

Preschool

The child is beginning to cruise; he explores himself and his surroundings and has a truly new awareness of himself and of others. Trusting his human contacts and his environment, he wants to be a person in his own right, asserting himself and his independence. He wants to button his own clothes, feed himself, climb, touch, run, do what he wants to do. He wants freedom; he wants to find himself; but he still wants to be loved and to feel safe. He will want to be held

---

[3]Harold W. Bernard: *Human Development in Western Culture.* Second edition. Boston: Allyn and Bacon, Inc. 1966, p. 91.

close when he is tired or hurt, and can even sense the security which comes by being near those who stand for love and safety.

After about three years of age, he is aware of himself as an individual; he may be ready to branch out. He observes what others do in the family; he likes to imitate. He asks questions and likes to act out adult roles, especially those which are part of his family. Brother likes to watch his father shave, while sister tries to make cakes alongside of mother. Identification is important. Little girls need good identification with their female role; little boys need to find their places as males, according to the culture in which they will later assume full membership.

The preschool training period is important in establishing emotional adequacy. Readiness for school is important for success in school. A child should be socially ready for this new experience. He has related himself to home and to his peers in the neighborhood; now he should be able to participate in give-and-take associations at school.

Even though the emotional needs of children are similar, variations in progress occur. A sensitive mother of several children will observe that each child develops his own personality. He is himself. One child may need to be held for long periods of time, will get off his parent's lap for a short period of time to explore some area, and then clamber back to the enclosing arm. Another child will shrug off a hug and escape to play. Each needs to be accepted, appreciated, and trusted. Each needs to feel strong within himself. He needs to have the feeling that all is well.

Some children are full of energy and attack every experience with zeal. Others are quiet and observant. Some are sensitive to life; others are obtuse. Just as there are variations in patterns of physical growth, there are variations in emotional growth. No two children are necessarily handled alike.

Elementary Grades

Entering school may be as traumatic an experience as weaning, unless a child is ready. Elementary teachers need to recognize the importance of this experience. In being sent to school a child should not feel that he is being rejected at home. Some children are perfectly ready for school; others are not.

Entry into school is based upon chronological age. Normal patterns of emotional maturity vary widely. A child may be six years old and perfectly normal but still be too immature to bridge the gap between home and school. He should be kept home another year. His parents should understand that such a postponement would not be a reflection upon them nor the youngster. One school psychologist relates the incident of a mother who sat each morning for four months outside the door of the first-grade room to reassure her little boy who walked out every hour to make certain she was still there. That child had not been socially weaned. Parents should "give up" their children in preschool days and provide them with many experiences which will prepare them for the give-and-take relationship at school. Emotional maturity is necessary for success in school.

School systems should resist the pressure of parents who are anxious to start their children in kindergarten at an early age. This has its disadvantages, for the youngsters come to school with inadequate social skills and are so immature that the teacher is occupied with control of behavior rather than teaching unless curriculum changes are made.

In the first three grades a child is learning basic skills. He becomes interested early in social studies through the avenues open to him today—television, magazine pictures, and even newspapers. He begins to develop concepts early. Next to the parent, the teacher is the most important person in his life. A pupil learns to identify with the teacher; he is entitled to a friendly, well-adjusted teacher. Problems at school at this age may result from (1) illness, which makes him feel insecure, (2) inability to share, (3) disturbances arising from separation from home, and (4) unhappy homes.

In the third or fourth grade, a child is introduced to an increasingly complex curriculum in the social sciences and other subject areas and to subjects which involve more abstract concepts. A wider world is opened to him, and he asks questions. The customs and living habits of other countries and other parts of his own country challenge his curiosity and his way of life. If the Chinese eat rice almost exclusively, why don't we? Eskimos do not eat vegetables; how do they get their vitamins? Some countries have presidents, some have kings. Why?

Beginning about the third grade, there is identification with the peer group—the gang stage. What the gang says and does is of paramount importance. The gang's beliefs and activities may challenge or put a strain on the family relationships.

Curriculum planning ought to be based upon emotional development at these ages. Frequently it is based upon key concepts or organizational schemes of the several academic disciplines. Unless the teacher remains sensitive to the pupil's emotional maturity, the rigors of the school tasks, so based, can result in anxiety and frustration. Wisely handled, these intellecual challenges can open a whole new world that is healthful and stimulating. There is release of pent-up energies through self-expression in skills. The child needs to experience successes all along the way in order to sustain his interest and to develop his self-confidence. He needs to have a fine feeling of accomplishment. He needs to repeat and repeat until he is good at track events and at riding a bicycle. He collects the most butterflies and bugs. Girls jump rope and play hopscotch by the hour.

Children whose patterns of physical growth and emotional maturity are slower may be faced with dangerous situations. Developmental delay in learning can produce grave problems in emotional, social, and educational adjustment. A girl or boy who cannot follow the leader of the gang, or one who "cries like a baby" or is slow at acquiring skills, feels a sense of criticism or failure and may tend to withdraw from the group. This is a danger signal. Children who do not hear or see well, or belong to groups with different cultural or religious backgrounds, will run into difficulties with their peers. A boy or girl who cannot see the batted ball soon enough to catch it will not be selected for a team. Children who have not played much with others, who have suffered upsetting experiences before entering school, or who for various reasons have been objects of derision of their classmates—these children need help in order to adjust to school life.

Children do not like to be different from their classmates. Those who have been teased or laughed at can suffer emotional upsets which leave scars for years. Any deviation in appearance, such as strabismus, harelip, red hair, or a limp, may provoke ridicule. An irrelevant answer from a hard-of-hearing child, a stuttering response, reading and learning difficulties—these can make a child upset, unhappy, and hate school. Children who are harassed with too many extraclass activities which fill all of their days can begin to fidget, chew on their nails, look pale and tired, and suffer from chronic fatigue. When parents exert pressure for superior academic achievement of their young and set standards too high for their children's abilities ("if you make all A's, you can have a bicycle"), or when there is a rigid upbringing with unexpressed resentment, the result can be psychological chaos. A broken home may arouse a sense of shame and daydreams to bring the parents together.

So many problems beset children. They need help in order to live in peace. Much of this help can come from understanding teachers. Good schools and good teachers are alert to help each youngster achieve skills and some triumphs. A good teacher observes the interests of each child, whether scholastic, social, or with tools, and helps him to self-respect and self-confidence. A child must believe in himself and feel that he is important. Otherwise, he turns his back on others and their opinions.

"Ideally, each child should be educated according to his ability to learn so that he may experience the sense of satisfaction which comes with success. For the superior child this would require classes in which he would have the opportunity for more intense study and work in wider fields; for the dull child, classes in which he could learn good work habits and progress at his own rate; for the creative child, classes in which he could become competent in his special area of interest; for the hard of hearing, the blind, and others, classes specially suited to their handicaps."[4]

---

[4]Harry Bakwin and Ruth Morris Bakwin: *Behavior Disorders in Children.* Third edition. Philadelphia; W. B. Saunders Company, 1966, p. 340.

Adolescence

With junior and senior high school students, new problems arise. There are rapid changes in mental and emotional life. Physically, boys and girls are experiencing quite a spurt in growth. Sexual maturation is taking place. Interest in the opposite sex is gradually developed. Dating and courtship patterns are being established. Many couples are married before graduation yet may elect to continue school. These young people have already accepted responsibilities and usually are sobered into a more mature emotional pattern.

Adolescence is a time of transition when a youth looks to the future and anticipates his place in an adult society. The basic needs are still the same. If they have been met all along the way, he should have been prepared for a mature life. A failure to meet these needs will show up more at this time. A pattern which has been developing for years may not be detected until the teens, when the youngster is now a big boy or a big girl, and abnormal behavior is more noticeable. Undesirable behavior patterns do not occur spontaneously with the onset of adolescence. A boy of 17 insists that his mother accompany him to the dentist's office; she leaves him there for a short while to attend to an errand; he throws a temper tantrum. Such behavior did not develop suddenly; it is noticeable because we do not expect a 17-year-old to act like a child of three. A personality disorder in an adult is the result of a progressively developing condition which should have been identified in his earlier personality and behavior.

Since birth a child has been driving towards independence. During adolescence the drive is dominant; still, he is dependent. He is dependent for shelter, clothes, food, medical care, and money. With a physical handicap he is even more dependent. He needs the warmth of love and understanding from his oftentimes bewildered parents. He still needs to belong to the family. However, through increased socialization, he is influenced by his peers, his teachers, and others outside the home. He adopts new patterns and shows them at home. A boy or girl at this age is sensitive to group thinking and actions, develops fads in dressing, haircuts, eating, and social behavior. Independent thinking on religion, politics, or any other aspect of life may produce conflicts at home. Parents may demand too much and increase responsibilities to the point of resentment—a sober adult pattern of behavior, too much care and supervision of younger children in the family, too much housekeeping, too many chores.

The raucous laugh, sarcastic remarks, and arguments are not necessarily to be interpreted as brashness or resistance to learning. Rather, they often serve to cover up a young person's feelings of inadequacy and may be his cry for direction without his admission that he needs help.

Young people still need overall direction and fulfillment of basic needs at home and school. They need freedom to make their own decisions and must have time for living their own lives. Such provisions require a nice balance which can be discussed glibly but is not so easy to carry out in everyday living.

Serious problems at this age develop from an insecure background in childhood. If an adolescent has not felt secure or developed self-confidence, the lack will show up in personality problems.

Contributing seriously to this insecure background and creating confusion is lack of self-identification. A child must know who and what he is. With the living patterns today in an urban society, as a child grows up identification is often quite difficult. When father leaves home early for work and comes home late after traveling for miles, and when his weekends are devoted to the golf course and other adult pursuits away from home, children do not have the opportunity to associate with the leading male in the family. When mother goes to work also, and occupies all of her attention at home in catching up on housekeeping, the problem of identification is compounded. With a divorce in the family, or the death of a father, a boy may have no opportunity to know closely an adult male unless he is fortunate to have an understanding older brother, uncle, grandfather, or brother-in-law. Girls also need to have fathers and mothers and understand their own roles in society.

Division of a child's emotional growth by school level is to a small degree arbitrary. And there will be overlapping of behavior patterns. Some youngsters are more sophisticated at an earlier age. Some are still somewhat immature at graduation from high school. Nevertheless, the discussion on emotional growth describes development in general. Cultural influences and educational media have modified the patterns. Television viewing has promoted greater knowledge and sophistication. This observation is important to teachers; in fact, teaching is not the same as it was a generation ago. New curriculum materials are being introduced, and methods of teaching are being altered. Family living has changed in many homes. When the mother and father work and have little time to spend with their children, when baby sitters and nursery school teachers are the most intimate contacts, when children are familiar with only one parent because of a broken home, when story plots on television impress a kaleidoscope of cultural ideas, one can expect alterations of emotional developmental patterns. Lack of self-identity and gradual stabilized growth, and failure to appreciate sexuality can be associated with today's living.

MENTAL HEALTH PROGRAM AT SCHOOL

Emotional development follows a general pattern from infancy to adulthood. This development, however, is not necessarily a matter of chronological age. There are variations at each age level. Children vary in their capacity to withstand discipline and the pressures of living. Every child, regardless of whether he is handicapped, has his own basic needs and must be understood as an individual. Every child has his own personal problems, whether it be a cleft palate, a chronic illness, a poor complexion, a history of prolonged hospitalization, a broken home, a knowledge of adoption, or a shiftless parent. There is not a single experience in his life that does not have emotional implications.

Detection of the Emotionally Handicapped

The school occupies the most strategic position in the mental health program because "public school services are available to all children in the community; public schools employ professional personnel educated to understand the personality development of children; the relationship of the school to its children is a natural and positive one; teachers have opportunity to work with parents; teachers observe children over a longer period of time and in agreater variety of situations than persons in any other profession; and schools employ mental health specialists to assist in providing services to the more vulnerable child and his family. Schools provide organized social experiences which have a powerful formative influence on the personality of the child."[5]

Moreover, the mental health of a child is of profound importance in the learning process. With it, he can develop his capacity for effective mental performance. Without it, his progress will be impaired, if not rendered impossible. The school does have a responsibility in the mental health program.

Common Deviations in Behavior Patterns

More children are entering school who are already emotionally disturbed. Some kindergarten children are actually being treated with tranquilizers, and others have developed sufficiently severe emotional problems to require placement in special classes. Even well-adjusted ones are subjected to pressures outside of school, especially in underprivileged areas of cities. Teachers are confronted with much more difficult behavior problems ranging from violence to complete withdrawal.

Except in flagrant cases there are no guideposts which may be marked in precise fashion to facilitate the detection of emotional illness. Teacher education institutions incorporate courses into the curriculum which give some understanding of children and their emotional development. This knowledge, coupled with sensitiveness, should enable a teacher to pick out the pupil who is emotionally

---

[5]Eli M. Bower, et al.: "A Process for Early Identification of Emotionally Disturbed Children." Bulletin of the California State Department of Education, August 1958, p. 1.

disturbed. If he studies a child, and knows the family and environmental influences, he should have no difficulty in assaying the child's emotional maturity. Teachers should be observant, understanding, and free from intolerance. They will gradually develop a sixth sense which rarely fails. An elementary child who begins to suck his thumb, or an adolescent who suddenly becomes boisterous and aggressive is suspect. A youngster may be overt in his actions to call attention to himself because he needs help. Sometimes the manifestations are more subtle. In the earlier grades under the constantly vigilant eye of a teacher, emotional difficulties should be detected early.

Adolescents are the neglected group. No one teacher or counselor has much contact with the older student. Since one expects expressions of independence, his behavior must be quite unusual before it is called to the attention of those in authority. Overt patterns of thievery, smoking and drinking, belligerence, refusal to join the groups, and disregard for school may be interpreted offhand as "juvenile delinquency," when actually a boy who expresses himself in this fashion may have been suffering from schizophrenia for several years. On the other hand, a student may show by his sulkiness, brooding, resentment, or withdrawal that he is responding to nagging, overdiscipline, or insecurity. Such a pattern does not necessarily indicate a psychosis, but it should be investigated. The death of a parent can produce sudden and marked personality changes. A handicapped individual may come to realize that he cannot achieve the usual adult potentials.

Listen to the students. They want to talk about their feelings toward their homes, their schools, and themselves. Sometimes children speak more with actions than with words. There are reasons for what they do. Watch them. What are their needs?

Common behavior signs which may lead a teacher to suspect emotional difficulties are:

1. Changes in appearance. An abrupt change to a constant slovenly, unkempt appearance, or the opposite, unusual neatness, leads one to suspect alterations in personality or in home influence.

2. Changes in attitudes towards one's self or towards other children. A child who has always been pleasant and cooperative may begin to push and shove others, grab the possessions of others, and refuse to eat his lunch. Inquiry into one such sudden change elicited a confession from a mother that a divorce was pending.

3. Behavior, such as:

   a. Excessive nervousness as shown by picking or biting cuticles or nails, constant fidgeting, tearfulness, and tics; worried expressions, reactions from anxiety, overtalkativeness, stuttering, voicing of fears or worries; outbursts of anger or sullen and resentful responses; excessive negativism shown often by deliberate dawdling, pretending not to hear, and complaints of inability to perform; repetitive actions, such as washing the hands again and again, going over the answers to examination questions again and again, clearing the throat each time before recitation.

b. Over-interest in sex matters or complete absence of interest.

c. Marked hostility to other children, bullying, destructiveness, derision of handicapped, excessive aggression. Deprecation of others makes one feel superior.

Cruelty is considered to be a serious disorder. A child enjoys hurting others and seeing them suffer. He lacks sympathy, and since cruelty is usually associated with cowardice, he picks on smaller children and helpless animals. He may have been subjected to torture himself, maybe through sadistic though righteous discipline on the part of his parents.

d. Anxiousness to secure approval.

e. Observations of rigid rituals in daily life. Everything must be just so. Articles around him must be in a certain order. Behavior repeats a rigid pattern. Serious obsessions and compulsions.

4. Unusual manner within the group. Is the child too withdrawn, too quiet, timid, or brash? Does a bright child deliberately underplay in order to avoid seeming superior to his peers? Is a child so far advanced in her work that she becomes bored and daydreams a great deal? Is she too conforming and docile in her manner?

5. Exhibitionism. Does the child call attention to himself by clowning, wisecracks, and being the "life of the party"? Conversely, one who is ignored by the group deserves attention.

6. Infantile behavior patterns, such as thumb-sucking, lip- or tongue-biting, lack of control of bladder and bowels, and temper tantrums.

7. Escape mechanisms, such as fantasies or daydreams occupying a large percentage of the child's time and energy. Fantasies of little children involve wishes to fulfill some immediate desire—a toy, a visit. In the preteenage group they usually concern self-glorification, an award, excellence in some sport. During adolescence, when the peak of daydreaming occurs, the process is an escape or produces a feeling of success and satisfaction.

These patterns need to be detected and evaluated. The child should be helped to find satisfactions in ordinary everyday living so that resort to escape mechanisms is unnecessary. Such fantasies should not be permitted to become a child's only means of coping with a problem.

8. The "smiling mask." A child does not express his feelings. Is the smile sincere, or does it serve as a mask? Can he relax, or is he always tense?

9. Preoccupation with use of drugs. Young people, even in junior high school, are experimenting with psychedelics, depressants, stimulants, glue sniffing, alcohol, and other drugs. Motivations involve curiosity, conformity to peer group practices, a desire to

escape from reality, or beliefs that one can understand one's self better and excel with his talents.

10. The "too good child" may begin to show a drastic change in personality, sometimes associated with temper tantrums. Heretofore, the child may have been characterized as a "perfect little lady" or a "real gentleman." Underneath the polite, obedient, friendly surface may simmer a rigid, immature, and even sadistic personality. The mildest criticism may provoke an outburst of tears, rage, or frustration. Children do not have reserves of maturity; and too heavy demands by teachers and parents on the "good," supposedly mature child, "older than his years," may break a dam of self-control, manifested as a temper tantrum. Do not exact adult personality patterns in a child. He has a right to be childish.

Suicidal Behavior

A 12-year-old boy, subject of a custodial battle between divorcing parents, is found hanging from a rafter in the garage. A senior in high school commits suicide. His closest friend contemplates taking his own life because of intense grief. Months later, he sobs as he relates the incident.

When a person takes his own life, or attempts and fails to do so, those in close contact cannot help but be affected. Teachers and parents of a teenager speculate: "Could I have anticipated this tragedy?" "Were there any warning signs?" "Why didn't I realize he needed help?"

Suicide is often a rational, even if unjustifiable act. Very few are explained by serious mental illness. About one half are linked with emotional instability. Suicidal behavior refers to threats and attempts at suicide. The ratio of attempts at suicide to a successful outcome is estimated from 120 to 50 attempts to one death. Statistics on attempts show a rise beginning at age 14; most occur between 3 p.m. and midnight. Almost six times as many girls attempt suicide as boys. Boys, however, are more aggressive and successful in their efforts. Their common means are firearms and hanging; girls tend to use poisons. Of course, many attempts are not reported or may not be suspected; therefore, statistics are not reliable.

The incidence of suicidal deaths for 1967 is reported as follows:*

	TOTAL	5-9 YEARS	10-14 YEARS	15-19 YEARS
Female	6,138	–	27	212
Male	15,187	–	94	624

*Public Health Service, National Center for Health Statistics.

Suicides rank fourth as a cause of death in youth of 15 to 19 years. Superseding causes are motor vehicle accidents, malignant neoplasms, and drowning. They occur more in young people in urban areas than rural, and more in families of professional people.

Signs of Depression. Little children do not have a realistic conception of death. Their fantasies involve running away, and they do run away. "You will be sorry when I am gone." They are often fearful of punishment or have been badly treated at home.

During the prepubescent period the depressive behavioral pattern may manifest such emotions or actions as temper tantrums, disobedience, truancy, feeling that no one cares, running away from home, and masochistic and self-destructive activities. A youngster feels rejected; he may not be permitted to identify with a loved one in the home; he protests against lack of parental guidance; he may consider himself as evil, bad, or unworthy—any of which may lead to unsocial behavior. He may feel inferior to his classmates. Boys, especially, may wish to hide any soft, sentimental feelings which may reflect upon their manliness.

The adolescent may show his depression by boredom, restlessness, outbursts of irritability, search for new avenues of excitement, delinquent behavior, psychosomatic illnesses, sexual promiscuity, and may even attempt to escape his feelings through the use of alcohol and drugs. He may complain of excessive fatigue, exhaustion, difficulty in concentration, and many hypochondriacal health problems. Adolescents who attempt or commit suicide may act because of fear of punishment, loss of self-esteem, thwarted ambition, or from a desire for revenge on a punishing parent, teacher, or other person in authority. Personal factors may be feelings of inferiority as a result of physical defects, hormonal and physical changes accompanying adolescence, worries concerning sexuality, sex experiences, social maladjustments, personality disorders, or low intelligence. Family clashes, difficulties with the opposite sex, fears of being unloved, failures at school, worries over school work, and anxieties concerning living up to expectations of parents are impelling forces. A youth who is unloved or thinks he is unloved, particularly if he has a physical handicap, may attempt suicide as a bid for more love. Life may seem unbearable and he may see no other way of handling a problem except by suicide.

The common denominator for suicidal behavior seems to be a disorganized home. Only about one third of these sufferers lived with their parents. Some were first children who may have had too much responsibility or too much blame, may have felt rejected or unloved with the advent of siblings. Those who actually commit suicide or make a serious attempt apparently cannot cope with parental indifference or rejection and lack of cooperation between home and school.

The suicidal note in an attempted suicide or suicide will probably provide a clue as to the underlying problem.

Suicidal Crisis. Only when the pressures of life become intolerable does a person contemplate suicide. This phase is referred to as a *suicidal crisis.*

Depression manifests itself in various ways and is the most constant sign of an impending disaster. Depression is common to all ages. It is often associated with insomnia.

Hopeless, profound despair in which the young person feels that life is no longer worthwhile is an overwhelming depressing emotion. It takes time to get over this feeling, and professional help should be secured.

Impulsive suicidal behavior is one type of crisis. It may precipitated by anger, disappointment, frustration, or a feeling of unworthiness. A boy, rejected by a girl friend, may use a firearm. A girl, after a quarrel with her parents, may swallow a quantity of pills or slash her wrists. This type of emotion is usually transient. If support can be given to a depressed youngster until the pressure passes, he can carry on. Suicidal crises are painful and acute.

The Teacher's Role. A threat or attempt at suicide is a *cry for help.* Eight out of ten people who kill themselves discuss their intent, and this talk is a warning sign which must be taken seriously. Even a half-hearted attempt at self-destruction indicates a desperate need for sympathy and understanding. Without help, more serious and efficient suicidal activity may follow.

"The suicidal child and adolescent are victims—whether of their early life experiences, their biochemical or chromosomal makeup, or the world around them is not yet clear. It is not your job to treat them, only to teach them. It will be unfortunate if they seek you out—and you ignore them."[6]

The teacher listens and spots the depressive reaction. He is acquainted with the background of most of his students. The counselor and the principal may know the student well. Warning signs may be there to be heeded.

For example: during a faculty discussion concerning a student who had committed suicide several days before by taking poison, an English teacher commented that the girl had recently written in an assigned theme such a vivid and moving description of her own exhaustion that she was awarded an A grade. It was evident that the teacher felt absolutely no sense of guilt that she had not acted to help the girl personally. To her the dead girl represented an A grade. How can any teacher, in any disciplinary area, be oblivious to the needs of a student as a human being!

Family, friends, and teachers who know a student well may give emergency assistance. Professional help should be requested without delay. Every effort should be made to get at the cause of the unhappiness and resolve the situation, if possible. Hospitalization may be necessary to remove the student from a trying situation; such a move

---

[6]Dean Schuyler: "When Was The Last Time You Took a Suicidal Child to Lunch?" *J. Sch. Health* 43:8:506, October, 1973.

will make him feel that his problems are being interpreted seriously. If there has been an attempt at suicide, the individual should be watched for at least 90 days after a suicidal crisis, to anticipate a repeated attempt.

Psychosomatic Problems

A disturbance in either physical or mental well-being produces many characteristics which at times are typical. Each affects the other until a vicious cycle is established. For instance, conflicts can produce inner tensions and personality changes which probably contribute to the development of an "ulcer" (duodenal ulcer). The resulting discomfort produces still more nervousness and tension which aggravates the ulcer. A youth whith acne becomes unhappy, self-conscious, and nervous, which worsens the complexion. A fat girl finds satisfaction in eating. A deafened person is shy. A disturbed, insecure youth begins to stutter. A child becomes excited and develops an asthmatic attack. The mental health aspects of various physical defects have been discussed and will be presented again in the next chapter.

Severe shock can produce unusual behavior patterns. A little boy of eight was confronted unexpectedly with a dead member of his family. He lost his power of speech (aphonia). He attended class, would touch people and smile in greeting. After a year some speech returned, but two years passed before he was able to speak freely again.

Follow-up

Not only can a well-trained, emotionally mature teacher anticipate and prevent emotional disturbances in his classroom, but he can handle most of them himself once they have appeared. He should know his limitations, however, and not do harm as an amateur psychologist. He may need to consult with the principal or guidance personnel in his school. It is good for a teacher to talk over the problems of his pupils with trained counselors. In this way he receives practical experience in guidance and can help an individual child. One approach to follow-up is to ask, "What does this child have in the way of assets?" Assess his abilities, his likeness to other children, and the areas in which he can be helped. In regard to the epileptic or the brain-damaged child or any afflicted child, think not only in terms of handicaps, but also in terms of positive assets.

Channels for more extensive follow-up are gradually being established in large school systems. In-service training is given to teachers and counselors by working with psychologists and psychiatrists, sometimes in workshops which involve these and other specialized personnel. For evaluation or consultation, or for referral of serious disturbances, a youngster may be sent to the school psychologist, the psychiatric social worker, or other designated consultant. The latter will have interviews with the boy or girl concerned, will call in parents for consultation, and proceed further as indicated. Interviews with parents should mirror humane and considerate attitudes with no hint of criticism. The social worker, the nurse—either the school or public health nurse—and the family doctor are valuable resource people. They can provide information and advice and make contact with the proper agencies in the community.

One must keep an additional fact in mind. Help for one child in the family usually has a beneficial effect on the mental health of siblings and parents.

Mental health programs are frequently well organized in large school systems and in cities, especially those containing medical schools. Administrators and counselors in schools should work effectively with personnel in child guidance centers or mental health clinics in the community. The principal, counselor, and referring teacher should have concern all the way through the follow-up and therapy, since the child is still in the school and in the classroom. Suggestions as to how they can cooperate will further the progress of that child. There may be an attempt made in group therapy for parents whose children have similar problems.

Education of the greatly disturbed child poses a problem. If funds are available for tuition in a private school, more attention under supervision of the child's psychiatrist is possible. In a large school system provisions may be made for these children to attend special schools or special classes in regular schools part-time. The last makes them part of the school community, enables them to share the routine of other children, distracts them for a while, yet spares the teachers the strain of keeping them the entire school day.

A child who returns from hospitalization for emotional problems needs special attention. Planned experiences which culminate in success and praise offer proof of worthiness. This self-estimate is vital. Acceptance by the peer group is important. Physical activities through games draw him away from introspection and offer an opportunity for achievement.

The whole mental health program is still being expanded. Organized assistance and federal funds are increasingly available. In some rural districts, facilities for consultation are being taken to the communities. Traveling or itinerant clinics consisting of a psychiatrist, clinical psychologists, and psychiatric social workers have visiting schedules to distant areas, sometimes reporting as often as once a week. They can help with evaluations, give advice for guidance of parents and school personnel, and even offer direct psychotherapy on a weekly or semi-monthly basis. These clinics may be sponsored by medical schools, departments of health, or private organizations. Sometimes other specialists travel with them, such as audiologists and speech therapists. More clinics of this type are sorely needed.

The problems involved are finances, lack of trained personnel, and public ignorance.

It is estimated that one school psychiatrist or psychologist should be available for 2000 children and youth; one counselor should be provided for each 250 (White House Conference on Children and Youth, 1960).

Health Education – Mental Health in the Classroom

Promotion of good mental health and prevention of emotional disturbances in children should be paramount objectives of the school program.

"Hopefully all children will have a solid background to work from as they tackle the social and academic challenges of school and of life in general. Most children will learn to cope with these challenges without our help and without long-lasting emotional scars. It is our thesis that we can help them handle emotions by making them a legitimate part of the curriculum in health education."[7] Teachers have a major responsibility for the personality and character development of each child.

Approaches towards development of a healthy personality are:

1. Provide the basic needs of children. Feeling secure and feeling that one is important to one's self and to others are fundamental emotional needs. Children must develop a sense of responsibility towards others. They need kindly direction which does not threaten their growing independence.

2. The emotional climate of the school and the classroom should evoke a feeling of warmth and security. A sensitive person can frequently judge the predominant feeling of a school by walking through the halls. A principal who is a rigid disciplinarian will breed a cowering fear. Every teacher has an effect on a youth's personality, intentionally or unintentionally. Some teachers are emotionally unfit for the classroom. A teacher who is ridden by fears or worries, or is suffering pain, or is much disturbed and poorly adjusted himself can produce a class of nervous, tense, fearful children. They are entitled to happy, well-adjusted, understanding adults in their school environment.

3. The physical environment of the school and the classroom should encourage peace of mind and relaxation as well as opportunity for activity. Beauty is necessary in all lives. Well-landscaped yards which stir a child's pride and welcome him to the doors of the school, well-lighted, pleasantly decorated halls and rooms, adequate ventilation and heating, potted plants on the window sills, lively little animals in the elementary classrooms – all of these make a child comfortable in his home away from home.

---

[7]Herb Jones: "Exploring Emotions with Young Children." *Sch. Health Rev.* *4*:4:19, July/August, 1973.

4. Guidance and counseling of parents are necessary so that they may understand and help an emotionally handicapped child. Such an effort involves at least the teacher and principal, and psychiatric counselors at either school or community levels.

5. A well-planned mental health program and curriculum which is designed to help the child understand his physical and emotional changes at all ages will give him the knowledge and insight for handling his own personal problems and for living harmoniously with others.

Tables 1 and 2 at the end of Chapter 2 list the emotional, social, and intellectual characteristics and needs of children and youth. As the eyes scan the page, a teacher notices the pattern changes with increase in age. Such information can form the basis for a program of mental health in the classroom.

SUMMARY

Emotional development and physical development represent two interrelating aspects of a child. Teachers are familiar with the accepted, usual emotional behavior patterns at various age levels. Deviations from normal patterns should not be difficult to detect. A teacher needs to identify the maladjusted personality early, in order to secure help for the child. Occasionally, a severe depression culminates in suicidal behavior. Some description of the latter is offered here. Psychosomatic problems occur frequently.

Various mental health programs are followed in managing the child who is seriously disturbed. These depend upon the professional personnel and facilities in the community. Management involves directly the teacher, principal, counselor, parent, and private physician (with help at times from the school nurse or social worker) to secure professional guidance from private, school, or community services.

DISCUSSION QUESTIONS AND ACTIVITIES

1. Discuss the teacher's role in referring a suspected emotionally disturbed child. Should he follow up this referral?

2. Keep a record of your "ups and downs" for a week and record the actions you take to alleviate the "downs."

3. Discuss the factors that make the adolescent susceptible to mood changes and feelings of helplessness.

4. Discuss the indications that a person may be considering suicide. Have you ever thought of committing this act? If so, what made you realize your life's worth?

5. Discuss the reasons for approaching mental health from a positive point of view. Are there times when one's viewpoint on mental health should be negative?

6. Describe what depression means to you and the different levels of depression.

7. Discuss what you would believe to be the most desirable suggestions that one could offer you when you are in a bad mood.

8. Discuss the teacher's influence on the promotion of good mental health in the classroom.

9. Discuss the importance of goal setting and attainment.

10. Discuss the parents' and home environment's role in the shaping of a child's personality. Is there a big influence?

ADDITIONAL SOURCES OF INFORMATION

READINGS

American Medical Association: "Mental Health and School Health Services" (1965).

American School Health Association. Report of Committee on Mental Health: "Mental Health in the Classroom." Revised edition. *J. Sch. Health* 38:5a, Special issue. May, 1968.

The Association of State and Territorial Health Officers, The Association of State and Territorial Mental Health Authorities, and the Council of Chief State School Officers. Joint Statement. "Mental Health in the Schools." Washington: National Education Association, 1966. Excellent.

Bakwin, H., and Bakwin, R. M.: *Behavior Disorders in Children.* Fourth edition. Philadelphia: W. B. Saunders Co., 1972.

Bentz, W. K., et al.: "Attitudes of Teachers and the Public Towards Mental Health." *Ment. Hyg.* 55:324–330, July, 1971.

Blaine, G.: *Emotional Problems of the Student.* New York: Appleton-Century-Crofts, 1971.

David, H. P.: "Mental Health and Social Action Programs for Children and Youth in International Perspective." *Ment. Hyg.* 54:503–509, October, 1970.

Hymes, J. L.: "Teacher Listen. The Children Speak." Mental Health Materials Center.

Irwin, T.: *How to Cope with Crisis.* New York: Public Affairs Committee, 1971.

Johnston, M. K.: *Mental Health and Mental Illness.* Philadelphia: J. B. Lippincott Co., 1971.

Joint Commission on Mental Health of Children: *Crises in Child Mental Health: Challenge for the 70's.* New York: Harper and Row, 1970.

Joint Committee on Health Problems in Education of the American Medical Association and the National Education Association: "Mental Health and School Health Services." 1965.

Kaplan, L.: *Education and Mental Health.* New York: Harper and Row, 1971.

Kauffman, J. M.: "School and Family as Potential Change Agents in the Mental Health of Children." *J. Sch. Health* 40:443–446, October, 1970.

Lawrence, M. M.: *The Mental Health Team in the Schools.* New York: Behavioral Publications, 1971.

Martins, C.: "Poverty and Mental Health." *Can. Psychiat. Assoc. J.* 15:159–166, April, 1970.

National Association for Mental Health: Valuable pamphlets and audiovisual aids. Write for current catalog.

National Education Association: "Drugs Abuse. Escape to Nowhere." A Guide for Educators. 1967. "Mental Health in the Classroom." 1966.

Sawyer, J.: *Psychology of Adjustment.* Boston: Allyn and Bacon, 1971.

Senn, M. J. E., and Solnit, A. J.: *Problems in Child Behavior and Development.* Philadelphia: Lea and Febiger, 1968.
U.S. Department of Health, Education, and Welfare:
"A Healthy Personality for Your Child." Publication 337, 1966.
Bulletin on Suicidology. National Institute of Mental Health.
"Hooked." 1966. Published by National Institute of Mental Health.
"Mental Health of Children. The Child Program of the National Institute of Mental Health." Public Health Service Publication No. 1396, 1965.
"The Protection and Promotion of Mental Health in Schools." Mental Health Monograph 5.
"Your Child from One to Six." Publication 30, Revised 1962.
"Your Child from Three to Four." Publication 446, 1967.
"Your Child from Six to Twelve." Publication 324, 1966.
U.S. Government Printing Office, Washington, D.C.

AUDIOVISUAL MATERIALS

Conscience of a Child

30 min. Black and White *sh,* adults National Education Television*

Shows ways that psychologists are studying growth and development of personality and emotional behavior in children.

Dangerous Years

27 min. Black and White *sh,* adults Kemper Ins. Co. 4750 Sheridan Road Chicago 40, Illinois

Reveals on-the-spot juvenile offenders and efforts of the police and others to stem the tide of juvenile crime. Explores new bold approaches to rehabilitation and prevention.

If These Were Your Children

Two parts 28 min. each Black and White Metropolitan Life Insurance Co.

Designed to help teachers, parents, nurses, and others understand basic needs of children, recognize their emotional problems, and work out ways to meet their needs. Part I is set in a second-grade classroom. Part II presents four authorities who discuss the film.

Jamie: Story of a Sibling

27 min. Black and White adults, teacher education National Film Board of Canada

Shows emotional development of children affected by parental attitudes and by competition for parental attention. Excellent.

A Long Time to Grow

Part I. Two- and three-year-olds in nursery school, 37 min.
Part II. Four- and five-year-olds in school, 37 min.
Part III. Six-, seven-, and eight-year-olds – society of children, 27 min.
New York University Film Library*

The New Baby

20 min. Black and White National Film Board of Canada

Shows family preparation for the new arrival, infant care, and emotional preparation with other children in the family.

*See Appendix A for addresses of film companies.

Roots of Happiness

25 min. Black and White *sh,* teachers, parents Bailey Films, Inc.

Points out elements necessary for a happy family atmosphere. Illustrates theories by comparing two families.

Sixteen in Webster Grove

47 min. Black and White *sh,* adults Carousel Films, Inc.

Explores attitudes of 16-year-olds growing up in an affluent society. Contrasts desires of the youth to the stereotyped patterns considered as being right regarding education, dating, and social functions.

Who Cares About Jamie

17 min. Color parents, teachers, schools nurses, social workers Association Films, Inc.

Depicts a day of normal school age boy. Interrelates home, school, and interpersonal relationships. Demonstrates importance of preventing emotional illness before it occurs.

Series of films on Emotional Development (partial list)

Child Development Series	Encyclopaedia Britannica Educ. Corp.
Child Development Series (see list at end of Chapter 2)	McGraw-Hill
Guidance Series	Coronet Films
Personality Series	Pennsylvania State University, Audiovisual Aids Library
Social Behavior Series	Pennsylvania State University, Audiovisual Aids Library

Write for catalogs.

Also, McGraw-Hill offers a number of excellent films regarding the social problems confronting the young people of today, as follows:

You Can Go a Long Way	Dropout from school
Narcotics: Why Not?	Drug use
You're No Good	Stealing
The Game	Premarital relations
Phoebe	Pregnancy of a high school girl

U. S. Department of Health, Education, and Welfare:

Write for most recent, selective guides on mental health motion pictures.

"Selected Mental Health Films." Public Health Service Publication 1591 (1967), 119 pp.

MATERIALS FOR TEACHERS' USE IN SCHOOLS

AUDIOVISUAL MATERIALS

A wealth of material is available for presentation to junior and senior high school groups. Films can be secured from the libraries of state and local departments of health and education, from universities, various local resource agencies and from film distributors (see Appendix A). Some have been produced for use with particular textbooks.

Films on Drug Dependence

Drugs and the Nervous System

16 min. Color *jh, sh,* adults Churchill Films

Surveys the effects of drugs on the nervous system (even aspirin). Explains disruptions caused by narcotics.

Hooked

20 min. Black and White *jh, sh,* adults Churchill Films

Drug addicts tell of experiences and how they became addicted. Voices of experience rather than authority. Excellent.

L.S.D.: Insight or Insanity

28 min. Color *jh, sh,* adults Bailey Films, Inc.

Documents dangers of capricious unsupervised use of L.S.D. Explains psychological and physiological effect. Shows proven ill effects. Excellent.

Marijuana

26 min. Color *jh, sh,* adults Bailey Films, Inc.

Narcotic: Pit of Despair

20 min. Color *jh, sh,* adults Film Distributors, International
223 South Olive Street
Los Angeles, Calif.

Shows dangers of drug-dependency, even after limited use. Instills a desire never to experiment.

RESOURCES

American Institute of Family Relations
American Medical Association
Child Study Association of America
Hogg Foundation for Mental Health
Mental Health Materials Center
National Association for Mental Health (state associations and local chapters)
Public Affairs Committee
National Education Association
Science Research Associates, Inc.
U.S. Department of Health, Education, and Welfare

Chapter 15

SOME SPECIAL PROBLEMS WITH SIGNIFICANT EMOTIONAL IMPLICATIONS

INTRODUCTION

The preceding chapter is concerned with primarily emotional problems, their detection, and the mental health follow-up program at school. However, in the follow-up on any disturbed child, the explanation may ultimately be found to have a physical basis. This chapter should be viewed as a continuation of the foregoing presentation and is concerned with frequently encountered problems in which physiological or physical defects have significant emotional implications.

The regular classroom seems to be the best place to secure their education for most children with physical impairments. This means that every teacher from kindergarten to twelfth grade will have from time to time a handicapped child in his class. He will have to teach this child. Moreover, he will meet handicapped children in corridors, in the auditorium, and on playgrounds.

Detailed attention is given in this chapter to various handicaps. If a teacher comes in contact with a child who suffers from an intermittent or chronic health problem, he is entitled to know a little of the medical explanation of the disease and the usual emotional responses to it. He can then formulate his own guidelines in his management of the youngster in his classroom, as well as in his relationships with other afflicted ones in the school.

The deaf student may tend to become paranoid because he suspects that others are talking about him. A crippled youngster turns away with a downcast countenance from a physical contest of his peers. A particularly trying situation may trigger a vicious headache. A lone child of perfectionist parents writhes on the lawn with the gnawing abdominal pain of a duodenal ulcer. A hyperactive, nonconforming child becomes resentful. Delay in maturation of those areas of the brain involved with language or with motor development may produce serious emotional and educational consequences. Such problems with emotional overtones must be understood and managed at school to meet a child's needs and prevent the development of undesirable secondary emotional characteristics.

General Discussion

The White House Conference on Children and Youth held in 1960 defined the handicapped youth as a "child who cannot play, learn, work, or do the things other children his age do; or who is hindered in achieving a full physical, mental, and social potentiality; whether by a disability which is initially mild but potentially handicapping, or by a serious disability involving several areas of function, with the probability of life-long impairment."

Many of the defects described in previous chapters fall into this category, e.g., the hard-of-hearing or partially-seeing child, or the one with heart disease. There are other handicapped—the child who must walk with braces or crutches or remain in a wheel chair, the one who must remain home with a prolonged illness from kidney disease, the youth with slowly mending fractures who also is homebound for months, the epileptic, the bright child with cerebral palsy, the youngster with repaired cleft lip and/or palate who is haunted by the derisive yell "old split-lip" from his classmates. Speech disorders of various types are handicaps—stuttering, lisping, the denasalized voice of the mouth breather, the difficult speech of the person with cleft lip and cleft palate.

The physical and emotional well-being of a child are interrelated. They form a total personality and cannot be separated. The emotional, social, and intellectual needs are the same, regardless of age or handicap. The axiom to follow in handling a sick or handicapped youngster is, "Do what is best for the child." What is best may not necessarily be what is pleasing or what is comfortable.

Emotional reactions to illness or handicapping conditions depend upon whether the child recovers completely. He accepts complete disability rather well and learns to adjust. He should be told the truth, as much as he can comprehend at his age. He has no conception of time in his earlier years and the statement that he must be confined to a wheel chair for a lifetime means very little. He will need day-to-day interpretation, even throughout adolescent development. If a handicap is permanent, he must adapt to reality.

A child develops interesting patterns of response to illness and crippling conditions. He may resort to fantasies concerning his disease and deny its existence. He is placed in a dependency role and may regress to a level of emotional development far below his chronological age. It is difficult to progress again. Sometimes, if he recovers, he will develop other physical illnesses in order to continue his dependency. He needs to be stimulated to think for himself and use his mind, so that he can escape his physical handicaps and so become independent. A youngster may become hostile, resentful, jealous, and vengeful. He sees others riding bicycles, playing ball, watching sound movies, or playing in ways denied him. Adjustment to a handicap is not necessarily proportionate to its severity; rather it is dependent upon the response of others, especially parents and peers, and upon the extent of the child's frustration. There must be means in which he can develop skills and prove his self-worth. Parents and teachers are challenged to exercise their ingenuity in stimulating his daily living activities.

A child may have been overprotected at home or he may have been ignored. He may have been unable to get around much because of a wheelchair or a brace or because of spasticity. His experiences will have been limited; consequently, his intelligence may be questioned.

Severely handicapped youngsters do need special instruction. Various arrangements for giving this instruction have already been described in previous chapters. A few large school systems are managing special children in a number of ways, both in elementary and secondary schools. The New York City Board of Education through its Office of Special Education offers instruction to 40,000 handicapped children of all ages in a variety of special classes, special schools, and in classrooms set up in medical treatment centers. Even these provisions are considered inadequate for the needs of the city. Special facilities for special children are indeed limited in the United States.

There are special children in all communities. Most of them attend regular schools. Our immediate concern is for the classroom teacher.

The Teacher's Role

What can a teacher do? Maybe there are no specific answers. Teachers give support and help children function at their best. Each child is influenced in his responses by his physical handicaps. There is no blueprint for handling each difficulty. The teacher must understand; he manages the problem child and meets his needs in his own way, not necessarily as done by his predecessor. He appreciates the fact that a child with a cleft palate or epilepsy is as worthwhile as any other child. He looks beyond the wheelchair, the brace, the stutter and sees the individual. He considers strengths. This child must be made to feel that he is perfectly acceptable and worthy of love and consideration.

A teacher conveys this interpretation to parents and to classmates. He creates feelings of acceptance and helpfulness in the classroom. By respecting a handicapped child as an individual, he can influence a parent's attitude. If a mother suffers a feeling of guilt or blame concerning her child's handicap, she can be encouraged to do something constructive and to appreciate that something can be done.

Teachers and classmates can include these children in many activities. One teacher watched an interesting relationship develop between a very bright boy who could not use his lower extremities and a brawny youngster who was more deliberate in his actions. The strong boy would lift the mate astraddle his shoulders and stride forth. The bright boy did much of the thinking; the muscular boy did all the fighting. With this symbiotic arrangement, they were ready to take on all comers.

The attitude towards a handicapped child should never be one of overprotection or pity. He should be held to his potential intellectual capacities, with gentle firmness and understanding. A child who does not consider himself too different from others will relax and learn more readily.

This general discussion of the teacher's role in management of all handicapped children is, of course, applicable to the special problems which follow. Of necessity there will be some repetition in the discussions of psychological reactions.

Some Special Problems

A few particular problems are presented here which require special emotional, social, and intellectual guidance at school. The teacher will probably not be too interested in their physical bases, but since he will surely have contacts with children who are afflicted with them, he must know how to fulfill their needs and do no harm.

The following problems are considered to have significant emotional implications and are being brought to a teacher's attention: hyperactivity, epilepsy, cerebral palsy, mental retardation, learning disabilities, superior intelligence, headaches, the battered or neglected child, and management of the child with a malignant neoplasm.

HYPERACTIVITY

Hyperactivity is not a disease; it is a behavior pattern.[1] Reference is sometimes made to the hyperactive child syndrome. A syndrome is a pattern or complex of symptoms which occur together.

---

[1]Synonymous terms for hyperactivity include hyperkinetic behavior, minimal brain dysfunction, and organic driveness.

Hyperactive Child Syndrome

A child who carries out activities at a higher rate of speed, who is always in motion, disregards disciplinary regulations, suddenly shoves the child sitting next to him, and pays no attention to the teacher has a disrupting influence in the classroom. Unless a teacher has understanding and patience, he finds himself frustrated and irritable and will soon demand withdrawal of the child from class. The defensive parents, the principal, social worker, and nurse become involved, along with the physician, psychiatrist, counselor, neighbors, and relatives. Ultimately, it is the child who often suffers permanent damage from the development of secondary emotional disturbances. In contrast, the shy, withdrawn youngster who sits quietly in his seat and "causes no trouble" may be seriously disturbed emotionally, but some teachers wish for more like him.

There are many hyperactive children, quite a number in each elementary school. They constitute a high percentage of those attending child guidance centers.

One child psychiatrist gives this sketch of a typical hyperactive child:

> Charles was nine years old when first seen, and the chief complaint was that he was doing badly in school. He vomited a lot as a baby, banged his head and rocked in his bed for hours, and cried much more than his sister. He walked at eleven months, talked first at two-and-a-half years, did not talk in sentences until four. Always very active, he has broken a bed and a trampoline and wears out the double knees in his jeans before the second washing. At age five, he was constantly turning off the furnace and water heater. He does not learn from punishment, is afraid of nothing, wanders from home and gets lost, dashes into the street without looking. He never completes projects at home and never finishes work at school. Hard to get to bed at night, he takes two hours or more to go to sleep and gets up at six a.m. Neighbors 'live in quiet terror' because he has run water into their basements through the hose, ridden his bicycle over their gardens, and blocked their sewers. He fights all the time with the neighborhood children and has no friends. In school he is 'creative' in avoiding work, he hides his books, eats crayons, tears papers, and pokes the other children. Every teacher reports that she has to stand over him to get him to do any work. Though bright, he has had to repeat second grade twice and is now in a special school.[2]

The parents are beset by an impulsive youngster who darts here and there, is almost always in motion, sleeps poorly, conforms to no routine, ignores discipline, tolerates frustration poorly, is always talking, always squirming, is tired because of excessive activity, is constantly over-stimulated, and is an ever-present source of anxiety.

---

[2]Roger Signor: "Hyperactive Children." *Washington University Magazine,* Winter 1967, p. 21.

About 10 per cent are perceived by the neighbors as "little demons." They are severely hyperactive children who set fires, commit acts of violence, and are a physical danger to themselves and their families.

People are disapproving of a child with the hyperactive behavior pattern. He is a constant storm center. He is squelched at home, at school, and at Sunday School. Sometimes a parent rejects him. Teachers may ask that the child be removed from school because he is a distracting influence; discipline cannot be maintained. He is easily distracted and unable to concentrate. Attention span is brief. He is considered stubborn, stupid, mean, bad, noncooperative. Yet, he cannot help or control himself. He is not primarily and basically an emotionally disturbed individual.

A significant number of hyperactive children are labeled as delinquents later in life. At about eight years of age the chances are that a child has been impulsive in his lying and stealing. If he is not held to strict standards at home, when he has quieted down in his physiological development at about 12 years or so, he may persist in antisocial behavior and become a prospective delinquent. A hyperactive child brought up in a disorganized environment may suffer a poor prognosis.

Let us consider this behavior in the child's defense. From the earliest understanding of language, the hyperactive child hears such admonitions as: "Be quiet." "Sit still." "Stop shouting." "Don't run." "Stop fiddling with those books." "Finish your work." "Why can't you be like other children?"

From less restrained adults, he hears tirades about his many faults and dark prophecies about his probable unsavory future. There is great danger that such a child, originally as warm and affectionate as any child, will finally answer society, "If you hate me, I hate you, too!" He may give this answer during the conflicts of adolescence in his unsuccessful attempts to adjust to a hostile society.

Hyperactive behavior may be associated with physiological or developmental delay, neurosis, brain damage and mental retardation. In order to determine the cause of hyperactivity, a complete neurological and psychological study should be done on each child suspected of this behavior.

Physiological Hyperactivity

The best acceptable theory in explaining most cases of hyperactivity is that these children suffer from a delay in the physiological development of the brain. The cause is not known. The extent of delay is variable. There is no evidence of brain damage. The breathless drive of the brain-damaged individual is absent. These hyperactive children are immature psychologically and follow a younger pattern. This pattern was previously described. Management at schools is similar to that for other developmental problems. Time must lapse. Most of these hyperactive children seem to achieve a more quiet behavior pattern when they are 11 or 12 years old.

Hyperactivity Due to Neurosis

The child subconsciously uses his excessive activity for neurotic purposes. The purpose may be either a defense against intolerable stress in his environment or it may be an outlet for his unresolved emotional conflicts. Hyperactivity is not so intense, is more variable, and develops later.

Obviously, management of the problem of neurotic hyperactivity depends on treatment of the underlying neurosis. The teacher or counselor may be the first to suspect a serious disturbance. The school nurse will probably be asked to make a preliminary home visit and to communicate with the child's physician. The school social worker can offer assistance in evaluating the interpersonal relationships within the home and becoming the liaison officer between the home and the school. Referral for psychiatric evaluation and treatment should be considered. Establishing a constructive program of evaluation and management would go far to eliminate the teacher's frustration in working with the child.

Hyperactivity Due to Brain Damage

Brain damage manifests itself as one of several disabilities or combinations of disabilities: cerebral palsy, epilepsy, mental retardation, and a behavior pattern which stems from minimal brain damage. The latter has been designated as the brain damage behavior syndrome. Children with any of these disabilities may be hyperactive. When children do not learn from experience, the possibility of brain damage should certainly be considered.

The child whose most obvious diability from brain damage is hyperactivity will probably be in the ordinary classroom because his intelligence has not been affected. He may have normal or even superior intelligence. Proportionately few hyperactive children fall into this category; but because their presence in regular elementary classrooms creates problems, detailed discussion follows.

The brain-damaged hyperactive child creates disorder. He does have learning disabilities.[3] He follows the pattern described above; may impulsively pace up and down the room; learns concrete facts well; has conceptual blanks in the area of abstractions, e.g., arithmetic; gives bizarre answers to questions; is unable to concentrate

---

[3]U.S. Department of Health, Education, and Welfare. Public Health Service: "Learning Disabilities Due to Minimal Brain Dysfunction." Publication 1646 (1967), 21 pp.

or pay attention for very long; is unusually reactive to sensory stimuli in his environments, looks up at sounds to which his classmates will pay no attention; is absolutely unpredictable in his behavior; tends to be creative and cannot follow routine tasks. Speech is not too clear and may be slow to develop. If he is psychologically tested in a group, he will perform poorly and be considered retarded. If examined individually, he will perform surprisingly well.

If he tends to be a little spastic, he will be awkward and will not be adept in group physical activities. Often he can perform the gross motor acts of running, jumping, and drinking but has trouble with the finer movements of writing. He has difficulty acquiring skills, such as bicycle riding, catching balls, dancing, etc. With his peers he is likely to be aggressive and bossy. He cannot establish good relationships with classmates, disregards their rights, and is rejected by them.

If the brain-damaged hyperactive child is not managed wisely, he gradually develops secondary undesirable characteristics. At first, he does not understand the reactions which he evokes in others. He becomes frustrated and discouraged because of rejection and impatient treatment. As he grows into adulthood, he may become resentful, hostile, and antisocial, and take his place in society as a "delinquent." He may commit delinquencies because of feelings of guilt, inadequacy, and resentment evoked by the continual rejection he has experienced.

He develops *anxieties* and *vague fears* because of his failure to enjoy constructive relationships with others. He is emotionally immature because he has not enjoyed the success that would enable him to move steadily forward in his emotional responses.

He acquires many *compensatory mechanisms* to cover his distress from his social and scholastic failures and his inability to relate to others. Examples of these mechanisms are stubbornness, rebellion, lying, bullying, and boasting. Or, he may become withdrawn and shy.

He may *fail at school* because it has been hard for him to conform and achieve at school and because he has missed much of the instruction while his attention was on the fleeting activity. When his educational progress is carefully guided, this hyperactive child does improve as time goes on. Coordination improves. He quiets down. He may become a person who relates successfully with his group, is creative and intelligent, provided he has not become resentful and antisocial. Understanding management over the years is not easy. A stable and favorable environment at home and school is the key to progressively normal development.

Education of the Brain-Damaged Hyperactive Child

Many teachers do not have the personality to cope with this child. If he could be regarded as a nice person who cannot repress himself, with an unusually short span of attention and a normal intelligence which in some instances is obscured by blanks in his learning and difficulty in appreciating the abstract, including number concepts, then he can be accepted. He is alive, he is educable, he should be prepared to accept his place in society.

The teacher is confronted by problems in teaching techniques. The child is so distractable that he needs a quiet, bare, plain corner or booth or a screened-off area in which to work. It must be offered him as an opportunity; seclusion must not be punitive to him. He needs close supervision, help, and encouragement to establish necessary control and working habits. The teacher must be able to translate abstractions into concrete situations for him. Frequent opportunities to move about and to change activity must be provided. Perhaps special test situations must be created to check his achievement. Throughout all activities the pupil must be helped to accept limits and conform to essential rules. Firm constructive guidance is better than overpermissiveness. The help must be given so tactfully by a warm, accepting teacher that the child does not lose the respect of his peers. They must accept him also.

A very wise and accepting teacher wrote on the report card of a hyperactive second-grade pupil with minimal brain damage, "All children need love and understanding and encouragement. Bill needs even more love and understanding and encouragement than most children." Bill made excellent progress in this second-grade class. The teacher enjoyed excellent rapport with Bill's parents.

Management of the Hyperactive Child

The hyperactive child may respond favorably to psychological, drug therapy and educational treatment. The hyperactive child usually is not referred for medical consultation soon enough. Because of the intensity of the problems and the fact that hyperactivity occurs more often than has been appreciated in the past, a good deal of research is being conducted in child psychiatric centers. New drugs are being tried. "The drugs most commonly used are in three categories: central nervous system stimulants, tranquilizers, and anticonvulsants."[4] Early referral is desirable.

Some of the preceding suggestions for management of the brain-damaged can be used for all hyperactive children at school.

In addition, a teacher needs to structure a program that is less stimulating and more consistent than that required for normal children. There is a need for a clear-cut sequence in instruction and patient checking of mastery at every stage.

---

[4]Vivian K. Harlin: "The Hyperkinetic Child—His Management in the School Environment." *Sch. Health Rev.* March–April, 1973, p. 12.

In school systems which provide special education classes, the hyperactive child will be accepted. If such classes are not provided, there must be modification of the curriculum. Some parents have been advised to keep the hyperactive child out of school until he is about eight years old. By this time he has become a little more quiet, and life is not so stressful. Then he may enter school at the level in which he can achieve success. Perhaps he could attend one half day, rest, and then be tutored or be visited by a teacher in the afternoon. There is a tendency for his hyperactivity to become worse when he is tired. Also, the teacher and classmates are relieved of the strain of a whole day with him. In junior high school it may still be necessary for him to continue the half-day routine. Secondary behavior problems must be minimized. In senior high school he may be able to attend the whole day.

The education of each hyperactive child must be individually planned, with understanding from teachers and adjustment made to the facilities available.

EPILEPSY

Probably no behavior causes more concern in a school than the convulsive or epileptic seizure, "spell," "fit," "black out," "brown out," or convulsion. No other physical handicap has such a social stigma attached to it. An epileptic person may be ashamed and will not face his problem realistically in order to secure proper medical attention. Too many educators live in the Dark Ages as far as knowledge and attitudes towards epilepsy are concerned; their lack of understanding can add to the unhappiness and poor social adjustment of an afflicted child. Because of the attitude of society, a parent will refuse to accept a diagnosis in her own child and will delay medical care. The child is at first bewildered, then finally comes to feel inferior.

"Since epileptic students will be in the classroom in the future, it would seem imperative that teacher preparation for the management of epileptic students be comprehensive, that teacher attitudes be unprejudiced, that all services be promoted by school nurses, and that guidance procedures meet the needs of epileptic students. Both teacher-training institutions and public schools in which epileptics are enrolled need to develop more appropriate responses to the condition of epilepsy."[5]

Seizures

The word "epilepsy" means seizure. Epilepsy is not a disease in the traditional sense of the word. It is the outward manifestation of

[5]Jane W. Martin: "Attitude toward Epileptic Students in a City High School System." *J. Sch. Health* *44*:3:146, March, 1974.

an irregular and overwhelming neurological disturbance in some brain area. It is characterized by recurrent or spasmodic attacks of unconsciousness or impaired consciousness or control. There may or may not be rigidity or muscle spasm.

The seizure itself is explained by a chemical disturbance in the brain cell which causes irregularities in the brain wave pattern. This pattern eventually subsides in many instances, since epilepsy is temporary in more than half the cases. There may be a predisposition to this disturbance. The incidence in the general population is one in 200; the likelihood of its appearance in the offspring of an epileptic is one in 40. It is not advised, however, that epileptics forego marriage and parenthood.

Each brain has a wave pattern which can be recorded by an electroencephalograph. These waves vary a little in all people, but the electroencephalograms (EEG) of people with epileptic seizures show more alteration from the normal pattern; and still more marked changes occur during an attack. About 85 per cent of epileptics show some irregularity when free of seizures, while only 15 per cent of other persons show some irregularity, usually minor.

Causes of Epilepsy

1. Acute infections, particularly those with high fever, may produce convulsive seizures. This occurs more in infants and little children; in most individuals they will never happen again.

2. Profound emotional disturbances do not cause seizures but may precipitate them in a brain which already has an abnormal pattern. Emotionally disturbed children of all ages may have an occasional seizure.

3. Profound metabolic disturbances, such as those produced by low blood sugar, malnutrition, accumulation of toxic chemicals in advanced kidney disease, and severe exhaustion have been known to produce seizures. A person during insulin reaction may twitch or jerk during unconsciousness.

4. Brain injury may be a cause, owing to:
   a. Congenital defects, for instance, cerebral palsy;
   b. Brain tumor;
   c. Brain injury before or during birth;
   d. Brain injury from accidents – a skull fracture, a fall, or blow on the head from a fist or thrown ball;
   e. Acute infections of the nervous system, as in meningitis, encephalitis ("sleeping sickness"), or brain abscess.

Mental retardation may also be a complication; hence the child may suffer both seizures and mental retardation stemming from the same original brain injury.

5. Seizures of unknown cause occur (sometimes labeled "idiopathic," "cryptogenic," or "true epilepsy"). Fifty per cent of these

cases are first observed between the ages of four and eight years. Two per cent have a seizure before the age of two.

It has been observed that a rapid or intent perception of visual images, as happens in watching television, reading, or riding in a car, may precipitate seizures in some susceptible individuals. A report on one child describes his convulsive response to soft, smooth music. Seizures which occur with reading are now called "reading epilepsy." Reports on all of these precipitating factors are currently appearing in the medical literature.

In the past the fifth group was labeled "epilepsy"; seizures from known origins were referred to as "convulsive seizures" or some such title. The objective was to escape the emotional reactions created by use of the word "epilepsy." However, for the last two decades, there has been a concentrated effort by those interested in this problem to disabuse the public's interpretation of epilepsy as a dread disease; correct terminology should be used. Indeed, one pamphlet published by the Epilepsy Foundation of America is entitled, "Let's say it out Loud."

Incidence of Epilepsy

Epilepsy occurs more in children; a high percentage have their onset in preschool years. It is estimated that approximately two million people in this country suffer from epilepsy. Among the general population the estimate is one in 100. Any statistics will be inaccurate because the social stigma attached to this disturbance has induced people to hide it. Minor seizures may be unsuspected for years.

School Health Program

Detection

Identification requires knowledge of the various types of epileptic attacks.

Petit Mal Seizures. More prevalent in infancy and early childhood, these are momentary lapses from reality, usually without muscular jerking or spasm. Occasionally there may be a slight manifestation, shown by staring into space, rolling the eyes upward, moving the lips, twitching the eyelids or eyebrows, or a generalized trembling. The child returns to awareness of his environment fairly quickly; a lapse rarely lasts longer than 30 seconds. He is usually immobile during the seizure, rarely falls, but tends to drop any article he may have in his hand or mouth at the time. Such attacks may be referred to by parents as "dreams," "spells," "lapses," "black outs," or "absences." These seizures may occur only occasionally, or as often as a hundred or more times during a day and night. A child may not observe these lapses in his preschool days but notices them in time, particularly during classroom procedures. For instance, he awakens to the realization that the teacher has written more on the blackboard than he was last aware of seeing. If asked, he can usually make a record of the attacks occurring during the day.

No emergency measures need to be taken at school about petit mal seizures. One physical education teacher of a seventh grader was confronted with this problem repeatedly. His adroitness in handling it was interesting:

> Once, when the boys were marching around the gymnasium, this particular student stopped suddenly and stood quietly in position. The remainder of the boys marched on, returned to the original position and halted. When the student smiled and looked around, they all marched off together. This boy had not responded too well to therapy and was not permitted to take swimming nor cross a street alone. He would be likely to stop abruptly at any time, and arrangements were always made for a sibling to accompany him.

Each teacher in the school needs to be acquainted with the children who have petit mal seizures. By doing so, he can appreciate the lapses of attention and assume a sympathetic yet casual attitude. A child with petit mal seizures should be under the care of a physician. This disorder has been the object of a good deal of research and effective medication is being found to control the frequency of seizures. With full control, these children are permitted a full life with no restriction of activities.

Generalized Motor Seizures (Grand Mal). These may occur at any age and are sometimes preceded by an *aura*, a feeling of impending attack or warning. This aura, which may be either motor or sensory in reaction, appears from a fraction of a second to several hours or even days before the seizure. Some attacks occur without warning. The pattern of grand mal seizures is varied. Some individuals have many auras and no attack or only an occasional one; some lose consciousness and have only a mild convulsion; some stiffen but do not jerk the muscles; some seem to have repeated jerkiness without tension of the muscles. Some are confused afterwards, and others get up and resume their work. Some have a slight convulsion followed by a long period of somnolence. The commonly described attack is the typical abrupt seizure of unconsciousness with rigidity and jerking of the muscles. The tongue may be severely bitten and bloody froth issue from the mouth. Injury can result from these violent movements. With the closing of the glottis, breathing is suspended, and the face assumes a suffused bluish-purple color. The bladder and, occasionally, the rectum may empty. Finally, relaxation occurs, the color becomes pink, and breathing is stertorous; the child is weary, sleepy, and not too well oriented.

A child may have only nocturnal seizures, and a parent sleeps with one ear alert for sounds from the child's room. Eventually some seizures may occur in the daytime.

FIRST AID DURING A SEIZURE

Keep calm. There is almost an instinctive panic reaction when people observe the beginning of a seizure.

1. *Ease the child to the floor.*

Loosen clothing. Remove any furniture which child may strike.

Allow him to lie quietly until he recovers. Rarely is any other treatment necessary.

2. *Do not force any object between the epileptic's teeth.*

For many years it has been suggested that some firm object be placed between the individual's teeth so he will not bite his tongue. More epileptic individuals' teeth and gums have been injured by well-intentioned but misguided efforts to prevent biting than by the biting itself. Dislocated jaws have also been known to occur. The major injury to the tongue comes with the initial contraction and setting of the jaw muscles before anything can be done.

3. *If possible, turn him on his side to permit saliva to run out of the mouth.*

4. *Watch the child until his senses are clear and rational.*

Most persons who suffer from major attacks are confused for considerable periods of time after and they should not be left alone or expected to go their way without some supervision or friendly guidance. In minor attacks, not accompanied by complete loss of consciousness or falling, the person often becomes perfectly clear in a matter of seconds.

The remainder of the children in the school room should pursue their tasks. The teacher should remain calm and wait out the attack. If necessary, the exhausted child can be carried to a cot where he can recover at his own tempo. Later he can rejoin the group. Remember, an epileptic seizure is not dangerous to life unless a child injures himself in falling or becomes unconscious in a hazardous situation, e.g., in traffic or working with an electric saw in industrial arts class. Unless the attack lasts for a very long time (a half hour or more) and there is some danger from exhaustion, no particular treatment is needed.

5. *Notification of parents is a wise procedure.*

A *first* seizure is particularly significant. Parents should know that a seizure has occurred so that they may consult their physician.

In individual cases a child's doctor may have special recommendations for a teacher concerning care during a seizure.

Psychomotor Attacks. These are detected with more difficulty, because the pattern varies. This type of attack afflicts about one third of adults with epilepsy. With the seizure the individual is apparently following normal behavior, when actually the reflexes are automatic, and he is unaware of reality. The lapse usually lasts only a minute or two during which a child may move around aimlessly, finger objects, make chewing or swallowing motions, ignore directions, indulge in overt behavior, such as a temper tantrum—all of which activity is well-coordinated and breeds no suspicion of abnormality. When this behavior seems alien to a child's ordinary living pattern, and he has no recollection of its occurrence, discussion with parents is indicated.

Focal Epilepsy. In this type the abnormal electrical discharge can be traced back to one small focus or area or a number of areas of the brain. The type of motor or sensory involvement depends upon which part of the brain is involved. If one area of the brain after another is affected in sequence, the attack is labeled a *jacksonian seizure.* A classic seizure may start at the end of an extremity, possibly the fingers. The part begins to tremble or just feel numb. Trembling and numbness march sequentially on to involve the arm, the face, the whole side, may cross over to the other side, and may stop at any point along the march. If only one side is involved, consciousness is retained. If the disturbance spreads to the other half of the body, the person loses consciousness and suffers a grand mal attack.

First aid is the same as for any motor seizure.

Minor Motor Seizures. These are brief, may occur frequently, leave no after-effects, and may be unobserved. They may be associated with other types of epilepsy. There may be sudden loss of tone of the back muscles, and the person falls forward on his face or head. He usually recovers immediately. There may be a sudden abdominal pain and "black-out"; the child stumbles or falls and quickly regains composure. Sometimes a muscle or set of muscles may contract. If a person is holding a glass and his arm jerks, the glass can be thrown from his hand. If these jerks occur with increasing severity and frequency, a grand mal seizure may follow. There may be a tension of the muscles generally to produce a "jackknife" position. This is held for only a few seconds, but may be repeated rapidly within a few minutes and frequently during the day.

Distribution. The age distribution of the various types of seizures will interest a teacher. Petit mal frequently begins between four and eight years of age, rarely starts much before the age of three or after fifteen. It is more common in early childhood, decreases during adolescence, and is rare in adulthood. Children with grand mal may be observed in early childhood, also. The incidence of the latter seems to be uniformly distributed over the years. There is no peak or rise, as far as age is concerned. Sometimes a child will suffer a mixed pattern of grand mal and petit mal, a pattern which may start early in childhood. Psychomotor cases are rare in the early years, begin to appear before adolescence, and increase in frequency in adulthood. Mixed psychomotor and grand mal seizures in an individual occur mostly in adults.

Among known cases of epilepsy about 63.5 per cent suffer from grand mal, 17.5 per cent suffer from petit mal or focal seizures, 16.5 per cent have psychomotor attacks, and 2.5 per cent are unclassified.[6]

---

[6]Epilepsy Foundation of America: "Epilepsy: The Facts." Pamphlet, p. 3.

In most children the tendency to seizures lessens as they grow older. Attacks may disappear. Since such a high per cent occurs in preschool years, if the seizures can be controlled before a child starts to school, many psychological disturbances can be obviated.

With encephalograms and other examinations by the physician, epilepsy is not usually difficult to diagnose; and with modern medication the disease is not difficult to control. *Teacher observation* can contribute to diagnosis. Every epileptic seizure should be observed closely so that a teacher will be able to give an accurate description to a school nurse or physician. The events immediately preceding the attack, if any, are important. The pattern of the attack—the twitching or jerking, tension of body and muscles, clenching of jaws, biting of tongue, lack of orientation—all of this information is significant, especially if the seizure seems to begin in one part or one side of the body.

FOLLOW-UP

Management of the Epileptic Child at School. A child who has a *first known* seizure at school should be reported to his parents immediately. He deserves a thorough medical investigation. In many instances, medical or surgical treatment may result in a cure.

The following cases demonstrate the variety of causes of epilepsy and methods of handling them.

> A high school boy was hit on the side of the head with a baseball. Soon after, he suffered his first convulsive seizure with pronounced jerking of the muscles. The convulsions occurred with increasing frequency; his school work deteriorated in quality; personality seemed altered. Finally, he was examined by a neurosurgeon. Pressure on the brain was relieved by surgery, and the boy recovered completely.

> A freshman university student fell to the ground unconscious; there were a few convulsive twitchings of the muscles, but not many. He was removed to the Health Service. The parents were called and gave no history of any previous seizure. The boy remained unconscious and was taken to a hospital. After study, surgery was done, and a benign brain tumor was excised completely. The boy recovered and returned as a student.

> University Health Service personnel were called over to a classroom where a boy was said to be having an epileptic fit. The student, a known uncontrolled diabetic, was brought to the Infirmary, where he shortly recovered consciousness. He was accustomed to taking his daily doses of insulin, but often he did not take time to eat his meals. He even carried sandwiches in his pockets but ignored them. Students observing this student were heard to mention the word "epileptic."

> An older student was heard to moan; he arched his back, extended his arms rigidly, and his face assumed a purple color. The episode was momentary. He then relaxed and appeared

dazed. The professor walked over and pressed the student's head to the arm-lift of the chair and had him remain there until the lecture was over. After class both walked to the Health Service. The student had no recollection of this episode; there was no past history of such. He was working the "swing shift" in a factory several miles from town and had a morning eight o'clock class. His meals consisted mostly of cold sandwiches and were inadequate; he carried a full schedule of classes, was an officer in his fraternity, and was busy with campus elections; he had lost some weight and was tired. The explanation in this case is obvious. The remainder of the school year this student reported to the Health Service at regular intervals; his health improved, he planned more leisure time and had no recurrences of the above experience. A number of years later he visited the Health Service and reported no further unpleasant experiences.

Every child with epilepsy should be under competent medical supervision. If the child is subject to too many seizures and is under no treatment, the school administration should insist on medical supervision. This is particularly true of grand mal seizures when one or more attacks at school daily may have a disrupting effect. Modern drugs have wrought wonders in controlling the incidence and severity of attacks. Treatment is individualized. Focal epilepsy and grand mal are the easiest to control. The whole outlook for epileptics has changed. They do not need to be plagued with anxieties concerning an unexpected embarrassing situation. Thus psychic trauma can be avoided to a great extent. About 50 per cent of epileptics enjoy complete control of seizures. Another 30 per cent are greatly improved, so that they can lead normal lives. For those cases which cannot be controlled by medication, arrangements for education should be made, either in special classes or at home.

A person with epilepsy must take his medicine regularly. Teachers can encourage a child to be conscientious in following instructions. Even though a child has suffered only one seizure, he may be advised by his physician to take his medicine for an extended period. The full cooperation of parents and teachers is required to avoid the temptation of discontinuing treatment after a long period without a seizure. A teacher does not ordinarily administer medication; but he may remind a child who has brought his pills to school. Sometimes a child will forget to take his medicine during the day, or he does not want his classmates to observe him doing so. If taking medication during school hours presents a real problem and scheduled doses are being missed, the teacher or school nurse should notify the parents or the child's physician so that proper adjustments of the schedule may be made.

A word is indicated here about the possible side-effects from the use of anti-convulsant medication. Drowsiness may be noticed. A child may drop off to sleep in class. Another possibility is unsteadiness in walking or lack of coordination. A teacher should report to the family or to the physician or indirectly to them through the school nurse that these behavior patterns occur. The physician can adjust the dose of medication or change it to maintain control without these undue side-effects. A child who is overly sedated is not receptive to learning.

Epileptics are often the butt of quackery and receive much literature through the mail on "sure cures." This makes it even more important that scientific advice be secured. For those parents who ask questions and have not seemed to understand epilepsy, referral can be made to the local medical society.

Education. Elsewhere in this chapter references are made to behavior and intellectual achievement patterns associated with brain damage. Hyperactivity and learning and speech disabilities are described. These same youngsters may also suffer epileptic seizures (see outline). They are often hyperactive, irritable, erratic in behavior; academic performance varies.

Most epileptic children, however, attend regular classes and show no unusual deviations. Actually, there are fewer seizures when the brain is active. A child is not enevitably doomed to mental deterioration, as some teachers think. Many famous people, some of them geniuses, have had seizures. Young people with epilepsy should be exposed to firm, fair discipline at home and at school and fulfill the same expectations as others. Curriculum should not be changed, and they should be expected to complete their school assignments. One of the commonly used medications (phenobarbital) apparently does not affect school work.[7] Overconcern, overprotection, and anxiety weaken a child's opinion of himself. If he is subject to the same discipline as others, he will acquire habits of responsibility and independence, which will prepare him, the same as his peers, to accept his place in society.

> Physical activity has a favorable effect on epilepsy in a child. Such children may and should participate in the general physical activities of the normal child, although the use of some types of gymnastic apparatus should be restricted. The child does not need extra rest, daily naps, or a quiet and sheltered life. Unneeded restrictions and limitations may arouse the child's anger and resentment or encourage him to feel he is different from other children. Restrictions should be only those requested by the family physician, including usually avoidance of hot equipment, power machinery, climbing to a height, and swimming during school hours. Manual arts activities may usually be permitted.[8]

Young people from junior high school through high school have a vital interest in Driver Education and in securing a driver's license.

---

[7]Irwin Wapner, et al.: "Phenobarbital. Its Effect on Learning in Epileptic Children." *J.A.M.A.* *182*:937, 1962.

[8]Epilepsy League, Inc.: "The Epileptic Child in Your School." Milwaukee, Wisconsin: 1955, pp. 9–10.

> If the high school student with epilepsy feels he has no hopes of every getting a driver's license, he becomes quite discouraged; whereas if he understands that by remaining free of seizures for a given period of time he can qualify, this becomes one of the strongest motivations for regular medication that we have. Driver Education and driver's licensing is handled differently in different states; in general most states have provisions whereby people with controlled seizures can qualify for licenses. Inquiry should be made locally concerning the state law, with its policies and regulations, so that accurate information can be used as a basis for planning an individual's class schedule to include Driver Education.[9]

Health Education

A teacher will be shocked as he watches a grand mal seizure for the first time. He will feel helpless and await anxiously the relaxation of the victim. Children should be informed about such a health problem if there is a possibility of such an episode occurring to one of their classmates. They should be taught to accept these situations, make no derogatory personal comments, and show no discrimination. The child and his parents will appreciate such an attitude.

The teacher's *attitude* is of the utmost importance. The following two case studies are self-explanatory:

> A student teacher related the following incident in a shocked, unbelieving voice. She was assisting the sixth-grade teacher to whom she had been assigned when she noticed one of the girls quietly go into the cloak room. A few minutes later there was a thrashing sound from that region; and when the assistant looked perturbed, she was told, "Oh, she is in there just having a fit. She has them all of the time. She is such a nuisance. No one wants her in the classroom, so this year I have to suffer."
>
> An elementary teacher reported the following incident: When a youngster in her classroom had a grand mal seizure, she not only took care of the immediate situation but discussed the health problem with the class. Her fine understanding brought a letter of gratitude from the parents.

Continuous education about epilepsy among counselors and teachers is necessary. Special teachers, social workers, school and public health nurses, classmates, and all who come in contact with our epileptic youth have a role to play in promoting understanding and in eliminating the misconceptions which are so damaging to a child's welfare and future.

> A senior high student who had suffered psychomotor episodes since the age of eight found himself slipping in his classwork. He was confused, preoccupied, and dispirited, "faltering and beset with rejection." He was having trouble because of apparent aggressive, offensive, and antisocial behavior, which he

[9]Personal communication from Madison H. Thomas, M.D., Salt Lake City, Utah.

> did not remember. Classmates and teachers were ready to drop the student entirely. The father asked for a meeting with his teachers and listened to the complaints. At first, the attitude of the teachers was "strained and formal." He suddenly realized that the complaints were based upon his son's behavior during the time he was having a seizure. When the father explained the nature of the seizures, the lack of awareness and responsibility of his son at this time, the attitude of the teachers changed. They began to discuss the problem enthusiastically—how the episodes could be handled, how the student could be given help in his studies, how the attitude of classmates could be changed to acceptance and assistance. "If we got him to talk to his class about epilepsy, it might change their attitude.[10]

Parents, teachers, social workers, school nurses, and physicians need to communicate with each other.

Sociopsychological attitudes towards epileptics are important. They have suffered from discrimination by various state laws concerning marriage, sterilization, driving, employment, and even education. William G. Lennox, one of the world's authorities on epilepsy, described these restrictions and the current attitudes towards the disease as follows:

> The restrictions, justified and unjustified, that are placed on the person's activities seriously affect his prospects and accomplishments; however, the larger injury is not apparent. Repeated rebuffs lead to timidity or to irritations and anger ending in aggressiveness and antisocial behavior. But the most grievous injury is to the person's spirit, which assumes the furtive fear of the hunted, the guilt of the criminal, the sense of uncleanness of the patient with leprosy. Decay of confidence, ambition, and hope may follow . . .
>
> Every patient and every family confronted with epilepsy has apprehensions born of general misunderstanding. The physician can counteract these sentiments by words such as these: "Epilepsy is not a mysterious disease and certainly is no disgrace. Simple epilepsy, like diabetes, is a metabolic disorder. It is, perhaps, an enigma, but not a stigma. It does not tend to get worse with time. There are effective medicaments. The mind is rarely affected. A child should continue schooling, and the adult should work. Activity is an antagonist of seizures. Marriage and children are not necessarily precluded. Given social acceptance, the great majority of patients can lead normal lives."
>
> The epileptic person needs education as an offset to his handicap, as a stimulant to morale, and for social development—the largest difficulty is the complaint of teachers and the parents of other children that the epileptic child is a hindrance to the healthy. Yet the child whose seizures are reasonably controlled can be a positive asset in the classroom. Deft handling of convulsions is a lesson in first aid. Association with a person who carries on in spite of such a handicap is a lesson in brave living.

---

[10]Robin White: "The Battle for Understanding." *The Sat. Eve. Post* 236:62–64, (June 8) 1963.

> One must reconsider the effect of the sight of a convulsion on school children when the murder and mayhem that they view every night on television is remembered.[11]

Accordance with the preceding viewpoint is gradually being shown by recent actions of legislatures who have eliminated all restrictions on marriages and have adopted reasonable regulations on drivers' licenses. More individuals with controlled epilepsy are being employed.

Differentiation from Other Nervous Patterns

Not all cases of *apparent* unconsciousness, tenseness, or jerking muscles can be labeled as epilepsy. A differentiation should not be difficult.

Hysterical Conversion Reaction. This reaction is usually interpreted as an occurrence in which somatic behavior mirrors deep-seated emotional disturbances. One somatic pattern is an apparent unconsciousness, so-called "black out" spell. Convulsions are not a part of the picture, but the attack may resemble petit mal or be associated with fast, deep breathing or culminate in a generalized trembling of the body. There is no aftermath of stupor or somnolence. A regular epidemic may occur among teen-agers, especially girls. Visual and neurological complaints, paralyses, trembling, spasticity, tingling along nerves, meaningless laughter and sobs are other manifestations. This reaction may be described as "histrionic behavior." All cases of suspected hysteria warrant a thorough neurological and psychological examination. The school psychologist should definitely be used as a consultant.

> A school medical examiner was called down to the Dean of Women's office in a junior high school. A girl lay on a couch, immobile, tense, hands clenched, eyelids closed tightly, breathing regularly, color good. Any attempt to pull back the lids and expose the eyes was resisted by strong contraction of the muscles. Fingers could not be extended. The girl had maintained this condition for half an hour. There was no convulsive movement nor injury. The Dean of Women reported that the girl had been summoned for a reprimand and had proceeded to moan, drop to the floor, and assume a stiffened position. The most revealing information had been written on the back of the cumulative health record by someone in elementary grades. "This girl is very unhappy, unrealistic, and daydreams a great deal." After a while the girl arose and went back to class. A tentative diagnosis of hysteria was made and psychotherapy advised.

Fainting. A fainting episode is occasionally seen at school. A boy or girl may slump over while viewing a gory, colored film in a biology class. Fainting is not uncommon among adolescent girls. The body is relaxed and there may be a momentary unconsciousness.

---

[11]William G. Lennox and Charles H. Markham: "The Socio-psychological Treatment of Epilepsy." *J.A.M.A.* *152*:1690–94, 1953.

Causes are many: illness, impending menstrual period or menstrual discomfort, an uncomfortably warm room, no breakfast or inadequate food intake, or low blood pressure. Fainting is rarely due to heart disease. Any person who faints repeatedly should have a complete medical examination. The student who faints should be permitted to lie quietly until she wishes to move. If she is sitting in a classroom, all that is usually necessary is to place her head on the arm of the chair.

Tics. Tics are rather disconcerting to a bystander. One gesture or muscular pattern is performed over and over again. Examples are a grimace, shrugging of a shoulder, raising of the eyebrows, nervous cough or clearing of the throat, wrinkling of the nose, blinking of the eyes, or twisting of the head, repeated at regular, frequent intervals. The pattern is stereotyped and involves one or more muscles. A tic is probably produced by nervous tension, and the underlying causes need to be treated. The electroencephalogram shows no changes. Motions can be temporarily controlled, and there is no impairment of consciousness. Young children get into the habit of repeating a grimace, gesture, or sound; the more attention that is called to such action, the more pleasure that is derived from repeating it.

CEREBRAL PALSY

Reference has been made to cerebral palsy under the discussions of speech disorders, dyslexia, hyperactivity due to brain damage, emotional disturbances, and learning disabilities.

Cerebral palsy refers to the abnormality in that group of individuals who, as a result of brain damage, have trouble with movement. Muscles are involved. The result may be rigidity or spasticity, involuntary movements (athetosis), trembling, or inability to keep balance (ataxia). Muscles of the eyes, the throat, or any or many muscles may have impaired function. The extent will vary with the amount of brain damage. In some instances, sensory areas in the brain are affected. Hearing and visual disturbances are common. The condition occurs more in boys than girls.

About 68 per cent of children with cerebral palsy show delayed development early in life. Hyperactivity, learning disabilities, mental retardation, and speech disorders must be taken into account. Communication is difficult; therefore, assay of intelligence may be difficult. Almost one half of those in schools are mentally retarded. They join comparable achieving groups in school.

Some children will be in regular classrooms. These will be ones with minimal brain dysfunction, manifested by such conditions as a slight abnormality of gait, difficulty in speech or retarded speech, and various amounts of spasticity. Those children with normal or superior intelligence join their peer groups and participate as much as possible in regular activities.

Obviously, no blueprint is possible for explaining management in school. Each youngster must have individual adjustments and allowances.

> Conditions favorable to the development of a socially acceptable personality in the child with cerebral palsy include (1) A sustained emotional atmosphere in which the child experiences affection, friendship, and acceptance. He should not be too dependent, nor should he be expected to take too much responsibility. (2) A stable, permanent home, without moving and changing schools, thereby giving the handicapped child a chance to find his own niche and to discover the things that he can do well. (3) Opportunity for new experiences. Life must not be too monotonous; on the other hand, the child's powers of concentration may be slight and his experiences few, so that he may need help in adjusting to new situations. (4) Adequate scope for his abilities. Too much must not be anticipated, but the handicapped person should be permitted and expected to succeed within the limits of his handicap. (5) Adequate scope for his energy. He must not be restricted too much, but the impossible should not be expected.
>
> The aim for the child with cerebral palsy should be independence, courage, a sense of responsibility, and a well developed social sense.[12]

Depending upon the amount of handicap, he may become discouraged with what the future holds for him. Some individuals have overcome their speech handicaps, mastered their minimal muscular problems, and progressed to academic and vocational high schools. Some have gone to college and achieved satisfactions in the professions.

In most school systems children with cerebral palsy are found distributed through the schools in the community. They are usually being followed also in Rehabilitation Centers or by private physicians, with the physical therapist, school nurse, physician, speech therapist, and parents involved. Management of each child should be a team approach. Special Education personnel have a role to play. Some large school systems have special schools for the handicapped. Some children will have visiting teachers come to their homes.

MENTAL RETARDATION

The term "mental retardation" encompasses a large number of conditions, which in themselves are often unrelated but in the aggregate result in a low intellectual status which permits at best a low level of performance.

In recent years a surge of interest in the mentally retarded child coupled with funds for education and management has brought this child from the home and private schools and clinics to the attention of educators. Practically every elementary school will have mentally retarded children in classrooms.

---

[12]Harry Bakwin and Ruth Morris Bakwin: *Clinical Management of Behavior Disorders in Children.* Third edition. Philadelphia: W. B. Saunders Co., 1966, p. 153.

To what extent are there emotional implications? Parents of mentally retarded children have suffered an emotional, economic, and social burden. They may be ashamed; they may be troubled with a sense of guilt for having produced such a child; they may withdraw from social contacts because of these feelings. There is a tendency to overprotection of the afflicted one, with attention and money concentrated on him to the neglect of the needs of others in the family. Or, there may be rejection and indifference. Parents need guidance and should follow the counsel of personnel who are familiar with the various aspects of the mental retardation problem.

As for those who are qualified to enter school, all teachers have contact with them in one way or another—in study groups, in the lunch room, in the corridors, or on the playgrounds. Teachers trained in special education techniques for management of the mentally retarded may conduct segregated classes or act as consultants.

Those youngsters who are qualified to attend school, even at a low level of educability, do react to the emotional climate in their environment. There can be some reaction to harsh criticism and, unfortunately, some people voice their remarks in a child's presence.

Some observations can be made about the personality problems of mentally retarded children at school. "Many have gross feelings of inadequacy because they have faced failure at every turn. They are well aware of the differences between themselves and the nonretarded. Society has done a thorough job in emphasizing these differences to them. They can get depressed, show anxiety, and exhibit guilt feelings. Many of them have deep seated hostility for which they have no adequate outlet, a condition which often leads to antisocial behavior. A particularly nagging problem for the retarded child is the many hours spent in loneliness because peer group membership has been denied him."[12]

Behavior can be unpredictable, because of inability to adjust to routine in school. Hyperactivity can be a problem. If enough of these children justify a special school in a large school system, a child will feel more free from pressure. As far as management at school is concerned, expectations depend upon the mental rather than the chronological age of a child. Parents need to be reminded of his limitations.

Every child is studied carefully; a detailed report on his assets and his deficits should be made, with emphasis on strengths; predictions as to educability are formulated. "Assessment of the child's entire personality and interaction with those in the home, school and community should be included with an eye to improving adaptive skills in those areas."[13] The plan of management should be understood by all concerned. The team approach of teacher, social worker, school nurse, psychologist, physician, parent, and others is or should

---

[12]Richard L. Stafford and Roger J. Meyer: "Diagnosis and Counseling of the Mentally Retarded: Implications for School Health." *J. Sch. Health* 38:152 (March) 1968.

[13]*Ibid.*, p. 155.

be pursued in either regular schools or in special schools set aside for the mentally retarded.[14]

LEARNING DISABILITIES

Causes and Emotional Implications

Quite a fund of information is now available concerning learning disabilities. Analysis reveals the following explanations:

1. Developmental abnormalities in specific areas of the brain seem to account for most learning problems in reading (dyslexia), writing, arithmetic, comprehension and distinction of sounds (auditory verbal problems), and visual difficulties, and also for certain motor functions, such as handedness and hyperactivity.
2. Physical defects account for some learning problems. These may be visual and auditory defects, cerebral or brain damage, and chronic illness.
3. Emotional problems may precede or occur secondary to learning disabilities; in either case they complicate the learning situation.

The scope of this discussion is limited to the emotional aspects of learning problems. All three of the preceding broad explanations should be examined. In many instances they are interrelated.

1. The child who is expected to read or write before he is developmentally ready is in the same position as one who is subjected to training procedures prematurely. Parents may be in competition with other parents whose children do not have learning difficulties and may interpret the lag in learning as a personal affront or as a reflection upon their child's intelligence. Pressures are exerted. The child strains to keep pace. He can be frustrated and discouraged by the criticisms of parents and teachers and the laughter of his peers. (See discussion on dyslexia in Chapter 5.)

Overprotection at home before entering school seems to have no effects on language achievements because these children have learned to verbalize with adults and usually read extensively. Problems in learning arithmetic may occur, however.

Speech disorders may develop because of delay in articulation or because of pressures from school and home. (See discussion in Chapter 6.)

When sounds are blurred or indistinct, a child is unable to associate them with the written word. The result is retardation. This auditory difficulty may result from developmental abnormality in the brain and have nothing to do with the organ of hearing.

2. The second broad explanation is self-explanatory. Good vision and good hearing facilitate learning. Brain damage may be minimal

---

[14]Lorynne Cahn and Robert Petersen: "Education and Mental Health: A Need for Interdisciplinary Inducement." *J. Sch. Health* *18*:4:218–220, April, 1973.

yet affect learning ability. A child who is chronically ill does not have the endurance for peak academic performance.

3. Emotional problems may antedate learning difficulties. Consider such factors as lack of motivation, anxiety, negativism, emotional blocking, indifference and absence of stimulation from parents and home environment, or conversely the pressures to excel, and the daily disturbances resulting from hearing and visual defects.

Whether it be a developmental problem, a visual or auditory problem, an incipient or progressive stutter, or hyperactivity, the rebound reactions may be those described under behavior problems in the preceding chapter. These are referred to here as secondary undesirable emotional characteristics. The child may become aggressive and nervous, or discouraged, submissive and hypoactive. The unhappy child with his bravado or his resignation deserves understanding and proper management.

Management of the Child with Learning Disabilities

Serious emotional reactions can be averted if learning disabilities are detected early. Responsibility for recognition lies with the school. The problem may not be detected and evaluated until a child is several years behind; in the meantime he has been considered stupid.

Parents and child must know the nature of the disorder. All underlying causes need to be found and corrected as far as possible.

Patience is necessary until the developmental lag has been replaced by a more mature pattern, even though the lag may cover several years. The age at which a child begins to read depends upon instructional procedures as well as innate ability and experiential background. Most children begin to read at about six years of age, and by eight years most can read simple books easily. Some may not start to read until later, and a few never learn to read. Progress is variable.

For reading problems a child should be stimulated to read and learn. Remedial reading classes should be available. Provide reading at the child's level. Watch his interests. Emphasize strengths. Restore a child's confidence; let him demonstrate to himself that he is not stupid. Accept him for what he is with his abilities and limitations. Make him surer of himself in all his relationships.

Educators today are more flexible in their standards of learning for each grade school level and take into account developmental delays, mental retardation, physical abnormalities, and behavior problems in planning a curriculum. More and more, attention is focused upon the individual and his needs and interests rather than upon chronological age and the amount of knowledge to be possessed in advancing from one grade to another. Indeed, in elementary schools architects take into account this shift in educational approach in various ways. Booths, alcoves, and peripheral arrangement of rooms around a central area, with or without doors, are some innovations. One plan provides spacious rooms in each of which pupils in two or more grades may be dispersed into quite a number of working groups, assigned to various teachers. A child can move from one group to another, according to his ability to handle various subjects. This particular arrangement is sometimes referred to as a pod, in which the enlarged group is organized and reorganized into subgroups for instructional purposes.

Learning centers for the mentally retarded can be fit into such an arrangement. All of the mentally retarded follow their own pursuits but will join other children for common activities in the lunchroom, the auditorium, and on the playgrounds. In this way they do not stand out as an unusual group. One must not forget that at times a child in the mentally retarded group, regardless of cause, is promoted to groups who have more average academic achievement. He may show talent in some field, e.g., art, and join a more advanced group in art in the same room. Parents are particularly gratified by these considerations and deplore the time when their youngsters must leave elementary school. With proper acoustical planning, thick carpets, and subdued voices, movement and learning and individual expression are possible. Ungraded classes and team teaching are some of the educational approaches being tried today in regular schools. Handicapped children benefit from flexible arrangements.

SUPERIOR INTELLIGENCE

What about the gifted child, the child of superior intelligence, or the child with specific, ingenious talents? His needs are the same as those of any child. In addition, he may present characteristics which need to be understood, and he needs special guidance to reach his potential.

On the whole, the gifted child tends to be superior physically, socially, and emotionally. More than average, he possesses integrity, wholesome attitudes, and a warm personality. Of course, there are exceptions.

The bright child begins to have problems in elementary school, before the age of 12, and these should be recognized early. In elementary school he represents 1 per cent of the population for his school age.

His common faults probably stem from lack of challenge and from boredom. He may present himself as inattentive, impatient, argumentative, loquacious, troublesome, as making poor grades deliberately in order to underplay his intelligence or because he feels the task as unworthy of effort. He may irritate others by his cocky and know-it-all attitude. He may tend to correct others, including the teachers. Desirable traits are warmth, independence, originality, poise, trustworthiness, and superior talents along certain lines.

Because he considers that his school work offers little challenge, he may become lazy, superficial, and scornful. He may arouse the antagonism of peer group and teacher. Given a challenge, he is anxious to succeed, but may be reluctant to undertake sports or projects where he may not excel.

Management of the Gifted Child

If he is advanced rapidly in school, the gifted child must be watched carefully. Emotional maturity and peer group relationships are of prime importance. With his own age he may hear, "If you're so smart, prove it." If promoted to association with an older group, he is more likely to be respected for his intelligence. How will he adjust to this group? He should not feel inadequate socially or emotionally. Because he is known to be superior intellectually, he will often have trouble making friends. He may become withdrawn. Or, if his magnificent talent is focused to a narrow field, he may be annoyed with any distractions and become a loner. Occasionally, a teacher may be resentful of a bright child and will suppress or ridicule him.

Parents and teachers should not stand in awe of the gifted child; he needs understanding, but he should be held to reasonable guidance and discipline. Some children wish to be considered as special, however, and may become demanding, aggressive, selfish, and unable to participate in group activities.

A plan should be formulated which should involve the parents, teachers, school psychologist, and educators who can give advice in management of gifted children. This plan should be patterned especially for each child, and efforts made to have the parents understand relationships and objectives. If parents do not understand or cooperate, if they apply too much pressure to the child or exact adult behavior, or if they are mediocre themselves and do not understand or appreciate their child, the far-reaching result will be a maladjusted individual. Educators should take a leading, continuing role in management of a gifted child; they should enjoy the superior child in the classroom and create opportunities for intellectual challenge; the school and society must be benefited by the preparation of the gifted and highly gifted child.

HEADACHES IN YOUTH

Children in the elementary grades suffer from headaches. When these occur, they are likely to be premonitory of oncoming infection and may be associated with nausea and vomiting. If they persist or recur, they may be due to emotional disturbances, or occasionally to a serious organic disease. The child may have suffered a head injury. A youngster with a headache should be taken home. On the other hand, with the increase in tensions of adolescence, headaches occur in this age group with greater frequency.

A headache is a symptom, not a disease. It is uncomfortable and common, and its causes are many. If headaches persist and recur frequently, a thorough investigation is indicated. It is not always easy for a physician to ascertain the cause of a headache. Close questioning is necessary in order to secure an exact description—the site, the frequency, the time of day it occurs—and to secure an impression of the physical and emotional problems of an individual. Physical examinations must be done; often various neurological tests are performed; and always the physician keeps in mind that emotions play an important role.

POSSIBLE CAUSES

Pain-sensitive structures about the head are the scalp, skin, muscles of the forehead, blood vessels and nerves in this region (brain itself is insensitive), brain coverings, eyes, ears, nose, neck, and teeth.

Organic Disorders

Extrinsic diseases of the scalp.

Injuries (bruises and cuts) to the scalp and its nerves, muscles, or blood vessels.

Infections.

Neuritis.

Intrinsic diseases within the cranium (1 to 2 per cent of cases).

Brain tumors, anomalies of blood vessels, circulatory disturbances, including clots and hemorrhages, injuries to supporting tissues of the brain (as in concussion), infections of the coverings of the brain (as in meningitis), infections in the brain itself (a brain abscess).

These two categories will include the broad designation of head injury.

Systemic disease.

Extremes of blood pressure (too high or too low), too much or too little blood, too much alkali, kidney failure, low blood sugar (as with no breakfast), withdrawal of drugs (sometimes even from withdrawal of beverages containing caffeine, such as coffee), infections (influenza, common cold, etc.), spread of a malignant tumor from some other organ to the brain, allergies, or exposure to poisons, e.g., carbon monoxide.

Neck.

Arthritis of the vertebrae, neuritis, inflammation in the muscles (wry neck), and injuries, for instance, the "whiplash" injury.

Eyes.

Intrinsic eye disease of parts of the eye (iris, retina, optic nerve), including glaucoma.

Most refractive errors do not cause headaches. Headaches which seem attributable to refractive errors tend to occur in the latter half of the day. Actually, very few headaches are related to eyes.

Teeth (occasionally).

Infections, pressures, malocclusion. Not a significant source of headaches.

Nose, sinuses, and ears.

May cause acute headaches. Seen with acute sinus and ear infections.

Not a common cause of chronic headaches. Not as often as blamed.

FUNCTIONAL DISORDERS (NON-ORGANIC)

The word "functional" is frequently used as a designation to imply that no physical or organic explanation can be found for a disorder, and that after a process of evaluation the cause is considered to be on an emotional basis. Ninety-five per cent of all headaches are considered to be functional.

1. Vascular headaches (changes in blood vessels).
   Migraine headaches.
   Vascular tension headaches ("nervous" headaches, atypical, nonmigrainous).
2. Muscle contraction headaches.
   Steady contraction of muscles in neck and those attached to scalp.
   Produced by tension.

Migraine Headaches. Migraine headaches, the headaches of civilization, do occur in children. Symptoms may start at some time before the age of ten. They are more common in boys than girls; the converse is true among adults. They vary in intensity, duration, and frequency, even in the same individual. The tendency to this type of headache occurs in families, for it is noticed that about 50 per cent of the children of parents suffering from migraine develop headaches also. Of this number, 80 per cent receive the trait from the mother, 20 per cent from the father. Apparently there is a hereditary, constitutional tendency, and emotion or stress precipitates the headache.

Physiology. The physiological explanation of this particular type of headache is on a vascular basis. With the onset of the attack, there is first a constriction of branches of the external carotid artery on the affected side. They then relax and dilate beyond their usual diameters; as the vessels pulsate, the dilated walls stretch, producing the throbbing headache. Later, there may be tenderness with pressure over the blood vessels on the painful side. A typical migraine attack is characterized as having:

1. an aura or warning, consisting often of disturbances of vision in one or both eyes, starting with the visual center and spreading out slowly in circles until partial, one half of a field, or total vision is lost for a few moments. Some describe scintillating, jagged, or irregular bands of light surrounding a bright white, misty visual defect. In children the earliest symptoms and signs are usually lassitude, loss of appetite, and abdominal distress. Complaints of sensitivity to light may be heard.
2. a unilateral headache—usually only one side of the head is involved at a time, but a severe headache may spread to both sides. In young children headaches are less likely to be localized to one side.
3. nausea and vomiting. These may be more dominant than actual headache.
4. a history of such headaches in the family.

Usually several, if not all, of the above criteria exist. The pattern varies from person to person and varies in the same individual. The initial constriction of the blood vessels accounts for the visual disturbances. These headaches are sometimes described as "blinding headaches," "sick headaches," or as "bilious headaches" because of the nausea and vomiting. Initiation of the attack may be trigger-like, a result of sudden anxiety or worry, or the pain may develop gradually with some warning. A child may suffer a migraine headache the night before an examination, or may be tense during the examination only to suffer the attack after the tension is over and relaxation occurs. This child is usually an intelligent individual who does not have poor grades. Rather, a heavy study schedule and the drive for perfect performance are more than he can handle without tension.

Role of Emotions. Emotional disturbances account for most headaches. The emotional conflict may not be obvious; and the headache may appear before, during or after the crisis.

> A young girl dated the onset of her migraine headaches back two years when she had eloped, contracted a marriage disapproved by her parents, secured a divorce, and then returned to the family home, all within her senior year in high school. Several members of her family also suffered from migraine attacks. After she left home for college, the headaches became infrequent, only to return in full force when she went home for vacation.

A demand for accomplishing some unusual project which may reveal a person's inadequacy, such as making a speech or playing in a concert, may precipitate an incapacitating headache. A victim who is rigid in personality or a perfectionist may find that he cannot fulfill his own high standards or self-demands or those of his family and begins to suffer head pain.

Most individuals who suffer migraine headaches conform to a similar psychological pattern. They are intelligent, tense, striving, perfectionistic, orderly people who when under duress become more tense and more fatigued. They suffer guilt feelings with deviations from an orderly pattern, such as going to a show or taking time off to listen to musical records. Highly spontaneous situations worry them because everything must be planned just so and be under control.

These people with migraine headaches exact from themselves the highest standards and are frustrated, anxious, self-derogatory, and angry within when their demands upon themselves are not fulfilled. Bogged down by detail, unable to delegate tasks, sensitive to criticism, they will persist in doing things harder, longer, and better than others and are despairing when not permitted to do their best.

Perfectionists are their own worst enemies. There are not enough hours in the day to do everything perfectly; nor can one be consistently superior to his peers.

These sensitive children need constant reassurance that they are not inferior, that migraine headaches are a disorder of worthwhile people.

Not everyone with the above psychological pattern develops migraine headaches; but given a basic tendency towards migraine, they will probably develop. These headaches become a way of life.

Migraine headaches may occur quite early in childhood.

> One pediatrician relates the problems of a youngster who began to suffer disabling pain midway through her first year at school. She had one particular handicap which became an object of derision of her classmates. There was no history of migraine in the family.
>
> A little boy of eight years had suffered typical migraine headaches for some time. His mother had them also. What types of problems aroused tension? Trivial as they may seem to an adult, he worried if he had an ink blot on his paper while writing. Once, when he could not draw a turkey's feet satisfactorily, the pain started. His physician suggested an ingenious procedure for therapy. The boy was given a sheet of paper with three columns on it. On it he was to record whether a problem was truly serious, moderately serious, or only slightly so. The youngster sometimes recorded his reactions in the first column, changed his mind and shifted to the second, and with increasing frequency began to shift to the third.

Migraine headaches may start in the teens, at a time when there is increasing stress, increasing responsibility, increasing need to define future objectives, and a need to conform to a way of life. They may stop in middle age when presumably personal ambitions are not so strong and some compromises to living have been made.

Vascular Tension Headaches. Many of the attacks due to emotional tensions are characterized as "vascular tension headaches" or as "nervous headaches." They are not typically migraine-like in character but may respond to the same type of treatment. They may be troubling, affect both temples, the "top" of the head, the "whole" head, or just the forehead. They may be described as generalized, dull headaches or simply as discomforts. Sometimes they are hard to describe.

A headache often serves as a convenient escape mechanism. One cannot prove its presence or absence. There may even be some suspicion of malingering, as evidenced by the following episode:

> A new girl in the seventh grade was seen by a physician during routine health examinations at school. She had managed to avoid such an examination on several occasions, but was found this particular morning and escorted to the examining room in the gymnasium. About an hour later she reported to the physical education teacher, who incidentally was acting as a recorder during examinations, that she needed an excuse to go home because of a headache. Questioning elicited the fact that she had been requesting such a slip at ten o'clock each morning. Description of the headache was vague; the girl herself seemed lethargic and vague. Following a consultation of physician, physical education teacher, and the school nurse, the nurse visited the home immediately. After some delay the mother was awakened and questioned about her daughter's headaches. She evinced no interest in a medical follow-up because she herself had suffered such headaches for years and thought nothing could be done about them.

Muscle Contraction Headaches. Pains or discomforts in the back of the neck, forehead, or scalp, or a vise-like or band-like tightness around the cranium are usually caused by steady contraction of muscles from tension—contraction of which a person may be unaware.

The constant strain of daily life, with the accompanying persistent rigidity of all or some of the muscles of the body, the chronic anxieties which plague many people in their insecurities, the fears which may be deep-rooted and unsuspected—all these can account for most of our modern headache problems.

Child, adolescent, or adult, the mechanism and results are the same.

Follow-up

From the detailed outline above, it is obvious that the determination of a possible cause for persistent headaches may require extensive investigation. One must be sure that there has been no blow on the head. Children frequently forget an injury and do not mention it. A complete physical examination is usually necessary, and at times a special neurological study is undertaken. To delay a medical consultation may be a serious mistake. The vicious habit of self-medication with pain-killing drugs, tranquilizers, and drugs containing bromides not only may result in toxicity, but may delay an urgent investigation that might reveal a diseased condition which warrants immediate care in order to save a life. For instance, surgery for some types of brain tumors is often successful.

Contrary to general belief, the need for glasses for distant or close vision, or the prolonged use of the eyes rarely causes headaches.

If the conclusion is reached that a headache is psychogenic in origin, appropriate therapy should follow. A teacher can seek to learn what situations are causing stress at school and attempt to help. Teachers should lighten study loads, manage the perfectionist, modify intense straining or frustration, allay feelings of guilt or inferiority, offer opportunities for triumphs, and provide reassurances. This is a big order! Communications should be possible between counselor, teacher, school nurse, physician, and parent. It is possible that a student may be referred to a psychiatrist or to a mental health clinic.

THE BATTERED OR NEGLECTED CHILD

A parent, in frustration, anger, or to satisfy sadistic impulses, plunges his child's hands into hot water or holds them over a flame. A sixth-grade boy runs away from home again and again; each time he is beaten by his step-father; the last time he was beaten with the buckle end of a belt; his teacher noticed bruises along the ribs and reported the injury. A second grade girl wears a long-sleeved blouse to cover the marks of whiplashes on the arms. Children are left abandoned at home for days without food or care. There is no end to the tales of brutality suffered by children, from neglect to murder. The term "battered child syndrome" refers to their physical abuse by parents.

Until children are old enough to defend themselves, as with a senior high school boy, mistreatment occurs at all ages, more so in infants and in the preschool group. Still, school nurses, teachers, principals, police officers, and juvenile court personnel can relate unbelievable stories for all ages, including high school. Most of these do not receive publicity until a flagrant episode catches the newspaper's attention or a child dies.

Many cases of assault and neglect are not reported. A mother who is a bystander usually will not report the father or stepfather. Indeed, she will lie to protect him. Other contacts may suspect maltreatment but do not want to become involved, testify in court, or participate otherwise in the routine of follow-up. A neighbor may feel that he does not have sufficient evidence. And, there is reluctance to believe that parents could intentionally abuse their own children.

Children themselves usually do not complain at school. Surprisingly enough, some of them take it for granted that all children are punished in similar fashion by their parents. Some are afraid to report. The spirit can be beaten down; home does not offer a haven of security; they believe the tirades concerning their unworthiness. Only when they are in pain, or when evidence of injury or neglect is observed by others, will the extent of the abuse be determined.

Blows on the head may produce skull fractures, headaches, nausea and vomiting, convulsions, or combinations of these; cuffing over the ears may puncture ear drums and impair hearing; blows to the abdomen can cause pain, especially if an organ is ruptured; blows to the chest can produce pain with breathing; bones can be broken and x-rays may show evidence of previous healing or healed fractures; bruises can hurt.

Neglect is not necessarily correlated with assault. A child may be well-nourished and attractively clothed, yet suffer many injuries.

Abuse does not necessarily need to be physical. A vicious, mean parent who visits her neuroses and her sadistic feelings on her little girl, whether natural or adopted, by demeaning her spiritually and intellectually until the child sits dispirited and parrots everything the mother says is murdering a personality.

What moves parents to beat or abuse or neglect their children? The answer varies. A child may irritate his family by mannerisms, defiance, refusal to "mind," insults and abusive words, or the many manifestations of rebellion. More often, severe abuse can be accounted for in the personality of parents. Here are some general observations on parents and on the family situations:

> A defect in the character structure of a parent permits impulsive, aggressive behavior upon the slightest provocation. Most parents suffer from such psychological deviations as neuroses, immature or inadequate feelings of unworthiness of self and child, alcoholism, mental retardation, or combinations of these.
>
> A guilty parent may justify his behavior on the basis that he received similar treatment in his own childhood.
>
> There may be conscious or unconscious rejection of a child for various reasons.
>
> The battered or neglected child usually lives where the marriage is unstable or in a broken home. He usually lives with parents in the lower economic bracket, although this does not always hold. There can be serious marital conflicts in any level of society, even in apparently stable, financially secure homes.
>
> The child is usually the object of parents' frustrations, anxieties, and hostilities.
>
> In general, parents show little remorse or feelings of guilt or even concern about an injury unless motivated by fear of discovery. They are quick to deny any blame for injury or neglect. These parents are preoccupied with themselves and not with their children.

Follow-up and Management

Legal Liability

Almost every state has a statute regarding the welfare of the battered or neglected child. Provisions vary on the method of handling a case. Either a law enforcement agency, sheriff's office or local police, or a child protective agency, or both, should be notified. Under the last provision, where both are involved at once, complaint has been made of confusion and delay in rehabilitation of the parents and child.[15] The child protective agency is usually placed under the organization of the juvenile court.

Provisions of the law in one state[16] make it mandatory that "Any person having cause to believe that a minor has had physical injury as a result of unusual or unreasonable physical abuse or neglect shall report or cause reports to be made." *Confidentiality is important,* and the person making the report "in good faith" should be protected from suit. "Any person or institution making a report in good faith pursuant to this act shall have immunity from any liability, civil or criminal, that might be otherwise incurred or imposed."

A teacher needs to know the channels organized in his school system for reporting suspected cases of neglect or assault. The Department of Health Services of the Denver Public School reported for 1967–1968:

> Battered children reported through the school health services and therefore initially detected by school personnel such as teachers, principals, nurses, or social workers, totaled 46 during the school year.

Just reporting a suspected case to either the school nursing office, the social worker, the sheriff, a child protective agency, or to the juvenile court is only the beginning of a long road of readjustments. Parents do not change overnight. Their conduct must be under observation for a long period of time; sometimes divorces occur. Agencies take time to investigate cases. Decisions as to placement in foster homes must be made. Progress depends upon the family and upon the facilities in the community for protecting children. The approach is a combined medical, social, and legal one. The home situation is evaluated. The final disposition of a child depends upon the rehabilitation, if possible, of parents. Prosecution may be necessary.

The concern of the teacher is with the child in his classroom—a child who has been subjected to trauma, both physical and emotional, who is threatened with separation from his parents, who has been subjected to questioning by strangers, and who may have been the object of a good deal of publicity. Every attention of the school should safeguard the child.

MANAGEMENT AT SCHOOL OF THE CHILD WITH A MALIGNANT NEOPLASM

The term "malignant neoplasm" refers to a growth of cells within the body, which is invasive, destructive, "malign," and tends to spread to other parts of the body.

---

[15]Lenore C. Terr and Andrew S. Watson: "The Battered Child Rebrutalized: Ten Cases of Medical-Legal Confusion." *Amer. J. Psych. 124*:1432–1439, 1968.

[16]Law passed in Utah in 1965.

Children with malignant neoplasms do attend school, at least for a while, or intermittently. A child with a malignant bone tumor may return after amputation of an extremity. How should his teachers and peers approach him? "First, the child with cancer who is well enough to be in school can still learn, and can, and should, enjoy learning."[17] A child with leukemia gradually becomes weaker, yet is spirited and insistent upon participating in all activities. How may he be handled wisely?

Malignancies in childhood constitute the second leading cause of death in children one to 14 years of age. The common sites are: the lymphatic system (including leukemia)—47.6 per cent; the nervous system (including the eyes)—22.9 per cent; and other organs and tissues, namely kidneys, bone, adrenal glands, and soft tissues.

Leukemia is a disease of the blood-forming tissue, characterized usually by a persistent and uncontrolled production of white blood cells and their precursors. In childhood the disease tends to be acute. As the disease progresses, there is anemia, internal hemorrhage, and increasing exhaustion. With modern treatment there may be several remissions during which the child looks and feels better and may resume his school and play activities. Current drug therapy holds great promise for prolonging life.

In many instances the removal of an extremity because of a malignant bone tumor assures a long survival rate. With an early diagnosis while the growth is localized, a probable cure is effected. It is not unusual to interview a student in college who suffered an amputation years before, is apparently well, and has adjusted to the efficient use of a prosthesis. Children adapt well to the loss of an extremity.

A child prefers to attend school and remain with his classmates. His parents and his physician wish him to lead a "normal" life as

[17] Frederick R. Cyphert: "Back to School for the Child with Cancer." *J. Sch. Health* *43*:4:215, April, 1973.

TABLE 9 Deaths from Malignant Neoplasms 1967 (United States)*

ALL CAUSES	TOTAL (ALL AGES)	AGES UNDER 5 YEARS	5–9 YEARS	10–14 YEARS	15–19 YEARS
Male	169,164	797	866	680	840
Female	141,819	682	634	531	500
LEUKEMIA AND ALEUKEMIA					
Male	8,222	363	459	285	276
Female	6,114	321	342	193	135

*U.S. Public Health Service, National Center for Health Statistics.

TABLE 10 Leading Causes of Death in Children 1–14 Years—Rate Per 100,000 Children. (Cancer kills more children in the United States than any other illness. Approximately 4,000 children under 15 years of age die of cancer annually.)*

1936		1966	
1. Accidents	40.1	1. Accidents	41.5
2. Pneumonia	38.6	2. Cancer	12.2
3. Diarrhea and Enteritis	16.1	3. Congenital Malformations	8.6
4. Influenza	11.0	4. Influenza and Pneumonia	8.0
5. Appendicitis	10.6	5. Meningitis	1.5
6. Tuberculosis	9.7	6. Heart Diseases	1.4
7. Heart Diseases	8.8	7. Homicide	1.4
8. Diphtheria	7.6	8. Gastritis	1.3
9. Cancer†	5.3	9. Cerebral Hemorrhage (Stroke)	1.3
10. Scarlet Fever	5.1	10. Meningococcal Infections	1.2
11. Diseases of Ear and Mastoid	4.7	11. Cystic Fibrosis	1.1
12. Diseases of Buccal Cavity and Pharynx	4.5	12. Cerebral Spastic Infantile Paralysis	1.0

*Courtesy of the American Cancer Society. Source: the vital statistics of the United States.
†Includes leukemia and Hodgkin's disease.

long as his physical capacity permits him to do so.[18] He probably has no conception of his health problem; when he does acquire a dim understanding, he will be likely to adopt an unrealistic attitude.

On the other hand, sometimes a child does suspect or actually know the nature of his illness. This is particularly true of an older, intelligent person. He overhears a conversation of nurses or other adults on the ward; he returns to a clinic or to a physician's office time after time for blood tests and examinations. Even if he knows that he has a fatal disease, if his parents do not wish him to be aware of the diagnosis and prognosis, he usually plays the game.

As far as the school and the teacher are concerned, the same philosophy holds here as in the discussion of the handicapped or crippled child. He has the same needs as other children. He should be held to reasonable standards. Ask him to participate and contribute. Expectations are based upon the pupil's ability level. The school nurse, the patent, the principal, and the teacher need to confer at intervals and plan management.

SUMMARY

The trend is to place youth with physical handicaps, nervous manifestations, or mental deficiencies in regular schools and in regular classrooms. This means that teachers will have contact with these young people in teaching situations and in the school environment. Teachers need to have some scientific information concerning the nature of a child's handicap or disorder, should appreciate the

[18]Lawrence Elliott: *A Little Girl's Gift*. New York: Holt, Rinehart and Winston, Inc., 1963. The story of an eight-year-old girl with leukemia.

general and unique emotional implications of each problem in order to pursue intelligent management, and, of course, must be familiar with educational techniques. This chapter endeavors to explain the scientific bases of handicaps and disorders which a teacher is likely to encounter. The detailed descriptions of the emotional aspects of these problems will serve to clarify interrelationships, benefiting both pupil and educator. Specifically described are hyperactivity, epilepsy, cerebral palsy, mental retardation, learning disabilities, superior intelligence, headaches, the battered or neglected child, and management at school of the child with a malignant neoplasm.

DISCUSSION QUESTIONS AND ACTIVITIES

1. Discuss the problems and solutions of a hyperkinetic student. What kind of understanding is needed in dealing with his medication?
2. Discuss the first aid for a grand mal seizure. If this happens to a student in class, what should the teacher tell the other students?
3. Write the Epilepsy Foundation of America and request materials that a teacher could use concerning epilepsy.
4. Inquire at a large school system to find what they are doing with students who have learning disabilities.
5. Discuss how you would handle a student with superior intelligence.
6. Inquire as to the procedure a teacher would use to report a child neglect case. Are social workers involved?
7. Explain why cancer has risen from the ninth to the second leading cause of death in the past thirty years for children from 1 to 14 years of age.
8. Discuss what should be done with a child with recurring headaches. What causes are associated with this problem?
9. Organize a group interested in collecting donations for one of the charity research agencies in this area. Make sure they know what disorder they are collecting for.
10. Visit a cerebral palsy clinic and report on this to the class. Could you apply anything you learned there to teaching?

ADDITIONAL SOURCES OF INFORMATION

READINGS

Bagley, C.: *The Social Psychology of the Child with Epilepsy.* London: Routledge and Paul, 1971.

Bierbauer, E.: "The Educationally Handicapped Child." *J.A.M.A.* 217:482, July 26, 1971.
Birenbaum, A.: "The Mentally Retarded Child in the Home and Family Cycle." *J. Health Soc. Behav.* 12:55–65, March, 1971.
Chasey, W. C.: "Effects of a Physical Development Program on Psychomotor Ability of Retarded Children." *Am. J. Ment. Defic.* 75:566–570, March, 1971.
Chess, S., et al.: "Behavior Deviation in Mentally Retarded Children." *J. Am. Acad. Child Psychiat.* 9:282–297, April, 1970.
Dykman, R. A., et al.: "Children With Learning Disabilities: Conditioning, Differentiation, and the Effect of Distraction." *Am. J. Orthopsychiat.* 40:766–782, October, 1970.
Fassler, J.: "Performance of Cerebral Palsied Children Under Conditions of Reduced Auditory Input." *Exceptional Child.* 37:201–209, November, 1970.
Harlin, V. K.: "Experiences with Epileptic Children in a Public School Program." *J. Sch. Health* 35:20–24, 1965.
Holmes, L.: *Mental Retardation: An Atlas of Diseases with Associated Physical Abnormalities.* New York: The Macmillan Co., 1972.
Ives, L. A.. "Learning Difficulties in Children with Epilepsy." *Brit. J. Disord. Commun.* 5:77–84, April, 1970.
Loehner, C.: *Learning Disabilities and the Educationally Handicapped Child.* Upland, California: Phalarope Pub. Co., 1971.
McGrady, H. J.: "Learning Disabilities: Implications for Medicine and Education." *J. Sch. Health* 41:227–234, May, 1971.
Mitchell, R. G.: "The Prevention of Cerebral Palsy." *Develop. Med. Child Neurol.* 13:137–146, April, 1971.
NEA Journal: Vol. 56 (November, 1967) has a number of articles on what the classroom teacher can do for "The Handicapped in the Regular Classroom," "The Child with Speech Defects," "Crippled and Health-Impaired Children," "The Asthmatic Child," "The Child with Impaired Vision," "The Child with Impaired Hearing." Also, "The Surge in Special Education."
Pond, D. A.: "Psychiatric Disorders Accompanying Epilepsy in Children." *Rev. Neuropsychiat. Infant.* 18:517–521, 18:505–510, July–August, 1970.
Tarnopol, L. (Ed.): *Learning Disorders in Children: Diagnosis, Medication, Education.* Boston: Little, Brown and Co., 1971.

AUDIOVISUAL MATERIALS

Care of the Young Retarded Child

18 min. Color *sh,* adults International Film Bureau

Training aid for parents and teachers of retarded children.

Handle With Care

28 min. Black and White *sh,* adults U. S. Department of Health, Education, and Welfare

Shows a variety of activities coordinated to provide comprehensive services to mentally retarded children in a metropolitan area.

Rafe: Developing Giftedness in the Educational Disadvantaged

120 min. Color teacher education Bailey Films, Inc.

Portrays Rafe—a gifted child in three situations—his home, his school, and neighborhood. Provides stimulus for action toward establishing adequate programs for the gifted child. Excellent.

The Gifted Ones

22 min. Black and White *sh,* adults International Film Bureau

Presents views of educators regarding challenge presented in education for the gifted child. Shows some in their regular classroom activities.

All of the following films listed are available from the Epilepsy Foundation of America.

Blueprint for Epilepsy

25 min. Black and White

Deals with vocational problems of the adult with epilepsy.

Boy in a Storm

30 min. From "Medic" TV program.

Dark Wave

24 min. Color

Excellent for showing to teachers, students, P.T.A. Illustrates problems of children with minor seizures.

Modern Concepts of Epilepsy

25 min. Color

For doctors, nurses, social workers, educators. Demonstrates actual seizures.

On the Go

20 min. Color

An interview type of film.

Seizures

21 min. Black and White

Illustrates major types of seizures.

RESOURCES (Partial list)

American Association on Mental Deficiency
American Cancer Society
American Medical Association
American Public Health Association, Inc.
Council for Exceptional Children
Epilepsy Foundation of America (state and local chapters)
International Council on Exceptional Children
Muscular Dystrophy Association of America, Inc.
National Association for Mental Health
National Foundation
 Catalog. "Publication, Films, and Exhibits"—current edition.
National Society for Crippled Children and Adults, Inc.
 (State and local affiliates—Easter Seal societies)
 Catalog of Publications. Films, film strips, slides.
 The Crippled Child—magazine.
Offices of Vocational Rehabilitation (state and local)
Ohio Youth Commission, 2280 West Broad Street, Columbus, Ohio 43223, publishes a "Directory for Children with Special Needs." This lists schools, agencies, and institutions for children with a variety of handicaps.
Public Affairs Committee, Inc.
 Up-to-date pamphlets on many health problems.
Special Education departments of teacher training institutions
The American Cleft Palate Association
United Cerebral Palsy Association, Inc.
U. S. Department of Health, Education, and Welfare
 Social and Rehabilitation Service—information about obtaining financial assistance for a special child. Various bulletins on health problems discussed in this chapter.
See Appendix A for names of organizations. Names designate health interest.
See footnotes in this chapter.
See readings and resources at end of each chapter on health problems.

Part II

THE SCHOOL HEALTH PROGRAM

School Health Program

HEALTHFUL SCHOOL LIVING

HEALTHFUL PHYSICAL ENVIRONMENT

- The plant
  - Selection of site
  - Design for educational needs, adaptability, comfort
    - Organization of space
    - Basic considerations
      - Visual, thermal, acoustical
    - Esthetic values
  - Design for safety, health facilities, sanitation
  - Operation and maintenance
    - Custodial services
  - Community use
- School bus

HEALTHFUL SCHOOL DAY

- Educational aspects
- School organization
  - Schedule
  - Extraclass activities
  - Safety program
  - Lunch program
- Classroom experience
  - Emotional climate of school and classroom
  - Discipline
  - Methods of teaching

HEALTH OF PERSONNEL

- Provision of favorable conditions for physical, emotional, and mental well-being

HEALTH SERVICES

HEALTH APPRAISAL

- Health history
- Health observations
- Screening tests
- Special surveys
- Psychological tests
- Health examination
- Cumulative health record

FOLLOW-UP SERVICES

- Individual
  - Referral for correction of remediable defects
  - Adjustment to classroom and school environment
  - Special programs
    - Speech correction
    - Auditory training
    - Mental health
- Health counseling of child and parents
- Nursing services for detection and follow-up

OTHER SERVICES

- Communicable disease control
  - Immunizations
- Emergency care of injuries and sudden illness

HEALTH OF PERSONNEL

- Appraisal of health status
  - Periodic health examinations for teachers and employees
- Health services for personnel

HEALTH EDUCATION

HEALTH INSTRUCTION

- Development of health concepts by means of planned and incidental health teaching experiences
- Curriculum based on student needs and interests and the needs of community and social groups
- Organized classes in health science and healthful living
- Utilization of various educational media, library resources, and community facilities

INTEGRATION

- Health information integrated with experiences of daily living and personal achievement
- To build wholesome attitudes towards health
- To establish sound health practices
- To appreciate responsibilities for health in the home, school, and community

GUIDANCE

- Individual and group counseling

Chapter 16

DEVELOPMENT OF THE SCHOOL HEALTH PROGRAM

Interest in the health of the school child did not spring full-grown from the minds of a group of educators or public health officials. The gradual awareness of the importance of health—health for the general masses and specifically for the school child—covers hundreds of years, and has gathered impetus in this century as our knowledge of the causes of diseases has been placed upon a scientific basis. To appreciate the present status of the school health program, a brief review of the development of the public health movement is indicated.

GROWTH OF THE PUBLIC HEALTH PROGRAM

It is not too far a cry from the health rules laid down for participants in the Olympic games in ancient Greece to the present day emphasis on physical fitness. The objectives of the leaders were the same: a physically fit young generation, the hope of the future for a nation. The Greeks were devoted to Hygeia, the goddess of health, and most of the precepts of hygiene observed then are perfectly acceptable today. From the athletic fields of Greece and the clean streets of Rome with its sanitary codes, pure food laws, good water, and clean public baths, from the devotion of the Greeks and Romans to bodily perfection and cleanliness, one turns to the dismal centuries of the Middle Ages, the dark ages indeed of personal hygiene.

The Middle Ages had many public health problems. A series of plagues decimated the population of Europe. These plagues were considered as manifestations of the disfavor of Divine Providence, and the prevailing attitude was one of submission. Some attempt was made, however, to combat them by isolation or quarantine, a public health technique which was effective for the plague of leprosy.

This technique was not successful in the control of bubonic plague, a disease spread by the fleas which infested rats.

Europe was confronted with almost insurmountable health problems as it emerged from the Middle Ages. Changes in the way of life, such as the transfer of population from the feudal lands to the larger towns and cities, and the transfer of industry from the homes to the factories, resulted in deplorable living conditions. Whenever people live in communities, questions arise concerning sanitation, water supply, sewage disposal, food supply, and spread of communicable disease. During the Industrial Revolution, as exemplified by the development of the textile industry in England, not only did these public health problems arise, but the plight of child labor aroused the concern of governing bodies and thoughtful people. Communicable diseases, commonly typhoid and typhus fevers, dysentery and diphtheria, were rampant in Europe and in the United States. Since the only explanation of disease at that time was the *miasmic* theory, i.e., something in the air causes diseases, attempts were made to improve sanitation. The Era of Sanitation in public health began in the middle of the nineteenth century.

Sanitation and Communicable Disease Control

The preceding explanation of disease and attempts founded upon it to combat and prevent disease could prove only partly effective. A more accurate explanation of the causes of disease and methods of prevention and control was necessary. The modern public health era became firmly established with the patient, scientific research of Louis Pasteur (1822–1895). He proved that many diseases are caused by microbes, actual organisms which can be grown in culture media and seen through a microscope. He not only developed the theory of *parasitology*, i.e., disease is due to living parasites, but also evolved our modern concepts of immunology. His work opened up the whole field of study of communicable diseases. Scientists in Europe and in the United States began investigation of communicable diseases, their causative organisms, methods of spread, and control and prevention. The 1890's were indeed the golden age of bacteriology.

With the turn of the century, and for the next two decades, public attention was focused by public health officials upon the control of communicable diseases, and the problems of sanitation were gradually solved by departments of health. With good water supply, adequate disposal of sewage, pasteurization of milk, regulations on foods, isolation techniques, immunization procedures, and emphasis on health education, the incidence of the common communicable diseases was greatly reduced. Such scourges as typhoid fever and childhood dysenteries, the latter once a cause of high infant mortality, were controlled. With the pasteurization of milk and high milk standards, tuberculosis in children dropped amazingly. Diphtheria no longer killed entire families of children.

In more recent times the advent of the antibiotics and the development of effective vaccines have greatly reduced the incidence of communicable diseases. Research in the diseases caused by the viruses is being pursued in many laboratories today. The incidence of poliomyelitis and measles fell dramatically after mass inoculations in the last decade. See Figures 44 and 49. In general the communicable diseases are well under control and no longer present a dominant problem in a child's life.

Interest in the Individual

With the advent of the first World War, health-minded officials in this country were confronted with a different type of problem. From 1916 to 1918 physical examinations of the men being drafted between ages 21 and 31 directed attention to the health status of the individual. Approximately three and one-half million men were examined. On the first draft 2,510,706 men were examined. Almost one third (730,756) were rejected for health reasons. Such a high percentage of rejectees and defects gave rise to much discussion of ways and means for promoting healthier future generations. Could the schools have prevented or corrected many of these defects by conserving or improving the health of children?

After World War I, the school administrator and teacher were still interested in the prevention and early detection of communicable diseases; but their attention shifted to other areas, such as child growth and development, nutrition, condition of teeth, emotional disturbances, mental hygiene, and the effects of physical and mental defects upon learning processes. Interest, in other words, shifted to the health of the individual.

Since World War I various criteria have been applied to any evaluation of the health status of American youth. The results of the preinduction health examinations for Selective Service provide one criterion. Although the objective here is military fitness, we obtain an overall review of the health defects of the group over 18 years of age.

The next opportunity after 1918 to measure the results of mass examinations of youth began just before World War II. By May, 1944 more than 13,000,000 preinduction health examinations were conducted on registrants between the ages of 18 and 37. About 4,000,000 were disqualified for physical and mental disabilities. Physical defects accounted for 58 per cent; mental disease accounted for 16 per cent.

What are the disqualifying physical problems? By far, the leading physical cause of rejection has been musculoskeletal or orthopedic defects. Apparently, our youth suffer from the cumulative effects of injuries in their childhood. Back trouble and poor function of knees and shoulders are common complaints. Other causes of rejection are hearing and visual defects, allergies, heart diseases, ulcers in the digestive tract, severe disfiguring acne, overweight and underweight, and, in diminishing incidence, other problems.

A most embarrassing situation centers around teeth. At the beginning of World War II a man was expected to have 12 teeth which met in a bite six in front and six on the sides. Despite this modest requirement, defective teeth was the leading cause of physical disqualification. Finally, all dental standards were abolished. Today if a man has "anything in his mouth," he is accepted and supplied with dentures.

A summary of medical disqualifications, covering two decades, is shown in Table 11.

Perhaps a few words of explanation are indicated here to clarify the tabulation in Table 11. There are examinations conducted other

TABLE 11 Selective Service Registrants Not Qualified (September 1948 – September 1967)*

AGENCY AND REASON FOR NON-QUALIFICATION	NUMBER OF REGISTRANTS		
Not Qualified by Local Boards upon Medical Interview at Request of Armed Forces			1,605,578
Total Examined – Preinduction			11,878,249
Not Qualified by Armed Forces at Preinduction Examination			4,937,220
Not Qualified, Mental Test Only	1,683,592		
Not Qualified, Medically Only	2,764,843		
Circulatory System Diseases		314,466	
Bones and Organs of Movement Diseases and Defects		429,172	
Psychiatric Disorders		357,737	
Digestive System Diseases		188,424	
Eye Diseases and Defects		245,761	
Ear and Mastoid Process Diseases and Defects		173,528	
Allergic Disorders		154,831	
Congenital Malformations		106,654	
Neoplastic Disorders		54,813	
Infectious and Parasitic Disorders		133,162	
Neurological Diseases		121,169	
Skin, Cellular Tissue Diseases		49,834	
Endocrine System Diseases		58,028	
Respiratory System Diseases		32,212	
Genito-Urinary System and Breast Diseases		36,772	
Metabolic Diseases and Avitaminoses		4,113	
Blood and Bloodforming Organs Diseases		6,566	
Failure to Meet Anthropometric Standards		140,938	
Miscellaneous Diseases and Defects		156,663	
Not Qualified, Mental Test and Medically	306,108		
Administrative Non-Qualifications Including Moral	182,677		

*Courtesy National Headquarters, Selective Service System.

than the preinduction ones. The local Selective Service Boards carry out some cursory interviewing upon request for manifestly disqualifying medical defects, e.g., blindness, deafness, and permanently crippling conditions. Other examinations are also conducted: for enlistees for reserve or regular duty (probably in better physical condition because of self-selection), for commissioning, for advanced R.O.T.C., etc. Some of these were not qualified, but they are not included in the statistics in Table 11. "Mental Test Only" refers to intelligence tests.

Should the military statistics be accepted as a reflection upon the progress of the public health movement, since interest first centered upon the individual? The answer is, "yes, to some extent." The following observations must be kept in mind, however.

Statistics on health disabilities of those examined for the draft in World Wars I and II are not comparable. The same is true for succeeding years. Medical knowledge and improved diagnostic techniques have dictated increasingly higher standards. Alertness in detecting and screening out nervous and emotional disturbances has been a saving factor for both the armed services and youth. If the improved diagnostic procedures and knowledge of today had been applied to former generations, undoubtedly the number of rejectees would have been proportionately greater in many of the categories.

Another vital fact has not been emphasized sufficiently. Medical science in the United States has preserved the lives of many handicapped children who otherwise would have died. It follows that there will always be in our population a high incidence of children and youth with defects, probably proportionately higher than in other countries.

Nevertheless, the situation concerning teeth has been deplorable. Surely, a more effective dental health program, including funds for free care, when needed, would have saved plenty of teeth. Some hearing problems could have been prevented with early medical care. Overweight and underweight are nutrition problems. School health services could have been more effective over the years.

The preceding observations give food for thought. In addition, while evaluating the results of preinduction examinations, one is reminded that physical fitness should not be equated with military fitness. A young man may be disqualified because of a missing trigger finger and yet be a fine physical specimen. A professional athlete may be considered in fine health and fail his preinduction examination because of a musculoskeletal problem. Very commonly, the problem involves a knee.

The fact is that the strides made in public health over the decade are reflected in the better health of successive generations of youth. They are taller and weigh more; they are fairly free from serious communicable diseases; their life expectancy is greater. Nevertheless, attention is given here to the results of health examinations on millions of youth. These findings cannot be ignored. They designate the kinds of defects which exist; they remind us that youth must be ready in each generation for military service; and they should be studied continuously with an eye for improvement.

Where do we begin improving the next generation? The time to start worrying about a child is before it is born; the public health program today starts with prenatal care. Each child should be followed through infancy, the preschool period, and through his whole school life. Every person who comes in contact with that child is part of a public health team: the parents, the physician, dentist, school nurse, social worker, psychologist, school custodian, teacher, and administrator. All should appreciate their respective roles, and a health program which will involve all of these specialists needs to be planned. All the past efforts in promotion of effective prenatal, preschool, and school health programs must be continued and intensified.

DEVELOPMENT OF THE SCHOOL HEALTH PROGRAM

The school health program embraces all procedures which seek to maintain and improve the health of children and school personnel —through healthful living at school, health services, and health education.

No one event or study stimulated the development or organization of a school health program. Glimmerings of interest in the school child date back to early in the last century. William A. Alcott (1798–1859), pioneer in school health who wrote an "Essay on the Construction of School Houses"[1] in 1829, suggested the attendance of a physician in schools and wrote the first health book for children. Horace Mann (1796–1859) refers to school hygiene in his "First Annual Report" as secretary to the Massachusetts Board of Education in 1838. As editor of the "Common School Journal," he wrote in the first issue:

> "When physical education is mentioned, that is a knowledge of the laws by which health and strength are attained and preserved, many people start and ask in surprise whether every man is to be a physician. The answer to this is easy. Physicians must understand the laws and symptoms of the diseased body. It is enough for common men to understand the laws and functions of the healthy body. . . . That knowledge respecting air, exercise, dress, and diet, which is requisite for the preservation of health, may be acquired with a far less amount of attention and expense, than are commonly necessary in a three month's sickness. . . ."[2]

---

[1]William A. Alcott: "Essay on the Construction of School Houses." *Lectures Before the American Institute of Instruction.* Vol. II. Boston: Hilliard, Gray, Little and Wilkins, 1832.

[2]Horace Mann (ed.): "Physical Education." *Common School Journal 1*:10–11 (November) 1838.

Early interest was shown not only in health knowledge and in healthful environment, but in the introduction of health services. For example, during an epidemic in Boston in 1894, record is made of medical inspections to detect the presence of diphtheria in the school population. The Department of Health of New York City in 1897 assigned medical inspectors to several schools with the specific duty of asking the teachers whether any of the children appeared ill. Suspected cases of communicable diseases could then be checked. The first school nurse was assigned to help these medical inspectors in 1902.

Between 1880 and 1890 most of the states had laws requiring the teaching of hygiene and physiology, with particular emphasis on uses of alcohol and narcotics. Physical education was gradually incorporated into the curriculum during this time.

The state of Connecticut passed a law in 1899 requiring that the teachers in public schools check the vision of children. In 1903 the first school dentist served in Reading, Pennsylvania. In 1906 medical inspections were required in the public schools of Massachusetts; by 1910, 337 cities required such inspections. In 1910 the first school lunch program was promoted in New York City.

Various professional groups, too many to discuss here, have become involved in child health programs over the years. Some have merged into stronger organizations. They all exert great influence today.

Beginning in 1909, the American Association for the Study and Prevention of Infant Mortality, later known as the American Child Hygiene Association, carried on programs of education for better child health in a period of 13 years. The work continued after the organization merged with the Child Health Association to form the American Child Health Association, a group which promoted health education through its publications and projects to integrate education and public health. In 1935 this organization was dissolved; its responsibilities were transferred to the National Education Association and the American Public Health Association.

The Joint Committee on Health Problems in Education of the National Education Association and the American Medical Association had its beginning in 1911. The philosophies, policies, and basic information sponsored and promoted by this group, founded upon its broad interests and knowledge in the area of school health, have been published in reports, pamphlets, and books. These are incorporated into the reference lists at the end of many chapters in this text.

The American Association for Health, Physical Education, and Recreation, which had its origin in 1885, has played a vital role in the development of the health programs in the schools of this country.

The first White House Conference in 1909, the second one in 1919, and subsequent ones held each decade beginning with 1930 demonstrate the persistent interest in child health and the widening explorations by leaders into all aspects of life which touch upon the child.

What are the trends in the school health movement today? Conferences and workshops held, singly or cooperatively, by professional, voluntary, and educational agencies command popular support and attendance. Objectives emphasize such areas as "Physicians and Schools," "Rural Health," "Physical Fitness of Youth," "Smoking and Youth," "Use of Drugs," and "The Juvenile Court and the Dropout." Interest in a progressive sex education or family life education curriculum fluctuates in intensity but is always present. Emphasis on the effects of smoking has been the result of a concerted attack by various federal and voluntary agencies.

The federal government has acknowledged its responsibility to children by furnishing funds and helping to establish standards for use of these funds. Much of this money is available for health problems of youth, with an eye on the deprived child. In the 1930's surplus commodities were made available for the school lunch program. Congress has continued this generosity and has passed legislation from time to time, allotting funds for various educational and antipoverty projects. Most federal legislation concerning youth has a health component. Attention has centered upon underprivileged preschool children, upon children of migrant workers, and upon adolescents who need training for employment or need encouragement to continue in school. Medical services include health examinations in clinics or in mobile health units, often provide comprehensive dental services, and in general seek to improve the health of "disadvantaged" youth. Physicians found that the most pressing problems in the Head Start group of four-year-olds were malnutrition, dental defects, and emotional disturbances.

In addition to direct medical attention, federal funds are available for improvement of educational services. This means more resource material in science and health teaching.

One especially significant recent event, initiated in 1961 by the Joint Committee on Health Problems in Education of the National Education Association and the American Medical Association, has been intensive research in health education through a nationwide study of health instruction in public schools. This study evolved into the gradual development of curriculum materials for health education, kindergarten through twelfth grade;[3] it has provided stimulus for strengthening health education in schools in many states.

One also observes a realignment of bureaus and agencies at the government level. These reorganizations should serve more effectively the modern-day needs of children.

Another change which affects the school program has been the shift in services of many voluntary health agencies to meet current

---

[3]School Health Education Study: "Health Education: A Conceptual Approach." 1965, 63 pp.

health problems. The National Tuberculosis Association has become interested in the respiratory diseases. The National Foundation is still concerned with poliomyelitis, toward whose conquest it can proudly take a great deal of credit, but its funds are now being allocated for study of birth defects. These are only two examples of public health interest in the health problems of children.

The spectacular increase in emphasis upon Special Education and upon preparation of teachers in this area is another manifestation of expanding interest in the health of the individual child. Funds have been generous for care and education of the mentally retarded. Some teachers look forward to working with hearing-impaired or visually-limited or with crippled children. We are just beginning to meet the demands of handicapped children.

Appreciation of the role of the teacher in the school health program has been emphasized repeatedly. He is considered to be in the first line of defense for promoting good health and detecting defects in the school child; his knowledge, alertness, and cooperation are absolutely essential. In 1924 a pamphlet to this effect was written by Dr. James Frederick Rogers, Consultant in Hygiene of the United States Office of Education, "What Every Teacher Should Know about the Physical Condition of Her Pupils."[4] The practical information presented here as a guide in constant observation and appraisal of the child is an example of subsequent material brought forward in this area by publications, demonstrations, workshops, and formal courses in teacher education institutions. The values of teacher-nurse conferences and the maintenance of adequate health records by teachers were later demonstrated in the Astoria Plan.[5]

Boards of education, administrators, teachers, and all who are interested in the school child acknowledge that the school has some responsibility for the health of that child. As far back as 1918 there was recognition of the importance of health. In its statement of objectives, referred to as the "seven cardinal principles," the Commission on Reorganization of Secondary Education (1912–1918) designates the first objective as:

> The secondary school should provide health instruction, inculcate health habits, organize an effective program of physical activities, regard health needs in planning work and play, and cooperate with home and community in safeguarding and promoting health interests.[6]

An acknowledgment of this responsibility was indicated in a statement produced at a meeting in 1951 of the National Council of Chief State School Officers and the Association of State and Territorial

---

[4]Pamphlet No. 68. Federal Security Agency. United States Office of Education.

[5]Dorothy B. Nyswander: *Solving School Health Problems.* New York: The Commonwealth Fund, 1942.

[6]National Education Association of the United States: "Cardinal Principles of Secondary Education." U.S. Department of Interior, Bureau of Education Bulletin No. 35, 1918. Superintendent of Documents, Government Printing Office, Washington, D.C.

Health Officers on "Responsibilities of State Departments of Education and Health for School Health Services." This statement was re-emphasized in 1959.

Every school is involved in a health program to some extent. Some programs are slipshod and ineffective; others are well-organized and comprehensive. Any program revolves around the child, with the objective of promoting his good health through preventing health problems and by detecting and correcting them as early as possible.

International Health Programs

No discussion on development of the school health program would be complete without some mention of progress being made in the world, particularly in the developing countries. Among the powerful forces for improving the health of all people in these countries are the agencies related to the United Nations: Education, Scientific, and Cultural Organization (UNESCO), United Nations Children's Fund (UNICEF), and the Food and Agricultural Organization (FAO). These groups have their own individual responsibilities, but they also act jointly on some projects. Some of the activities which have been undertaken are: emphasis on health education, teacher preparation for health education, and provision of health education resource materials; study of school health services; distribution of food commodities to children; and medical care, including mass immunizations.

A number of international educational organizations, such as the International Council on Education for Teaching and the International Council for Health, Physical Education, and Recreation, promote in various ways and according to their prime interests the health of children. Each of these organizations meets at intervals in different parts of the world with representatives attending from many countries. In their assemblies they exchange ideas and discuss their problems and methods of approach in solving them.

The International Red Cross and the Organizations of the Red Crescent and the Red Lion and Sun, all three of which are in agreement and have similar functions in the world, conduct various health programs. In some places they operate hospitals; they distribute clothing and food; they may sponsor mass immunizations; and, of course, they provide extensive service during disasters.

Volunteers of the Peace Corps of the United States and their counterparts from other countries have been excellent health educators, through what they teach in the classroom and community and by the example they set with their own living habits.

To bridge the hunger and nutrition gap around the world, some commercial companies have been conducting research and propose some eventful changes. One seed company has developed a corn with a high protein content. The seed can be planted in countries that utilize corn in their diets, as in Central and South America and parts of Africa. Such a product can combat protein deficiency in children. Another exciting development has been the research sponsored by a number of commercial firms with international distribution of beverages. Soft drinks are popular all over the world. Protein foods are now being included in the contents of some name products. In countries where youngsters have little or no protein in their dietary, these fortified drinks should prove a nutritional boon.

SUMMARY

The public health program developed slowly through the centuries. The historical background which has just been outlined, from early Greek history to the present, should give the impression of a gradual evolution, one that acquired momentum with scientific advances and eventually fostered a humanitarian spirit focused upon the individual.

The school health program developed slowly and naturally as interest in the individual centered upon school-age youth. First manifestations of concern for the school child appeared in the last century, when interest was aroused in the architecture and improvement of school buildings, health services performed at school, and in health instruction. Exposure of defects in the millions of physical examinations done in times of war and peace from World War I to the present has given stimulus to the promotion and conservation of the health of children and youth through programs which include those developed by schools. Federal aid in recent decades has contributed invaluable assistance. The teacher, as a participant in the school health program, is a part of the great public health movement; he gives his services to further the objectives of such a program.

DISCUSSION QUESTIONS AND ACTIVITIES

1. Discuss how the world wars of this century helped us to realize our poor health status.
2. Make a list of organizations and their functions with regard to helping to solve the international health problems of our lifetime.
3. Describe the relationship desirable between the school health program and the public health program.
4. Discuss the role of vital statistics in planning and evaluating health programs.
5. Devise a list of professional agencies which help to promote the school health program.

6. Review recent legislation of school health programs and find how states differ in health teaching status.
7. Discuss your opinion on the following topic: should health be a subject-oriented study or a child-oriented study.

ADDITIONAL SOURCES OF INFORMATION

READINGS

Means, R. K.: *A History of Health Education in the United States.* Philadelphia: Lea & Febiger, 1962.

Rich, R.: "A Century of School Health in Los Angeles." *J. Sch. Health* 41:323–328, June, 1971.

Simon, J. E.: "An Historical and Philosophical Analysis of Dual Professional Preparation in Health and Physical Education." *J. Sch. Health* 41:365–371, September, 1971.

Smith, R. E.: "Great School Doctors and the Evolution of Adolescent Medicine." *Practitioner* 206:183–186, February, 1971.

U.S. Department of Health, Education, and Welfare: "National Organizations with Interest in School Health." Washington: The Department, (1968).

Veselak, K. E.: "Historical Steps in the Development of the Modern School Health Program." *J. Sch. Health* 29:262–269, September, 1959.

Chapter 17

ORGANIZATION AND ADMINISTRATION OF THE SCHOOL HEALTH PROGRAM

INTRODUCTION

Health has been defined by the World Health Organization in positive terms as a "state of complete physical, mental and social well-being." It is more than simply the absence of a diseased condition. To promote or preserve this well-being in school-age youth, a concept of a school health program has gradually been developed which encompasses all the health needs of the whole child. Such a program is concerned with providing a safe, comfortable *healthful environment* in which the child lives for a number of hours each day—an environment which should make him contented physically, prevent emotional strain, and permit him to progress toward his physical, social, and mental potential. It offers him *health services* which aim to detect and correct or improve any health problems he may have. Such services should also enable him to maintain his good health by providing well-trained teaching and medical personnel as well as other specialists. This program stresses *health education* which affords him an opportunity to learn how to live healthfully and motivates him to assume gradually more responsibility for his own health.

Such a program is not isolated and confined within the school. From the time of birth to five or six years of age the well-being of a youngster has been affected by the environment in which he has been reared, by the health knowledge, attitudes, and practices of his parents, by the health and health facilities of the community, and by all of these working together for his best interests.

HEALTH IN THE HOME

Regardless of a child's age, his well-being depends largely upon his parents. Theirs is the primary responsibility. The role of the parents is dominant in handling health problems. There is need, however, for cooperation with the principal, teacher, social worker, nurse, dentist, physician, and other interested personnel. The school can point out a pupil's defects and make recommendations, take a child home who has sustained a head injury, or sponsor an immunization program, but it is up to the parents to seek medical consultation, to have defects corrected, and to promote a better health status for their children. If parents do not believe in calling a physician until a child is desperately ill or think that filling a tooth is a waste of money, reasonable persuasion should be tried. If a father whose family is subsisting on public welfare is too lazy to go down to the clinic for his child's free medicine or to take his little cross-eyed boy to the oculist for the free examination already arranged by the public health nurse, what is to be done? On the other hand, most parents are sincerely interested in the health of their offspring and appreciate the help of the school. Many do arrange periodic dental and medical checkups without prompting.

Parents must be motivated to secure the best for their children. Their viewpoint must be appreciated also. The impact on the family of new ideas and suggestions proposed at school may require a change in eating habits or discontinuing home remedies. Recommendations for examinations or for correction may involve expenditure of money which the family cannot afford; the school, through the principal, school nurse, or social worker, may arrange for this service within the financial ability of the family.

When a child enters school his health status and his feelings about health have been molded by his parents, by the environment in which he has lived, by the type of medical care he has had, by what he has learned through advertising media, and what he has gathered from his playmates. Parents and children must keep up-to-date on health information and practices; so should the school personnel who strive to educate parents.

The home is the strongest force in influencing the physical, mental, and emotional life of a child. If the school and community are working together, they will assist the home.

HEALTH IN THE COMMUNITY

Larger cities have established efficient health departments whose functions are performed by the divisions of sanitation, milk and water supervision, communicable disease control, laboratories, and all the other bureaus necessary for maintaining a healthy community. Associated with the health organizations are adequate medical personnel, hospitals, and local branches of social welfare and private health agencies. Small towns and rural areas may not be so fortunate. There may be no local boards of health. There may be no dentist or physician available and people must travel miles for medical care. With today's transportation, such a situation ordinarily is not too great a handicap, but emergency care is still a problem. To remedy the paucity of medical facilities, services are often offered by traveling clinics sponsored by medical centers, departments of health, and voluntary health agencies for the handling of such health problems as hearing education, mental health, crippling conditions, and nutrition education. In our country health services should be accessible to everyone. The community can analyze its needs and secure help. Leaders in the community must take the initiative.

HEALTH IN THE SCHOOL

The school health program is integrated with that in the home and community, but the responsiblity for the program lies with the school.

ORGANIZATION

The various phases of the school health program have been categorized as Healthful School Living, School Health Services, and Health Education. (See chart on page 340.) There is some controversy over nomenclature; nevertheless, the three approaches indicate the intent to include all the encompassing features which will promote the physical, social, and mental well-being of a child. The three phases are by no means rigidly demarcated. One supports the other, and the interrelationship involves coordination. For instance, a child discusses daily food requirements in class, discovers when he steps on the scales that he is underweight, and applies what he has learned in class about nutrition at the cafeteria counter.

The three phases of the school health program reach outside the school. A discussion on the values of immunization against some specific disease is carried on in class, and is followed by a similar one in a PTA meeting, where a public health official has been invited to speak. It finally culminates in a mass immunization project sponsored by the local medical society.

ADMINISTRATION

School systems have various ways of administering their health programs. Two aspects of living are involved—health and education. Each has its professionally trained people and auxiliary personnel. Authorities from each field must understand the goals, techniques, and problems of the other so that a smoothly working operation may be achieved.

National Level

The government maintains the Department of Health, Education, and Welfare which is represented by a member in the President's cabinet. Among the divisions in this department which are concerned with a child's health are the ones under the Public Health Service. Two of these which are closely involved are (1) The Institute of Child Health and Human Development and (2) the Health Services and Mental Health Administration.

For years the federal government, through various agencies, has taken a deep interest in the welfare of children. The lunch program has been with us since the 1930's; through the Department of Agriculture surplus food commodities are supplied free to state boards of education and are incorporated at local levels into lunches which are available at low cost or free. Federal aid for vocational education and vocational rehabilitation have existed for years. More generalized aid in academic areas was offered in 1958 with passage of the National Defense Education Act.

The underprivileged child has been the object of Congressional attention. The Economic Opportunity Act of 1964 recognized the needs of deprived youth through development of the Head Start program, concerned with ages four to six, and the Job Corps for adolescents. Both programs recognize the need to detect and correct health problems.

A most important commitment for the improvement of education was passed by Congress in 1965—the Elementary and Secondary Education Act. Among the provisions of this act were funds for services to cope with all types of problems of children, particularly the problems of the educationally deprived in low income areas. Money was made available for supplementing or strengthening the academic offerings in local schools through improved curricula, more equipment, expanded library facilities, and other services. Health education should benefit from these provisions. No doubt the future will offer more federal help. Educators need to familiarize themselves with the various provisions of federal legislation, know what money is available and how to secure it, and then utilize it. Part of this assistance should be devoted to the improvement of health of school children.

Also at the national level, there has been a meeting of minds of two professional organizations, the American Medical Association and the National Education Association, with the establishment of a joint committee on school health policies.

Frequently, volunteer and official groups combine to hold conferences for similar purposes. This cooperative planning aims to define values and formulate policies. The various White House conferences on the welfare of the child and on physical fitness have similar objectives, also.

Since the leading cause of death in school children is accidents, emphasis has been given to the various aspects of safety education.

Some of these are driver and pedestrian safety education, environmental health and safety, emergency care of injuries and illness, legal responsibilities, curriculum planning, and coordination of activities of those organizations in educational, professional, and community circles, school and nonschool agencies, whose efforts are directed towards the safety of children. To mention a few of these active organizations—the National Commission on Safety Education of the National Education Association, The National Congress of Parents and Teachers, the National Safety Council, the International Association of Chiefs of Police, and the United States Public Health Service. Organization and coordination of their combined efforts starts at the national level and extends to state, district, and school levels.

State Level

Legislation

The health of the state and school health education have been major concerns of state legislatures. The tendency now is to leave the administration of education to the State Department of Education (Instruction). Curriculum is defined by the latter, rather than specified by legislation. Money is allotted by the legislature.

Nevertheless, many states have statutes which require health teaching on the effects or harmful effects of alcohol, tobacco, and narcotics. Some states specify the duties of a teacher in inspecting children for health problems.

State Department of Education

A board of education, consisting of elected or appointed members, is responsible for the department of education and selects a superintendent. In some states the superintendent may be an elected officer. This board is responsible for enforcement of statutes, administers funds allotted to it, and acts in a policy-making capacity. The superintendent serves as the executive officer of the board.

Requirements for certification of teachers are defined. These may specify health qualifications of teachers and health education courses in preservice training. In some states school nurses must also have teaching certificates. Sanitary standards are established for the school plant and for food services. One division, cooperating with the State Board of Health, handles the school lunch program. In-service education of administrators and teachers through workshops and conferences should provide current information on all phases of the school health program.

State boards of education appoint specialists to direct many phases of the program. A health and physical education supervisor or director may also be responsible for the safety education program, including driver and pedestrian training. Or, the safety education division may be an autonomous division of the state department of education. Usually, the director of school planning must approve the architectural plans for all new school buildings in the state. Considerations are given to environmental safety and provision of health facilities. (See Figure 63.)

A close working relationship should exist between the personnel in the state departments of health and education. In some states the heads of these two departments, acting as co-chairmen, have cooperated to formulate policies, develop curriculum guides in health education, and coordinate services which directly and indirectly affect the health of the school child.

Community Level

Board of Education

Members are elected from the community. The board is responsible on a policy-making, value-defining basis for the school health program. The appointed superintendent, as executive officer of the board, carries out the details.

Administration of Local School Health Program

As far as the school health program is concerned, administrative patterns vary according to personnel, facilities, finances, traditions, and inclinations of those in authority. Some phases of the health program are more distinctly the province of the educator, e.g., health instruction. Others involve educator and professional medical personnel. For instance, it would be wise to have the school physician and dentist serve on the committee which passes upon the authenticity of all health textbooks and health curriculum materials.

Basic patterns for administration of a school health program may be outlined as follows:

1. Administration as a joint responsibility of the boards of health and education is one adopted pattern, with the heads acting as co-chairmen and sharing responsibility for coordination. The advantages of having public health officials on a planning committee are:
    a. There is a balance between the two interests—health and teaching—and both are concerned with the same child.
    b. The health department has supervision over certain areas, such as sanitary regulations and construction codes, which involve health in all schools of the community. This provision assures conformity of health standards and practices.
    c. The interest of the health department is more comprehen-

sive. It is concerned with the health of the individual from prenatal life to old age. Public health people know the gaps in health education as seen in prenatal and preschool clinics and can offer valid help with curriculum planning and health instruction.

d. The public health nurse is familiar with health problems in the community and family. She can be a valuable consultant.
e. The health department has a close working relationship with hospitals, clinics, and health agencies and can expedite services.
f. The health department has the personnel to carry out its part of the program.
g. Small school systems or a single school may not be able to afford a full-time physician or nurse. Part-time help may be secured from the local board of health.
h. Duplication of health facilities is avoided.

2. Administration primarily by the board of education with various modifications of the above plan and use of health personnel is the more usual arrangement. A school physician may be hired by the board, while the nurses may be provided by the department of health. Such an administrative set-up may not prove too satisfactory, however, because the physician has no official authority over the nurses. There may be no board of health in a community or the board may not have the money to furnish medical help. In small towns the county medical society or the one doctor in the area may act as consultant working with principals and teachers on the many health projects of the school and community.

Whatever plan is most feasible and efficient is the one to be implemented. There is no hard and fast rule.

Some large school systems have established Health Services Divisions which are dynamic and comprehensive in their functions, e.g., Chicago, Denver, Los Angeles, and New York. Their annual reports describe their many research efforts, projects, and services. These reports are well worth reading.

School Health Councils

Councils have been organized on a city or district basis, which bring together representatives of parents, teachers, school administrators, physicians, dentists, public health officials, civic organizations, community groups, and the voluntary social welfare and health and safety agencies. One of their objectives is to develop in the community an understanding and appreciation of school health procedures. Another is to evaluate pertinent problems and plan future programs which will improve the health of children and youth. They usually serve in an advisory capacity to departments of education and health.

Superintendent of Schools

The superintendent works closely with the board and with his administrative personnel in policy formation and in seeing that all schools under his supervision function to optimum capacity. His own attitude towards health will be mirrored in the efficiency and effectiveness of that program. His functions as an administrator should be:

> "1. To direct and coordinate all phases of the school health program under the school's jurisdiction. To see that adequate funds are secured and budgeted for the health program administered by the school, and to cooperate with the health department in obtaining and budgeting funds for medical and nursing services which may be administered by that department.
>
> 2. To be responsible for seeing that all functions of the school health program are performed, and to cooperate with the health department if the latter is responsible for the health or medical service program.
>
> 3. To assume administrative responsibility for providing and maintaining a safe and healthful school environment.
>
> 4. To set up a health curriculum in which health education is coordinated with all other features of the school program, and to see that health education is broadly conceived, based on the best scientific authority, and truly functional.
>
> 5. To set up a procedure for the continuous appraisal of the school health program in terms of improved status, improved individual and group health behavior, and adequacy of school plant."[1]
>
> 6. To develop good school-community relationships and interpret the health needs and resources of the school to the community and vice versa.
>
> 7. To recommend selection of teachers and personnel involved in the school health program.
>
> 8. To plan in-service programs in health education for teachers and interested personnel, including medical people.

School Level

Principal

The principal has similar functions to those of the superintendent, only at a more immediate level. He is the key person in the school to administer the school health program. His attitude towards health will either deter or spark an active, stimulative participation on the part of those who serve the school. Principals are chosen for their educational experience, their executive abilities, their wisdom and kindliness, and for their ability to develop the best public relations. Occasionally a rigid disciplinarian stirs up fear, tension, and anxiety in the climate of a school. A principal should be healthminded and inter-

---

[1]Metropolitan Life Insurance Company: "The School Administrator, Physician, and Nurse in the School Health Program." A report sponsored by the National Conference for Cooperation in Health Education. Pamphlet, pp. 28–30.

ested in workshops and refresher courses on the health of the school child. He should be interested in health instruction in the classroom. If he is afraid to call the custodian's attention to his sloppy housekeeping and storage of waste material in the basement because the latter's brother-in-law is on the board of education, the school plant will be unattractive and a fire hazard. If he allots the visiting physician a poorly ventilated cubbyhole in which to do health examinations, he is not lending dignity to an important part of the educational program.

On the other hand, a progressive administrator promotes all phases of the school health program. He is responsible for health instruction in his school. He comes to know the children, their families, and their backgrounds. He knows the leaders of the community through church and civic organizations and can wield invaluable influence in promoting good school health.

The principal is the center of all activities in a school. He is the educator-consultant when crippled or handicapped children are brought to the building. In the elementary schools he is called for major first-aid decisions. He frequently decides whether a child should be taken home for health reasons. He is an important member of the health team, and his cooperation is absolutely essential.

Teacher

Discussion of the role of the teacher in school health forms the introduction to this book. This is done to emphasize the objective of this text: to acquaint each teacher, either elementary or secondary, with his responsibilities in the school health program.

Health Educator

Standards in professional training have been carefully formulated for the health educator. The health education major program in teacher education institutions should prepare such an individual to understand children and their health problems, give counsel to students and parents, and assist in curriculum planning. He is ready to teach the health education courses offered in a well-organized curriculum. If much health counseling is assigned to him, the teaching load should be lightened.

Although the standards for professional training have been agreed upon, there has been a good deal of evidence that health instruction has been inadequate in our schools. This is due to several factors, but poor teacher preparation is certainly one of them.

At a teacher preparation conference in 1968, J. H. Haag outlined a remedy for the certification requirements of health teachers at the secondary level.[2] These recommendations encompassed the *pro-*

---

[2] J. H. Haag: "Certification Requirements for the Teachers of Health Education in the Secondary Schools." *J. Sch. Health* 38:7:438–443 September, 1968.

visional and the *professional* certificates. The *provisional certificate* should include (1) three semester hours of methods in health education; (2) six semester hours of student teaching; (3) 24 semester hours in an academic minor; (4) 24 semester hours in the academic major; (5) content should include: current health problems, school health program, first aid, safety education, community health, nutrition, disease prevention and family life education.

The *professional certificate* should include: (1) 24 of the 36 semester hours of graduate study in health education; (2) content should be taken from: consumer health, mental health, misuse of alcohol, tobacco, narcotics, and other stimulants and depressants, supervision of health education, safety education, family life education, community health, international health, health and aging, disease prevention, research in health education, and a thesis or project in health education.

The present joint or dual patterns of preparing teachers of health and physical education are hindering rather than promoting effective health education programs in the schools. These joint certification programs in health and physical education should be abolished. Most of the instructional preparation for this joint major is in the physical education portion, usually leaving the individual with far too little training in the health field to be an effective health instructor.

Oberteuffer[3] points out that most physical educators really do not ask to teach about health and would be most happy to have this responsibility taken over by someone else. Nevertheless, as they perform a task which would not be done at all if not for them, they should be kept up to date through various types of in-service education programs until adequately trained health educators are ready to take over.

Though similar in long-range goals, physical education and health education differ significantly in subject matter and methodology. Because of the health science "knowledge explosion," preparation in physical education no longer equips a teacher to function in the health instruction area beyond a very low level. Therefore, the time has come to implement the standards for educational training and certification that have long been recommended.

Health Coordinator

One person should be delegated at the central administrative level and also in each school to serve as coordinator. The functions of a coordinator should be:

1. To organize and supervise all aspects of the school health program.
2. To coordinate the activities of such a program with those in the

---

[3] Delbert Oberteuffer: "Health and Education—an Appraisal." Report of the Ninth National Conference on Physicians and Schools, American Medical Association, October, 1963.

community—working with health departments, civic and professional organizations, parents, police, safety specialists, physicians, dentists, private and voluntary health agencies, and school and community health councils.

3. To serve as consultant on health activities to professional and nonteaching personnel.

4. To maintain a continuous evaluation program.

5. To plan for in-service education.

6. To help develop a progressive well-coordinated health curriculum, including safety education.

7. To counsel with individual students after recommendations have been made by a physician.

In large school systems the health coordinator is frequently a physician with educational experience. He is usually placed in charge of the whole school health program. In a large district an assistant superintendent may be assigned to special services and special education and act as health coordinator. The physician in charge of school health services works under him.

A health educator in a school or in a small school system may serve as coordinator. In preparation for such a position, the health educator should have administrative experience and some work in various fields of public health.

There is increasing recognition of the need for health coordinators in the educational field. Such a trained person needs time to fulfill the functions required of this position and may spend very few hours in a classroom. If there is poor understanding of the role of a health coordinator in a school, pressure will soon be applied for this individual to accept a regular teaching load in addition to the services mentioned above.

Physical Educator

The physical education teacher (and often the coach) are in strategic positions to observe a child's health behavior and offer counsel. Except in big high schools, where the coach is restricted to interscholastic activities, the men as well as the women instructors in the field of physical education come in contact with a majority of the children at school. They may teach health facts in the gymnasium and on the playing field. Health topics on weight, nutrition, posture, phsyical fitness, muscular development, fatigue, and endurance may be discussed. Physical educators must be alert to detect a skin infection, poor physique, fatigue, and the shy withdrawal behavior of nonparticipants. The informal friendly atmosphere of the gymnasium invites relaxation and the divulgence of confidences. Emotional disturbances and odd behavior patterns may be detected more readily.

First aid measures are usually carried out in the gymnasium where supplies are kept. Or, the physical education teacher may be the first summoned when an injury occurs. Physical education teachers are expected to know more about health. They work with counselors, school nurses, and physicians. They might assist during health examinations at school by doing the preliminary measurements of height and weight. They work with physicians in adapting the physical education program to the handicapped child. They may interpret the physician's communications to the school. Because of these duties, physical educators need to have a good background in physiology and health education. As indicated earlier, more attention must be given to better preservice and in-service education in the health area.

Physical education teachers and coaches serve particularly as examples to young people who are inclined to imitate their mannerisms, speech, haircuts, and posture, repeat their comments, and quote them on health facts. The coach is frequently the idol and inspiration of his athletes. Our social and ethical values are applied in practice to physical activities where sportsmanship and fair play are emphasized. This is even more true in interscholastic competitions. Physical education teachers and coaches have repeated opportunities to influence the ideals, behavior, and character of a whole student body.

Counselors

Every school has one or more counselors who are specially trained to handle behavior problems. With the emphasis today on early detection of emotional disturbances, and with the many overt problems which occur in every school, their time is fully taken. They act as consultants to the teaching staff, work with parents, physicians, nurses, social workers, and not infrequently with police and courts, as well as official and voluntary service agencies. Their contributions to the school require versatile abilities, immense tact, and a fine understanding of children. They should take the initiative in planning a mental health program in the school.

At times the counselor is the person who receives physicians' notes, sees sick students and makes the decision as to whether one should be taken home, and acts as a liaison with teaching personnel on the health of a student.

Physician

Almost all physicians have contact with school children in some capacity. They need to know the health program of the school, the training of teachers in school health, and the adaptations which can be made for individual health problems. "What cannot be denied is that many of the problems that loom as most formidable for educator and physician alike can be found at the interface to be shared by both disciplines."[4] When the child enters school, the family physician and

---

[4]Philip R. Nader, and Gregg F. Wright: "School Health: The Teacher-Doctor Interface." *Hosp. Practice* February, 1973, Editorial.

parents join the classroom teacher, school nurse, and other school personnel in their program of health education and health supervision. State and county medical societies have special committees who work with administrators and teachers.

A full-time or part-time school physician has specific responsibilities. The more time he can devote to his school duties, the broader the field of his activities. The minimum requirements for a part-time school physician have been delineated by the Committee on School Physicians of the American School Health Association.

> Consults in matters of establishing policy concerning health of school personnel.
>
> Advises where medical-legal considerations arise.
>
> Serves as liaison with the community especially with its health agencies.
>
> Consults on validity and appropriateness of various health programs proposed for introduction into the school.
>
> Advises on health and safety of the school physical environment, usually in collaboration with building inspectors and public health sanitarians. (Makes periodic surveys of the school building and grounds for possible health or safety hazards and supervises the hygienic aspects of handling, preparation and storage of food in cafeterias.)
>
> Assist with the planning of parent-education meetings concerning school health problems.
>
> Arranges for medical appraisal of pupils who show signs of health problems and whose parents are unable to pay for such service.
>
> Compiles reports of the services rendered by the school medical program and of the health problems identified.
>
> Most authorities in school health currently agree that much of the time and effort of the part-time physician should be directed to the promotion of health education in the schools, rather than entirely to the health appraisal of individual pupils. He would assume the leadership in planning programs with his school coworkers to achieve the optimal results in the health and health education of the pupils. He can participate actively by talking to groups or individually at the time of his examinations regarding health problems. Health education in many schools is presently both sketchy and poorly coordinated.[5]

Large school systems have organized health services branches, with full-time physicians in attendance. Their attention is directed to every aspect of the school health program and to school-community relations. A school physician is a specialist.

Beginning with 1947, sponsored by the American Medical Association, national conferences on physicians and schools have been held at about two-year intervals. Reports are available from the sponsor. The goal has been to analyze the problems in the school health program and the physician's contributions.

---

[5] A Report of the Committee on School Physicians of the American School Health Association. *J. Sch. Health* 37:395–399, 1967.

Dentist

The duties of a dentist, whether in private practice or attached to a school system or to a state board of health, are comparable to those of a physician. The dental health program is vital; its interpretation of scientific information and needs for dental care should occupy a prominent part of the school health program. The dentist is a specialist and a resource person who may serve as a guest speaker at PTA meetings and in the classroom, inspiring action to develop a meaningful program in dental health.

Dental Hygienist

The dental hygienist follows a prescribed course of study in a dental school and is trained to perform an important role in dentistry. This person is qualified to recognize gross abnormalities in the mouth, take dental x-rays, give prophylaxis and fluoride treatment to teeth, and teach proper oral hygiene techniques. The dental hygienist occupies an increasingly important role in school dental health, may be employed to work solely in schools, can serve as a consultant in special education, and as a resource person for health education.

School Nurse

Large schools may be fortunate enough to have the services of one or more full-time nurses. More commonly, however, in small schools, a nurse has assigned hours at several schools and reports there daily or several times a week. Public health nurses supported by state, district, county, or city may be serving in a generalized program for a community and visit the school occasionally or when summoned on a special case. All school nurses are in daily, intimate contact with pupils, know their needs, and are familiar with the health problems of the community and of many families. Their assistance is particularly vital in contacting families in the low socioeconomic bracket.

The number of board of education nurses is increasing. The school nurse is indeed a specialist—nurse, health educator, and liaison with the home and with health personnel of the community. In addition, she will view the child in the school as a physical being who is a candidate for learning. One nurse should be available for each 1000 to 1500 students, depending upon the size of the area from which the school population is drawn. The distances traveled for home visits, the weather, traffic, terrain, and time required for travel must be considered in determining the ratio.

The functions and activities in current nursing practice may include:

1. Participating in obtaining a health history;
2. Performing a physical appraisal;
3. Evaluating developmental status;
4. Advising and counseling children, parents, and others;
5. Helping in the management of technologic, economic, and social influences affecting child health;

6. Participating in appropriate routine immunization programs;

7. Assessing and managing certain minor illnesses and accidents of children;

8. Planning to meet the health needs of children in cooperation with physicians and other members of the health team.

School nurses also may serve as health consultants to administrators, teachers, and the community. In association with physicians and others, school nurses may participate in the formulation, implementation, and coordination of standards, policies, and procedures for school health services and health education programs; assist parents in identifying and utilizing appropriate private and community resources for health care; provide in-service education for teachers and other school personnel to increase their knowledge and skills in the area of child health maintenance; and engage in defining their role with other members of the school health team.[6]

In recent years much has been proposed, written, studied and discussed about a new breed of school nurse called the school nurse practitioner. A study in the Denver elementary schools compared conventional school nurses with the school nurse practitioner. Their findings demonstrated that the school nurse practitioners:

1. Tended to be more sharply focused and specific in their management of pupils' health problems.

2. Excluded only about half as many pupils from school.

3. Referred only about half as many pupils for consultation, care, or further evaluation.

4. Were more likely to provide clear, specific advice to parents of excluded pupils.

5. Were more likely to have parents of excluded pupils agree with and follow their advice.[7]

The conventional school nurse, to be sure, will continue to provide an invaluable service. However, the school nurse practitioner will also become a valued addition to the health service team in many areas.

Many nurses have teachers' certificates and serve a dual role (school nurse–teachers). More are being encouraged to qualify; their contribution to the school health program will be enriched.

Social Workers

Some school systems employ social workers. One may have a full-time assignment in a single school, or his services may be divided

---

[6]American Nurses' Association and American School Health Association, a Joint Statement; *Recommendations on Educational Preparation and Definition of the Expanded Role and Functions of the School Nurse Practitioner* (Kansas City, Missouri: American Nurses' Association, September, 1973).

[7]Norman A. Hilmar and Patricia A. McAtee: "The School Nurse Practitioner and Her Practice: A Study of Traditional and Expanded Health Care Responsibilities for Nurses in Elementary Schools." *J. Sch. Health 43*:7:440–441, September, 1973.

between several schools, depending upon student population and need. This specialist possesses skills in investigating problems, interviewing members in a child's home, and promoting favorable school-family-community relationships. A principal should utilize this particular type of training and achieve a fine working arrangement. When information on family resources is necessary in order to help a child, the social worker can help the physician, the school or public health nurse, and the counselor. The capacity of the family for adjustment is assayed. A social worker counsels the parents of a handicapped youngster, strives to correct their negative attitudes and motivate them to help the child. Many parents plead for help, and every principal is confronted with needs which can be served by this specialist.

Health Aides

Other members of the health team have been very helpful in larger school health services. Because of the shortage of qualified personnel to serve an increasing student population, nonprofessional assistants are being used, working under supervision of the school nurse. Health aides or health clerks can relieve nurses and teachers of many tasks. They can carry out screening tests, keep records, contact parents, type correspondence and reports, keep track of follow-ups, assist in research, and, in general, provide invaluable help in a health office.

Other Specialists

Other specialists are in contact with the schools and make their contributions to the health program. These may be the clinical psychologist, those in charge of special hearing and speech services, architects, engineers, sanitarians, lighting experts, and many others.

Custodian

Arrangements for custodianship depend upon the size and location of the plant. A several-million-dollar city high school may well have an engineer with a large budget and a number of maintenance men under his supervision. (See Chapter 18, Healthful School Living.) Some of these men will care for the grounds; others work in various capacities within the building. Special knowledge on care of the swimming pool may be necessary. All of the expensive machinery for ventilation and heating must function well. Plumbing, painting, carpentry, proper lighting, fire prevention, and safety measures demand the attention of skilled help. There are gradations from such elaborate maintenance to the rural school where a neighbor starts the fire in the morning and returns in the afternoon to sweep the floors.

An average small school will have one custodian who is skilled in enough areas to keep the plant clean, safe, comfortable, and in good operation. He orders his supplies, cares for minor troubles in the building, and requests service for major projects from a central administration for maintenance. He takes care of the landscaping and should have pride in the appearance of his domain, both interior and exterior. He is constantly alert for hazards. Beyond all else he should be a man of fine moral character, a fit associate for little boys and girls and adolescents. He should be conscientious and cooperative in keeping the school comfortably warm in winter—ready when children come to school in the morning, and warm all day. He acts as the principal's right hand in providing a healthful environment. If he refuses to give the children toilet paper because a few have been throwing it around, sweeps dirt into the corners, and is indifferent to the fact that the teachers and children are shivering in their topcoats, his services are of little value.

The selection of a custodian should be based upon merit and possibly a civil service examination. He is a member of the school health team.

Other Personnel

Other nonteaching, nonmedical personnel are the bus drivers, food service personnel, and clerks. They themselves should be in good health, health-minded, and worthy of companionship with children. The role of the food handler in the communicable disease program has been discussed in Chapter 8.

Parents

The child still belongs to his family, and the final disposition of a health problem is the responsibility of a parent. Parents should be the constant factors in a changing world.

Parents can help the school to determine health needs of children. The National Congress of Parents and Teachers through its local councils is interested in preparation of teachers for special education in handling exceptional children. Attention is also focused upon assistance to pupils from families who are "too poor to pay for it and too rich to get it for nothing."[8]

Most parents are personally interested in school health, and this interest should be utilized to further needed projects—school lunches, immunization campaigns, surveys of various types, safety measures, and raising funds to purchase glasses for indigent children.

Parents need to be kept up to date on health information and practices by having guest speakers and pertinent movies at their meetings. Meetings should be stimulating. Pupils may present health plays. Exhibits may be displayed, and printed materials on various health

---

[8]Mildred Thompson: "The PTA Assists In Resolving Pupil Health Problems." *J. Sch. Health* 33:312–313, 1963.

topics may be distributed. Parents may be asked to serve as volunteer help during immunizations and screening tests. They may help to serve lunch, act as room-mothers, or interview parents bringing new children for enrollment. Mothers and fathers should serve on the school health council. One parent should be present when her own children, at least during their early years, are examined by the physician.

Pupils and Students

These are part of the school team. They participate in maintenance of a healthful environment, in the safety program, in the health services, and in many aspects of health education. They make surveys, put on demonstrations, prepare exhibits, help with school and community projects, teach the younger ones, and should be engaged in curriculum planning. They not only benefit from an effective school health program, but contribute to it.

School Health Committee

This important committee is concerned with the needs of its own school. Its make-up will vary somewhat with the problems to be handled. The principal, health coordinator, president of the PTA, teachers in fields concerned with health (home economics, physical education, physiology), and the nurse and/or social worker constitute a representative basic group which should work well together. Pupils and older students are frequently members and can make valuable contributions. If the problem to be considered involves the food service, the individual in charge of the cafeteria may be invited to participate. At times the custodian may be consulted. Guidance personnel may be included. Outside consultation is always available. Such a committee may meet regularly or be convened when the need arises. Organization of such an advisory, problem-solving committee follows democratic principles and should evoke a wider interest and cooperation in the health program.

COMMUNITY-SCHOOL RELATIONSHIPS

Working Together for Healthier Children

The roles of the school personnel closely associated with the health program have been described. Since this program is not an isolated one but is correlated with health in the home and in the community, fine community-school relationships are necessary. Many organizations in the community are working to promote good health for youth.

Professional Organizations

These have a predominant role to play in the school health program. Such groups as the American Medical Association, the Academy of Pediatrics, the American Dental Association, the American School Health Association, the American Public Health Association, and the American Association of Health, Physical Education, and Recreation are intimately and actively concerned with the health of the school child. Most of the medical organizations have appointed school health committees at the local levels, who can be of greatest assistance.

Medical Centers and Departments of Health

Mention has been made of the responsibilities of state departments of health in holding clinics throughout the state for dental health, mental health, crippled children, speech correction, and other health problems. Units from medical schools also hold clinics for similar purposes at the medical center or travel through the state either independently or in conjunction with department of health personnel. Community needs and facilities can be studied and attempts made to establish efficient treatment centers.

The interrelationship of state departments of health and education is necessary in viewing the many aspects of school health – for the formulation of health policies, provision of scientific information, health regulations in school planning and maintenance, and availability of consultants.

Vocational rehabilitation centers for the handicapped have been established by the states. They handle all types of crippling conditions, pay for medical services and supplies, and arrange for an education. They coordinate their services with those of school, voluntary agencies, special schools, and community health centers.

Public and Voluntary Social Welfare Agencies

Family and children's service agencies and settlement or neighborhood houses as well as tax-supported welfare departments have a part to play in the life of a school child. By helping families stay together, providing marriage counseling, placing children in foster homes, providing recreation, and sponsoring clinics, they make a big contribution to the life of a community.

Voluntary or Private Health Agencies

There are many organizations which are concerned with specific health handicaps, namely, heart disease, cancer, tuberculosis, crippling conditions, blindness, mental retardation, deafness, epilepsy, and with health education in general (see Appendix A and lists of resources at ends of chapters dealing with health problems). They are supported by public or private subscriptions and are accepted as part of our culture. Branches are located in most large cities from which representatives may travel to regions nearby.

The responsibilities of these agencies are:

1. To provide resource people who are specialists in their field. Their personnel frequently are experienced teachers who may act as consultants on health councils, attend workshops, contribute to in-service education, and serve as speakers and discussion leaders.

2. To promote health education. They act as resource agencies and supply many excellent teaching aids—exhibits, demonstrations, audiovisual and printed materials. The pamphlets and reprints which they distribute free or for a nominal sum provide a wealth of information. Many of these agencies are mentioned as resources in this book.

3. To identify the health needs of a nation and of the community and provide the service. This involves the support of basic scientific research on a given health problem and providing the appropriate primary health care when an answer to the problem is found. Scores of agencies work in their quiet way on important health problems and provide services.

Private Industry

Some companies, particularly those which handle foods (citrus fruits, bakery goods, meat, milk, and dairy products), and insurance companies that are interested in better health and longevity have established departments which assist in health education. Information attractively presented in posters, charts, pamphlets, and audiovisual materials is offered. Catalogs are available. See Appendix A. See the discussion on criteria for selection of resource material in the chapter on School Health Education.

Youth Groups

Youth organizations in the community involve a high proportion of the nation's young people, beginning usually before the age of 12 and continuing through high school. From their ranks are also prepared the future leaders of youth. Boys and girls are engrossed in the many activities of Boy Scouts, Girl Scouts, Camp Fire Girls, Boys' Clubs of America, 4-H Clubs, and similar groups. Practical considerations of health problems are a part of their educational programs—nutrition, camping, sanitation, lifesaving, emergency care of accidents and illnesses, the inculcation of ideals of mental health.

Civic or Service Clubs

Clubs, such as Rotarians, Kiwanis, and Soroptimists, create an interest in civic health projects. Club leaders become familiar with the health needs of a community and even of a particular family. They may work separately or join together to accomplish a goal. They may work through a community council or health council. Generous scholarships have enabled worthy individuals to become trained in handling the deaf or blind. Many organizations supply glasses and hearing aids for needy children.

Pooling of resources, both in adult leadership and in funds, can accomplish worthwhile health purposes. In one semi-rural area specialists from the state board of health screened the children at school for hearing defects. The survey stimulated the teachers to attend an extension course on hearing problems which was brought to the town by the state university. The children with hearing defects received medical care; and, as a culmination, the civic clubs added money to the funds available in the PTA, school, and municipal treasuries for purchase of an audiometer. This instrument was kept in the mayor's office.

Private, Religious, or Fraternal Groups

Private, religious, or fraternal groups and their auxiliaries sponsor or contribute to worthwhile undertakings. Crippled children's hospitals may be built and maintained by a religious or fraternal group. A private family may organize a school for hard-of-hearing or deaf children.

SUMMARY

The organization and administration of the school health program has been outlined. No one school system will encompass all of the organization or personnel described. The roles of the many members in a school who are responsible for a child's health and the contributions which can be made by auxiliary groups have been discussed at some length. Scores of organizations outside the school are involved. A child's health seems to be everyone's business. There must be a team approach in which each organization and each member fits into a part with as little overlapping of functions as possible.

DISCUSSION QUESTIONS AND ACTIVITIES

1. Write to your state department of education and ask for copies of the state statutes for health teaching. Are there new bills being introduced to require health teaching?
2. Develop a philosophy of health education which could be used in defending a school health program.

3. Discuss how health and education are compatible. Is there a balance between them in the school system you attended?
4. Develop a flow chart illustrating the responsibility chain from the national level to the student level.
5. Describe how a counselor can be a very important "middle man" among parents, student, and teacher.
6. Interview a school nurse and make a list of her most enjoyable functions.
7. Discuss the importance of good rapport between the PTA and the health educator, and between the public and the health educator.
8. Discuss the phrase, "A child's health seems to be everyone's business."
9. Discuss the duties, aside from direct education, of the health educator.
10. Discuss the relationship that exists between the public health department and the school health program.

ADDITIONAL SOURCES OF INFORMATION

READINGS

American Academy of Pediatrics:
Report of the Committee on School Health. (1966).
Emphasis on physician's role.
American Association for Health, Physical Education, and Recreation.
American Dental Association.
American Medical Association:
Department of Health Education—reprints, consultants.
Publishes *Today's Health.*
Reports of the National Conferences on Physicians and Schools.
American Nurses' Association.
American Public Health Association.
American School Health Association: Publishes Journal of School Health—excellent articles.
American Association for Health, Physical Education, and Recreation: *School Nursing for the 70's,* AAHPER, 1972.
Aubrey, R. F.: "Health education: Neglected child of the schools." *J. Sch. Health* 42: 285–8, May, 1972.
Council of Chief State School Officers: "Responsibilities of state departments of education and health for school health services." Washington: N.E.A. (1959). For school physicians and administrators.
Esty, G. W.: "Health education in our schools and the health manpower shortage." *J. Sch. Health* 40:11–4, January, 1970.
Hardind, F. K.: "Teachers and teams—Their importance to mental health in the classroom." *J. Sch. Health* 42:120–1, February, 1972.
Herberg, E. W.: "Sociological perspectives on school health programs." *J. Sch. Health* 42:10–5, January, 1972.
Hicks, D. A.: "Professional preparation of health educators in the seventies." *J. Sch. Health* 42:243–5, April, 1972.
Hoyman, H. S.: "Health ethics and relevant issues." *J. Sch. Health* 42:516–25, November, 1972.

Jacobson, R. F., and Siegel, E.: "Comprehensive health planning in the space age: The role of the school health program." *J. Sch. Health* 41:156–60, March, 1971.

Joint Committee on Health Problems in Education of the National Education Association and the American Medical Association. Write either organization.

Metropolitan Life Insurance Company. Health and Welfare Division. Publishes *Health Bulletin for Teachers.*

Miller, D. B.: *Introduction to School Nursing Curriculum.* AAHPER, 1973.

Miller, D. F.: "Legislative action, health education, and curriculum change." *J. Sch. Health* 42:513–5, November, 1972.

National League for Nursing, Inc. Publishes *Nurs. Outlook.*

Reed, C. E.: "An analysis of the perceptions of high school principals in public and Catholic schools relative to the importance of sex education in the curriculum." *J. Sch. Health* 43:198–200, March, 1973.

Turner, C. E.: "Editorial: International developments in school health education." *J. Sch. Health* 42:381, September, 1972.

U.S. Department of Health, Education, and Welfare: "A directory of national organizations with interest in school health." Washington: The Department 1968.

Professional, voluntary, and private health resources have catalogs. A great variety of reprints are available, dealing with various aspects of school health, such as health education, roles of various personnel mentioned in this chapter and their interrelationships, and school health policies. Some have published brochures or texts. Each organization will have somewhat specialized interests, but each is interested in the overall school health program. Excellent material is presented in their publications—up-to-date, dynamic, and offering practical suggestions for use in schools.

AUDIOVISUAL MATERIALS

Recommended grade levels are designated *pri, int, jh, sh.*

Community Health and You

10 min. Black and White *jh, sh,* adults McGraw-Hill*

Health in Our Community

13 min. Black and White, Color *int, jh* Encyclopaedia Britannica Educ. Corp.

Shows how local agencies help protect the health of the community. Over-view of public health programs on level of elementary children.

Journey in Health

15 min. Black and White teachers Coronet Films

Emphasizes the role of the physician, working with parents and the school in the continuous medical supervision of children.

Our Community

11 min. Color *int* Encyclopaedia Britannica Educ. Corp.

Illustrates important community institutions and their services by portraying a day in the life of a ten-year-old boy.

---

*See Appendix A for addresses of film companies.

Chapter 18

HEALTHFUL SCHOOL LIVING

DEFINITION AND PHILOSOPHY

The term healthful school living designates that aspect of the school health program which is concerned with providing a healthful physical and emotional environment, a healthful school day, and healthy school personnel.

Just as curriculum planning or educational specifications are based upon the physical, emotional, intellectual, and social development of a child, living at school is based upon the same considerations. The physical plant and grounds are also fitted to the characteristics, needs, and educational plans at each age. The environment must be healthful, safe, comfortable, and promote a warm feeling of security and contentment. To accomplish these objectives requires serious consideration of the physical and emotional environment and the planning of an efficient school experience.

HEALTHFUL PHYSICAL ENVIRONMENT

The Modern School Plant

A school plant—and in this term are included the site, the building with its furniture and equipment, and the grounds—should be a part of the educational process, and not just a shelter. The plant is the environment in which a child grows, develops, and learns. Living in it not only should be an educational experience in itself but should permit opportunities for other experiences. Its effective use depends upon how well it is planned, designed, and constructed to fulfill the preceding interpretation of healthful school living, and meet current and future educational needs.

The following discussion is important to every teacher. He should be consulted by the architect, especially during the preliminary design phase of a new building. He should have constructive suggestions for remodeling an old plant. A great deal of research and thought goes into the planning of a school. A teacher who walks into a new building and into a new classroom should not take the physical plant for granted. He should understand the basic considerations in its planning, design, and construction, and notice the unique features which indicate a recognition of the fundamental needs of children and youth in their school environment. He will have a keener appreciation of his good fortune, the opportunities he has to carry out an effective teaching assignment, and his role in maintaining a safe, efficient plant.

The physical plant controls to some degree the success or failure of teaching efforts. Good administrators and teachers are not drawn to unattractive, uncomfortable, cramped quarters. Neither are children or their families. An inadequate, unpleasant plant is hazardous; and if it is located in an environment which is being invaded by industry with its accompanying noise, fumes, smoke, dust, and increased traffic, the results of the educative effort will be poor. Deficiencies in mechanical provisions, inadequate spatial offerings, and outmoded plumbing, heating, and visual facilities are not suitable for comfort, modern curriculum, or modern teaching methods. All types of obsolescence are interrelated, including the teaching process. Substandard schools encourage substandard teaching.

Children like to attend an attractive, comfortable school. They will want to attend. A school should be an interesting, worthwhile place to be, where there is opportunity for creative, intensive work on the part of every student.

With the recent increase in school enrollment and great shifts in population, communities are striving to keep pace with needs by construction of additions and new buildings, as far as economy will permit. Never has there been such an opportunity for combining the finest of educational processes with research, esthetic considerations, utilitarianism and healthful living.

A new school building is a community project, designed to care for the education of the community's children. The local board of education, the educational staff, including teachers, the architect, and the construction staff, work together to produce an acceptable plant.

A modern school should satisfy all of these requirements:

1. It must meet definite educational specifications. These are based upon the characteristics and needs of school-age youth at each level. The educational needs are defined by the educators and must be understood by the architects.

2. It must be adaptable to tomorrow's educational program with its innovations and revisions of teaching techniques and new equipment requirements. Many new schools are prematurely obsolescent because they are unadaptable to changing educational philosophy and methodology.

3. It must be healthful, safe, and comfortable for its occupants.

4. It must be built for minimum cost and maintenance and with the least political and social controversy.

5. Future expansion of the structure with additions which fit an architecturally pleasing exterior should be possible.

6. It must lend itself to community use, because the interrelationships of school and community are close.

Design for Educational Needs, Adaptability, and Comfort

There are three basic factors to be considered by the educator in the construction of a school: organization of space; basic considerations of environment—visual environment (lighting, colors), acoustical or auditory environment (control of sound), thermal environment (heating, ventilation, air conditioning); and the esthetic values which make a plant attractive. These are interdependent.

Organization of Space

The first question to be asked is, "What educational offerings are planned for this school?" Since the curriculum varies throughout the school years, planning the overall dimensions and space within a building is dependent upon needs. Organization of space both indoors and outdoors will depend upon a study of educational specifications.

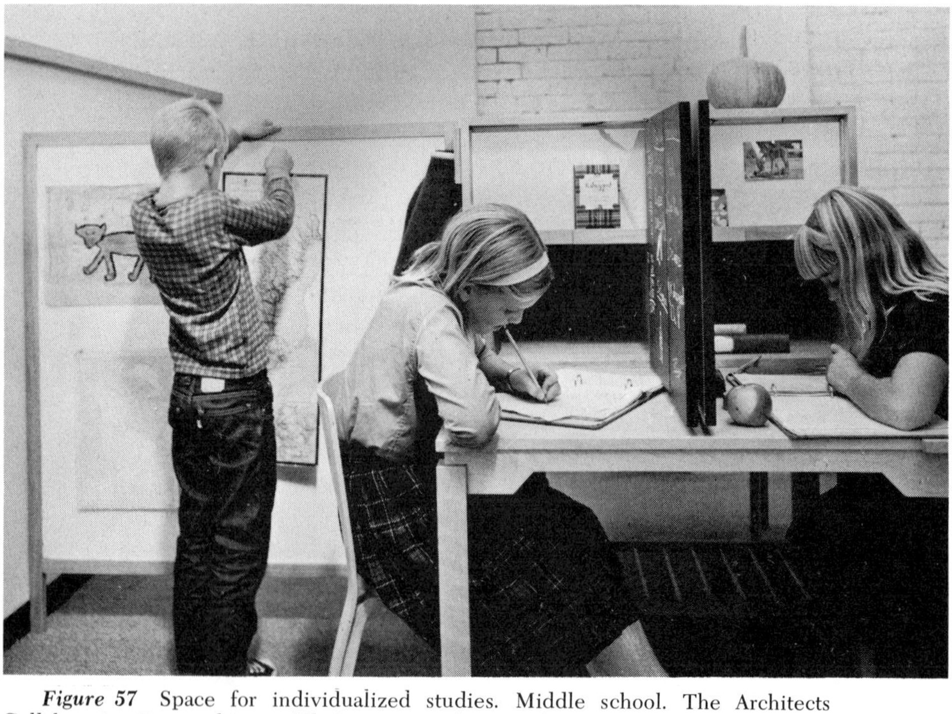

Figure 57 Space for individualized studies. Middle school. The Architects Collaborative, Inc., architects. (Phokion Karas, photographer.)

Changing teaching techniques require adaptable space for such activities as team teaching; group teaching; combining of classrooms; viewing television; listening to records; storage of audiovisual aids, supplies, equipment, and specimens; preparation of materials in social science and science classes; holding conferences and student meetings.

To meet current and future educational specifications, structural design and campus planning are providing and testing multi-purpose rooms, divisible classrooms and auditoriums and gymnasiums, ungraded schools, consolidated schools, complexes of elementary and secondary schools on one campus, educational parks, open-plan schools, windowless schools, carpeted rooms without doors, and various other interesting features.

At the same time it is necessary to evaluate the psychological responses of teachers and pupils to the school. Educational psychologists are evaluating these responses. What about windowless rooms? Is the peripheral arrangement of classrooms about a central concourse or court conducive to socializing and intimacy?

Structural design should allow for easy and inexpensive alterations of spaces within a building and for multiple uses of a space. For instance, a movable partition in the gymnasium will not only provide separate play areas for boys and girls but will permit one large hall which may be used for parties, dances, and athletic events, or serve as an auditorium for school assemblies and community gatherings. Auditoriums are the most expensive and least used facilities in a school. Some have been constructed with operable walls which create several enclosed areas that are suitable for lectures, team-teaching, films, assemblies and other group uses.

When space is designed for varied uses, there should be mobile furniture, partitions, and equipment for flexibility and for diversified activities to take care of individual needs, special group interests or instruction and to satisfy the interrelationship of school and community. Multipurpose rooms may not be the most ideal for one particular need or service, but they are cheaper to build and more economical to maintain.

Some school systems arrange for elementary, junior high, and senior high schools on the same campus, forming a complex which may be joined by walkways, patios, bridges, or similar connections. Only a single cafeteria, library, and auditorium are then necessary. Such an arrangement is economical, avoids identical facilities, and permits better equipment, more books and supplies.

One or more educational parks are being tried in some large cities. The park is a centralized meeting place where all high school students will attend one of several schools on one large site. The plan does not need to be confined to high school grade levels, however. Many children are transported for miles to this central place. Perhaps this arrangement can counteract the ghettos in both concept and reality. Again, a centralized system provides a central administration unit, a health center, a large library, one cafeteria, and one gymnasium. These could be in separate buildings which serve as a complex for the park.

Considerations for Elementary Schools. The basic unit is the child. The next large unit is the classroom. A child identifies himself socially with his class, then with his school.

Classrooms should be large enough with centers to care for the many interests and activities of small children: reading, writing, rest, painting, caring for pets and plants, games, construction with blocks and clay, making models, and other busy work for youngsters. There must be well-planned storage facilities. Elementary schools are designed so that supervision is easy.

Considerations for Secondary Schools. In the secondary schools the interests and needs of a student demand a varied curriculum of subject matter and extraclass activities. He has become a social being interested in his many relationships and must have space for clubs, committee meetings, group conversation, and play. A high school not only contains administrative offices and various utility spaces, but must provide room for classes of all types—art, music, gymnasium, laboratories, industrial crafts, and other activities not found in an elementary school. Play grounds usually contain various play courts, a football field and stadium, and possibly a swimming pool. There must be space for parking bicycles and automobiles.

Schools should not be too large. The transition from home to school, particularly in elementary grades, should not offer such a contrast that the child is overwhelmed. Small one-story schools of informal design, in which a child will not be confused and will be able to keep his self-identity and esteem, are recommended. This concept holds true, as much as is feasible, through high school. If it is necessary for a school to be large, an attempt is made to reduce the psychological impact of its bigness by such means as the campus plan where a student walks from building to building with enclosed corridors and colorful courts. There are architectual means of relieving bigness and a barracks appearance by the use of multiple buildings interspersed with courts and activity centers.

A few schools with one or two classrooms are still being constructed. These are placed in settlements with sparse school populations, and care must be taken in planning and utilizing space to satisfy educational specifications.

Basic Environmental Considerations

Every aspect of the physical environment should contribute to the health and comfort of pupils and school staff. The following discussion of basic environmental factors is not intended to provide technical information. It is not necessary that a teacher understand the intricacies of a heating and ventilating system. He should know how to cooperate in its use, however. The physics of light is the consideration of the lighting engineer; a teacher strives to utilize the light in his room for seeing ease. A teacher or administrator may be called into

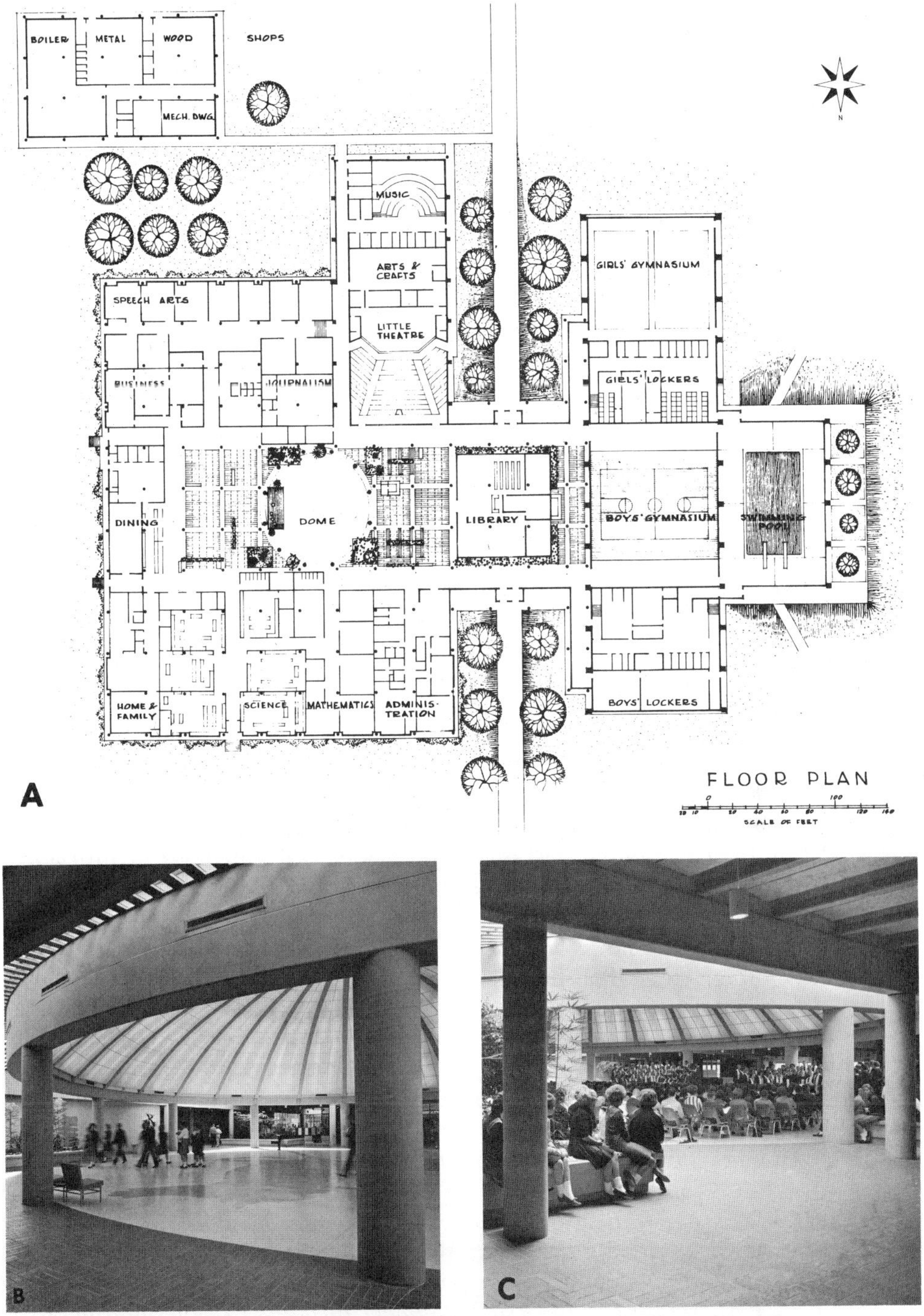

Figure 58 Andrews High School, Andrews, Texas. *A*, building plans. Floors are covered with carpet whose color matches the color of the soil outside the plant. One striking feature is the dome and concourse area (detailed views presented in B and C). The entire area under and adjacent to the dome is open and serves for traffic, gatherings, assemblies, social activities, and rallies, and also permits expansion of dining space. For assembly purposes it seats 1200. *B*, the dome and concourse area can be used for traffic and as a gathering place between classes. *C*, the dome area can be used for an assembly. (Reid and Tarics, architects. Roger Sturtevant, photographer.)

consultation on such plans as organization of space, color, or lighting, but basic technical provisions are the business of the experts. Occasionally, a teacher and/or nurse must learn the principles of good lighting and ventilation in order to urge needed changes in old buildings.

Visual Environment. *Physical Aspects.* Vision is a tool of learning. Ideal lighting enables an individual to sit anywhere in a classroom with visual comfort. To achieve this goal involves planning the quantity, the quality, and the distribution of light. We are interested in supplying the amount of light necessary on all working surfaces for efficiency and comfort. The desired result is twofold: (1) brightness on various surfaces in a room with acceptable contrasts (brightness differences or balances) to assure comfortable vision and (2) light distribution from either artificial or natural sources to avoid direct and reflected glare. In other words, acceptable school lighting implies a satisfactory intensity and avoidance of high brightness and intolerable glare.

Years of research have been devoted to the problem of school lighting. There is no uniform solution. Various techniques are being used by architects and illumination engineers. Each plan must be considered individually.

The lighting engineer is primarily concerned with providing adequate levels of illumination. Another consideration is the quality of light and its effect upon colors, textures, and furnishings. The exclusive use of fluorescent light throughout a school plant can be monotonous and sterile. Where the performance of visual tasks does not require uniformly high levels of light as in corridors, lobbies, and auditoriums, incandescent light can be used successfully. Because this light source is directional in character, it enhances texture and form. The warmth of incandescent light is more closely related to sunlight. When used effectively, it can lend interest to a space in contrast to non-directional, shadowless, fluorescent light.

Some general observations are presented. In new buildings teachers do not rely upon windows or adjustments of shades or blinds for illumination of interior spaces. When daylight is used, it is complemented by electric light with the use of a control which automatically keeps the electric lighting satisfactory. Some new designs for schools do not consider windows in the visual environment. There are two schools of thought concerning this provision. Absence of windows permits more wall space for instructional facilities and greater flexibilities in the utilization of space. On the other hand, windows are for views, for avoidance of claustrophobia, for a feeling of projection with the outside. Distracting? Encouraging daydreams?

Esthetic Values and Psychological Concepts. Good lighting provides physiological comfort. A cheerful, relaxed atmosphere with rooms in attractive colors should also be an objective.

Colors are not only important in controlling brightness balance and reflection, but they evoke psychological effects as well. For a school, color selection is also relevant to the environment. When students move from room to room, colors should be varied to avoid monotony. When children stay in one room, interest can be created by introducing limited areas of bright color in panels, pictures, and other furnishings. All four walls need not be the same color.

Small rooms need lighter colors with higher reflectances. Large rooms can tolerate more intense colors. Interest is created by variations in texture and color. Selection of color is dependent upon the activity planned. Stronger hues can be considered in assembly areas, including the cafeteria, where lively color schemes can produce a feeling of excitement and interest. A library should be an inviting, pleasant room to enter. Books provide color; good illumination here is a prerequisite.

In brief, even though emphasis is placed upon the engineering aspects of illumination, considerations should be given to some variation in lighting within the school with a possible mixture of incandescent and fluorescent lights, and variation in hues, tonality (brightness), and texture. The objective is to avoid the extremes of monotony and indiscriminate use of too many materials and colors. It is here that a consultant in color and interiors can make a contribution to school planning.

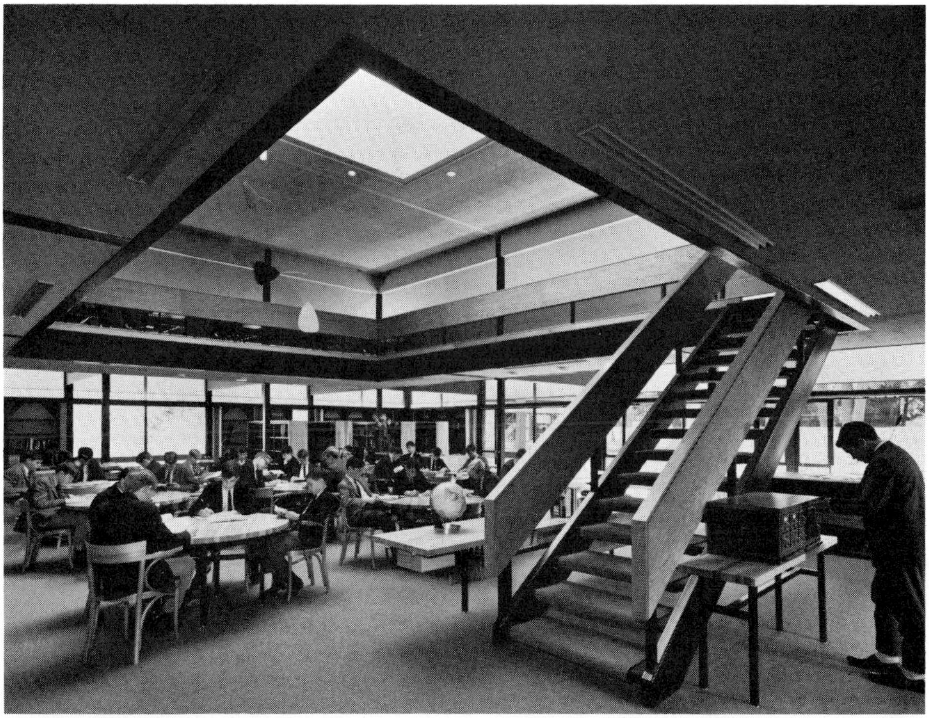

Figure 59 A library should be an inviting space. The Architects Collaborative, Inc., Architects. (Louis Reens, photographer.)

The cost of choosing paints with regard for the psychological aspects of environment should not increase the cost of a building. Selecting pleasing colors does not cost any more than selecting unpleasant or unsuitable colors.

Thermal Environment. Warmth is essential for well-being; shivering youngsters are in no mood to learn. A comfortable temperature is obtained with an efficient heating and ventilating system. The temperature should be steady, optimum, and uniformly distributed throughout a given space.

A heating and ventilating system should be designed by a competent engineer. The type will depend upon the size and architecture of the plant, its geographical location, the available source of fuel, and plans for future expansion. An automatic control is desirable, with a thermostat in each room. In some control systems a teacher can adjust the temperature for his own room; in most instances, however, this is not possible. Fahrenheit temperatures are recommended as follows:

Classrooms	68° to 72°
Corridors	66° to 70°
Gymnasiums	60° to 70°

A range of several degrees takes into account the humidity. If the air in the room is dry, the temperature should be higher. The converse is also true; the greater the humidity, the lower the requirement of heat.

Since their metabolic rates are higher, children do not require as high a temperature as adults. Teachers should don sweaters and wear warmer clothing in order to be comfortable, rather than increase the heat in a room. A room that is too warm induces drowsiness. When children are more active, they are warmer and require a cooler room. If the thermostat is set for a lower temperature in a gymnasium, the physical educator should leave it alone. Investigations by heating and ventilation experts show that in too many instances the Fahrenheit temperature of a room is set at a higher level than is recommended for children's comfort and learning efficiency. The teacher's comfort seems to be a prime consideration. As a matter of fact, children are not too critical of room temperature except for extremes. They are critical only if the teacher or parents are complaining and making an issue of a few degrees in heat.

The type of ventilating system is dependent upon the heating system selected. A mechanical system is usually installed with special arrangements for ducts which separately exhaust kitchens, toilet rooms, and laboratories.

Whenever a part of a building is to be used in the evenings, it should be possible to provide heat only to the part being occupied without heating the whole structure.

The thermal conditioning of school buildings includes the installation of an air conditioning system, preferably in the original plans. A new school without such an installation will soon be rare. Many school districts report an increasingly high enrollment of regular students for summer school sessions. This enrollment can be accounted for by the attendance of the student who needs to catch up on his studies, by those in accelerated programs, and by those who do not enjoy a summer's idleness. With an air-conditioned plant, school should be inviting. Future educational schedules may involve using the school 12 months a year. Moreover, if provisions for "fall-out" protection are incorporated into the school building design, as recommended by the Office of Civil Defense Mobilization, air conditioning will be necessary, and the systems must be shielded.

Acoustical (Auditory) Environment. A child who does not hear well does not learn readily. A room and a school should be acoustically comfortable. Achieving this involves two considerations: optimum hearing of speech, and the elimination, as much as possible, of noise. Speech should be perfectly understood in every part of a room or auditorium, without effort and without echoes, reverberations, or overlapping of sounds.

Noise is distracting; it affects the powers of concentration. Some children are particularly sensitive to extraneous sounds. In the selection of a building site, consideration is given to the possibility of outside noises, usually those from highway and train traffic. Noises within the building should be kept at a minimum with proper acoustical treatment and placement of noisy activities as far away as possible from classrooms. Noisy areas to be considered are: playgrounds; rooms for band, chorus, business machines, and shopwork; large spaces, as gymnasiums and auditoriums. Other sources of distracting sounds may be mechanical equipment (radiators, grills, motors, fans), the scraping of furniture, and the pounding of feet in corridors. Corridors may be efficient conductors of sound and should be acoustically treated. Audiovisual teaching aids may be a problem because their sound power is often much greater than a person's voice and may be transmitted not only to adjacent rooms but to some distance away.

Not only should noisiness be minimized, but sound should be well-transmitted in spaces which are used as auditoriums, music rooms, and gymnasiums. The medley of sounds which reverberate from the walls of a large space, and the straining to hear well, can produce excessive fatigue.

Research has produced vital information on acoustics and materials to be used in acoustical control. Such research should be utilized in every school. Carpeting is proving practical, economical to maintain, and comfortable; it contributes to dignity and reduces sound. The combination of carpet, acoustical ceiling, and the subdued voice of a teacher promotes a quiet environment in which several activities or classes can be conducted at one time.

Above all, teachers should know this: If a teacher's voice is loud, the children tend to answer with the same degree of loudness. If his voice is quiet, the response will be in similar vein.

Esthetic Values

Utility and beauty can be combined at little or no extra cost. Appreciation of the importance of an attractive interior and exterior comes first; then creative ideas follow. What is appealing, beautiful, and comfortable will be used more. This is true whether the facility is a library, an organization room, or rooms in the first-aid or health service unit with coverlets in attractive designs on the beds. What is inviting becomes functional.

Beauty is planned in the landscaping, in the design of the exterior of the building in terms of mass, form, scale, and use of varied construction materials, and in the appearance of the interior. Color has a major influence in decoration. Every room should have individuality yet form a part of the whole school. Planting-boxes or recesses can be placed outside or inside the building to add green color and "life" to the environment. Tile work, floors, woods used in the interior finish, and the selection of pictures and their frames can add to beauty yet serve their original purposes. Outdoor areas, when related to rooms, should expand the feeling of space.

The mental health of a child is affected by the feeling tones in the environment. A relaxed, contented child is in a mood to learn.

Design for Safety, Health Facilities, and Sanitation

After consideration has been given to the basic factors mentioned above, the architect and engineering staff automatically care for the painstaking details of school planning. Only health features which should be of interest to teachers will be discussed here—safety, health facilities, and sanitation.

Safety

All planning for building and grounds gives primary consideration to safety—structural safety, safety to prevent panic, and safety against accidents.

Structural safety means use of good and adequate materials to form a strong foundation and superstructure which will carry both a structural and live load and will withstand jolts of earthquakes and pressures of tornadoes. The opportunities for spread of fire should be reduced to a minimum. This means avoidance of fire hazards in the basement and use of fireproof materials in screens, partitions, and curtains. Automatic sprinkler systems or similar protection should be installed. One-story buildings permit quick evacuation during a hazardous crisis; they are especially desirable in earthquake belts. Multistoried buildings should have convenient fire escapes which open on avenues and not into blind alleys or courts. The exterior doors used for student traffic should be equipped with panic bolts which work. More than 40 fires occur each school day in schools of this country.

A study of the incidence and location of accidents within school buildings will direct safety in design. Accident reports filled out at school provide excellent information. Possible hazards are: narrow corridors which will not handle peaks of traffic; projections and obstacles as with dividers, water fountains, nails and clothes hangers on walls; steep or narrow stairs; dead-end halls; slippery floors. Entryways from the outside should be sheltered and covered with materials which prevent slipping. Fountains should be recessed in walls. More discussion on safety follows in the next chapter.

Any discussion on safety in design will be remiss unless a reminder is included on the possibility of nuclear disaster. Some school buildings are being constructed with facilities for decontamination not only of students but of all members of the community. Self-containment of utilities in case of emergency, and the conversion of space for assembly of the general population are considerations.

Health Facilities

No new school of any size should be constructed without a specially designed health service unit. This unit should fulfill a number of functions so that it can be used every day of the school year. If possible, there should be several rooms planned as a suite with bathroom facilities and comfortable beds or cots where young people who need rest periods will feel free to visit. Those who are below par physically and need to relax, convalescents, and even some who simply need more sleep, should have such beds available. A child who becomes ill or is injured and must await the arrival of a parent or the return bus can be kept here. Ideally, each room should contain very few beds in order to assure little distraction. See Figure 60.

One or two rooms of this unit may be used for health examinations and for health counseling. A nurse should have one room where she can inspect and counsel students, store records, reference books, and medical supplies. Somewhere in the unit, either in a corridor or consultation room, a twenty-two foot clear path should be provided for vision testing. The examination-health counseling room should be situated near boys' and girls' rooms, furnished with cots and adjacent toilet rooms. A receiving and waiting area should be planned, which should seat a number of students. See Figure 60.

In new school buildings health facilities are placed in the administrative area, so that close supervision is possible. A health service unit should be attractive and should be quiet, placed as far away as possible from music rooms, band practice, gymnasiums, flushing toilets, and noisy playgrounds. The set-up may be elaborate in large schools which have a full- or part-time physician and a full-time nurse. Health units are usually more simply planned in elementary schools.

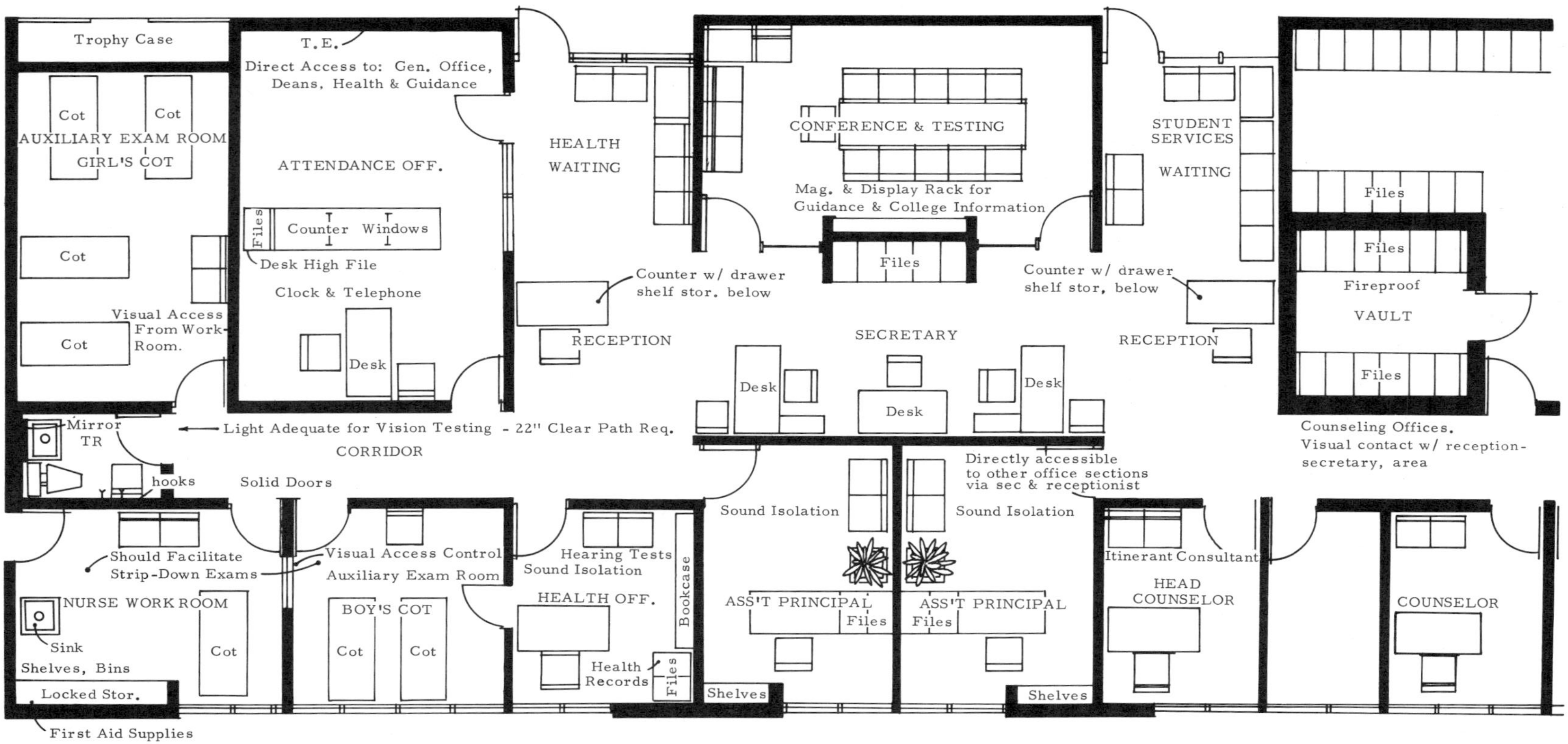

Figure 60 Health service unit. Placed in administrative area. Cottonwood High School, Salt Lake City, Utah. (Edwards and Daniels and Associates, architects.)

Sanitation

The problem of sanitation includes the provisions for water supply, sewage disposal, and plumbing installations. Designs for lunchrooms, shower and dressing rooms, swimming pools, laboratories, and classrooms require careful consideration.

Water supply, sewage disposal facilities, and lunchroom design should comply with state board of health regulations and any existing applicable building codes. Contaminated water can be a source of spread of typhoid and paratyphoid fevers, dysentery, amebiasis, and possibly infectious hepatitis.

Wherever hot and cold water are dispensed from a faucet or shower outlet, the water should be tempered first by installing mixing valves, in order to prevent burns. And there should be an adequate supply of shower stalls in the gymnasium.

Toilet Rooms. Toilet rooms should be conveniently placed near traffic flow—near the play space in elementary grades and near the library in high school—as well as in other locations. An ideal arrangement supplies a toilet room adjacent to kindergarten and first-grade classrooms or at least one between the two classrooms. The advantages of such an arrangement are: the class is "self-contained," toilet facilities are conveniently nearby and children can be encouraged to use them, conditions are similar to home, fixtures are adjusted to necessary heights, and the young children do not need to associate with older ones in the same toilet rooms.

Drinking Fountains. Drinking fountains should be sufficient in number so that children need not stand in line too long. A minimum of one fountain for every 75 students is recommended. A greater number is desirable, placed at points of greatest use. If placed in a corridor, they should be recessed in order not to impede the flow of traffic, and also in order to discourage scuffling, spraying water, and "bops on the head" of the drinker. The last practice has accounted for many a split lip and broken tooth. The fountain head should be placed to one side of the fountain rim with a guard which prevents the mouth from touching the source of water (angle-jet type). The water issues as a "jet stream," in contrast to the bubble type which permits contaminated water to flow back over the opening. The stream of water should always be running, with sufficient pressure to enable a child to enjoy a satisfying cool drink.

The Old School Plant

Not every teacher teaches in a modern school. The little red school house may be memorialized in nostalgic terms, but it was scarcely a comfortable, healthy place in which to teach or learn effectively. Unfortunately, too many of these schools still are being used. With the shortage of classrooms many will continue to be occupied.

Surveys of school buildings in various states reveal findings which are incredible and deplorable—conditions showing a lack of electric lighting, running water, indoor plumbing, or central heating. Many buildings are badly in need of repair. Some communities have had to close schools because they were too dangerous for use.

The demand of an increasing school population and the shifts of the peoples to various parts of the country are draining the funds available to boards of education for construction purposes. Heroic efforts are being made to meet educational needs. Many old plants are being modernized. A sound structure sometimes may be salvaged and remodeled to incorporate many of the features placed in new structures. An attractive addition may be built; patios and courts can produce beauty and intimacy. An attractive school building gives stability to a community and may revitalize an old neighborhood. Families will want to stay. This could be a partial answer to a deteriorating area of a city. If a community is determined to care for its educational needs, concerted effort and contribution of labor can make a school livable. Consultants from the state board of education or a school architect can provide valuable suggestions.

Using the School Plant

Operation and Maintenance

It costs money to run a plant efficiently. A school system usually hires a trained person as a supervisor of all buildings and grounds. He is responsible for hiring and training custodians for the schools under his jurisdiction. These employees plan their own budgets for supplies and request outside skilled help when basic services fail.

The operation and maintenance of a large plant sometimes requires the services of an engineer who will plan help for both indoor and outdoor needs. On the other hand, occupants of a small rural building will be fortunate to have the part-time services of someone nearby. All gradations of custodial services can be found.

Custodian

The custodian is an important member of the school team. His role has been fully described in the discussion on the Organization and Administration of the School Health Program. He should be capable of operating and maintaining a school plant. He should enjoy the association of youth. He should be fit to deserve their companionship.

No one person in a school can undertake all responsibility for a healthful physical school environment. First, there must be a desire to maintain such an environment. A well-kept plant in itself should sup-

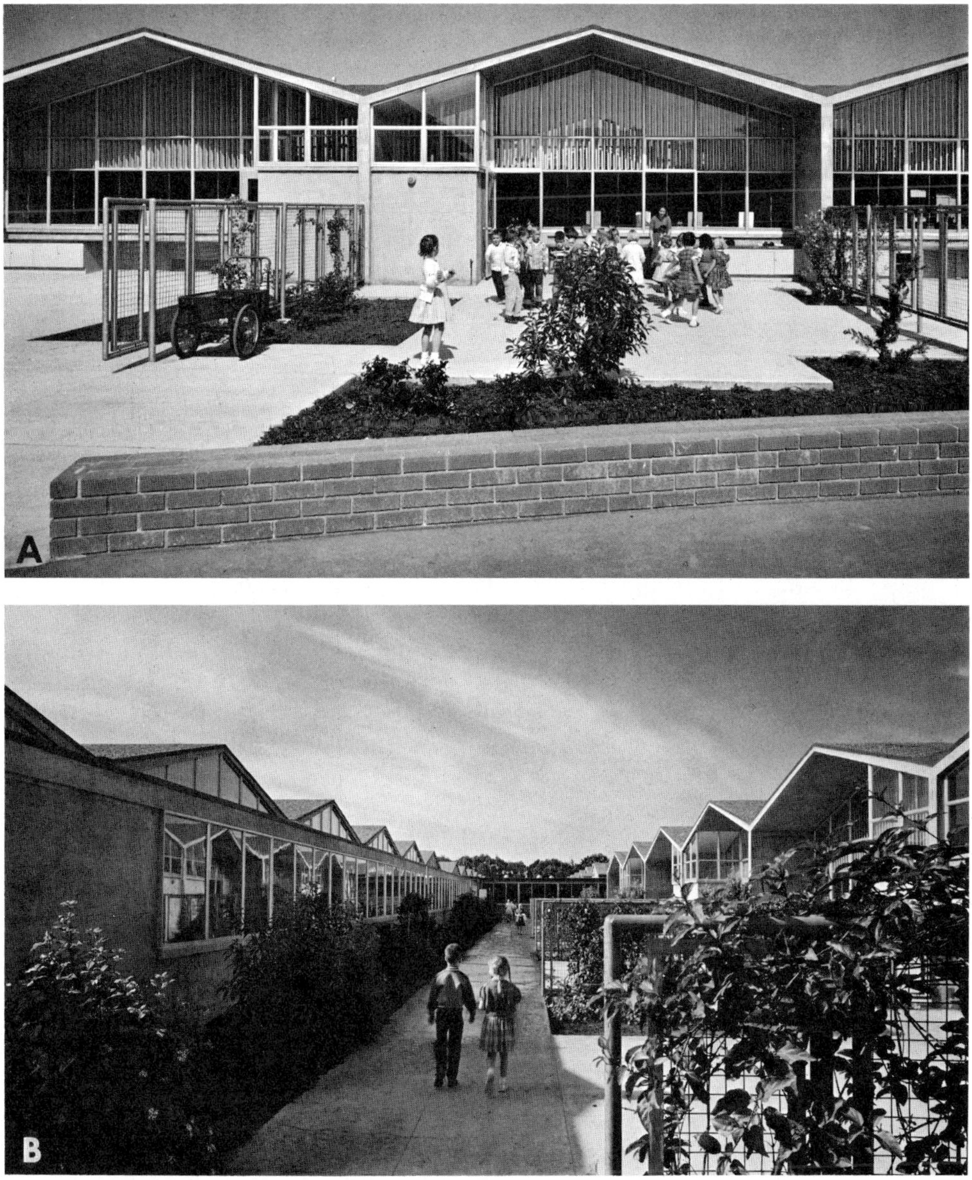

Figure 61 Frederick Burk Teacher Training School, San Francisco. *A*, south wall of the kindergarten rooms. The walled-in area at left center houses toilets for these rooms. *B*, area between building wings is used as outdoor classroom. (Reid and Tarics, architects. Roger Sturtevant, photographer.)

ply such motivation. The cooperation of all in the school is necessary. Children should understand their responsibilities. To emphasize this fact, one school assigned various sections of the grounds to groups of students and developed a lively competition with awards for keeping the sectors clean. Teachers can emphasize the phases of operation and maintenance in their own classrooms.

Community Use

If a community's investment can serve more than one function, there is a feeling that money is well spent. Some of a school's facilities can be used for night classes in adult education, for public meetings, for music and theater groups in the auditorium, and for sports events in the gymnasium. Physical education classes have been held for adult groups who wished to keep up activities and have fun.

The School Bus

While the school bus is not a stationary part of a plant, in many communities it is essential for long-distance transportation and is an integral part of the school system. About 20 million children are riding buses. Regulations on their use and the qualifications of the driver vary from state to state. Minimum standards are specified in a code recommended by the National Conference on School Transportation (available from the National Education Association). School bus fatalities occur from time to time, and such minor injuries as cut lips and bruised knees and elbows are commonplace in overcrowded vehicles.

The following observations are pertinent. The bus should be soundly constructed, be safe mechanically, and be comfortable and well-heated. Every child should have a seat. These seats should be sturdy and firmly anchored to the floor, have adequate protective padding, be supplied with lap safety belts, and have high backs to protect heads. The latter provision should also prevent noisy interplay. There should be no protruding structures, such as grips and rails. If present, they should be padded.[1] Overcrowding is an unsafe physical hazard and is a health menace. Respiratory infections can spread rapidly.

The driver should be mature enough to exercise good judgment and should qualify as a licensed chauffeur. Many tasks have been foisted upon a bus driver. He is not only asked to act as chauffeur, but is expected to maintain discipline (no mean chore, see Figure 62),

[1]Ralph Bugg: "Danger Rides the School Bus." *Today's Health* 45:21–23, 84–87, 1967.

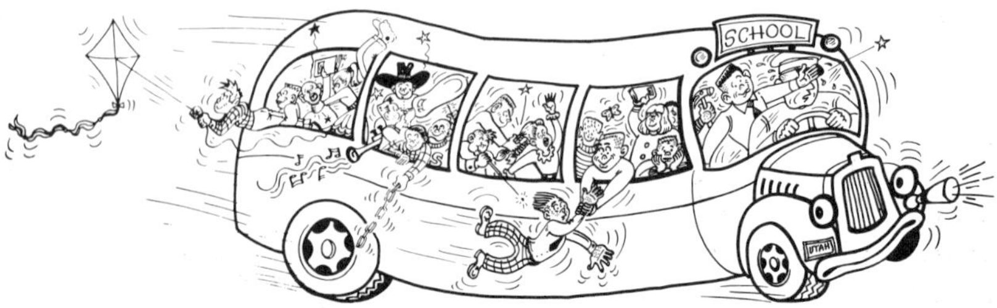

Figure 62 (Drawn with permission to reproduce by Johnny P. Pappas.)

administer emergency care, watch the children cross the street, and be a delivery man for the families on the route. No one person can fulfill all of these demands, especially the disciplinary problems, and watch the road. A parent or other responsible adult should ride the bus, watch the children, make sure that seat belts are fastened, and prevent rowdyism.

A HEALTHFUL SCHOOL DAY

After all precautions have been taken to provide a healthful physical environment, other factors are considered which will make the child comfortable and safe and permit him to learn most efficiently. A teacher may have little or no influence in planning or controlling the physical environment, but he certainly has immediate control of many of the factors to be described. In his own classroom he is alert to the physical and emotional welfare of those who sit before him, and he works with his colleagues to promote a healthful day at school.

Educational Aspects

Living in a school should be an educational experience.

> "The school is health education for good or for ill, depending upon what it is. Is the building overcrowded? Is it attractive? Are classes too large? Is bus transportation a wearing experience that jangles the nerves? Are admissions policies realistic in terms of child development? Are promotion practices in keeping with what is known of emotional needs? Is the school a demonstration of the way people ought to live and work together? Are classroom activities marked by warmth and pupil participation? Are the teachers paragons of creativity, maturity and understanding? Is the school schedule flexible and the curriculum rich in variety of opportunity? Is there a balance of work and rest and pursuit of excellence without tension and with pleasure? Are there specially trained personnel and professional resources available to supplement and reassure, as well as to insure expert advice and consultation?
>
> "These are modifiers within the school situation, just as the presence or absence of a safe water supply, loving parents, and genetically sound ancestors have implications for individual growth and development."[2]

One purpose of the physical environment is to provide an educational experience in healthful living. Teachers can use the school building in which they are housed as a health education laboratory.

---

[2]Ruth Abernathy: "Health Education Implications." From the report of the eighth National Conference on Physicians and Schools. Chicago: American Medical Association, 1961, pp. 34–35.

"Entering pupils can be taught how to use the drinking fountain and the lunchroom. They can be taught how to use the toilets and hand washing facilities. Older pupils can learn how the building is heated, ventilated, and lighted and how school personnel dispose of garbage and rubbish. They will be interested in fire precautions and the equipment available for fighting fire. They can learn the source of the school water supply and the measures taken to safeguard it. Understanding of problems related to sewage disposal can be learned by finding out the means taken to dispose of school sewage. Pupils can easily be involved in the study of reports of school building inspections and can exert an influence in securing needed improvements.

"School kitchens are excellent laboratories for health education. Pupils can observe how food is stored and prepared. They can learn how dishes are washed, about regulations designed to protect food from contamination, about the temperatures maintained in refrigerators, and about the methods used to keep flies, rodents, and insects away from food. Many will be impressed with the numerous procedures used to prevent food from becoming contaminated.

"Teachers of many subjects have unusual opportunities to emphasize healthful school living in relation to their particular interests. Science teachers inform pupils regarding the safe use of chemicals. Home economics teachers help pupils learn how to avoid burns. Teachers in shops point out the importance of machine guards, the value of eye goggles, and the proper use of sharp tools.

"Teachers of physical education are faced with special opportunities and responsibilities in teaching pupils to live healthfully. Attention should be given to helping pupils learn how to avoid accidents during participation in various types of activities. The role of proper protective equipment needs explanation as well as the importance of acquiring basic skills in different games and contests. Water-safety instruction is needed wherever there is a swimming pool. In addition, pupils should learn the precautions taken to maintain the safety of a swimming pool's water. They need answers to such questions as: Why is the water filtered? What chemicals are added? How is the quality of the water determined? Who checks the quality of water? What records of inspection are kept? Who keeps them?

"We can do more in the future than we have in the past to use school facilities and school equipment to help pupils learn about sanitation and safety."[3]

School Organization

Given a healthful, safe environment, the next step is to place the child in it and arrange his program so that he can function with maximum efficiency. He is in school to live and learn for many hours each day.

With the basic facts on his physical, emotional, intellectual, and social development in mind, and the educational specifications

---

[3]Charles C. Wilson: "Healthful School Living." *Ibid.* pp. 48–49.

evolved to meet his needs in these areas, the organization of his day can be planned. This is an area to be handled by the administrator and his professional teaching staff.

Schedule of the Day

No attempt will be made here to specify how long the school day should be, or what subjects should be given at what time. It is accepted knowledge that difficult subjects should be studied when the mind is fresh and free of accumulative fatigue products. The morning hours are more desirable. Again, sitting for long hours is tedious. Concentrated study should be interspersed with physical activity and some opportunity to rest. This routine can be followed in the elementary grades. Each school plans its own recess periods and its breaks for rest and activity within the classroom.

At the secondary level students do get some physical exercise with movement from class to class, and from their physical education activities. They are not as prone to fatigue as the youngsters. Their programs are individually planned; there should be provision for study periods. Many work in the afternoons and concentrate their studies into the morning hours.

With the shortage of classrooms and the crowding of school population today, modifications in the day's schedule in both elementary and secondary schools have been mandatory. Many schools have two shifts of teachers and students. Some teachers like such an arrangement; others deplore the unconventional schedule with its concentration of effort and lack of leisureliness.

Regulation of Extraclass Activities

Regulation of these activities is essential, as far as the school has control of them. Parents are anxious for their children to be accomplished and to fit into an intricate pattern in society. Even at considerable financial sacrifice, they will plan for instructions in many areas: tennis, skiing, ice-skating, swimming, dancing, instrument playing, singing, and other activities. Added to this may be scouting, church work, and chores at home. With the expanding social interests of the junior and senior high school students, participation in debating clubs, drama, choral groups, and other organizations naturally follows. It is no wonder that the child today has little time to relax and enjoy some leisure time. It follows often that he will be tired, tense, chew on his nails, and fidget. Too many extraclass activities breed fatigue and tension, a pattern which may persist through the year.

Administrators and teachers know these facts. They attempt to regulate the number and types of organizations a student may join at school. In a small school better observation is possible. But no control is possible over activities outside the school except by indirection. When considered necessary for a child's welfare, the principal, counselor, teacher, school nurse, or social worker may consult with a parent. The family doctor is often the first person to put on the brakes.

Safety Program

(Tables 12 through 14)

Deaths

Among persons of all ages, accidents are the fourth leading cause of death in the nation. In the ages one to 37 accidents are the leading cause of death.

Injuries

During the 1968–69 school year, school jurisdictional accidents numbered over 35,000 among the school population. At least, these were the total number of accidents reported on the Annual Student Accident Summary forms of the National Safety Council. These were the accidents which required a doctor's attention or caused one-half day's absence from school. Reporting them was voluntary.

The motor vehicle has become a major killer. Economic loss from traffic accidents reaches astronomical figures. Other losses cannot be calculated in terms of money. Traffic accidents can be cut and the flow of traffic improved only through adequate official programs, and officials can do only as much as citizens are willing to accept and support. Thus, traffic becomes a problem for all individuals.

Driver education is definitely paying off. The Department of Motor Vehicles of New York reports one-third fewer violations and one-fifth fewer accidents among a group who had driver education in contrast to a comparable group who had not had such training. All had drivers' licenses for at least 18 months.

TABLE 12 The National Accident Fatality Toll

	1972	Change From 1971
ALL ACCIDENTS	117,000	+2%
Motor vehicle	56,600	+3%
Public*	23,500	+4%
Home	22,000	−2%
Work	14,100	−1%

*Excludes motor vehicle and work. Includes recreation (swimming, hunting, etc.), transportation except motor vehicle, public building accidents, etc. National Safety Council: *Accident Facts,* 1973 Edition, p. 3.

TABLE 13 Accidental Deaths by Age, Sex, and Type*

Age	All Types	Motor Vehicle	Falls	Fires, Burns	Drowning	Fire-Arms	Ingestion of Food, Object	Poison (Solid, Liquid)	Poison by Gas	% Male–All Types
All Ages	116,385	55,791	17,827	7,163	7,699	2,309	3,712	2,967	1,549	69
Under 5	6,973	2,077	325	1,012	800	80	1,012	245	45	58
5 to 14	8,186	4,045	184	655	1,560	375	141	55	69	69
15 to 24	24,668	17,443	389	396	2,190	777	256	676	405	80

*National Safety Council: *Accident Facts*, 1973 Edition, p. 14.

TABLE 14 Accidental Deaths of School-age Children 5 to 14 Years (1969) per 100,000 Population*

	Deaths	Rate
TOTAL	8,186	20
Motor vehicle	4,045	10
Drowning	1,560	4
Fires, burns	655	1
Other	1,926	5

*National Safety Council: *Accident Facts*, 1973 Edition, p. 8.

Some facts on injuries in children are significant and interesting:

Definitions[4]

School Jurisdiction. From the time the child leaves home for school or school-sponsored activity until he returns home.

Injury. Any injury sufficiently serious to cause a one-half day absence from school, or requiring medical attention.

Accident. Any occurrence in a sequence of events which usually produces unintended injury, death, or property damage.

Under School Jurisdiction. More than 90 per cent of injuries occur in the school plant, in various parts of buildings, in physical education classes, in unorganized play on the grounds, intramural sports, etc.

High school boys have substantially more accidents than girls do.

About 7 per cent occur on the way to and from school, involving school bus accidents (a low incidence), motor vehicle accidents, bicycles, and accidents on sidewalks.

In Nonjurisdiction Accidents. The home accounts for about 50 per cent, from falls, cuts, scratches, burns, etc., more frequent in younger children.

Any statistics on injuries or accidents in school-age youth will be incomplete. Unless injuries are called to a physician's or teacher's attention, or require absence from school, they will be unrecorded.

Preventive Safety Program at School

Since accidents rank high as a health problem and cause the most deaths in school children, how can they be prevented? A preventive safety program will involve a study of the records to evolve plans for plant safety, traffic safety, placement of responsibilities, and school-community relationships.

Use of Records. A study of the statistics reveals clearly where the emphases must be placed.in preventing injuries and deaths in school-age children. Every year in July the National Safety Council issues an edition of "Accident Facts" which summarizes reports. Current data on location of accidents and the types of activities which are associated with them are published by the Council.

A few words about the National Safety Council: It is a private, nonprofit, noncommercial organization chartered by the Congress of the United States to prevent accidents of all kinds. It is supported by labor, civic, business, school, and church organizations.

A compilation of statistics on school accidents from many school systems can be helpful for local application. A reprint of the school section from "Accident Facts" is sent annually to every cooperating school system. Comparisons can be made with hazards and mishaps in an individual school. For instance, if organized athletics is under scrutiny at the secondary level, those concerned with this phase of

[4]National Safety Council.

TABLE 15 Deaths from Accidental Poisoning by Solids and Liquids by Agency of Poisoning, United States, 1965*

Agency of Poisoning	Males*		Females*		Total Persons at Ages						
	Number	Percent of Total	Number	Percent of Total	Under 5	5-14	15-24	25-34	35-44	45-64	65 and Over
Total	1,159	100	951	100	379	25	166	275	365	638	211
Barbituric acid and derivatives	212	18	332	35	13	1	28	67	117	257	60
Drugs and medicines (except barbiturates)	464	40	382	40	176	6	105	147	124	205	83
Aspirin and other salicylates	89	8	86	9	113	5	2	7	8	28	12
Other sedatives, analgesic and soporific drugs	202	17	148	16	18	–	53	82	63	110	24
Morphine, other opium derivatives	59	5	10	1	1	–	27	30	8	3	–
Other and unspecified drugs	114	10	138	14	44	1	23	28	45	64	47
Alcohol	161	14	40	4	1	–	7	21	57	96	19
Caustic alkalies, acids	24	2	23	2	11	1	2	2	8	10	13
Lead and its compounds	41	4	24	3	46	1	1	3	4	9	1
Other and unspecified	257	22	150	16	132	16	23	35	55	111	35

*Source of basic data: Report of the Division of Vital Statistics, National Center for Health Statistics.
†Includes deaths at unspecified ages.

school life can analyze their own problems in light of national occurrences. If accidents in the classroom and auditoriums occur frequently, and if these have the highest incidence in the first eight grades, attention should be directed to this part of the elementary school plant. Also, since elementary schools report a large number of accidents on playground apparatus, the questions would logically revolve around the type of apparatus and how it is used. In junior and senior high schools, two thirds of the accidents involving play apparatus occur in physical education classes.[5] If the rise of injuries in the shops begins with the eighth grade and continues through high school, many safety factors and detailed instructions for students who use the equipment should command the observant care of those who teach in this field. If falls, cuts, and scratches in the home demand the most emphasis in health education for the elementary years, a teacher has his teaching unit clearly indicated. Safe use of knives and scissors can be discussed at school. An analysis can be made in class discussion by the children themselves on causes of falls and how they can be prevented.

Local school records provide resource material in a safety program. First, the principal of a school is urged to see that the Standard Student Accident Report Form, formulated by the National Safety Council (see Figure 63), is filled out for every injury requiring a doctor's care or absence from school. These are filed permanently in the superintendent's office, for reference in case further information concerning the circumstances of an accident is needed or for reference in case of a possible law suit or in determining permanent disability in childhood. A summary of these cases should be placed on the Student Accident Summary Form published by the National Safety Council and a copy sent once a year to the Council. These reports make it possible to compile the valuable statistics presented in "Accident Facts." Such statistics in turn may be used as a baseline from which a local school may compare its own status and evaluate its progress in the safety program.

In addition, some principals keep a daily log of minor injuries which require first aid. One visual informative device is to place a map of the school plant on the wall and designate locations of accidents by pins with colored heads.

Of equal value, analysis of local school accidents will reveal pertinent information: which steps outside a building become icy or slippery and cause many falls, where collisions occur in hallways, where steps are too steep, where projections in halls or rooms cause injuries, whether laboratories are poorly ventilated, whether unsafe equipment is used in the shops, and whether students in chemistry classes have received proper instruction on the technique of inserting glass tubing through corks. Are the students in these laboratories wearing safety goggles?

Records on equipment checks, fire drills, sanitary inspections,

[5]*Accident Facts*, 1973 Edition, pp. 90–91.

(check one)
☐ School Jurisdictional
☐ Non-School Jurisdictional

RECOMMENDED
STANDARD STUDENT ACCIDENT REPORT
(See instructions on reverse side)

(check one)
Recordable ☐
Reportable Only ☐

School District:
City, State:

General	1. Name			2. Address	
	3. School	4. Sex Male ☐ Female ☐	5. Age	6. Grade/Special Program	
	7. Time Accident Occurred Date:	Day of Week:		Exact Time:	AM ☐ PM ☐
Injury	8. Nature of Injury				
	9. Part of Body Injured				
	10. Degree of Injury (check one) Death ☐	Permanent ☐		Temporary (lost time) ☐	Non-Disabling (no lost time) ☐
	11. Days Lost From School:			From Activities Other Than School:	Total:
	12. Cause of Injury				
Accident	13. Accident Jurisdiction (check one) School: Grounds ☐ Non-School: Home ☐	Building ☐ Other ☐		To and From ☐	Other Activities Not on School Property ☐
	14. Location of Accident (be specific)			15. Activity of Person (be specific)	
	16. Status of Activity			17. Supervision (if yes, give title & name of supervisor) Yes ☐ No ☐	
	18. Agency Involved			19. Unsafe Act	
	20. Unsafe Mechanical/Physical Condition			21. Unsafe Personal Factor	
	22. Corrective Action Taken or Recommended				
	23. Property Damage School $	Non-School $		Total $	
	24. Description (Give a word picture of the accident, explaining who, what, when, why and how)				
Signature	25. Date of Report			26. Report Prepared by (signature & title)	
	27. Principal's Signature				

This form is recommended for securing data for accident prevention and safety education. School districts may reproduce this form adding space for optional data. Reference: *Student Accident Reporting Guidebook*, National Safety Council, 425 N. Michigan Avenue, Chicago, Illinois 60611. 1966. 34 pages.

Figure 63 (Courtesy National Safety Council.)

and use of check lists on various safety aspects of school living can be helpful in a safety program.

Plant Safety. *The Building.* Basic considerations for safety in design, construction, operation, and maintenance have already been presented in this chapter. Alertness for detection of trouble spots is the responsibility of everyone in the school. Regulations help; e.g., rules prohibiting running in the corridors, and having teachers on duty in the halls at recess time and during free periods.

The Grounds. In elementary grades it may be necessary to stagger the times for recess. There should be adequate supervision while children are outside. At all levels there should be instruction on use of equipment and the proper way to play. Playground apparatus should be inspected daily; its maintenance is the responsibility of the custodian. The ground should be clear of all hazards, which may vary from poison oak to an open irrigation ditch.

Fire Safety. We teach by doing. Safe living must be an experience. Fire drills should be held at frequent intervals. The elementary children should at first be led through the channels of escape so that they can memorize them. Fire fighting equipment should be available in laboratories and all designated areas. A fire marshal or chief should make regular inspections and instruct on fire safety.

Inspections. Detailed checks of the physical environment can be made by groups of pupils. Is the plant safe? They study about safety in the classroom and can then go forth with their check lists on an evaluation tour. They can check stairs, doors, fire equipment, and under stairways for inflammable materials. They inspect the custodian's housekeeping. They look for sharp projections and slippery floors. The toilet rooms can be viewed critically. Inspection of swings and other playground equipment will be part of the tour. They come back to the classroom, analyze their data, and make recommendations. Such a procedure affords an opportunity to learn and develop desirable attitudes towards safe living.

Literature is available from the National Safety Council and from the National Commission on SafetyEducation of the National Education Association on practically every phase of living which involves a school. Check lists also serve as guides and are available from the National Safety Council. Excellent teaching films on the many aspects of safety have been produced for the various grades.

Traffic Safety. Since such a great number of accidents in the United States are motor vehicle casualties, a most careful program should be established at school to lower the incidence.

Elementary School. In the lower grades school boy and girl patrols have a protective function; but the principal objective is educational—children are taught to be intelligent pedestrians.

Children learn "safe practices in the use of streets and highways at all times and places."[6] Pupils wearing the wide, white or orange

[6]National Safety Council: "Standard Rules for the Operation of School Safety Patrols." Chicago: 12 pp. Rules were formulated by a committee of representatives from the American Automobile Association, International Association of Chiefs of Police, National Commission on Safety of the National Education Association, National Congress of Parents and Teachers, National Safety Council, and United States Office of Education.

Sam Browne belt are familiar figures at intersections during the school year. They are on duty at the times children cross streets or highways going to and from school. Their function is not to direct vehicular traffic, but to hold the children back on the sidewalk until there is a break in the line of motor traffic. A pupil-patrolman stands on the curb and steps aside when a break occurs to permit the children to cross over to the other side. If his vision is obstructed, he steps down from the curb, checks on traffic, motions the children to cross, and then resumes his position on the curb. At hazardous intersections a police officer or adult crossing guard may be present to supervise the crossing and direct traffic. When children are transported by bus, patrols are assigned to protect them.

A first-grade teacher may take her class to the nearest street intersection and practice crossing it. This will not only serve as a realistic experience but assist the school patrol boy in his duties. Those children who violate patrol directions are disciplined by their peers, possibly through the school safety council.

Such a program not only protects youngsters, but it serves to develop a respect for authority and regulations. Members of the patrol benefit in terms of leadership from the authority delegated to them.

Organization and administration of the safety patrol system is the responsibility of the school authorities. They work closely with the community traffic offices and with the PTA.

Some school systems in densely populated areas with heavy traffic do not sponsor such safety patrol systems. Adults, both men and women, are hired for this responsibility. They escort the children across the streets adjacent to the plant before and after school.

Upper Elementary and Junior High School. Children at this level are interested in bicycles. Communities and schools have devised various programs to promote their safe and efficient use. Bicycle clubs may be established. Riders learn traffic regulations and use of signals. They pass a skill test. Police may be invited to administer the examination and issue a license for operation of a bicycle. Sometimes the PTA sets up a training course. It is hoped that the knowledge, attitude, and experience gained in using a bicycle will carry over into the use of an automobile.

Senior High School. Driver education programs have been established in high schools throughout the country. Since a high percentage of automobile accidents occurs with drivers in the 16 to 25 year age group, and the resulting automobile insurance coverage for this group is relatively more expensive, steps are being taken to instruct senior high school students in safe driving. Legislative help is being secured. Money obtained from the additional cost of license plates is one source of revenue for financing this program. A specified number of hours in classroom instruction on traffic regulations and use of a car, with additional hours of observation in a dual control car, plus a number of hours behind the wheel of the dual control car are required. Students who pass this course may be allowed a deduction in premium on their car insurance policies. Much of the success of driver education depends upon the attitude of the student. Frequently those who have accidents have no regard for themselves or others.

Responsibilities for the Safety Program at School. Emphasis is placed upon the team approach in handling school safety problems. All professional teaching personnel and nonteaching individuals have a responsibility. So does the student at each age level. The National Safety Council has an excellent slogan: "Make safety their responsibility, too." Students are taught to assume responsibility for their own as well as everyone else's safety—the "Golden Rule."

In this discussion on safety, suggestions have been made about how a child can participate in safe living. Various types of councils and clubs may be organized. In the elementary grades, classroom and school safety councils have definite roles. Later, specialized phases are stressed through such organizations as those for bicycle, automobile, and shop safety. In the secondary schools there may be a student traffic court and committees responsible for traffic regulations and parking permits, for planning programs and publicity on safety, and for reporting and analyzing accidents.

The first aid program is presented in the next chapter.

School-Community Relationships. Safe living is everyone's business. A safety program involves every activity of living in our country. From the national to the local school level, private and public organizations are concerned with the prevention of accidents and the preservation of lives. Any local plan which involves a school child will include the school, but will also command the attention of parents, branches of the city and state governments (Fire, Police, Boards of Health, Building Codes), and organizations devoted to safety problems (see footnote 6).

Lunch Program

Eating lunch forms a part of a child's school day. Each school system and school plans its own program. If children live in the neighborhood, they may go home for the noon meal. If the weather is bad, they may bring a lunch. For those who come from more distant areas, provisions are made for a lunch at school, or for some beverage or hot dish to supplement the food brought from home. Many working mothers plan on their children's having a well-balanced lunch at school.

Some schools also provide an opportunity to buy milk or fruit juice in midmorning or midafternoon recess. If a child is indigent and if some sort of food is being sold at school, arrangements should always be made to feed the youngster at no cost.

If a school is large enough, a separate area should be set aside for cooking and lunch purposes. This area should be bright and cheerful, quiet and clean—in other words, socially attractive. There should be faculty supervision during meal time, when children should be encouraged to sit and eat in leisurely fashion. In the absence of a lunchroom, the classroom itself serves as a dining area, particularly in inclement weather. Such a period permits the teacher to observe the quality of the lunches brought from home.

With a large school population students may have assigned lunch periods so that all may have an opportunity to eat quietly without any rush. If children go home for lunch, they should have time enough to walk both ways, without a feeling of being rushed.

The lunch program with its many benefits has been discussed under Nutrition. Provision of sanitary facilities have been emphasized earlier in this chapter. The importance of preventing spread of disease in the kitchen and lunchroom has been stressed in the discussion of communicable diseases. The health of food service personnel must be a major concern.

Classroom Experience

Human interrelationships are important during the hours of living in a classroom. The emotional development of a child is affected by his experience here. Harsh words, sarcasm, tension in the teacher, undesirable techniques of discipline, too much stress on grades or on attendance, too much competition, noisiness and tiring activities—all these can make a pupil uneasy and nervous.

> Aside from the home, growing children spend more time in school than anywhere else. What they observe and do in school may reinforce the teachings and examples of the good home or help to correct harmful influences if they come from poor homes in which standards are low and conflict prevalent. If the school environment is not conducive to effective personality development, the children in the community are indeed underprivileged, no matter what their economic status. The examples set and attitudes shown by school-board members, superintendents, principals, and teachers are of key importance in the development of healthy personalities in young people learning to live by democratic principles in a crowded but free world.[7]

We are interested in the physical environment of the classroom. We are more interested in the basic concepts of teaching which should help formulate well-integrated personalities in children. An emotionally stable teacher who maintains a cheerful and calm emotional climate in the classroom is a jewel beyond price. Farnsworth presents the following guides with the comment, "They are somewhat philosophical and idealistic, but so is teaching":

> 1. The teacher should know himself well, accept his own shortcomings and determine to overcome them when possible,

[7]Dana L. Farnsworth: *Mental Health in College and University.* Cambridge: Harvard University Press, 1957, pp. 204–205.

and be able to recognize in himself when emotional reactions begin to displace reason. In this way he should not have to work out his own problems at the expense of his students.

2. He should understand his students in terms of their being products of all their previous experiences, as well as heredity. Each one is therefore different, and hence treating them all alike is frequently futile.

3. The teacher cannot cause growth in his students but only influence and direct it to a limited extent. He can remove obstacles, furnish material to make greater growth possible, and aid in every way possible to help the child achieve self-realization of his own potentialities.

4. Immaturity in all its forms—lack of knowledge, misconceptions, prejudice, sensitivity, tensions between individuals and groups, and unreasonable fears—is the reason for the existence of the teacher as a professional person.

5. Next to mastery of subject-matter, the teacher's own attitude toward students is the most important factor in his success. If he likes them, is consistently firm and patient in applying pressure toward achieving high standards, and can wait patiently for favorable results, his teaching will be successful.

6. What the teacher is and does is more influential on students than anything he may say. It is sometimes a shock to teachers to realize how much their students are concerned with what they do, say, read, wear, enjoy, and their manner and behavior generally.

7. Discipline is a slow process of transferring authority from without (parents, teachers, law-enforcement officers) to within the individual's own personality (self-discipline, self-control, maturity). The older the student, the greater the proportion of reason and explanation and self-participation in enforcing discipline. Without definite external standards in the young child, self-discipline is nearly impossible in the older child.

8. A permissive attitude balanced with firm discipline is the quickest route to responsibility and self-control, especially when discipline is applied with consistency, kindness and thoughtfulness.

9. Authoritarian, inflexible, and impersonal attitudes in the teacher encourage and perpetuate rebellion, negativism, and hostility in the pupil.

10. The good teacher should have a personal philosophy that will tolerate frustration and defeat. He works for the long-term goals. He has the habit of reasonable expectation rather than wishful thinking. He has a respect for, but does not worship facts. He can be uneasy without being unhappy. He can tolerate uncertainty without being paralyzed by anxiety. He can show joy and enthusiasm as well as righteous indignation.[8]

HEALTH OF PERSONNEL

Professional Teaching Personnel

Teaching is not easy work. Regardless of what level or what subject is being taught, a good teacher is always expending energy. The

[8] *Ibid.*, pp. 206–207.

impact of many personalities upon each teacher and the impact of his personality upon many in the effort to stimulate intellectual growth requires physical and emotional stamina. It is not true that "anyone can teach" or that an individual with debilitating physical handicaps will find a comfortable niche in the teaching profession. One must be physically fit to undertake an assignment in the professional education field and should strive to remain that way. As an employee, each teacher has an obligation to the board of education and to the students to preserve his health.

FROM THE LONDON "WOMAN TEACHER'S CHRONICLE," FEBRUARY 13, 1925

1. Thou shalt have other interests besides thy school-room.

2. Thou shalt not try to make of thy children little images, for they are a live bunch, visiting the wriggling of their captivity upon you, their teacher, unto the last weary moment of the day; and showing interest and cooperation unto those who can give them reasonable freedom in working.

3. Thou shalt not scream the names of thy children in irritation, for they will not hold thee in respect if thou screamest their names in vain.

4. Remember the last day of the school week, to keep it happy.

5. Humor the feelings of thy children that their good will may speak well for thee in the little domain over which thou rulest.

6. Thou shalt not kill one breath of endeavour in the heart of a little child.

7. Thou shalt not suffer any unkindness of speech or action to enter the door of thy room.

8. Thou shalt not steal for the drudgery of many "papers" the precious hours that shall be given to recreation, that thy strength and happiness may appear unto all that shall come within thy presence.

9. Thou shalt not bear witness to too many "schemes of work" for much scattered effort is a weariness to the soul and a stumbling block to weary fingers.

10. Thou shalt not covet thy neighbor's room, nor her children, nor her manner, nor her system, nor anything that is thy neighbor's, but work out thine own salvation with fear and trembling—only don't let anyone know about the fear and trembling.

11. Thou shalt laugh—when it rains, and wee, wooly ones muddy the floor, when little angels conceal their wings and wriggle, when Tommy spills ink, when visitors appear at the precise moment when all small heads have forgotten everything you thought they knew.

Again I say unto you, LAUGH for upon these commandments hang all the law and the profits in thy schoolroom.

The board of education and the administration have an obligation toward the teacher. Any help which will provide comfort and relieve tension in a teaching situation should be given. A teacher is entitled to a financial compensation which will permit a standard of living commensurate with his education and prestige and which will permit time for graduate study. There should be reassurance of adequate retirement benefits. Sick leave should not entail such a financial sacrifice that a teacher will attend classes anyway, do a half-hearted job, and, in case of a communicable disease, expose many individuals. Members of the board and administration in a small town should introduce new faculty members to the community and make every effort to integrate them into the social and civic life of the people whose children they teach. A lonely teacher who must depend upon the companionship of pupils and students is not an asset to school or town.

The administration should strive to make teaching a pleasure. The teaching load should not be excessive, in terms of numbers of students to a class, or in numbers of classes. Demands for supervision of extraclass activities should not be an imposition. For instance, an English instructor may carry a full teaching schedule of classes and yet be required to spend many extra hours with the editors of a school paper. Teachers should have a separate lunch area. A teachers' lounge should be provided where they may relax and converse with each other, away from the energetic throng. Such a lounge should adjoin restrooms and a kitchenette. These rooms are for adults.

Most teachers live to a comfortable old age; their life expectancy is slightly longer than average. Their most common illnesses are the respiratory diseases. They fail to use sick leave when needed. For longer absences from school, nervousness and emotional problems are the usual causes.

Nonteaching Personnel

The philosophy to be applied in hiring other personnel, as far as health is concerned, is expressed in the last few paragraphs of the next chapter on School Health Services. If the emotional climate of a school is important, then all nonteaching personnel not only should be physically fit but should be emotionally and morally fit. By their satisfactory performance of assigned tasks, they should contribute to the objectives of the school health program.

These employees should enjoy benefits comparable to those in industry. They should be required to have periodic health examinations and x-rays of the chest as well as health evaluations after extensive leaves of absences for illness. No employee should be assigned to a job which taxes his physical capacity. All employees should strive to follow the health precepts taught children.

SUMMARY

The environment at school is described in its relationship to healthful living. One factor to be considered is the school plant itself with the emphasis placed upon comfortable living which permits fulfillment of educational specifications and promotes ease of learning. Organization of space, environmental conditions (visual, thermal, acoustical), and esthetic values are discussed in some detail. An equally important factor is the experience of the child at school during a healthful school day. The health of teaching and nonteaching personnel also has an influence upon the child's living at school.

DISCUSSION QUESTIONS AND ACTIVITIES

1. Explore the building requirements for a school in your community. Why are these standards set?
2. Obtain a copy of the yearly budget for a school system and compute the amount of money spent on health and safety activities.
3. Investigate (with permission) the health files of a local school. What kind of information is kept on file?
4. Explore and discuss the legal meaning of "in loco parentis" when it is applied to the first aid actions of a teacher for a student.
5. Discuss the importance of the custodian on the school health team.
6. Discuss who is responsible for making the school lunch program possible. Who makes up the menus?
7. Discuss the ethics involved in a teacher's taking sick leave; should he take off when he just feels ill or wait until sure signs of sickness are evident?
8. Discuss the importance of esthetic values in the building of a school.
9. Take a poll of several school districts to see how widespread the practice of hiring a school nurse is; is this only done in large cities?
10. Discuss the issue of community use of the school. Would you be willing to let your room be used for night classes and the like?

ADDITIONAL SOURCES OF INFORMATION

American Association for Health, Physical Education and Recreation:
"Health Aspects of the School Lunch Program." (1962).
Offers suggestions for planning and conducting school lunch programs.
"Health of School Personnel." (1964).
"School Safety Policies with Emphasis on Physical Education, Activities and Recreation." (1968).
"Teaching Safety in the Elementary School." (1962).
Anderson, C. L.: *School Health Practice.* St. Louis: The C. V. Mosby Co., 1972.
Callan, L. B., and Rowe, D. E.: "The role of the school sanitarian." *J. Sch. Health* 42: 360–3, June, 1972.

Englehardt, N. L., Englehardt, N. L., Jr., and Leggett, S.: *School Planning and Building Handbook.* New York: F. W. Dodge Corporation, 1956.
Florio, A. E., and Stafford, G. T.: *Safety Education.* Third edition. New York: McGraw-Hill Book Company, Inc., 1969.
Gordon, J., et al.: "Classroom ecology and safety." *J. Sch. Health* 42:178–81, March, 1972.
Haag, J. H.: *School Health Program.* Philadelphia: Lea & Febiger, 1972.
Hanlon, J. J.: *Design for Health: School and Community.* Philadelphia: Lea & Febiger, 1971.
Joint Committee on Health Problems in Education of the National Education Association and the American Medical Association: *Healthful School Environment.* Washington: The National Education Association, 1969.
Konopa, V. O.: "Noise–The challenge of the future." *J. Sch. Health* 42:172–6, March, 1972.
Larson, L.: *Lighting and Its Designs.* New York: Whitney Library of Design, 1964.
National Education Association, Department of Classroom Teachers and Research Division: Discussion pamphlets on such subjects as "Teachers' Leave of Absence," "Teacher Retirement," "Teacher Tenure," "Salary Scheduling," "School Marks and Promotion," "Teacher Rating," and "Democracy in School Administration." Washington: National Education Association.
National Education Association, National Committee on Safety Education:
Numerous publications on such topics as school safety, traffic safety, driver education, civil defense, standards for buses, and check lists on school safety education. Write for catalog.
National Safety Council:
Accident Facts. Current annual edition. Issued in July. Complete catalog of school materials.
School Safety. A monthly magazine for teachers in elementary schools. "A school safety education program." (1966).
School safety information packets can be ordered on numerous topics. Write for catalog.
S.C.S.D. (School Construction Systems Development): the Project and the Schools. Published by Educational Facilities Laboratories, Inc., a subsidiary of the Ford Foundation. 477 Madison Avenue, New York 22, New York, 1967. Result of research and experiment regarding educational facilities.
U.S. Department of Health, Education, and Welfare:
Bulletins on various aspects of healthful school living, sanitation, school plants, school buses, custodial services, fire safety, etc., published by Joint Committee on Rural Sanitation and Office of Education. Available from Superintendent of Documents, Government Printing Office, Washington, D.C.
"A Guide for Teaching Poison Prevention in Kindergartens and Primary Grades." 1965.

Planning guides, surveys, and check lists for elementary and secondary schools and for special facilities have been published by the U.S. Department of Health, Education, and Welfare and by many state departments of education.

AUDIOVISUAL MATERIALS

Recommended grade levels are designated *pri, int, jh, sh.*

Community Health and You

10 min. Black and White *jh, sh* McGraw-Hill*

Role of average health department in maintaining sanitary standards.

Safety on Our School Bus

11 min. Color *pri, int* Encyclopaedia Britannica Educ. Corp.

How a popular bus driver and his riders have maintained their fine safety record.

---

*See Appendix A for addresses of film companies.

Your Health at School

11 min. | Black and White | *int, jh* | Coronet Films

Children, teachers, and other school personnel must work together for healthful school living. The children learn that they also can help keep the school tidy and comfortable by observing good health practices and reporting illness or injuries to their teachers.

A wealth of audiovisual materials has been prepared in the field of Safety Education. Films, film strips, and posters are used. A good source of information on films is the "National Directory of Safety Films," published by the National Safety Council. Local chapters of the Council at city, state, or district levels will lend films from their libraries. State and local departments of education and of health can provide assistance. Film distributors (Appendix A) have produced films at appropriate grade levels in their Safety or Safe Driving Series. Write for catalogs from Association Films, Inc., Bailey Films, Inc., Coronet Films, Encyclopaedia Britannica Educational Corporation, McGraw-Hill Text-Film Department, and Modern Talking Service.

Chapter 19

SCHOOL HEALTH SERVICES

OBJECTIVES

Health Services represent one part of the school health program and are interrelated with the other two areas of healthful school living and health education. A division of the school health program into these three areas clarifies thinking and makes possible a delineation of their basic functions; however, there is no rigid demarcation. The various aspects support each other and merge at times. The objective is still the same—to promote and maintain the health of the school child. Here are some examples. Maintenance of a healthful environment helps prevent and control disease and serves as an educational experience. Health education, in turn, promotes healthful school living and utilizes student participation in various health services as a practical application of basic health principles. The service of tuberculosis detection assures a healthful environment and is abetted by class discussion. A school safety program involves a safe environment, care of injuries, planning an accident prevention program, and teaching safety not only by classroom procedures, but in almost every phase of school living.

School health services are those designed:

1. To appraise the health status of pupils and school personnel.
2. To counsel pupils, parents, and others concerning appraisal findings.
3. To encourage the correction of remediable defects.
4. To assist in the identification and education of handicapped children.
5. To help prevent and control diseases.
6. To provide emergency service for injury or sudden sickness.[1]

[1]New Definitions: Report of the 1972–73 Joint Committee on Health Education Terminology," *Health Ed. Monographs* Society for Public Health Education, Inc., 33:63–70, 1973.

And in addition:

7. To plan services which will provide a healthful environment.

8. To adjust individual school programs to meet the needs of children with health problems.

The patterns for administration of health services vary. A survey of 230 cities in 50 states indicates that they are administered predominantly by boards of education. They have allocated to themselves this responsibility for a number of reasons: "(1) efficiency and simplicity in single agency administration; (2) greater success in obtaining funds for school health services; (3) better understanding of the total school situation by the health service personnel; (4) more complete integration of health services and health education; (5) more emphasis placed on school health; and (6) larger and better service to school-age children."[2] See Figure 64.

Another possible pattern for administration is a joint organization of departments of health and education. More likely, one agency may be charged with specific responsibility (usually the board of education), but the administration of that responsibility should be the result of joint planning of education and medical professions.

HEALTH APPRAISAL

Health appraisal has been defined as "the process of determining the total health status of a pupil through such means as parent, teacher and nurse observations; screening tests; physical fitness tests; study of information concerning the pupil's past health experience; and medical and dental examinations. This concept recognizes that medical examinations include mental and emotional evaluation and that dental examinations are important in appraising pupil health. Such examinations, however, need to be supplemented by the other procedures mentioned."[3] Special surveys, reports from parents, and studies of adequate cumulative health records will also reveal pertinent information for appraisal.

Health History

A health history on a child supplies pertinent information which may be secured from preschool records, from conferences with parents or other children in the family, and from questionnaires. Forms for the latter (inventories) are available for elementary and secondary schools

---

[2]James M. Woolf and Howard C. Pritham: "Administrative Patterns of School Health Services." *J.A.M.A. 193*:195–199, 1965.

[3]Joint Committee on Health Problems in Education of the National Education Association and the American Medical Association: *Health Appraisal of School Children*, Fourth Edition. 1969, p. 2.

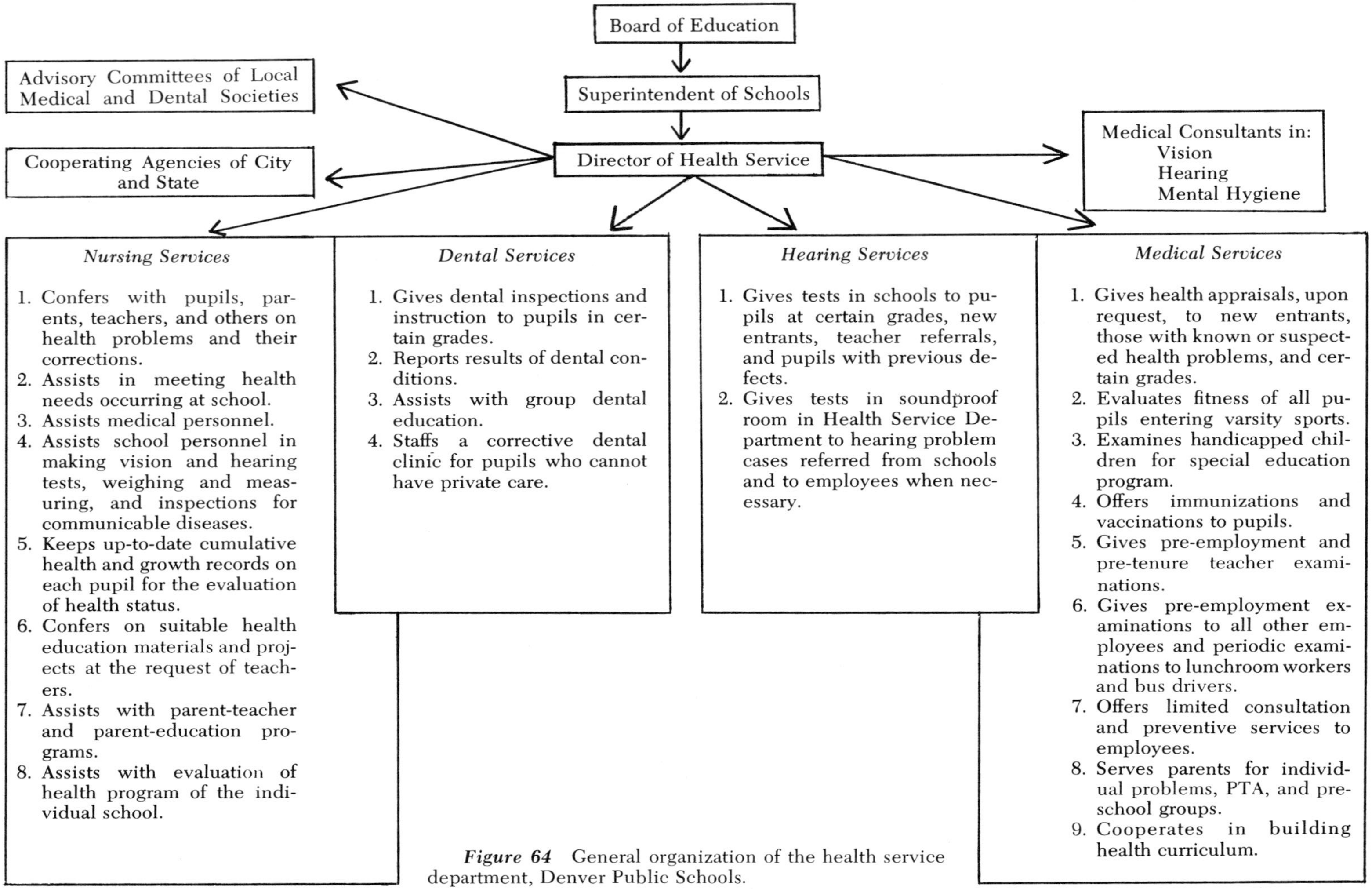

Figure 64 General organization of the health service department, Denver Public Schools.

with variations in emphasis at the two levels (see Appendix B). They may be filled out at home or during a conference with a parent. An older student should be capable of answering most of the questions concerning his own health.

Health histories provide information on past illnesses and operations, injuries, physical handicaps, immunizations, and habits of living. Questions should be asked on chronic complaints and about symptoms which may have a psychosomatic implication. Direct questions on "nervous breakdowns," nervousness, emotional upsets, crying spells, temper tantrums, bed-wetting, and moodiness are important as clues in the area of mental health.

These histories identify those with serious problems, such as diabetes, asthmatic attacks, epilepsy, and tuberculosis contacts—problems which will not usually be detected in a routine school health examination. Health histories serve as guides for further questioning. They should be valuable for research purposes. The history, which may be attached to the cumulative record, should always be available for study before the health examination.

Health observation is "a fundamental procedure in appraising pupil health involving sensitivity to changes in the way a pupil behaves or alteration in his color, gait or general appearance, which may be the first indication of physical and emotional problems."[4]

The observations of teacher, principal, physician, school nurse, social worker, and counselor are important in appraisal of a child's health status. Brief comments should be placed upon the cumulative health record or upon a separate form (Appendix B). A nurse may have consulted with a welfare agency concerning a crippled youngster. A siege of a serious illness deserves to be mentioned.

These observations should in most instances be of immediate value in handling a child. Occasionally they lie dormant upon the record and become meaningful at a later date. This is particularly true with comments on emotional behavior.

Teacher Observation. The tendency now is to avoid a formalized type of inspection during which each child is scrutinized in ritualistic fashion by the teacher each morning upon first entry into the classroom or shortly thereafter. Some teachers in the past have required that a clean handkerchief be placed in view and the hands be arranged upon the desk for criticism of cleanliness. They then proceeded to walk up and down the aisles for morning inspection. Many pupils religiously kept the same clean handkerchief for display and possibly another of dubious status for actual use. "One for blow and one for show." Stress now is laid upon continuous observation, all day long and not just in the morning. The constant day-to-day contacts and observations of elementary and secondary teachers will reveal findings which would probably not be noticed in a periodic health examination and may even escape a busy parent's notice.

---

[4]*Ibid.*, p. 2.

Because the teacher has become such an important individual in the school health program, pre-service and in-service courses in school health are designed to provide the necessary information for fulfilling a most essential role. Teacher-observation skills need to be improved. Detailed information is presented in the first part of this book which will familiarize a teacher with normal behavior and with the abnormal patterns of common health problems, thereby permitting early detection and subsequent correction. Symptoms and signs to be watched for are described in their proper settings under specific health topics. They become more significant when interpreted in terms of their underlying causes. However, they are presented here in condensed form as a review:[5]

Signs of Health. The teacher knows if a school-age youth is healthy:

He has an abundance of energy.
His eyes are clear and bright.
His skin is clear and pink.
He is relatively well-coordinated for his age.
His posture and other body mechanics are reasonably good for his age.
His hair is clean.
His muscles are firm.
His appetite is hearty.
He is free from all remediable disabilities.
He grows in weight and height in accordance with age, body type, sex, and maturation level.
He is full of good humor and gets along with himself and others.
He looks well.
He has purpose and a positive outlook on life commensurate with his level of maturity. (See Tables in chapter on Growth and Development.)

Symptoms and Signs of Acute Illness. The teacher knows that a combination of some of the following suggests the presence of a communicable disease:

Fever—a temperature of 102° F. or more.
Flushed or pale face, "glassy" appearance to eyes.
Nausea, vomiting.
Diarrhea, complaint of abdominal pain.
Headache, generalized aching.
Stuffy or "running" nose, sore throat, coughing, tearing.
A rash.
Unusual sleepiness, unusual irritability.
Swollen lymph nodes (glands) in the neck.
Stiffness of neck.
Lethargy or listlessness.
The child looks sick.

---

[5]Modified from: Elsa Schneider and Simon A. McNeely: "Teachers Contribute to Child Health." U.S. Department of Health, Education, and Welfare, Office of Education, Bulletin 1951, 8:6–8, Revised 1962.

If any of these signs or symptoms are present, the teacher knows that the child should be isolated from the classroom to protect others from exposure. He may be kept in the health room until a parent comes. Or, he may be taken home by a responsible adult, with the assurance that a responsible adult is there to receive him.

Additional signs and symptoms which demand prompt attention and are considered acute are:

Drowsiness with pallor or flushing of face in a diabetic.
Complaint of abdominal pain of any type.
Earache.
Toothache.

Symptoms and Signs of Other Possible Health Needs. The defects listed below, observed by the teacher, require medical or dental treatment. They are important but not acute. The teacher notices the presence of any of these health problems and plans the follow-up which has been designed for his grade level. An elementary teacher plans the follow-up in guidance and health instruction which will encourage a child to seek improvement. Secondary teachers may plan their own follow-up or refer through the personnel directly concerned with health problems of students.

Eyes. Styes, crusted lids, crossed eyes (strabismus), complaint of inability to see well (blurring).

Ears. Earaches, discharge from ear, cotton in ear canal, inability to hear discussions or questions, irrelevant answers, a tendency to tilt or turn the head to one side, a look of "watchful waiting," monotone or poor inflection of voice, pulling at or picking in ear, or covering ear with palm of hand.

Teeth. Toothaches; sensitivity to cold, hot or sweet foods or beverages; unclean, discolored, decayed, protruding, or crooked teeth (malocclusion); bleeding, puffy, or tender gums; inability to chew hard foods, such as apples, carrots, and celery; too many missing teeth; persistent foul breath.

Respiratory tract. Mouth breathing, recurring colds and sore throats, constantly stuffed-up nose, unusual noises made in nose and throat, nasal discharge, chronic swollen lymph nodes (glands) in the neck, persistent cough and expectoration, wheezing, shortness of breath or difficult breathing.

Skin. Unusual pallor or flushing, rash, boils, cracks at corners of mouth, blisters, crusty sores, persistent sores, cracks and rough skin between toes (may be fungus infection), rough, scaling patches suggestive of "ringworm" or eczema, persistent flush of cheeks associated with bluish lips and bluish finger nails.

Hair and scalp. Whitish little louse eggs that cling to hair (nits), actual presence of lice, grayish patches of baldness (possibly ringworm), excessive dandruff, sores on scalp, unclean hair.

General appearance. "Too anything,"—too fat, too thin, too tired, too drowsy, listless, or apathetic; peculiar gait, poor coordination, jerking gestures; does not "look well," a change from usual appearance; use of braces, crutches, wheelchair.

Behavior. Frequent loss of emotional poise, actions which indicate nervousness, such as the biting of fingernails or pencil, inability to concentrate, frequent accidents, continuous restlessness, languid interest, extreme shyness or boldness, constant desire to be the center of attention, inability to cooperate with others, frequent need to go to the toilet.

Health practices. Being unclean and unkempt, evidence of poor sleeping and eating habits, lack of interest in helping to maintain a healthful environment, apparent inability to put health knowledge into practice.

Attendance at school. Frequent absences because of allergies, colds, headaches, toothaches, upset stomach, accidents, feeling sick generally, feeling too tired to come to school, lack of interest in school.

Signs revealed during physical activity. Elementary teachers observe their pupils on the playgrounds daily. Physical educators have several contacts a week with each of their students. The screening of youngsters who react poorly to exercise should not be difficult. A teacher simply notes the reactions and requests a medical evaluation.

This means that a teacher is *alert* to the unusual reactions of an individual. This alertness does not involve conscious effort but becomes automatic. Observable signs are shortness of breath or excessive breathlessness with exercise, which does not return to normal as quickly as in his classmates, blue lips and flushed cheeks, pallor around lips, pale skin, poor endurance, quick fatigue, and unusual weakness or trembling. No attempt should be made in diagnosis. These signs may not indicate anything serious. A child may have been ill, may be ill at the time of the activity, or may not be "conditioned" to vigorous physical activity; on the other hand, some basic disorder may be revealed in a thorough medical examination.

Progress in school. Marked change in scholastic achievement—drop in interest and grades without apparent explanation.

Screening Tests

Screening tests, as a part of health appraisal, are those "procedures performed by teachers, nurses, technicians, nurses' aides or trained volunteers to provide a preliminary evaluation of the state of development or functioning of various body organs, and to uncover health problems not identified by observation of pupil appearance and behavior."[6] Tests for vision and hearing have already been described and evaluated under the appropriate topics. Technicians and even instructed parents can perform them. Speech difficulties can be detected. Heights and weights are taken. Results of screening tests should be noted on the cumulative health record. Tests should be done at regular intervals.

Special Surveys

Surveys may be conducted at regular intervals or when indicated. They may be made upon the incidence of immunization against a particular disease. Case-finding surveys for tuberculosis should be con-

[6] *Ibid.*, p. 3.

ducted as a routine program. Studies may be made on dietary habits, hours of sitting before a television set, or any other subject with health implications. Surveys should be carefully planned and administered in order to secure full cooperation and reliable findings. Results should be noted on the cumulative health record. They also offer opportunity for research studies.

Psychological Tests

These tests are important in evaluating mental and emotional development. The results should be significant to every teacher, and they will be meaningful to those who may need to handle a youngster in a mental health follow-up. Findings or conclusions should be placed on the cumulative health record.

The School Health Examination

The discussion which immediately follows pertains to the physician's examination at school. Much of this discussion will also apply to that performed in his private office.

"Ideally, all children entering school for the first time should have a medical examination and re-examination in grades four or five, eight or nine and eleven or twelve. Medical examinations done more frequently have been found to be unproductive and too expensive."[7]

The health (medical) examination is that phase of health appraisal which is conducted by physicians and dentists. The physician weighs all the health history available, uses the objective measurements and observations made by school personnel, and studies the cumulative health record to supplement his own clinical findings.

Any health program would be inadequate without information concerning the health of each child and a follow-up on his health needs. An examination is needed for a youth's protection. With the emphasis on physical fitness, the school must know each person's health status. Elementary teachers and the physical education staff, particularly, must have reassurance that no harm is being done a pupil or student who follows a vigorous activity program.

The Objectives

The objectives of a school health examination may be stated in order of importance as follows:

1. It should be an educational experience.
2. There should be a positive appraisal of health status (physical and emotional).
3. Defects are detected.
4. Communicable diseases are detected.

[7]Austin E. Hill: "School Health Services Today." *Clin. Ped. 10*:11:620, November, 1971.

5. Adjustments are made to the physical education program and to school life.

6. The findings serve as a basis for individual health counseling and for instruction in health education classes.

An Educational Experience. Children should be impressed with the importance of individual periodic health evaluations from a physician and a dentist. This approach represents the positive public health viewpoint. Discussions on this subject should be conducted in the classroom preliminary to the health examination regardless of whether it is done at school or in a private office. Many children have never consulted a physician since their entry into this world. They do not know what constitutes an adequate health examination. In many cases fear needs to be dispelled. The student-physician contact should be anticipated with intelligent interest. Since this experience should serve an educational purpose, it follows that every child should be examined and not a select few who are suspected of having defects.

Positive Appraisal of Health Status. The total child is evaluated. Most children are healthy and have few, if any, defects of importance. Positive findings deserve comment. It is an educational experience for a child and stimulating to his ego to be complimented on the cleanliness of his scalp, the good texture of his skin, the fine repaired condition of his teeth, his good nutrition, and his body build. The child learns that these positive findings are worthwhile; for instance, if a dentist or physician compliments him on his teeth, he feels that the time, expense, and discomfort of dental care are justified. Positive appraisal stimulates a child to health awareness. He goes home and brags to the family. Everyone has a good feeling, and parents are included as well in the evaluation. They too have a sense of satisfaction. Children talk over the doctor's comments among themselves later; again the examination becomes an educational experience. No child should ever leave the doctor's presence without at least one positive finding being emphasized. Interest is easily gained by a personal compliment, and thereafter, it is easy to arouse cooperation in discussing any defects which may be found. Discussion is a part of a health interview. No mysterious ritual is being held.

Detection of Defects. Assuming that eyes, hearing, feet, posture, height, weight, and urine have been checked before the physician's examination, either at school or in his private office, there is a wide range of clinical material available for study about each student by the end of the examination, brief though it may be. If a parent is present—and it is highly desirable, even at the junior high level, to have a parent there—additional information can be considered. Sometimes disturbances of an emotional nature are mentioned. The above data, coupled with the physician's own findings, should enable him to pick up many defects.

If routine examinations are done at school on an entire class, the faculty member who is most responsible for follow-up and counseling on health problems should be sitting near the physician to record findings and comments. The classroom teacher in elementary grades, the health or physical education teacher, the coach, the nurse, and the health counselor are usually the most vitally interested. A teacher has prepared the students during a classroom session for this examination. He is familiar with their health complaints and knows their anxieties in advance. A wise physician listens to this teacher as a consultant. The interview involves student, physician, and teacher, and if possible, parent. Again we have an educational experience.

If only a few students are taken from a room for a special examination by the physician, the teacher's presence is not necessary. A physician-teacher conference held later, at recess, noon, or after school, will probably be sufficient. A physician-student private conference is often rewarding.

Detection of Communicable Diseases. Since the physician-student contact constitutes only an occasional few minutes in a student's life, most cases of communicable diseases are detected by others. It is convenient, however, to have a physician's opinion about a rash or to have him differentiate between a callus and a plantar wart, or to determine whether the peeling of skin between the toes is due to fungus infection or to excessive perspiration.

Adjustments to the Physical Education Program and to School Life. The findings of the health examination should be utilized in adjusting the child to the physical education program. Sometimes the decision can only be made after a thorough study of an individual case.

We must keep in mind that as time goes on, more and more physically handicapped children will be present in our schools. Medical science has preserved their lives and prolonged their life expectancies. Moreover, the tendency now is to send these children to public school. The time should be past when a child sits in a study room while his classmates go to the gymnasium. Some physical activities do not require use of all muscles; if a child is well enough to come to school, he is usually well enough at least to "suit-up," keep the roll, and take a shower. Occasionally a teacher complains that there are too many children to keep the roll. Some sort of modified activity could even be given to a child who leans on crutches. Modified (adaptive) physical education activities for partially disabled students must be provided. The psychological factor is more important than the physical in the handicapped child, and time must be taken from a busy day to adjust each child to his physical abilities. In situations where parents refuse to take a child to a private physician for follow-up, the decision made during the examination at school concerning physical ability is particularly important.

As a corollary, the findings of the examination may be utilized as well in adjusting the child to his whole school life. Children with such handicaps as personality problems, defective vision, defective hearing, or heart damage are adjusted to living and learning at school.

Health Education Opportunities. The findings of the health examination should serve as a springboard for individual counseling and for classroom work in personal health instruction. The child's own health problems can become his projects for correction or improvement. Even the individual with serious heart disease gets recognition for his rest period. To this child, rest is physical education and health education. As a matter of fact, follow-up in the health class upon individual findings can be fun, because everyone is interested in improving himself. Care must be taken to prevent embarrassment. The health teacher reviews the findings of the health examinations and knows the common defects of his students. Thus, his health topics for class discussion are chosen for him. Health instruction becomes personal and positive.

Planning the Health Examination Program

One of the biggest problems in the school health program concerns health examinations of children. Many questions arise: What should be our policy? Shall we request the parents to take their children to private physicians? Or, shall we make arrangements to have all the children examined at school? If the latter, can we finance the project? Shall we select a few children who apparently have health problems and arrange to have them examined at school? What are our medical facilities in this community? What are our understandings with the local medical society? The role of the dentist in the medical examination program has been discussed in the chapter on Dental Problems.

Who is responsible for arranging health examinations at school? How often should we request health examinations during a child's school life? Should parents be present? What constitutes an adequate health examination? What is the routine for conducting it at school? Who is responsible for the health records? What constitutes a follow-up? Who should do it?

These are only a few of the questions which arise in planning the health examination program. There is no ideal solution.

Several avenues are possible in planning health examinations:

1. *All children are seen by private physicians in their offices.* A specific standard form should be filled out and returned to the school with pertinent health information for guidance. Parents pay a private fee. *This is the method of choice.* The private physician should understand the needs of the school and the importance of the health information he supplies. He is entitled to any observations and screening tests the school may have concerning an individual student in order to appraise more accurately.

Advantages:

a. A more thorough appraisal is possible.

(1) Medical facilities are available, so that x-ray and laboratory tests are possible. These may assure a more complete evaluation.

(2) One or both parents will usually be present, except possibly for senior high school students. The attitude here is that an indi-

vidual at this age should accept responsibility more fully for his own health. Information from parents is important in health appraisal, however.

(3) Frequently, the private physician is already the family physician, has probably ushered the youngster into the world, and is familiar with the medical history. This is an advantage.

b. Follow up can be immediate and direct. With the parent present, information and recommendations for follow-up can be given directly, thereby relieving the school of this procedure except in a few neglectful or resistant instances.

c. The atmosphere of the physician's office supplies a more educational, realistic medical environment than can be offered with a similar experience at school.

d. Responsibility for the health of a child is placed upon his parents.

e. Since our objective is to teach a child to assume gradually the care of his own health, he will best learn this responsibility if he learns to seek the guidance of a private physician.

Disadvantages:

a. Health information supplied to the school by the private physician may be too sketchy to be helpful or may not be meaningful to school personnel.

b. Human beings reacting as they do, there will be a hard core of children who will not be appraised because their parents (1) have no money, (2) have no physician and do not wish to make the effort to find one, (3) are indifferent to the whole proposal.

What should be done for the students who have not been seen by a private physician, regardless of urging? Some of these children are likely to have defects. Should a physician be invited to the school to examine this group? Should some type of fund be established from which, if necessary, the private physician may be paid? Every child should be examined. The poor children need attention also.

2. *All children are examined at school.* Such a program is planned carefully. A school nurse, the physical education teacher, health coordinator, or the principal may accept responsibility for this undertaking. If a school physician serves the system, he may plan the schedule and secure the help of other physicians in the community. The school district or school system pays an agreed fee.

Advantages:

a. All children are examined. All of the objectives of the health examinations can be applied to each child.

b. Needed re-checks can be done on heart, tonsils, and other known defects. These are particularly needed for children who have not consulted a physician in spite of school recommendations.

c. The physician may act as a consultant to the health teacher and to administrative personnel while at the school.

d. Health needs are probably discovered earlier than by waiting for teacher or nurse referral.

Disadvantages:

a. The school health examination is not a substitute for that made in a private physician's office. Nevertheless, with an experienced physician, it is more than a screening procedure. The latter implies superficiality, and a physician's examination at school can detect defects as a result of the information provided him combined with his particular professional skill.

b. The school medical examiner does not prescribe; he can only recommend referral. Such delay in securing treatment or correction does not usually occur in a private office.

3. *The teacher selects students to be referred to a private physician or to the school medical examiner.* The trained alertness of many teachers will result in early detection of many defects with good referrals for follow-up. Teacher-nurse conferences produce many referrals also. However, to confront a school health examiner with only a selected group of students suspected of having defects and to ignore all others is to defeat the first two objectives of a school health examination: educational experience and positive appraisal. Even if the school examiner spends a whole hour with one youngster and is satisfied with his conclusions, he still must recommend the care of a private physician and is in no position to give clinical treatment. There is a question whether such expense and time is justified, when the teacher can refer these same students for private medical consultation.

It must be emphasized that these selected students do need immediate follow-up, and recommendation for private care should be made to parents. Repeated urging may be necessary before a child receives deserved attention.

Many teachers do not wish to accept the responsibility of selecting students for referral to a physician. Moreover, this policy implies well-informed teacher observation, which exists to variable degrees.

4. *Some school districts offer periodic examinations to all children whose parents ask for it.* Parents are first urged to visit a private physician. See Appendix B for form utilizing this arrangement.

Frequency of Examinations. It is recommended that each child have at least four examinations during his school years: just prior to entering school, third or fourth grade, and upon entrance to junior and to senior high schools. The fourth examination may be given before graduation. Some states require by law a specified number of health examinations during a child's school career. Children who have health problems will be directed by their own physicians to return at more frequent intervals. All new pupils should be examined. Members of varsity teams should be examined each year. The health records of each child in the special education program should be reviewed annually and appropriate referrals made to specialists, if indicated.

Time Required for an Examination. Complaints that school examiners see too many students in one hour are valid. A few minutes devoted to each child will not be sufficient for a satisfactory appraisal. Moreover, an opportunity to impress each one with the value of a health examination by a physician will be lost. A clear understanding of the objectives of the health examination will determine the time to be devoted to each child. If abnormalities are present, such as a heart murmur, or if a parent is present, more attention will be required. Examinations conducted in private offices, because of the opportunity for more thoroughness, will require variable lengths of time.

Should Parents Be Present? Parents have a good deal of information which will enable a physician to form a satisfactory evaluation. This is particularly true if the youngster has a health problem. Parents should be encouraged to attend examinations of their children through junior high school. If the parent attends a health examination *at school,* the process may be slowed up because of time consumed in consultation, but the parental contact and the satisfactions usually expressed make such provisions worthwhile. If defects are found or follow-up is necessary, the presence of a parent eliminates the need for contacts or written notes. Most parents appreciate the interest shown in their children. If a mother is interested enough to report for her child's examination, her presence should be recognized; she should not be required to wait long for the examination. She should be consulted and given information of a positive nature as well as a review of defects. Thus the educational experience extends to the parent, who is expected to support the school health program. Moreover, she will feel that the expense incurred by the school in connection with these examinations is worthwhile. During the examination, while the parent is present, a medical examiner may call in one or more assistants—the school nurse, teacher, social worker, principal, or guidance counselor—and hold a conference. Everything should be done which will benefit a child.

The Extent of the Examination. Whether a child is seen at school or in a private office, his *whole health status* is appraised. As has been explained, the facilities in a private office permit a more thorough investigation. A thorough health examination will likely include:

General appearance	Thyroid
Body structure	Lungs
Musculature	Heart
Posture	Abdomen
Facial expression	External genitalia
Skin	Hernia
Cleanliness	Orthopedic problems
Eyes and lids	Height
Nose	Weight
Tonsils	Vision
Throat	Hearing
Teeth	Urinalysis
Gums	Hematocrit
Lymph nodes	Tuberculin test

Any mannerisms (tics, chewing nails, evidences of nervousness).

The school medical examiner should note common defects and questionable conditions, if any, and must refer the child to the private physician for a more detailed diagnosis.

Conducting the Examination

Health examinations should be conducted in a quiet, attractive place where the feeling tones are easy and comfortable, where a door can be closed, and absolute privacy assured.

At School. The examination at school should be conducted quietly and leisurely, in an atmosphere of seriousness and dignity. The logical place for holding it is in the health suite. Many older buildings have no facilities for medical consultations. Sometimes a basement room may be hastily cleaned before the physician arrives. Principals have been known to vacate their offices during examinations. Not infrequently the only available space will be the office of the physical education teacher or coach, next to the playing floor and dressing rooms. In order to assure quiet, physical education classes must be dismissed or sent out on the grounds, and elaborate efforts made to hush all within earshot of the examining office. Since noisy activities are grouped together, music rooms and auditorium are frequently adjacent to the gymnasium. Heart sounds mixed with the strains of the national anthem as they float through the stethoscope produce an interesting effect.

In the examining room, only the physician, pupil, parent, and recorder should be present. The child should be at least partially disrobed. The physician will determine the extent. Some children are exceedingly modest and must be handled gently. In the elementary grades the classroom teacher, health counselor, or health aide should be the recorder. Such a process is dignified and confidential. Pupils and parents resent others being present, particularly when health problems are being discussed. Older students and parents should not be used as recorders, since a suspicion may be raised concerning breach of confidence. At the secondary level, ideally, a designated person who is responsible for health counseling and follow-up should be present to make notes on the cumulative health record. A health aide may assist.

Before the physician arrives, the results of all screening tests and any pertinent observations should have been placed on the cumulative health record. The health history card should be at hand. Both of these medical records not only supply needed information, but serve as entries for conversation and questions with parent and child. Frequently, physical education teachers have already examined posture and feet; these additional findings are valuable to the physician.

The physician then proceeds with his examination. A child should be examined from head to toe; any abnormal findings in gait, mannerisms, or nutritional status, and changes in appearance of the skin, eyes, or bony skeleton are noted. Other parts of the body will be checked—ears, nasal passages, throat, mouth, lymph nodes, thyroid gland, heart, lungs, and abdomen. Emotional disturbances may be suspected and referred for further investigation. All findings, normal and abnormal, should be recorded on the cumulative health record. The physician's recommendations for handling a health problem should be made part of such a record.

In a Private Office. If a personal physician conducts an examination in his own office, he should have the benefit of all school records on a child's health. He should also have the supplied examination form, which can be returned to the school. It is the responsibility of the administrator to plan channels for exchange of information. The school health education committees of the local dental and medical societies will be of assistance on this matter. The personal physician must be assured that the confidential nature of the health report is appreciated by the school, and that only authorized personnel may consult the records. If a private physician seems reluctant or refuses to divulge health findings, he is observing his legal, liable restrictions. Public health nurses must also preserve the same confidence. If necessary, parents may sign a release so that privileged information can be given to the proper school authorities.

The Cumulative Health Record

Medical records at school consist of the health history and cumulative health card. Frequently, for convenience both are placed on the same form. Many forms have been used, all essentially the same as far as basic findings are concerned. (See Appendix B.) There may be a standard form for all the schools of the state or for a school system. The school physician and other medical personnel should have a prominent voice in formulating it. Some records provide ample room for observations of non-medical personnel; others are too brief and permit no space for cumulative information. The latter are worthless. A stark diagnosis of "epilepsy" spread across the surface of a card can be startling and evoke a feeling of disgust at such poor medical procedure. Such a record does not do a child justice. Some medical records state only the "positive findings" (defects) noticed by the physician.

Health records should be filed where they will be available for reference. They are usually kept in the principal's office, along with the academic history, and form part of the whole school record. A principal may elect to use a different system of filing, however. For instance, in one junior high school each homeroom teacher is given all the records for his group (about 35). It is assumed that he will have the most contact with each of these students and be in a more favorable position to make observations, receive confidences, and counsel on health. He may consult with parents and with other teachers. He is called into conference if a problem should arise concerning the health of an advisee. The principal of the school considers this advisory system more satisfactory than having all records in one large file with only one counselor or no one person responsible for health counseling. With the whole student body under the particular observation of homeroom teachers, he feels that a better quality of health service is possible. In addition, more time and effort can be devoted to each child as an individual with his own problems.

Health records are valuable to the physician, nurse, health counselor, social worker, principal, and teacher. The performance of a child or a disciplinary problem may be explained by consulting the results of a vision and hearing test or other appraisals.

All observations of interested personnel, findings from screening tests and surveys, all progress notes on health happenings, possibly a serious accident, a bout of rheumatic fever, or an epileptic seizure, should be recorded on the cumulative health record. The history of past immunizations is important. The results of all previous health examinations can be reviewed quickly. Records should be kept up-to-date. If all teeth have been repaired, a notation should be made. If a physician specifies that activities should be limited because of heart disease, this fact should be recorded. If a child's decayed teeth and diseased tonsils remain throughout the years, in spite of repeated requests for referral, the deductions are obvious. He is usually the rejectee from a preinduction health examination later on.

Such a record, with the accumulated information from various sources, should be a valuable document. It tells a child's health story and mirrors his parents' attitude toward corrective procedures and health protection. Such a document can be used in the evaluation of the health service and health instruction in a school. It can be used for research purposes. It should follow the child from school to school until he graduates and then be kept in permanent files. The White House Conference on Children and Youth (1960) observed that 25 per cent of all the children in the United States will move out of a county by the age of ten. A continuous health record should follow each child.

How long should cumulative health records be kept by a school system? The answer probably should be, "Indefinitely." There are two reasons for this answer. A child himself can institute a law suit within a specified length of time after reaching his majority, if he thinks he has a claim against anyone. This can happen regardless of parental consent. A parent cannot sign away his child's rights. Second, amendments in 1967 to the social security law provided that "monthly disability payments are now payable to persons severely disabled in childhood (before 18) who continue to be disabled. These benefits are payable as early as age 18 when a parent receives social security retirement or disability benefits or when an insured parent dies. Insured mothers now have this protection for their children even though they have not worked recently."

If an insured worker should die in his late years and leave a disabled child in his twenties, thirties, or forties, etc., the latter could well claim that he had a childhood injury. A note on a cumulative health record will help substantiate his claim. On the other hand, absence of a comment, particularly if an examination was done after the claimed date of disability, could be quite significant. No doubt federal representatives will ask to consult school health records. Information may be given, *provided the individual concerned gives written consent.*

The confidential nature of the health record must be emphasized. At school only teaching personnel and a few other trustworthy people should have access to the files. The administrator is responsible for their care. If information is given to indiscreet individuals, there may be damaging repercussions which affect the child. It is understood that the code of ethics of the medical, dental, and nursing professions does not permit release of health information without consent of a parent or guardian. There may be reluctance to give information because of social reactions. For instance, a student may have had electrical shock therapy for an acute "breakdown." The private physician may not know just how the information provided will be used, either by a school or an agency. The interchange of health information is not as simple as it sounds.

In addition to all the cumulative health information on each child's record, there should be an attached permit (Figure 65) signed by a parent, indicating the names of two physicians and two dentists

SALT LAKE CITY PUBLIC SCHOOLS FORM 410B (REVISED)

Parent's or Guardian's Authorization for Emergency Medical Aid

Name of Child.. School..................................

In the event of illness or accident to a child or children of mine attending school, which in the judgment of the principal of the school, would seem to demand medical attention, I hereby authorize the said principal to summon medical help at my expense if I cannot be promptly reached by phone. I further authorize the principal to cause the child's transportation to a place where appropriate medical aid can be rendered, if in the principal's judgment such transportation is necessary. I would prefer that the principal call:

Dr.. Phone.........................., or

Dr.. Phone.........................., if available, but otherwise he shall use his own judgment as to the doctor to be called.

In my absence the following persons are authorized to act for me in the above respect in behalf of my child:

Name.................................Phone.................... Address..............................

Name.................................Phone.................... Address..............................

Signed.. Date..................................

Home Address.. Home Phone..........................

Father's Business Address.................................... Phone..........................

Mother's Business Address.................................... Phone..........................

Figure 65 Sample form.

(first and second choices) who may be called in case of accident or sudden illness, and the names and addresses of other people who may be notified in the parents' absence. A hospital of choice may also be mentioned. A clinic or welfare agency may be designated. This permit is valuable when a parent cannot be reached. Sometimes both parents work, or the mother may not be home at the time of an urgent call. The place of employment (with phone number) of one or both parents is valuable information. Most school systems have instituted the policy of having these signed forms, and the response of parents has been quite satisfactory. Even so, it is better to contact a parent before making a referral to a physician in case of emergency.

To *summarize* the values of cumulative health records, they should serve:

1. Health records and the statistics collected from them help educators plan health education curriculums.
2. Health records enable the school to provide examining physicians with a past history of a student.
3. Health records aid the school psychologist to understand better a child's mental health in the light of his physical condition.
4. Health records enable safety personnel to pinpoint hazards in the school environment.
5. Health records provide a means of helping to control communicable disease.
6. Health records permit the health counselor to follow up on remediable defects.
7. Health records aid the coaches to understand the student's past and present health status.
8. Health records are a valuable aid in an emergency. We can find the family doctor's name, special medications, or other health information pertinent to a student's health.
9. The health record aids the trained observor to anticipate a student's future health needs.
10. The health record permits us to protect the abnormal child from himself (e.g., a child with a heart problem who registers for physical education class without informing anyone of his condition).
11. The health records save human resources by spotting children in poor health who are potential drop-outs or repeaters due to illness.
12. Spotting health problems may help to prevent excessive absence due to poor health.
13. The health record in the hands of a trained person indicates when special adjustments are needed for a student.
14. The health record can reduce school costs by keeping the unfit out of regular school.
15. The health record can serve to assure the student he is healthy.[8]
16. The health record may be a source for referral in case of disability which justifies social security compensation.

---

[8]Stephen M. Schneeweiss and Addison Locke: "New Horizons in School Health Services: The Computer." *J. Sch. Health* 37:349–350, 1967.

HEALTH COUNSELING AND FOLLOW-UP

Health counseling should enable pupils and parents to understand the appraisal findings and their significance. Follow-up involves both counseling and an attempt to secure correction of defects and improvement in health. Particular effort must be made for follow-up on indigent children and for those with problems which require adaptation to the school program.

The specific aims of health counseling are:

> 1. To give pupils as much information about their health status, as revealed by appraisal procedures, as they can use to good advantage.
> 2. To interpret to parents the significance of health conditions and to encourage them to obtain needed care for their children.
> 3. To motivate pupils and their parents to seek needed treatment.
> 4. To promote each pupil's acceptance of responsibility for his own health, in keeping with his stage of maturity. . . .
> 7. To contribute to the health education of pupils and parents.
> 8. To obtain for exceptional pupils educational programs adapted to their individual needs and abilities.[9]

Once the health appraisal has revealed problems, the next step is one of action. To place a health record in a file and forget it is inexcusable. Some type of organization for counseling and follow-up should be planned for each school system and school. How this will be handled in any school depends upon the personnel available in the school and upon community resources. Workable methods must be sought. In a poorly prepared district a principal, teacher, and nurse will battle great odds to help a child, especially if the parents are indigent or indifferent. All of those involved in follow-up must be familiar with federal legislation which provides money for physical examinations and follow-up.

The type of health problems which require follow-ups ordinarily fall into the following groups: those which require (1) more detailed examination in order to establish a diagnosis, such as tuberculosis contacts, heart murmurs, "blackouts," and chronic fatigue; (2) treatment, correction, or constant medical supervision, such as dental caries, diseased tonsils, and allergies; (3) altered or improved home care, such as malnutrition, insufficient sleep, too many chores and not enough play, too many worries and tensions produced by conflicts and anxieties in the home; and (4) mental health studies.

Many people may be involved in counseling and follow-up; the physician, school nurse, social worker, counselor, health coordinator,

---

[9] A Report of the Joint Committee on Health Problems in Education of the National Education Association and the American Medical Association. *School Health Services.* 1964, pp. 111–112.

principal, and teacher, either individually or working with others in this group, and working with parents and children.

Follow-up procedures are discussed in detail in association with each health problem presented in the first part of this text.

The Role of the Classroom Teacher

The *elementary teacher* is in a strategic position to watch his pupils throughout the day. He watches deviations from normal in behavior or appearance. He listens to complaints. He conducts surveys. He is familiar with health needs. He watches the growth in height and weight and the emotional development of his charges. He is acquainted with their parents. He counsels with them and knows whether there has been a follow-up with the physician or school nurse or whether there are improved health practices in the home. He works with principal, social worker, and school nurse, and with physician and dentist. Sometimes, the principal will take over responsibility for counseling and follow-up.

The *secondary teacher* has an opportunity to counsel, as well, even though there may be established channels for health counseling in a school. A good rapport between teacher and students invites confidences, and such a fortunate teacher will be most influential in helping a student to handle a health problem.

All teachers should have basic health information which enables them to understand the health problems of children.

The Health Counselor

Some school systems have regulations which require the position of health counselor. The administrator should provide adequate time and funds for such service. Policies and procedures should be established. Health counseling should be considered an important function. A haphazard follow-up relies too much on printed notes to parents and throws the burden on teachers who are too busy to make the necessary contacts. No consistent efforts will be made, and no evaluation of results is possible. A regimen in which only one person is responsible for planning the contacts with a parent prevents too many people from descending upon a mother and spreading confusion.

A health counselor should possess two attributes. He should be familiar with counseling techniques and be prepared in health education. He may be a professionally prepared health coordinator, a health teacher, or someone equally qualified. A counselor never makes a diagnosis, never prescribes or suggests methods of treatment. The health counselor may be the school nurse.

An interesting study was made to determine the value of a "health assistant" working with the school nurse and the physician. Results indicate this person can play an important role in health counseling as well as in other health service activities.[10]

At the secondary level in large schools one qualified person should be assigned the responsibility of follow-up. He should have a pleasant office which invites relaxation and confidence. In the course of follow-up, he may discuss health problems with student and parent. Regardless of referral practices in his school, he should be the key person who watches the progress of management of each child called to his attention. He works with school and medical personnel and with the appropriate community resources.

The School Nurse – A Counselor

The school nurse is a fine health counselor. With her medical and educational background, her association with medical and public health personnel and with health agencies in the community, and her opportunities to visit homes, she occupies a strategic role in guiding the management of health problems of school children. She can arrange for medical care. She counsels the handicapped and their parents. She consults with teachers and principal, and should be a consultant in the guidance program. When one contemplates the many activities of a school nurse, her many associations require her to assume a prominent position as health counselor.[11]

Contact with Parents

Face-to-face contact with a parent, either at school or at home, is the method of choice in follow-up. Notes sent home may never reach there or may be ignored. It is impossible to know the reaction of parents. There is always the question of how much information should be written and how it should be stated. Parents must understand the health problem clearly; it should be explained in their own language. Some of the difficulties which impede understanding are: low comprehension, lack of knowledge, fears, prejudices, cultural differences, and poor grasp of the English language. When there are many children in a family and funds are limited, correction of some defects will have higher priority than others. Children from homes where ties are weak may also suffer from limited finances. Parents are reluctant to seek medical consultation as long as a child seems active and well and does not complain. The aching tooth will be more apt to receive attention than a quietly decaying one.

Some parents are unconcerned and accept health problems as inevitable. The response can be discouraging. One principal found

[10]Philip R. Nader, Anne Emmel, and Evan Charney: "The School Health Service: A New Model." *Clinical Pediatrics* 49:6:811, 1972.

[11]School Nursing Committee of the American School Health Association: "The Nurse in the School Health Program." *J. Sch. Health* 37:2a:15–16, 1967.

himself completely frustrated by the attitude of a family whose children were infested with head lice. His own personal contacts with the family and the nurse's visits were met with complete indifference. Having head lice was a way of life with these people. He could not keep the children in school; yet barring them evoked nothing but enthusiasm from the victims. To invoke police aid would produce a transitory clean-up and no change of attitude. When last consulted, he had reached an impasse.

The higher the intelligence of the student and the better the educational background of the mother, the greater will be the cooperation in securing correction of defects. Teachers and counselors must be careful not to talk "down" to an intelligent, conscientious parent. They are partners sharing the same interest.

Some interesting studies have been made on the success of referrals to parents. The most fruitful single contact involves personal interaction, either by telephone or a home visit. Two contacts may be more effective than one. More than two does not seem to increase effectiveness. An excellent combination is a note by a physician and a telephone call by a nurse. Another is a telephone call by a physician and a visit or phone call by a nurse. Personal contacts by visit or telephone give an opportunity for interaction. Notification should depend upon more than one contact technique and should be by more than one professional individual.[12] The response of the parent more than likely will be to take the child to private sources for medical and dental care. So many families carry health insurance now; this is a prompting factor in parental response.

Another study[13] on the attitudes of parents is significant. If parents thought that a health problem was urgent, response was good. If they thought that the problem was self-limiting (would get better anyway), response was poor. The best response occurred when parents thought that the problem would interfere with school work. This attitude explains the high response to notification on vision (92.3 per cent), dental problems (75 per cent), and mental problems (65 per cent). These same parents were prone to delay referrals for chronic diseases.

OTHER HEALTH SERVICES FOR THE CHILD

Health services not only include identification and care of individual health problems but also provide broad programs, notably, services for the handicapped, control of communicable diseases, emergency care, services which will insure a healthful environment, and experiences for health education.

---

[12]Joy Cauffmann: "Factors Affecting Outcome of School Health Referrals." *J. Sch. Health* 38:333–339, 1968.

[13]Ira W. Gabrielson, Lowell S. Levin, and Margaret D. Ellison: "Factors Affecting School Health Follow-up." *A.J.P.H.* 57:48–59, 1967.

Services for the Handicapped

Services for the handicapped which should be offered by each teacher and by the school are detailed under the discussions of health problems in Part I of this text. For instance, the hard-of-hearing child may need auditory training or training in lip reading. Partially-sighted children need special equipment but may remain in the classroom with their peers. Malnourished, indigent children are provided with free lunches. A child with surgical repairs of cleft lip and/or cleft palate needs speech training.

Orthopedic problems may handicap children. A child may have a limping gait from many causes—a club foot, a shortening of one leg, an artificial leg, or affected muscles from a neurological problem, e.g., cerebral palsy. A child may use crutches or braces. He may be confined to a wheelchair because of an injury to the spinal cord. He may come to school with a cast on. He may return after an amputation of an extremity.

Teachers and administrators need to know the exact nature of a physical handicap. The school or public health nurse, the physician, or the parent may provide necessary information and interpret needs in order to fit the child into the school. This interpretation is necessary so that the teacher and school can meet the child's needs. There may be problems of transportation, braces, activities, and toileting.

Adaptations of school routine may involve:

1. Helping the child to make up missed work.
2. Physical activity adjusted to handicap.
3. Avoidance of stairs, or arranging transportation from one floor to another at school. Use of elevator passes.
4. Individual health counseling to impress the importance of continued medical care, e.g., speech therapy, physical therapy.
5. Consultation with public health nurse and/or physician on special cases.

Many of these youngsters attend special clinics for treatment and special education. Crippled children's services are available in most communities, either in hospitals or clinics, or in itinerant clinics sponsored by various public and private agencies. Speech therapy classes may be available only at a central location in the summer, possibly a board of health clinic, or may be offered at special centers throughout the year. Speech correctionists are now being employed by many school systems; their specialized assistance helps many handicapped children. Physical therapy can be secured in the outpatient department of hospitals, where parents are given instructions for continuing exercises at home. The latter arrangement helps those families who live at a distance. Special classes for children with cerebral palsy may be located in a service center or may be integrated into a large school system.

Some large school systems, for example the Los Angeles city

schools, have special schools for handicapped children. Whether a child enters a special school, if available, or a regular classroom, depends upon the individual evaluation.

Occasionally, a child does not have the endurance to stay in school a whole day. He should be encouraged to attend for as long and as often as he can. A visiting teacher can supplement his deficiencies.

If a child cannot attend school, then instruction is taken to him at the hospital or home. Preparation of teachers in Special Education has been an important addition to the curriculum in teacher education institutions. Visits from a teacher should be scheduled at least twice a week. He works with the parent and physician in this home situation. If at all possible, the child should be admitted to school in order to secure more normal socializing experiences.

The visiting teacher has a task in encouraging school attendance of the emotionally disturbed child who is withdrawn, resists school, and prefers to stay home.

The State Vocational Rehabilitation Department and its local representatives enter the picture where older students are concerned.

Communicable Disease Control

Detailed information on the communicable diseases likely to be seen at school is presented in the first part of this text. Material as outlined covers: a general discussion, a description of individual diseases, the immunization possibilities, and the school health program for control and prevention of each disease.

Because of improved knowledge on immunology and treatment, in time the incidence of communicable diseases should be lessened; but some will always be present. The same type of program for control and prevention should be maintained continuously. Early detection of infectious diseases is essential for protection of others at school; the immunization procedures require routine planning. The tuberculosis-detection program should be an established routine also.

Health education should be the keystone of the whole program. Parents, pupils, and teachers should have the information necessary to promote alertness in early detection of an infection. Parents need to be impressed with the importance of keeping their sick children at home. This is particularly important where they are transported distances by bus. There should be an established policy for acceptance of a child into school once he has been absent because of a communicable disease. Reassurance to the school may be provided by a note from the attending physician, or the school nurse may interview the child upon his return.

Many schools make it a practice to notify the parents of all children in a classroom when one child has a diagnosed serious contagious disease.

The program for control and prevention of communicable dis-

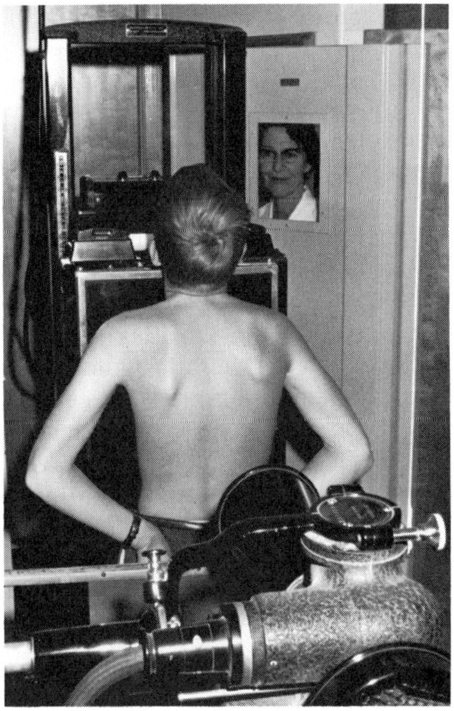

Figure 66 Tuberculosis-detection program. Chest x-ray of a junior high school student is being taken.

eases applies to employees as well. A food handler or custodian with tuberculosis, or a bus driver with a streptococcal sore throat is a dangerous contact. A sniffling, coughing teacher is hardly setting a good example. Provisions should be made by the administration for sick leave with adequate pay, so that a sick employee can afford to take time off without much economic loss or anxiety. Employees need to have periodic health examinations and maintain general good resistance against infections. They are more exposed than other adults to the common communicable diseases and need the same immunizations advised for the school child.

Emergency Care of Injuries

Every teacher at some time will be confronted with a child who has been hurt badly or who is seriously ill. A new teacher before ever starting his first class may have the problem of a youngster who has fallen out of a tree and broken an arm. Serious eye injuries can evoke a feeling of horror.

Every school, regardless of size, should have a carefully planned routine for handling these emergencies. This routine should be described in written standing orders for all concerned to read. These orders should be comprehensive and up-to-date. Policies and procedures will depend upon the organization of a safety education program at state, district, and school levels (see Chapter 17), upon the presence of medical or trained non-medical personnel at school, and upon such community resources as ambulance and hospital facilities. Each person must know his role and perform with calmness and good judgment. Orientation of new teachers to the school program should include information on the emergency set-up. Advance preparation offers better protection of children and may prevent serious complications of injuries or illness. Organization and administration of a program for emergency care is the responsibility of the superintendent and principal, who, as a matter of course, should have expert medical advice.

A teacher must know the regulations on emergency care of illness and injuries in a particular school, in the school system, and at the state level. Teacher education institutions should ensure that all persons preparing to teach have adequate knowledge of first aid. In some states a teacher is not permitted to perform a single first aid procedure. One wonders under those circumstances if a child will be permitted to die for lack of mouth-to-mouth resuscitation. For those schools where emergency aid is permitted, the following information is offered to teachers.

Emergency care of injuries involves (1) first aid procedures by trained personnel, (2) provision of needed supplies in strategic places, and (3) maintenance of records.

First Aid Procedures

Care of Minor Wounds. A minor wound of the skin is a *superficial* abrasion or laceration or scraping of the skin, in which the edges of skin do not gape and sutures (stitches) are not needed. In the elementary grades the classroom teacher stresses the importance of cleanliness. Soap and water are used to scrub the skin. The basic procedure to apply here is that one scrubs away *from* the wound to avoid more contamination. Dirty gauze or cotton should not be pulled over the wound. A sterile dressing may be used. Where regulations permit such first aid, the principal delegates this responsibility to the teachers. No antiseptics are used. At upper grade levels the student is referred to one of several places in the building where instructors can apply first aid measures. The bus driver should also be trained in first aid and have supplies handy. These responsible people should keep up-to-date in care of minor wounds by consulting a nurse or physician.

Care of Major Injuries. First aid for a serious injury is administered by a teacher or principal when a school nurse or physician is not immediately available. For injuries which will probably require the attention of a physician, one follows the established routine. Some school systems have detailed printed instructions on handling various problems. At least one person, preferably two or three, in the school should be skilled in administering first aid. The principal in an elementary school is usually the one called upon to handle serious emergencies. In high schools a number of persons may be available: the coach, physical education teacher, health coordinator, industrial arts instructor, and those in charge of various laboratories. One person is designated for overall responsibility. He should be interested enough to keep up with the latest advice on emergency care by taking refresher courses and by consulting with medical specialists. Since every single step in handling each injury can neither be spelled out nor remembered, this responsible individual should not only have special preparation for handling injuries, but he should be a person of calm judgment, unshaken by the sight of blood, who is acquainted with the legal implications.

The responsibilities of the school are to (1) give immediate care, (2) notify parents, and (3) see that the child is placed under responsible care, either that of the parents or a physician designated by them.

Immediate Care. First aid means first aid, not continuous care or responsibility. It does not mean caring for an injured swollen thumb by having a student sit in the dressing room a couple of periods daily, soaking the digit in hot water, with the instructor assaying progress from day to day. It does not mean repeated applications of bandages to major wounds, and it does not mean restrapping an ankle because the old adhesive tape is dirty. Teachers usually administer treatment because the student will complain that the family is either not interested in or cannot afford medical care. By assuming such responsibility, a teacher is mistaken and may be legally liable in case the treatment is not effective. A swollen thumb may be due to an infection rather than a sprain, and the strapped ankle may be fractured. First aid means first aid.

Notifying Parents. Parents are responsible for their children's health and injuries. An immediate phone call to the home or place of work will usually reach most parents. A calm voice which reassures will allay the quick rise of fear. Details should be given. Medical treatment should be firmly recommended. If hospitalization seems indicated, the fact should be stressed. The parent may come to the school and get the child, or he may wish him to be brought home where the physician will make a house call. In other instances, the parent may accept responsibility for having the physician go to the school, may have an ambulance sent to the school, or may ask that someone from the school accompany the child to a physician's office or emergency department of a hospital where the parent may meet him. The latter action saves time, which in some instances may be vital. In case a parent cannot be reached, the permit signed by the parent leaves the school free to call the designated physician or dentist directly. See Figure 66.

If a parent cannot be contacted and there is no signed permit, where available, a police ambulance may be called. The child will be taken to a city or county hospital or clinic where further emergency care and careful observation can be done, the damage assayed, and attempts made by the staff to contact parents. Most older students know the name of the family physician, who can be called. He will assume limited responsibility and may ask that the child be taken directly to his office or to the hospital. Radio appeals in rural communities may locate parents. In the absence of parental permission, if surgery is indicated *to preserve life,* as with a skull fracture where intercranial pressure must be relieved, it is common medical procedure to call a consultation of three physicians on a hospital staff. If they concur that delay in operating may be fatal, the surgeon and hospital are presumed to be legally protected. Otherwise, if the injury is not that serious, a physician will await the parent. For treatment of a minor, only the signature of a parent or legal guardian is acceptable for medical care.

See that the Child is Placed under Responsible Care. The parent assumes responsibility. Once the child has been handed over to the parent's care, the principal can sigh with relief. If the victim is taken home, to a hospital, or to a physician's office, a responsible adult escorts him. If a parent refuses to secure medical consultation, there is nothing the school administration can do as far as care is concerned. If unable to reach a parent, even though the designated physician (from parental permit) takes over, the school still should persist in making personal contact with the home.

Follow-up on Accidents. Whether an accident occurred at school or elsewhere, good public relations indicate that with a known case a phone call be made to the parents within 24 hours. The condition of the child can be ascertained; there can be assurances not only of interest but that plans can be made for an adapted program, if indicated.

SUPPLIES

Most schools need only a minimum of supplies both in types and amounts for immediate use. Supplies and equipment will vary with the size of the school and its trained personnel, and with the medical, ambulance, and hospital services available in the community. One person in each school should be assigned responsibility for ordering and keeping up supplies. Consultation with medical personnel should offer some guidance. Some boards of education both at state and local levels provide lists of suggested first aid supplies.

There should be at least one place in a school building where these materials are kept. In an elementary school they will probably be under the principal's care. Classroom teachers will have access to soap and water and may keep small dressings for minor wounds. In high schools, supplies are usually found where accidents are more likely to occur: the laboratories, workshops, homemaking rooms, gymnasiums, and school buses. A stretcher, splints, and blankets should be kept in one place known to all interested personnel. A health consultation room or health suite may provide storage for stock supplies and major equipment.

Various lists of first aid supplies may be consulted. The amount ordered will depend upon enrollment. There should be plenty of small dressings for minor wounds. Again, provision and use of small dressings depends upon policies of the school system and of the school. The following list is offered for a school with non-medical personnel:

SUGGESTED SUPPLIES	USE
Tincture of green soap.	Should be diluted with water. To wash dog bites, cuts, and abrasions. (See Chapter 10—Health Problems of Skin.)
Hand brushes.	For scrubbing dirt from shallow wounds. Should be sterilized after use.
Hospital cotton, sterilized. Small (preferable) or large rolls.	For washing wounds.
Dressings. Various sizes of gauze pads in sterilized, individual packages. (Nonmedicated.)	Applied on wounds. Fasten with adhesive tape.
Special types of dressings—individual packages—for fingers and eyes.	Not necessary, but easier to apply.
Adhesive tape. One inch roll. Or a roller containing various widths, can be attached to wall.	To fasten dressings. (Not to tape injured joints.)
Cotton swabs—sterilized—in packages.	To clean wounds.
Bandage scissors.	
Tourniquet.	To stop *major* hemorrhage. Apply between wound and heart. Not to be used if pressure over bandaged wound will stop bleeding. Avoid use, if hand pressure is adequate. *To be used only if necessary to save life,* as with an amputation.

Triangular bandages. Some sterilized in packages.	Many uses. For arm slings, to keep splints in place, or to support a sprained ankle. Sterilized ones may be used on large areas of injury or burns.
Rolls of gauze. 1 and 2 inches wide.	Over sterile dressing to fix it in place. Not used often. Should never be used as a circular wrap for sprains.
Small strips ½ and 1 inch wide of adhesive tape with sterile gauze pads attached. (Nonmedicated.) Can or package of 100.	Easy way to protect small injuries which have been cleaned.
Elastic bandages. 2 and 3 inches wide.	Used for support in sprains, and to hold large dressings in place. Should be returned to school.
Blankets.	For warmth. For shock or chills. Also for improvised stretcher.
Splints, plastic air splints highly recommended, and pillows.	To immobilize parts where fracture is suspected.
Stretcher.	

First aid supplies should contain no medication. The simpler the care, the easier for the physician to continue treatment. Individuals may be allergic to the pink or red mercurial antiseptics, iodine, medicated dressings, and burn or sunburn ointments. Keep in mind that large dressings, elastic bandages, and triangle slings are used temporarily, until the injured person can be seen by a physician.

Records and Reports on Injuries

The cumulative health record should give data on the home address and place of employment of either one or both parents, or of the legal guardian. This information should be kept up-to-date. The signed authorization for calling a physician or dentist should also be attached. Any information on a major accident, regardless of where it may have occurred, should be noted on the record.

Reports should be filled out for injuries requiring a doctor's care or absence from school. Injuries on the athletic field, in the building, on the grounds, to and from school, and during school-sponsored activities should be written up.

A standard reporting system recommended by the National

Safety Council is widely used (see Figure 63). It consists of a summary blank on accidents and a form for reporting individual injuries.

Legal Responsibility

Mention has been made of the legal implications in giving medical care to a child. Only first aid procedures may be employed by the instructor. Until legal permission is obtained, the physician, knowing his liability, can only use emergency measures, unless, as has been explained, the life of a child is jeopardized.

The question of negligence arises, and laws differ in various states. "It is always a touchy subject to discuss how many 'rights' a teacher may have, but there is no question that he has the responsibility to safeguard his pupils from foreseeable harm as best he can, just as a parent would safeguard his child. Schools have a duty and responsibility to educate a child safely, a duty which falls most heavily upon the teacher. . . . *Perhaps the continuing decline of the immunity doctrine will force more school boards into serious consideration of this problem,* as removal of immunity will effectively render them liable for the sub-standard performance of their employee teachers. . . .

The law of teacher liability for negligence is complex and confused. The cardinal rule to remember, however, is that a teacher is liable in tort if a pupil is injured as a result of teacher negligence, the negligence being equal regardless of whether the failure was by omission or commission. Within the broad framework of existing law we may suggest that a teacher's legal responsibilities fall into the following broad duties:

1. Anticipation of foreseeable risk to students.
2. Reasonable steps to prevent those risks from occurring.
3. Warning and care addressed toward those risks that for whatever reason cannot be reduced or averted.
4. A duty to aid the injured.
5. A duty not to increase the severity of injury."[14]

"Some pupils may refuse to accept first aid because of certain beliefs which they or their parents hold. Constitutionally, this is within their right. In such instances the school should promptly notify the parents when an emergency occurs so that the responsibility is placed with them. Careful records of the case, attested by witness, should be kept. Local schools should anticipate such problems by obtaining legal advice in advance in regard to the school's responsibilities and powers."[15]

It may be of general interest to know that if a child's health or life is endangered, and if legal consent for treatment is withheld by par-

---

[14] Hillard J. Trubitt: "Legal Responsibilities of School Teachers in Emergency Situations." *J. Sch. Health* 36:23–24, 1966. Italics are author's.

[15] A Report of the Joint Committee on Health Problems in Education of the National Education Association and the American Medical Association. *School Health Services.* 1964, p. 231.

ents, a physician or anyone else interested in a child's welfare may appeal to the local prosecuting attorney or to any child welfare agency in order to initiate legal action. In some states the juvenile court may authorize necessary medical and surgical care.

The advice given below to physical education instructors should apply to all personnel in a school.

> When a student is injured while participating in the activities of a physical education class, the first task incumbent upon the teacher in all cases is to send for the principal and the school physician if one is on the premises. If it appears that the injury does not need immediate attention, the teacher should await the action of a medically trained person rather than attempt to do something. For example, if a pupil complains of head pains after being hit with a basketball or develops a swelling on the hand after being struck by a field hockey stick, the physical education teacher should see to it that the pupil is brought before a school nurse, doctor, or medical supervisor. Any aid can wait to be administered by a qualified medical person.
>
> But unfortunately, many of the injuries occurring to pupils during physical education class cannot await later treatment. When a pupil is injured to the extent that something must be done for him in the emergency, the physical education instructor is the person upon whom this initial task usually falls. If the injury is serious, such as broken bones, excessive bleeding, or severe abrasions, and the pupil is obviously in need of some assistance, the physical educator should administer first aid. In fact, the courts have implied that there is a duty or obligation upon the teacher to do something for the injured pupil, and that not to do so may be deemed negligence.
>
> Thus it may be set down as a general principle that when an emergency arises in which a pupil is seriously injured, and a school nurse, doctor, or other medically trained person is unavailable at the moment of the accident, there is a duty upon the physical education teacher to administer first aid. Failure to do so could very well make the physical education instructor liable for negligence in an ensuing lawsuit.
>
> A helpful guide to use in deciding if there is *an emergency is whether or not something must be done immediately to preserve the life of the injured pupil or to prevent further injury*. . . . The physical educator should confine himself to first aid treatment—preserving life and limb, alleviating the pain of the victim, and making him as comfortable as possible. He should not perform the functions of diagnosis, prescription, or treatment, for this is the practice of medicine and must be left to a duly licensed and qualified physician.
>
> An attempt by a teacher to administer treatment, in the absence of an emergency, will make him personally liable for negligence if the treatment proves harmful to the pupil.[16]

[16]Sondra Y. Gold and Gerald F. Gold: "First Aid and Legal Liability. What the physical educator needs to know about his responsibilities and liabilities in administering aid to injured pupils." *J. Health Phys. Ed. Rec. 34*:42–43, 1963. Italics are the author's.

Some school systems carry blanket insurance policies to protect all teachers against liability for accidents which may happen to children under their supervision. If there is no such liability coverage, a teacher should carry an individual liability insurance policy.

Insurance Plans

The administration should consider adoption of some form of accident insurance for children. Some plans have been formulated which insure against injuries in the building and on the grounds or on the way to and from school. These are available for a small sum. School systems should carry a policy which protects students in interscholastic activities.

Planning for Disasters

All organized units for care of injuries should wheel into action in the presence of catastrophe. These units should be organized in the school, the community, and at the state and national levels. This means careful planning on a standby basis so that there will be no delay should disaster hit. The school works with the community in this planning. Such events as fires, explosions, hurricanes, tornadoes, and earthquakes have occurred to damage or demolish a school and kill many children. The school and its young population should be considered in local civil defense plans to combat the results of possible nuclear warfare. The preceding chapter mentions how the school can be a shelter in case of nuclear attack. Responsible older children should have assigned roles both on the safety committees and in actual help should the occasion arise.

Standing First Aid Instructions for Serious Injuries

Everyone should be familiar with the basic principles of first aid. These have been widely publicized and demonstrated in Red Cross classes; schools usually include such classes.

If many have been injured, the lay person taking responsibility appraises the situation quickly, assigns onlookers who seem capable and willing to certain tasks, and cares for the urgent cases first. The latter would be cases of bleeding and shock. Broken bones and minor injuries can be given attention shortly after. The first aider should remain calm, ask someone to call a physician and an ambulance, and start his care. If the case is one of asphyxia, he starts artificial respiration procedures immediately. The cardinal rule is: *Stop serious bleeding; keep person breathing.*

The first aider:

1. Stops serious bleeding.
2. Administers artificial respiration, if needed.

3. Treats shock.
4. Splints bones before moving.
5. Does not move a person suspected of neck or back injury.
6. Leaves the unconscious person alone (no attempt to arouse him or give liquids).
7. Maintains an encouraging manner.
8. Does no harm.

Detailed specific emergency procedures for severe bleeding, shock, cessation of breathing, poisoning, head injuries, sprains, fractures, and dislocations of bones can be studied in any first aid manual.

Be cautious with *head injuries*. They may or may not be associated with unconsciousness. Headaches may be a complaint. Nausea and vomiting occur at times. The child may have forgotten the blow or brushed off the incident.

> One child pounded a classmate's head on the cement walk until the principal intervened. The injured child stood up, appeared a little unsteady on his feet, and then vomited. He seemed to recover and the principal permitted him to walk home alone. When the mother happened to look out of the window and saw her child approaching the house with a weaving gait, she was alarmed and took him to a physician. X-rays revealed a skull fracture. When this finding was called to the principal's attention, he protested that he did not know the skull was fractured. Neither did anyone else until x-rays were taken. There should be a strong index of suspicion with head injuries.
>
> One afternoon a fourth-grade girl called her teacher's attention to the fact that Arthur was acting funny and did not remember anything. Upon questioning, he remembered that he had brought a lunch to school and recalled its contents, but could not remember whether he had eaten it. He seemed dazed. His mother called for him at school and took him to a physician. Neurological examination revealed no damage; yet the physician suspected a head injury. Classmates were called at their homes and the story was revealed. A group of boys had been sliding on ice in a forbidden area at noon, and Arthur had tumbled and hit his head with quite a thump. After that, his behavior changed. Information concerning the injury was not elicited earlier at school because the boys kept mum, for fear of disciplinary measures.

The following recommendations have been formulated by the Committee on Accident Prevention of the American Academy of Pediatrics, in cooperation with the Surgical Section of the same organization:

> EMERGENCY CARE OF CHILDHOOD SKELETAL TRAUMA
>
> 1. Evaluate and splint where they lie before moving. Do not attempt reduction.
> 2. Move cervical (neck) injuries face up on a rigid support with manual traction applied gently by cupping chin at the time of moving. Sand bags on either side of neck to prevent turning, if possible.
> 3. Spine injuries should not be flexed in transportation.

4. Lower leg injuries transport in pillow strapped with belt.

5. Upper leg injuries with both legs and trunk bound to board without circulatory interference.

6. Lower arm injuries transport with splint, such as rolled newspaper, gentle compression wrapping, and sling.

7. Upper arm can be bound to chest with lower arm supporting in sling.

8. Open injuries or open wounds cover with sterile dressing.

EMERGENCY CARE OF BURNS

Burns may result from a catastrophic accident, such as an explosion in a laboratory or a fire in an industrial arts shop. Or, they may be minor in character.

1. Burns are due to thermal agents (scalds or fire); chemical agents (battery acid or lye); radiation (sunburn or nuclear); and electrical energy.

2. Even small burns may be followed by infection, lockjaw, excessive scarring and disfigurement. Large burns may represent an immediate threat to life from shock. Arrest of the circulation and respiration may occur following electrocution.

3. Flames should be smothered; children who have been scalded should have their clothing removed immediately; chemical burns (except phosphorus) should be washed with large quantities of running water. Chemical burns of the eye should be flushed with saline solution or water. Patients should be removed from source of radiant energy.

4. Fresh burns are relatively clean. They should be covered by a clean cloth immediately and should not be uncovered until the patient is delivered to a hospital emergency room or a doctor's office. Such covering should be loosely applied without constriction.

5. *Ointments, greases, powder, etc. should not be used in the emergency treatment of burns.* Leave this management to the physician who will care for the patient.

6. Shock may be combated by keeping the patient flat, reassuring him, and keeping him warm during transportation to the hospital.

7. Pain is usually not a serious problem in the emergency treatment of a burn and drugs for pain should not be administered except by the physician who will care for the burn.

8. Patients with burns of the face, hands, feet, or areas surrounding a joint as well as any burn equivalent to more than 5% of the body surface should be hospitalized after emergency treatment.

9. Electrical burns accompanied by electrocution and failure of respiration and circulation should receive artificial respiration for an indefinite period and until ordered to stop by a physician.[17]

A good deal of research has been done on the management of burns. Acceptable care today involves the use of cold water, either as an immersion of a part of the body or as cold compresses.

For minor burns: "Pain may be treated by intermittent application of cold. This can be accomplished by submerging a burned area

[17]American Academy of Pediatrics, Committee on Accident Prevention. Reprint. December 1956. Italics are the author's.

in ice water or applying cold compresses. As soon as the patient's pain has been relieved, the cold application is discontinued until pain recurs. Then the cold is reapplied. This therapy is employed until its discontinuation causes no discomfort."[18]

Emergency Care of Sudden Illness

Occasionally a child at school will "double up" with abdominal pain, with or without nausea and vomiting. A sore throat may become more severe, and the fever may rise during the day. An earache may become excruciatingly painful. A diabetic may show signs which worry the teacher. A sick child should be under the supervision of his parents. He should not remain at school.

Procedures should be the same as for handling injuries. First, an attempt is made to contact a parent. If this fails, reference is made to the permit attached to the cumulative health record, and the physician is contacted. Or, the child may already be under medical care. A description of the complaint will bring instructions on further handling. The physician may request that the child be taken directly to a hospital for observation and laboratory work, or be brought to the private office. In any event he accepts responsibility. There should still be an attempt on the part of the school and physician to contact parents. If no physician has been designated and the parent cannot be contacted and if judgment indicates that the child should be under adequate medical care immediately, the same procedures outlined for injuries should be taken. Under no circumstances should a diagnosis be made by a lay person, and *no medication*, not even an aspirin tablet, should be given at school.

Services Planned to Provide Healthful Environment

The objectives and achievements of health services are interwoven with those of the school environment. This interrelationship is particularly noticeable in the communicable disease program. Employees and students must be protected in their daily contacts with each other and in their environment, especially in the food services. Immunization procedures, the tuberculosis-finding program, detection of acute infections, inspection of the dining area and kitchen—these are all services which help maintain a healthful environment. It must be stressed also that both of these areas—services and environment—are interdependent with health education.

---

[18] Duane Larson: "Current Trends in the Care of Burned Patients." *Am. J. Nursing* *61*:319, 1967.

Services Which Provide Experiences for Health Education

Every health service at school is an experience which can be utilized in health teaching at each grade level. The converse is also true. Health education should prepare youth to develop favorable attitudes, which will be demonstrated as participation in many aspects of the health service program. Details of the services which are usually considered in selection of content for health instruction are discussed in the preceding and in the following chapters.

Health Services in Rural Areas

Detailed information has been given in the preceding pages for a comprehensive set-up which should care for a child's health needs. Such an arrangement includes a full- or part-time physician, a nurse, a health coordinator, social worker, and other personnel. Large school systems and large schools may well afford such personnel.

What about the small school in a small community? Rural schools usually do not have adequate health programs. Periodic health examinations and follow-up care are seldom required by the school administration.

Rural health facilities are improving, however. More hospitals and health centers are being established. Preventive health services are extended into rural areas. The provisions of a good school health program can be adapted to local facilities. The attitudes of the principal and teachers in a sincere desire to formulate and adapt a program are what is important.

In a small school the principal and teacher are more self-reliant. They tend to accept more responsibility in implementing the various objectives of school health services. They are not isolated, however. Every community has access to some type of medical care, even though a physician or dentist may be located miles away. The state board of health is concerned with the health of scantily populated districts and strives to provide services through visiting personnel, taking the services to the people. Services from visiting dental units, mental health teams, and speech clinics may be available. Leaders in the local community are concerned with the health of their children and should have a more intimate interest in working with the school and other agencies to provide the services needed.

HEALTH SERVICES FOR SCHOOL PERSONNEL

In considering the health of all personnel in contact with school children, the school administration is interested not only in whether an individual has a communicable disease, but also whether he is physically able to perform with reasonable efficiency the tasks required of the position.

Teaching Personnel

Good health of a teacher is a prerequisite for good teaching, for protection of children against communicable diseases, and for pleasant feeling tones in the classroom. Recognition of this fact should impel departments of education at state and local levels to establish pre-employment health standards.

Some states do have standards which must be met for certification. An applicant for a teacher's certificate receives a health examination form to be filled out by a physician. Information to the physician concerning the standards, both mental and physical, which may exclude the prospective teacher should accompany the form. These forms and standards should represent the consensus of a group of health-minded educators and education-minded physicians, all of whom are concerned both with the welfare of the applicant and the impact of a physical or emotional abnormality on school children. For instance, good hearing, good vision, and good speech are tools of the teaching profession. A teacher with active tuberculosis is a health menace. An example of the extensive damage which may be done is described in the discussion on tuberculosis. And it is agreed that a good personality adjustment is most essential.

Local boards of education may request an additional pre-employment health examination on an applicant, to be done by a private or school physician. The Los Angeles Board of Education maintains an elaborate health service which examines its own applicants. A board of education, as an employer, has a right to set its own standards. It may choose to accept only those examinations done by its own school physician. The reason for this policy is that the physician in doubtful cases will avoid personalities and lean toward the employer's advantage and viewpoint. If the state requires a thorough pre-certification examination, the local board may waive the requirement. Some boards are content with a physician's statement that an individual is in good health; a surprising number of teachers are hired without any type of a health examination. A shortage of teachers does not justify waiving health standards.

All communications from an examining physician should be sent directly by him to a state or local board of education, as required, and should be reviewed by a physician who represents the board.

Once a teacher has been employed, health examination requirements vary. Some boards of education require an examination each year, some every three years, and some ask for no further checkup. Some require a chest x-ray each year or at specified intervals; some will arrange to have x-rays taken. Some require another health examination only after a leave of absence for illness; some large school systems with elaborate health services require that a teacher who has been ill for a certain number of days report for clearance from the school physician before entering his classroom. Such a school health service maintains close supervision of the health of teachers.

A pre-employment health examination should not suffice for a teacher's professional lifetime. Interval appraisals should be required.

Health Standards for Teacher Candidates

The time to disqualify teacher candidates for health reasons is in preservice training. To permit a student to prepare for the teaching profession with known disqualifying abnormalities is a cruel waste of time and money and will eventually produce psychic trauma. All teacher education institutions should adopt objective health standards, and each applicant for formal entrance into the teacher certification program should be "processed" accordingly. These standards are formulated by educators and physicians in the institutions, with the welfare of both the prospective teacher and his prospective pupils taken into consideration. This "processing" not only serves to detect any defects or problems which may be present but should be an educational experience to the applicant as well. If defects are remediable, correction should be made before acceptance into the field of education.

The following statement serves to present the philosophy of most physicians and educators who are concerned about the health of teachers:

> Good health, mental and physical, is a prerequisite for efficient and wholesome teaching. In their hourly and daily contacts teachers probably more than any other professional individuals are the cynosure of many critical eyes. Their appearances, mannerisms, defects of speech, and emotional impacts on pupils can leave lasting impressions.
>
> Also, teaching at any level, from kindergarten through high school, requires considerable expenditure of energy. Constant association in the classroom with robust, active children for many hours each day as well as supervision of various physical activities on the playgrounds may be fairly strenuous for many individuals. One must consider the ability of the teacher to respond to such physical stress.
>
> An individual whose health prevents reasonably good attendance at school or who is suffering from a communicable disease, such as tuberculosis, certainly should not be employed as a teacher. An individual whose hearing or visual defects impede efficient teaching should not be placed in a classroom. One must remember that children are not only quick to detect such impairments but can devise means of adding to the nervous strain of such a teacher.
>
> On the other hand, it is possible that discrimination may be made to a minor degree in health standards for elementary and

> secondary teachers. For instance, a lisp or other speech defect, a tic, or a limping gait which would likely be imitated by a first grader will probably be ignored by a high school student. The reaction of children to cosmetic defects, such as artificial limbs, artificial eyes, or extensive visible scars, is difficult to evaluate.
>
> The emotional climate of a classroom should promote serenity of mind. Any observations or knowledge in regard to personality defects or emotional disabilities must be carefully evaluated.
>
> In all fairness to the prospective teacher and to his future pupils and school administration, certain standards of physical and mental health should be considered. In some instances acceptance into Education can be delayed until the applicant makes corrections or takes recommended treatment. . . . These are not rigid standards; it is to be kept in mind that in an occasional instance outstanding personality or mental ability may be considered to compensate for one or more health defects. . . .[19]

Teaching requires a great deal of energy. A teacher needs to be in the finest physical condition possible. When one elementary teacher was asked if she rested enough, this was her answer:

> As to whether I get enough rest—if the time ever comes when school is to be conducted twelve months a year, then I know of one teacher who will become a saleslady or a baby-sitter instead of a teacher. I put in eight hours a day at school and about an hour of homework regularly. And all day long when I'm teaching, I'm pushing to cover the material in the time allotted. In this state teachers are legally required to teach *nineteen* subjects in the elementary schools. By the middle of June those shrill little voices begin to abrade my nerves, and I count the hours and minutes until the semester will be over. Yet by mid-September ideas for new techniques and lesson plans crowd my mind and I look forward to starting the new school year, because I'm rested.
>
> Rest comes from change but there is little change during the day for a teacher who goes from classroom teaching to hall and bus supervision, to playground, to lunch patrol, to patrol during recess, noon, and after school. Coffee breaks and duty-free lunch periods are needed for teachers' mental health as well as physical health. Sabbatical leaves and travel should be encouraged for teachers instead of innumerable summer classes, institutes, workshops, etc. I find it restful to leave the city for vacations in the high mountains and to associate with non-teachers to avoid shop-talk.

Nonteaching School Personnel

Since good health is a prerequisite to good performance, health examinations of applicants for a job should be required. Delay in employment may even be necessary while the applicant makes corrections or takes recommended treatments. Also, in considering employment, the applicant's physical status must be evaluated in terms

---

[19]Alma Nemir: "Health Qualifications of Prospective Teachers." *J. Teacher Education 10*:297, 1959.

of the job requirement. A man with heart trouble, or a hernia, or of middle age cannot accept certain types of jobs. The examining physician should be alert for personality defects or emotional disturbances. In addition, special qualifications are mandatory; for instance, a bus driver should have normal color vision, visual acuity, and hearing.

Emphasis upon freedom *at all times* from communicable diseases, of course, is essential. Food service personnel prepare and serve hundreds of meals daily. The possibility of transmission of any disease, either from lesions on the skin or from respiratory, gastrointestinal, or other sources must be eliminated. Office personnel, custodians, bus drivers, and others are in daily contact with pupils. They must be free of communicable diseases.

A periodic health examination with annual x-rays should be required of all employees. An evaluation of health status will enable the school administration to place an individual in a job where he can serve to his best physical capacity. Such an evaluation has practical value. (See form—Appendix B.)

Employees are often retained after reaching the age of 65. The incidence of accidents is increasing in this age group. This is caused by several factors, including possible decreased physical vigor for the task assigned, poor coordination, or faulty vision or hearing. The findings of an annual health examination would reveal such defects and should guide the school in placing employees in the various jobs. If a school board required a complete health examination annually of every employee over 50 years of age, the regulation would serve as a protection for the individual himself, decrease strain and hazards on the job, and reduce the number of accidents.

SUMMARY

The school is vitally interested in the health status of every student. Most are healthy; a few have handicaps. The constant objective is to maintain, protect, and, when possible, improve the health of each individual.

The school should have in its files a record of a complete health examination on each child, done preferably by a private physician. Such an examination should be repeated at about three-year intervals during his time in school. Further knowledge concerning his health status should be acquired by means of health histories, continuous teacher observation, screening tests for hearing, vision, weight, height, etc., special surveys, and psychological tests. All of this information should be available for study on each student's cumulative health record. A satisfactory health appraisal of a child enables a teacher to understand him and his achievements.

Not only must a school have an appraisal of each child's health, but well-organized, routine services are planned for him. The handicapped need adaptive services. There must be programs for communicable disease control and for care of sudden injuries and illnesses. Health services should be extended to school personnel, whose health most assuredly influences the physical and emotional health of children.

DISCUSSION QUESTIONS AND ACTIVITIES

1. Discuss the ethics of required immunization before acceptance into a school system.
2. Discuss the importance of teacher observation in discovering health deficiencies.
3. Find out what screening tests are used for health appraisal in a specific public school system.
4. Discuss your reasons, as a teacher of health, for a recommended physical examination for every student in the school.
5. Discuss the importance of keeping accurate cumulative health records.
6. Make up a first aid kit suitable for a classroom teacher with your training.
7. Discuss the requirements for health standards for teachers. Why are these health requirements necessary?
8. Discuss what service you consider to be of most value in a school health program. Do most of the schools have this service?
9. Describe the parents' role in the school health service program.
10. Discuss the importance of having a health history on records. Are all teachers allowed access to these records?

ADDITIONAL SOURCES OF INFORMATION

GENERAL REFERENCES ON SCHOOL HEALTH SERVICES

American Academy of Pediatrics: "School Health Policies." 1966.

American Medical Association: Reports of the National Conferences on Physicians and Schools, approximately every two years, beginning with 1949.

American National Red Cross: *First Aid Textbook.* Garden City, New York: Doubleday and Company, Inc. Most recent edition.

Bourne, I. B.: "A pilot project for improvement of school health services." *J. Sch. Health* 41:288–90, June, 1971.

Bright, D., et al.: "What school physicians, nurses, and health educators should know about transcendental meditation." *J. Sch. Health* 43:192–4, March, 1973.

Chinn, P.: "A relationship between health and school problems: A nursing assessment." *J. Sch. Health* 43:85–93, February, 1973.

Coleman, J., and Hawkins, W.: "The changing role of the nurse: An alternative to elimination." *J. Sch. Health* 40:121–2, March, 1970.

Eisner, V., and Oglesby, A.: "Health assessment of school children. I. Physical examinations." *J. Sch. Health* 41:239–42, May, 1971.

Eisner, V., and Oglesby, A.: "Health assessment of school children. II. Screening tests." *J. Sch. Health* 41:344–6, September, 1971.
Eisner, V., and Oglesby, A.: "Health assessment of school children. III. Vision." *J. Sch. Health* 41:408–11, October, 1971.
Eisner, V., and Oglesby, A.: "Health assessment of school children. IV. Hearing." *J. Sch. Health* 41:495–6, November, 1971.
Eisner, V., and Oglesby, A.: "Health assessment of school children. V. Selecting screening tests." *J. Sch. Health* 42:21–4, January, 1972.
Eisner, V., and Oglesby, A.: "Health assessment of school children. VI. Height and weight." *J. Sch. Health* 42:164–6, March, 1972.
Eisner, V., and Oglesby, A.: "Health assessment of school children. VII. Heart sound." *J. Sch. Health* 42:270–1, May, 1972.
Eisner, V., and Oglesby, A.: "Health assessment of school children. VIII. The unexpected health defect." *J. Sch. Health.* 42:348–50, June, 1972.
Harlin, V. K.: "Help for the hyperkinetic child in school." *J. Sch. Health* 42:587–91, December, 1972.
Henderson, J.: *Emergency Medical Guide.* New York: McGraw-Hill, 1969.
Joint Committee on Health Problems in Education of the National Education Association and the American Medical Association. Washington: The National Education Association.
"Health Appraisal of School Children." Fourth edition. 1969.
"Health of School Personnel." (1964).
"Mental Health and School Health Services." (1965).
School Health Services. 1964.
"Suggested School Health Policies." Fourth edition. (1966).
Kaufman, J. M., et al.: "Part-time consultants in the schools: Observations of a research team for service to children with school problems." *J. Sch. Health* 42:446–9, October, 1972.
Lampe, J. M.: "A new approach to the delivery of health care to school children as instituted by Denver, Colorado Public Schools." *J. Sch. Health* 42:272–4, May, 1972.
Lampe, J. M.: "The school physician of the future." *J. Sch. Health* 42:197–8, April, 1972.
Miller, D. F., and Shunk, S.: "A survey of elementary school health services with emphasis on preparations for emergency care procedures of sick and injured students." *J. Sch. Health* 42:114–7, February, 1972.
National Education Association, National Commission on Safety Education: "A School Safety Education Program." 1966.
"Who Is Liable for Pupil Injuries?" 1963.
Patterson, M. G.: "Extending the role of the school nurse to migrant families." *J. Sch. Health* 41:421–4, October, 1971.
Schneeweiss, S.: "The computer in school health services." *J. Sch. Health* 40:145–8, March, 1970.
Yocum, P. B.: "The health-related tasks, where does the school nurse function?" *J. Sch. Health* 43:316–9, May, 1973.
See annual reports of medical or health services branches of large public school systems; e.g., Denver, Los Angeles, Chicago.

AUDIOVISUAL MATERIALS

Recommended grade levels are designated *pri, int. jh, sh.*

Breath of Life

16 min.	Color	All ages	Available local chapters—American Heart Association

When and where to use mouth-to-mouth resuscitation. Excellent.

Emergency 77

14 min.	Black and White	*sh*	Metropolitan Life Insurance Company*

Should create awareness of need for learning how to prevent emergencies,

*See Appendix A for addresses of film companies.

how to handle some emergencies, how to utilize community resources. Emphasis on the importance of avoiding panic through knowledge, planning and practice. A 12-page film discussion guide is also available.

First Aid on the Spot

11 min. Black and White *jh, sh*
Encyclopaedia Britannica Educ. Corp.

Features six common types of injuries or disabilities and the approved first aid technique. Demonstrates care of wounds, burns, and shock; techniques of splinting, controlling bleeding, and artificial respiration.

Journey in Health

21 min. Color Teachers, parents Association Films, Inc.
Free loan.

Stresses importance of periodic medical checkups to the mental as well as physical welfare of a child. Cites three cases in which both physical and mental illness, deformities, and operation can follow parental neglect.

Journey Into Health (Parts 1 and 2)

24 min. each Black and White *sh*, adults Smart Foundation

A physician discusses the question: "What Is Health Supervision?" Explains physical and emotional values of periodical health examinations.

Looking at Children

24 min. Color Teachers Metropolitan
Life Insurance Company

Health observations of teachers in the classroom. Teacher's role as member of school health team demonstrated.

Rescue Breathing

22 min. Color *int, jh, sh* American Film Producers
Available from boards of health.

Demonstrates mouth-to-mouth resuscitation technique. Other films on mouth-to-mouth resuscitation should be available locally.

The Things a Teacher Sees

19 min. Color Teachers International
Film Bureau, Inc.

An experienced teacher observes appearance and behavior of pupils and reports any problems which may affect their physical or emotional being to the school nurse. The teacher is a member of the community health team.

Chapter 20

SCHOOL HEALTH EDUCATION

WHAT IS SCHOOL HEALTH EDUCATION?

A fundamental purpose of education is helping people to do better the things they will be doing anyway. In the school setting, as elsewhere, this is accomplished by developing critical thinkers.

The President's Committee on Health Education defines health education as a "process that bridges the gap between health information and health practices. Health education motivates the person to take the information and do something with it—to keep himself healthier by avoiding actions that are harmful and by forming habits that are beneficial."[1] This definition by a, basically, lay group of distinguished individuals, is remarkably similar to a definition formulated by a group of professional health educators. A coalition of health organization representatives defined health education as "a process with intellectual, psychological and social dimensions relating to activities which increase the abilities of people to make informed decisions affecting their personal, family and community well-being. This process, based on scientific principles, facilitates learning and behavioral change in both personnel and consumers, including children and youth."[2]

School health education aims to conserve or improve the health of school-age youth and give them guidelines for healthful living all of their lives. A teacher presents the basic factors or concepts of health and disease as a continuum throughout the school years in such fashion that a youth is stimulated to strive constantly for the best personal health, including a healthy emotional life ("self-discipline, self-reliance, and self-direction"), and will "possess an awareness and sense of responsibility" for the health of his family, community, and nation.

---

[1]President's Committee on Health Education: *The Report of the President's Committee on Health Education*, October, 1973, p. 17.

[2]*Op. cit.*, Joint Committee on Health Education Terminology, pp. 65–66.

School health education is defined as "that health education process associated with health activities planned and conducted under the supervision of school personnel with involvement of appropriate community health personnel and utilization of appropriate community resources."[3] To be truly effective, these experiences should involve individual children and the group in situations which are meaningful to them.

It may be stated that health education is, unequivocally, an academic discipline which richly deserves attention as a school subject. Its content is timely, relevant, and of inestimable value in helping an individual lead a meaningful life.

"Health education is never the mere transmission of health information to students as measured by their ability to recite back facts or to score high on a pencil and paper test. The 'proof of the pudding' in health education is what people do about health, not what they know about health. Accordingly, evaluation of instruction in this area must be concerned with attitudes, practices and values, in addition to knowledge."[4]

THE NEED FOR SCHOOL HEALTH EDUCATION

Early in this century educators recognized the importance of health and designated it as first of the "seven cardinal principles."

> The secondary school should provide health instruction, inculcate health habits, organize an effective program of physical activities, regard health needs in planning work and play, and cooperate with home and community in safe-guarding and promoting health interests.[5]

Despite this philosophy some boards of education, some school systems, and disquietingly true, some teacher education institutions, do not recognize the importance of health education nor teacher preparation in health education.

What recognition is given health education in the schools? Is there a need? With the impetus provided by a group of physicians and educators, the School Health Education Study was established; during 1961–1963 two surveys were made by valid sampling on a nation-wide basis. One of these surveys was concerned with the status of health education in the curriculum. The companion study was

---

[3]*Op. cit.*, Joint Committee on Health Education Terminology, pp. 67–68.

[4]Fred V. Hein: "Health Education in the Schools." *Clin. Pediat. 10*:11:645, November, 1971.

[5]National Education Association of the United States: "Cardinal Principles of Secondary Education." U. S. Department of Interior, Bureau of Education Bulletin No. 35, 1918. Superintendent of Documents, Government Printing Office Washington, D.C.

designed to evaluate student behavior in terms of health knowledge, attitudes, and practices.

The results were not unexpected, but, nevertheless, they were cruelly enlightening. One hundred and thirty-five school systems of various-sized populations in 38 states were surveyed. This encompassed 1101 elementary schools with 529,656 pupils and 359 secondary schools with 311,176 students. The summary on instructional problems survey reads as follows:

> Examples of problems related to health education in schools that were cited by school administrators or a person designated by him included:
>
> Failure of the home to encourage practice of health habits learned in school
> ineffectiveness of instruction methods
> parental and community resistance to certain health topics
> insufficient time in the school day for health instruction
> lack of coordination of the health education program throughout the school grades
> inadequate professional preparation of staff
> disinterest on part of some teachers assigned to health teaching
> failure of parents to follow up on needed and recommended health services for children
> indifference toward and hence lack of support for health education on the part of some teachers, parents, administrators, health officers, and other members of the community
> neglect of the health education course when combined with physical education
> inadequate facilities and instructional materials
> student indifference to health education
> lack of specialized supervisory and consultative services.[6]

As for health behavior of students, evaluated upon the basis of knowledge, attitudes and practices, results of the study were equally depressing. About 50 per cent was the average score on answers to test questions. Girls performed a little better than boys. Comparatively few pupils followed the health practices which they did know. Their misconceptions strike at fundamental health information. After all, every individual needs to know certain health facts.

The following are examples of *misconceptions* that existed most frequently among high school seniors in the sample group:

> Commercial medicines are safe to purchase if the label clearly indicates the dose and contents, or if recommended by a pharmacist.
>
> The use of "pep" pills and sleeping pills does not require medication supervision.
>
> Legislation guarantees the reliability of any advertised medicine.
>
> Popular brands of toothpaste are effective in killing germs in the mouth and in preventing cavities and loss of teeth.

---

[6]Elena M. Sliepcevich: "School Health Education Study: A Summary Report." Washington, D.C.: The Study, 1964, p. 11.

> The purpose of fluoridating water supplies is to purify water and make it safe to drink.
>
> Unrefrigerated chicken salad is not a potential source of food poisoning.
>
> A high school girl who was once underweight should regularly take vitamin pills to ensure adequate nutrition or take calorie-controlled diet preparations if she begins to gain weight.
>
> Chronic diseases can be transmitted from person to person.
>
> Although increasing today, venereal disease has never been a major social problem.
>
> Venereal disease can be inherited.
>
> The World Health Organization is a part of the International Red Cross.
>
> Voluntary health agencies are supported by public funds and these groups have power to enforce necessary community health regulations.
>
> A full-time public health department provides complete medical diagnosis and treatment for any citizen.
>
> Physical fitness and endurance naturally increase as adolescents grow up.
>
> For a specific health problem the source of help selected as best by high school seniors was: (1) a persistent skin inflammation—a non-medical health advisor or pharmacist, (2) a persistent cough—a pharmacist.[7]

These two studies reveal that the health education curriculum is woefully inadequate. Testimony before the President's Committee on Health Education resulted in their stating, "Our findings are that school health education in most primary and secondary schools either is not provided at all, or loses its proper emphasis because of the way it is tacked onto another subject such as physical education or biology, assigned to teachers whose interests and qualifications lie elsewhere."[8] Without proper information and with poor attitudes and practices, the health status of children cannot escape being affected. Consider also the various remediable health problems, especially dental health and early diagnosis of streptococcal sore throat, which predisposes to heart damage. In these two areas alone great improvement is possible. The physical and mental health needs of children are not being met by the school, the home, or the community. "The content of health instruction belongs in the school curriculum because such knowledge is necessary, is most efficiently learned in school, and no other public agency provides such instruction."[9]

One of the most impressive pieces of legislation to meet youths' health needs was passed in New York in 1967. It established a requirement for health instruction in all grades in all schools of the state and stressed the need for coordinating this instruction directly with the need for solving the critical health problems of society.

---

[7]*Ibid.*, p. 6.

[8]*Op. cit.*, President's Committee on Health Education, p. 21.

[9]National Education Association, Project on Instruction, "Schools for the 60's." 1963, p. 31.

THE HEALTH EDUCATION CURRICULUM

Health has been designated as a quality of life more comprehensive than an absence of disease, as that state of well-being which will enable one to live most fully. Health education is a discipline in its own right derived from the health and behavioral sciences. It touches upon every phase of living. There will be times when the many facts of healthful living will be incorporated within other subject fields, and times when the health education materials will be organized into formal health education courses.

Who Plans the Health Education Curriculum?

Who is interested in formulating, implementing, and evaluating a well-integrated curriculum?

Many people outside and inside the school system are interested. There are a great many educational, professional, voluntary, and commercial organizations concerned with health, directly or incidentally. (See Appendix A.) This accounts for the abundance of material available for teachers, both in factual information and in planned teaching units. These agencies employ expert consultants who not only prepare teaching aids on various health problems but also are available for workshops.

Interest comes primarily, however, from those associated with education. Most commonly, study or planning groups closely involved in health teaching will gather in sessions, such as workshops, conferences, committees, or in-service classes. The theme may be any phase of the health education curriculum—commonly, content, sequence, methodology, evaluation, or review of new materials. The purpose may be to plan a progressive curriculum on some health problem—alcohol, the effects of tobacco, drug abuse, physical and emotional aspects of sex, nutrition, safety, family life education, or any pertinent question.

These study groups may be organized at any level—state, district, or in a local system ("the grass roots"). Such meetings should be fun and stimulating. Education and health specialists may be invited as consultants from departments of education, teacher education institutions, and official or voluntary health agencies. The "grass roots" approach considers local mores and should assure meaningful teaching. Indeed, teachers who participate in health curriculum planning should be better prepared to teach health education.

A group may spend a year or two on the particular aspects of health instruction which it has chosen to study. If its endeavors form part of a state-wide project, the results of deliberations may be compiled, edited, refined, checked for integration from kindergarten through high school and for overlapping of related fields. The printed proceedings may be sent back to individual planners for use, evaluation, and future revision. Eventually a guide or manual may be adopted. Such a procedure in formulating a health education program is slow, but it should produce far-reaching effects as an educational experience for participating teachers and administrators. They compare information with others in the group, understand objectives, and should improve their own roles in health teaching.

Group planning may be prompted by new legislation. To discuss implementation of the health education requirement passed in New York State in 1967, the first conference held was attended by 1200 educators. After that, a series of regional conferences was held. From these conferences an outline of curriculum (to be discussed under Content) and new health education syllabi were developed.

Impetus for planning a health education program or for evaluating it may come from a school health council or from a school health committee. Community needs may dictate some avenues of health instruction. A state legislature may require a course in driver training. A local PTA may decide that health teaching is inadequate in its school and demand not only a better quality of instruction, but also an increased amount of it.

Public health problems which reflect a stressful situation, as in the case of drug dependence and drug abuse, will dictate that all teachers must be alert and diligent in their observations and must possess sufficient scientific information in order to know what to teach and how to manage an individual student in trouble. Under these circumstances an efficient procedure in curriculum planning should involve the whole faculty of a school or all teachers in a system or in the district and should include some students. Specialists are invited to participate. A few concentrated hours should start to produce the results desired.

Sometimes appreciation of the need for planning or evaluation and replanning a health education curriculum follows the observations of health educators from teacher education institutions. A faculty member who goes out to supervise student teaching becomes well aware of shortcomings in health instruction. In one instance a supervisor noticed that a health teacher was repeating a course in personal health in all three years of junior high school. Ignorance of the law (which requires only one semester) plus poor preparation in course planning produced a group of bored students. Arising from this observation was the provision of a university extension course in curriculum planning which all health teachers of the district could attend one evening a week. Credit was given. Interest was stimulated, and in-service education paid dividends.

State departments of education employ the services of consultants or supervisors in health education. These authorities help in many ways. They are in a strategic position to know exactly what is being done in health education in the state. During their travels through the districts they are available as consultants. They can give advice on many aspects of the school health program, such as curriculum planning, formation of health councils, or school-community relationships. They are often instrumental in planning workshops or conferences in local areas of the state or in association with courses to be presented in teacher education institutions. They are responsible for the preparation of guides or manuals which offer valuable suggestions in planning a health education curriculum. Recognition of the need for authentic, current health information prompts the distribution of packets of teaching materials for each grade level. Out-dated health information may be dangerous.

These supervisors can interpret existing laws or regulations which concern the health of the school child. For instance, most states have laws requiring instruction on the effects of alcohol, tobacco, and narcotics on the human body. Most state boards of education specify how much time should be spent in teaching health education in the primary and intermediate grades, and suggest the health subject matter to be taught in health education in the high school.

A state supervisor observes the trends in health instruction. He will note the following: Who is teaching health education? Is it the physical educator? Or general science teacher? Are health educators being hired? He makes recommendations for preparation of teachers in health education according to his findings.

At a lower level in administration than the state supervisor should be someone who has been delegated the responsibility of the health instruction program in a district or a school system. He should have a recognized, authoritative position so that he can carry out such duties as: make sure that time is set aside for health teaching, "sell" the principal and teacher on the importance of this area of instruction so that it will not be slighted, and plan the curriculum with all the considerations which are presented below. He should be skilled in techniques for involving the whole faculty of a school in an appreciation of health learning and emphasizing the responsibilities of each member for the health instruction curriculum.

A district supervisor or a health education supervisor for a school system is not necessarily a health educator. However, if he has had specific preparation, he may be designated as a health coordinator. What is important is that he occupy a position in the administration. Other personnel whose training is in the area of health education carry out their responsibilities under his administrative supervision.

Health coordinators or health educators in a school system or school are in a position to act as consultants and maintain continuous supervision to assure an on-going program. They are prepared to work with all personnel involved in teaching health education and can help plan a well-integrated unified program.

Mention has been made of available curriculum guides from departments of education. Certainly they are not to be followed slavishly.

Any group planning a curriculum or a teaching unit will consider such resources literally as guides. Various commissions, committees, and professional and voluntary organizations have prepared materials which can serve to expedite development of a local health curriculum.

Finally, those who are concerned with development of the health education curriculum must involve the pupils themselves. The role of teacher-pupil planning and problem solving will produce favorable attitudes as well as information.

Even though all teachers are not involved in planning a health education curriculum, every teacher is involved in health education to some degree. *Every teacher is a health teacher.* Every teacher candidate should read the discussion in the first chapter of this text. Many teachers are directly involved with a health education curriculum—elementary teachers, health educators, and others in fields allied to health. But all teachers who associate with youth have a role to fulfill in health teaching and should be familiar with the health education curriculum.

A health curriculum is merely a guide and aid in the health education process. The effectiveness of the process will be measured in terms of changes in health behavior. "In order to produce results two components must be integrated: a relevant curriculum and a creative and committed health educator. When these two components are plugged into each other, there will be generated electricity, excitement, enthusiasm, and vibrations in the student to turn him on to health learning."[10]

Content

Health as a quality of life involves every aspect of living. Therefore, the content of a health education curriculum is wide and involves many and diversified areas of learning—a range from a healthful school environment and the health aspects of daily classroom living to subjects which deal directly with health and health information, e.g., physiology, biology, general science, physical education, to areas which contribute to a quality of living, e.g., marriage and family living, music, drama.

Since health education derives its content from the biological and physical sciences, health educators should have a general familiarity with such scientific areas as anatomy, physics, chemistry, physiology, biology, genetics, microbiology, and pharmacology, and with the application of such information to man's health in the fields of medicine and dentistry. Since health education also derives its content from the behavioral or social sciences, it is related also to such areas as sociology, psychology, anthropology, political science, and econom-

---

[10]Loren B. Bensley: "Five Cures for Dull Health Curriculums." *School Health Rev.* 4:4:38, July/August, 1973.

ics. Knowledge along these lines promotes understanding of man's needs and adjustments in his environment and can indicate means to be used in motivating desirable health behavior. The primary purpose of a health education curriculum is using this knowledge to provide learning experiences which will influence the attitudes and practices relating to individual and community health.

SELECTION OF CONTENT
(What to Teach)

Selection of content of a health education curriculum will be determined by many factors:

1. The physical, emotional, social, and intellectual needs of children.
2. The health interests of children.
3. The personal experiences of children.
4. The capacities and levels of comprehension of children at each age level.
5. The health needs of the nation, state, community, school, and the home.
6. The objectives of health education (desirable outcomes).
7. Use of basic concepts inherent in health education to serve as a framework for selection of content.
8. The knowledge available from the health and behavioral sciences.
9. The contributions of specialists in health education.
10. The background and experiences of the teacher.

All of these factors are interrelated and discussion of them will be overlapping.

Determination of Needs. How does a teacher determine the needs of children? *A knowledge and understanding of their growth and development*—physical, emotional, social, and intellectual—is essential.

A review of the developmental patterns in terms of characteristics and implied needs is presented in Tables 1 and 2 (pp. 30–35). As the eyes scan the page horizontally, a teacher can trace a characteristic from its first appearance as a significant factor. Observe that physical growth is a health factor throughout the years. This implies need for rest, supervised activity, adequate sleep, and good nutrition. Teaching units along these lines are indicated. In the early primary grades time is actually taken for rest and relaxation. Dental health is always a problem. Some characteristics and needs are more significant with sexual maturation. Mental health needs throughout the school years must be appreciated and met in various ways, graded to emotional growth patterns.

Teacher observation supplies information on health needs. A teacher observes the change in physique, the individual differences in growth and development, sexual maturation, the changes related to emotional development and awareness of social relationships. Children need to know what is happening at each age; understanding and explanation should be supplied. A teacher notices physical defects (possibly involving problems of nutrition, vision, or hearing) and discusses them. He watches children's reactions to various experiences which have health implications and can prepare a teaching project or unit which will be pertinent. What children read, do, or say, and their attempts at socializing offer clues to their needs and cultural background. Selection of content must be immediate to the needs of the children sitting before the teacher, and even to special children present. Instruction can be based on the social and emotional problems which are observed by teachers, guidance personnel, and other professional workers.

A study of the *findings of the health examinations* will reveal the common health defects of children in a classroom or at any age level. Perhaps more stress needs to be placed on posture, teeth, exercise, rest, or cleanliness. With adolescents attention may be directed towards posture, skin, scalp, nervousness, refractive errors of the eyes, and sexual maturation. Individual health counseling is also health education.

A review of the *health histories*, if good records are kept, offers a wealth of information on health needs of children. Some may not have been immunized against any or some of the communicable diseases. This gives opportunity for a discussion in class on immunizations. The hours of sleep, habits of eating, selection of foods, number of visits to the dentist—these are all topics for discussion.

A prepared *curriculum guide, manual,* or *textbook* will provide information on the health needs of children at each age level—information gathered from educators and medical people as a result of their experiences and observations. The suggestions in the manual should be modified to the needs of an individual classroom, school, or community. Health books or readers present health information based on needs and interests. Children usually enjoy them immensely, and teachers select topics based on this reading.

Consultations or *interviews* with parents, social workers, school nurses, and medical authorities will reflect individual, family, and community needs. Here again is a rich source of information which may be a springboard for selection of course content. Written or oral *expression of pupil interests* in health problems may imply a need, and the teacher again has his topic selected.

Health Interests. Success in teaching is dependent upon the interest which can be aroused or utilized. Children wish to understand themselves. "Will I be large enough to make the varsity?" "How can I improve my complexion?" "Why are girls larger than the boys?" "How can I become more confident of myself in class?" In addition, boys are particularly interested in strength and vitality. Many children of both sexes are interested in athletic achievement today. Girls have problems dealing with beauty and attractiveness. Both sexes gradually become interested in heterosexual relationships.

With maturation health interests expand into many new areas. It is important that a teacher recognize these interests as they appear, with the intent of giving an individual an insight into the problems which present themselves. Junior high school students are interested in physical development, personal appearance, and acceptance by others. As they enter senior high school, they are still occupied by their own reactions, but they gradually become more aware of their social relationships with their peers. As they approach graduation, they become more serious about future health problems—personal and family living, child care, housing, and care of sick people.

Children show interest not only in themselves but in such diversified areas as accidents, disease, emotional trauma, environmental health and safety, and the health needs of the older population. They are concerned about the health problems which may afflict their parents, relatives, or older friends. The skilled teacher can relate these problems to future health considerations for the student who will progress through the grades, and later will take his place as a member of a family and of a community.

How does a teacher ascertain the interests of children? The following technique may be used:

An *interest survey* is one means of determining the major health concerns of a particular class. This approach may be implemented by having the students submit a list of topics or questions, or a list of chapters from a text. Interests vary from year to year, and from class to class, even at the same grade level. They may be due to timely events in medicine, such as heart surgery, a new vaccine, or epidemic disease, or radiation fallout, and to the background knowledge of individuals. At the high school level, a teacher may look over the results of interest surveys which have been conducted by others, but he would be wise to conduct his own with the students in each class in personal health.

Again, listen to them. What are they discussing? What are they reading? Where do they look in the health books? What subjects command their interest? Are new words and new meanings being incorporated into the vocabulary?

Personal Experiences. The experiences in which children have participated form an excellent basis for instruction. A teacher, however, should not assume that all children have been exposed to similar experiences. Knowledge and understanding of their cultural backgrounds, the mores of the community, and family patterns of living are necessary. As an example of the latter, if a family is not interested in dental health, a child may never have used a toothbrush or visited a dentist. Again, a teacher cannot help but be aware of dietary restrictions in many homes. A pupil may be lucky to have a piece of bread smeared with lard for breakfast or lunch. A piece of bread dunked in coffee may constitute a breakfast. A child from a so-called home may have no concepts of cleanliness and use of soap, combed hair, or clean clothes.

We worry about family life education, early marriages before graduation from high school, and the exceptional divorce rate which follows these marriages. If a child comes from a home where he is beaten, where alcoholism is present, and where the values of marriage and family life do not exist, how can he understand any discussion about the close ties of family life? When he grows up and responds to the sex drive, to him fulfillment of this drive may be his only interpretation of marriage because he knows no better. Neither does his girl friend. Family life education at school with its inculcation of values should start when a child starts school. Few children come from homes where there is constant sweetness and light. Hence, a teacher should never assume that all of his pupils have been exposed to similar cultural patterns. This fact will hold true even in an apparently staid, stolid community.

As for mental health, a child's wholesome emotional growth may be almost entirely reliant upon the forces in the environment at school. Learning experiences which promote mental health must be planned.

To care for the gaps in wholesome life experiences, a teacher should deliberately plan activities in which all members of the class participate. Those activities described in Healthful School Living and in School Health Services are utilized for educational purposes.

Some health experiences, however, are universal. Every person in the room knows about the common cold. In primary grades selections of content may well start with such a mutual illness as a springboard. This should unite a class in a topic of conversation which is understood by all. Facts concerning the common cold are presented early in the semester, then can be touched upon later in the year when colds are prevalent.

Capacities and Comprehension. Selection of content for health instruction should be governed by capacities of children at each age level. There should be an awareness of the stage of maturity and level of comprehension. Allowing for individual differences in growth and development of children and for their educational backgrounds, authorities still have a satisfactory understanding of levels at which specific information and experiences can be introduced. When is a child ready for the hand-washing experience? How much information on reproduction is a child capable of understanding at each age level? Instruction in sixth grade on communicable diseases is entirely different from that offered in the first grade. The materials presented to the class or the experiences which are provided must be adjusted to the capabilities and competencies of the group and of the particular student.

Public Health Needs. A program in health instruction is constructed with the public health needs in mind. Our needs are many in our complex society. Crucial health problems in the decades to come must receive attention now. Health facts may be interpreted in terms of deaths and illnesses and in the evaluation of poor living practices which produce a low level of efficiency, lack of energy, poor appearance, and undesirable mental attitudes. Surveys indicate a high incidence of serious problems arising from uncorrected remediable physical defects. There is an impulsive dependence of young and old on commercial advertising, quackery, fads, and poor health guidance. Consumer education should teach scientific health precepts to prevent the creation of hypochondriacs with their self-diagnosis and self-treatment. The efforts of the Federal Drug Administration to safeguard the health of the American people have educational implications. In cities and rural areas there still exist environmental conditions which prevent the desired goals of healthful living.

Mental illness is on the increase in every stratum of society and in every community. Mental health programs deserve high priority in all public and school health planning. Why do some states and communities have a higher divorce rate than others? Venereal diseases in teen-agers are proportionately increased. Why? Tranquilizing pills and stimulants are not permanent answers to tensions and poor social adjustments. The so-called generation gap demands an interpretation of national, community, and family living values in order to modify to some extent adolescent rebellions.

The four major causes of death in this country are heart disease, cancer, "strokes," and accidents. Management of these problems goes beyond anatomy and physiology and involves sociological, behavioral conduct as well as safety education.

Health education can justify its instructional program if its goals are set in relation to the needs of the American people, and if its results are demonstrable in the lives of children.

The content of health education is planned also around the health problems of the community and the family. Is there need of a water purification system? A sewage disposal plant? Pasteurization of milk? Slum clearance? Traffic safety? A town health council? A new traffic signal at an intersection? Aid for an indigent family?

Objectives (Desirable Outcomes). The definition of school health education in terms of individual and community health implies objectives. What do we expect a child to know in a specific area, and what should we expect as an outcome? If a unit on the effects of smoking is planned and current scientific information is presented, it is hoped that the child will make a decision not to smoke. The same philosophy holds true for use of alcohol and drugs.

Use of Basic Health Concepts. Some thoughtful health educators have concluded that an effective way to teach health education is to utilize the conceptual approach. Analysis of the wealth of health facts considered necessary as guides for promoting and maintaining good health reveals that they can be incorporated into a number of basic ideas or concepts.

The Maryland State Department of Instruction has identified and formulated concepts for the various grade levels. (See Figure 67.)

external environment

*Levels	NATURAL CONDITIONS[1+]	MAN-MADE PRODUCTS AND SERVICES[2]	SOCIAL FORCES[3]
Scope and Sequence of Growth and Development	**Conceptual Statement** The impact of natural conditions on human health correlates with man's ability and efforts to utilize, conserve, adapt to, or control the environment. **Subconceptual Statements** Natural conditions have a beneficial and/or harmful effect upon health. Man utilizes, conserves, adapts to, and/or controls natural conditions to enhance life. Decisions concerning the use, conservation, adaptation to, or control of natural conditions should be based upon man's needs and the effect of his behavior on natural conditions. Man should utilize, conserve, adapt to, and/or control natural conditions to contribute to the optimal health of himself and society.	**Conceptual Statement** The production, selection, and utilization of man-made products and services affect man's health. **Subconceptual Statements** Man creates and uses products and services that can affect health. Constant interaction of natural conditions and social forces affects the creation, alteration, and/or elimination of man-made products and services. An individual's needs and environmental influences determine his decision about the selection and utilization of man-made products and services. An individual should influence the production, selection, and utilization of man-made products and services that contribute to the optimal health of himself and society.	**Conceptual Statement** Social forces affect the physical, mental, and social health of man. **Subconceptual Statements** Existing social forces influence man's health behavior. An individual's characteristics, the nature of a social force, and the existing conditions determine his interaction with that force. An individual's decision about interacting with a social force should be based upon information about himself, the social force, and its effect upon himself and others. An individual should interact with and/or change a social force in a manner that contributes to his optimal health.
1 (K-2)	**Behavioral Objectives** 1 Given a natural condition, the learner will be able to list ways in which it may be beneficial and/or harmful to health. 2,4,5 2 Given a natural condition, the learner will be able to describe how man utilizes, conserves, adapts to, and controls it to support life. 2,4,5 3 Given a family situation which involves a natural condition, the learner will be able to list ways of utilizing, conserving, adapting to, and controlling the condition that may be beneficial and/or harmful to the health of the family or to one of its members. 2,3,4,5	**Behavioral Objectives** 1 Given a man-made product or service, the learner will be able to list its uses and classify each use as beneficial or harmful. 1,3,4,5,6 2 Given a man-made product or service which affects health, the learner will be able to list natural conditions and social forces which affect the creation, alteration, and/or elimination of this product or service and to explain how this is accomplished. 1,3 3 Given a situation in which an individual uses a man-made product or service, the learner will be able to demonstrate the feelings and behavior which might result from its use. 3,4 4 Given a description of a family pattern and the family's practice concerning a man-made product or service, the learner will be able to explain why the family selected and/or utilized the product or service. 3,5	**Behavioral Objectives** 1 Given examples of selected family, school, and peer group practices, the learner will be able to identify those which may be beneficial or harmful to health. 2,4 2 Given a description of a situation which illustrates good health or safety practices, the learner will be able to list the social forces which contribute to this situation and to explain how they contribute to health and safety. 1,2,4,5 3 Given a group of which an individual is a member and the lists of roles that individuals within each group play, the learner will be able to select those roles which he believes he plays in each group. 2,4
2 (3-5)	**Behavioral Objectives** 1 Given a natural condition, the learner will be able to describe the long and short term effects it may have on man's health. 2,3,4,5,6 2 Given a man-made product or service, the learner will be able to explain how its use affects the natural conditions of the environment. 2,3,4,5,6 3 Given a description of a community environment, the learner will be able to describe those activities conducted by man that have altered or protected natural conditions and to explain the effect of the activities upon man's health. 2,3,4,5	**Behavioral Objectives** 1 Given a man-made product and/or service, the learner will be able to list the natural conditions and/or social forces which have influenced the creation, alteration, and/or elimination of the product and/or service, to explain how this has happened, and to describe the effect on health. 1,3,4,5 2 Given a description of a family attitude and practice, the learner will be able to explain how the family group influences an individual member's choice of man-made products and services. 3,4,5,6 3 Given a case history of a man-made product or service, the learner will be able to identify the natural and social factors which influence its selection. 1,3,4,5, 4 Given a man-made product or service, the learner will be able to explain how an individual's use, non-use, or misuse can affect personal and community health and safety. 3,4,5, 5 Given a list of ways of utilizing a man-made product or service, the learner will be able to distinguish between those ways which have a beneficial effect on health and those which have a harmful effect and to explain how each occurs. 1,3,4,5,6	**Behavioral Objectives** 1 Given the role of an individual in a group with which the learner can identify, the learner will be able to explain how his behavior in this role could affect his health and the health of others. 2,4 2 Given a description of a family pattern and life style, the learner will be able to identify factors which influence the behavior of individual family members in their relationships with each other and to explain how these factors influence this behavior. 1 2,4,5,6 3 Given a list of social groups such as family, peer, school, and religious, the learner will be able to list and to compare the functions of these groups that affect the health and safety of the individual and community. 1,2,4,5,6 4 Given messages from selected mass media, the learner will be able to state the intent of the message, to explain the process by which it attempts to convey this message, and to describe what the message purports to offer to the viewer. 1,2,4,5 5 Given an opportunity to observe a family situation, the learner will be able to identify the behavior of family members which influences the acceptance or rejection of an individual family member's identity. 4 6 Given a family or peer group practice which affects health, the learner will be able to explain how an individual's behavior can influence this practice. 2,4,5
3 (6-8)	**Behavioral Objectives** 1 Given a human endeavor involving natural conditions, the learner will be able to explain how man's actions have influenced the effects of natural conditions upon his health. 2,3,4,5 2 Given a social force or a man-made product or service, the learner will be able to explain how it influences man's interaction with natural conditions. 2,3,4,6 3 Given an example of an interaction between an individual and/or a community and a natural condition, the learner will be able to describe the influence(s) of the interaction on personal and community health and to predict possible consequences. 2,3,4,6 4 Given the function of an agency which is responsible for the utilization of natural conditions, the learner will be able to describe the operations which the agency conducts to accomplish its function and to recommend alternative methods, if necessary. 2,3,4,5,6 5 Given a natural condition that affects health, the learner will be able to list ways of altering the condition to improve health and to list the advantages and disadvantages of each way of altering it. 2,3,4,5,6	**Behavioral Objectives** 1 Given a man-made product or service, the learner will be able to explain how the interaction of natural conditions and social forces causes the creation, alteration, and/or elimination of the man-made product or service. 1,3,4,5 2 Given a peer group practice which concerns the use, non-use, or misuse of a man-made product or service, the learner will be able to explain how the practice affects the creation of the product or service, and how the creation and marketing of the product or service affects the practice of the group. 3,4 3 Given an environmental factor, the learner will be able to explain its influence on the selection of man-made products and services which may be beneficial and/or harmful to health. 1,3,4,5,6 4 Given a health product or service, the learner will be able to explain how social forces, such as family, community, and religion, attempt to control its use. 3,4,5,6 5 Given a health product or service, the learner will be able to make a decision about his use or non-use of the product or service and to explain the reasons for his decision. 3,4 6 Given a natural condition, such as air or water, the learner will be able to explain how the creation, alteration, or elimination of certain man-made products and/or services alters the natural condition, and how this alteration affects health. 1,3,4,5	**Behavioral Objectives** 1 Given a local, state, national, or international health agency, the learner will be able to describe its function and to list the services which it renders. 1,2,4,5,6 2 Given a health problem in the community, the learner will be able to list those groups which contribute to the problem and those groups which attempt to alleviate it and to explain how each accomplishes this task. 1,2,4,5,6 3 Given a list of personal characteristics, such as chronological age, mental maturity, socio-economic status, and a list of social pressures exerted on behavior by individuals, groups, and institutions, the learner will be able to explain how an individual with these characteristics may respond to such pressures and to explain why. 4,5 4 Given the viewpoints expressed by peers, parents, doctors, teachers, and other individuals about a specific health practice, the learner will be able to explain how these viewpoints might influence his own behavior concerning the practice. 1,2,4,5,6 5 Given the demand of a social force, such as an ethnic, economic, or political group, the learner will be able to list the beneficial and detrimental effects that may result from a decision to accept, reject, or compromise this demand, to make such a decision, and to explain the reason for making the decision. 1,2,4,5 6 Given a community health problem and a list of social forces in a community, the learner will be able to explain what each force could contribute to a cooperative program to solve the problem. 1,2,4,5,6
4 (9-12)	**Behavioral Objectives** 1 Given a description of an interaction between man and natural conditions, the learner will be able to identify the components of the interaction and to explain how the interaction affects man's health. 2,3,4,5,6 2 Given a description of an interaction which occurs between man and natural conditions and which has a detrimental influence on health, the learner will be able to develop a plan for coping with the problem and for reversing the negative aspects of the interaction. 2,3,4 3 Given a description of the relationship of a local, state, national, or international community with a natural condition, the learner will be able to develop a plan for utilizing and protecting the natural condition in a healthful manner which requires the cooperation of the communities involved. 2,3,4 * These levels serve as a basis for planning a sequential health education program from kindergarten through grade twelve. Number' coding 1,2,3,4,5,6 indicates correlation/integration of the behavioral objectives and the interrelationships of the concepts.	**Behavioral Objectives** 1 Given a man-made product or service, the learner will be able to explain how its use, non-use, or misuse by an individual can affect his health and the health of others. 3,4,5 2 Given the local, state, and federal laws which regulate the use of a man-made product or service, the learner will be able to list the potential benefits or harmful effects that may occur to an individual and/or community if the laws are disobeyed or changed. 3,4,5 3 Given a man-made product or service, the learner will be able to list the social and economic factors which determine individual and community usage patterns and to explain how each factor influences these patterns. 3,4,5 4 Given a local, state, national, or international public health problem related to the creation, selection, and utilization of a man-made product or service, the learner will be able to list the contributions that the individual and the government can make to the solution of the problem. 1,3,4,5,6	**Behavioral Objectives** 1 Given a health problem, the learner will be able to explain the social forces which contribute to the cause and to the alleviation of the problem and to explain how they do this. 1,2,4,5,6 2 Given a local, state, national, or international public health problem, the learner will be able to cite examples whereby social forces interact to help alleviate, aggravate, or eliminate this problem and to explain how this interaction occurs. 1,2,4,5,6

Figure 67 Suggested concept goals and behavior objectives for grades k–12.

These concepts are not taught as such, but they reflect major instruction areas and give direction to curriculum planning. With a basic or key concept in mind, objectives are defined, research is done, health information is collected, subconcepts fall into line, content for

internal environment

*Levels	SENSORY STIMULATION[4]	ASSIMILATED SUBSTANCES[5]	GENETIC PERPETUATION[6]
Scope and Sequence of Growth and Development	**Conceptual Statement** Sensory stimulation can affect human growth and development. **Subconceptual Statements** The individual perceives the world around him through the senses. An individual's response to sensory stimulation is dependent upon the type of stimulation, the characteristics of the individual, and the existing conditions. Response to sensory stimulation affects an individual's growth and development. An individual utilizes sensory stimulation in his relationships with other persons and in his interaction with his environment.	**Conceptual Statement** Substances assimilated by the body can modify human growth and development. **Subconceptual Statements** The individual assimilates a variety of substances which can be beneficial and/or harmful to his growth and development. The unique response of the individual to an assimilated substance is determined by the type and quantity of the substance, the characteristics of the individual, and existing conditions. An individual's decision about the use of an assimilated substance should be based upon information concerning himself, the substance, and its effect upon him and others. An individual should use assimilated substances that contribute to his growth and development.	**Conceptual Statement** Genetic perpetuation forms the basis for man's growth and development. **Subconceptual Statements** Most living things are capable of reproducing their own kind. Certain characteristics of living things are inherited. Patterns of growth and development are predictable within limits but are unique for each individual. Genetic endowment interacting with the environment affects man's growth and development.
1 (K-2)	**Behavioral Objectives** 1 Given the names of the sense organs, the learner will be able to describe the function and care of each one. 2,3,5 2 Given an array of objects in the immediate environment, the learner will be able to describe the characteristics of each object and to state which sense organs provide him with this information. 2,3,5 3 Given examples of sensations and perceptions, the learner will be able to distinguish between them. 2,3 4 Given a sensory stimulus which is perceived by two or more individuals, the learner will be able to describe the reaction of each individual to the stimulus. 3 5 Given the reaction of an individual to a sensory stimulus, the learner will be able to explain the effect of this reaction on other people. 3,5	**Behavioral Objectives** 1 Given models of substances that may be assimilated, such as food, medicine, and household solutions, the learner will be able to select those that are beneficial to growth and development and to state their purpose. 1,2,4 2 Given a list of assimilated substances, the learner will be able to identify those which must be used only under supervision and to explain why. 2,4 3 Given an assimilated substance, the learner will be able to describe or demonstrate feelings and behavior that may result from using it. 2,3,4 4 Given an assimilated substance, the learner will be able to describe safe handling and storage procedures. 2,3,4 5 Given a list or display of assimilated substances which includes items appropriate for human beings and animals, the learner will be able to identify those substances which are appropriate for human beings, those appropriate for animals, and those which may be appropriate for both. 2,4 6 Given a description of different family patterns, the learner will be able to describe a variety of practices in the use of assimilated substances. 2,3,4	**Behavioral Objectives** 1 Given a series of models or pictures of living things, the learner will be able to match the parents with appropriate offspring. 1 2 Given a description of a living thing at two different stages of development, the learner will be able to cite changes in physical size and in physical features which indicate individual growth and development. 1,5 3 Given a description of an individual, the learner will be able to identify characteristics which are important to total growth and development and to explain why they are important. 3,4
2 (3-5)	**Behavioral Objectives** 1 Given a stimulus, the learner will be able to explain the difference between what he senses and what he perceives. 1,2,3,5,6 2 Given the same stimulus under different environmental conditions, the learner will be able to explain the difference between what he perceives in each situation. 1,2,3,5,6 3 Given a list of body systems, the learner will be able to compare the effects of a sensory stimulus on their functions and structures. 5,6 4 Given a sense, the learner will be able to describe ways in which it may be conserved in order to function effectively and efficiently. 2,3,5 5 Given a situation involving interaction among individuals, the learner will be able to identify perceptions of individuals in the group and to explain how they influenced the interaction. 1,2,3,5,6	**Behavioral Objectives** 1 Given a list of foods, the learner will be able to classify each food according to its basic food group and to identify the function of each group. 1,2,4 2 Given a body system, the learner will be able to describe its function and its reaction to various assimilated substances. 2,6 3 Given a non-food substance, the learner will be able to list beneficial effects of proper use and harmful effects of misuse of the substance. 1,3,4,6 4 Given an assimilated substance, the learner will be able to explain how an individual's use, non-use, or misuse of the substance can affect his health. 2,3,4,6 5 Given a variety of foods, the learner will be able to select a balanced diet. 2,4 6 Given an environmental factor (either external or internal), such as family, peers, personality, or physiological condition, the learner will be able to explain how this factor can influence one's use, non-use, or misuse of assimilated substances. 1 2 3 4 6	**Behavioral Objectives** 1 Given a living thing, the learner will be able to describe the way it reproduces. 3,4 2 Given a description of a cell of a living organism, the learner will be able to explain how living things transmit inherited characteristics. 1,2,4 3 Given a list of human characteristics, the learner will be able to distinguish between those that are inherited and those that are acquired. 1,2,3,4,5 4 Given a description of individuals of the same chronological age, the learner will be able to identify their similarities and differences and to explain the possible reasons for any differences. 1,2,3,4,5 5 Given a description or diagram of the reproductive systems, the learner will be able to identify their parts and to describe their development and their function. 4
3 (6-8)	**Behavioral Objectives** 1 Given a sensory stimulus, the learner will be able to describe ways of developing his perception of the sensation. 2,3,5 2 Given an emotion, the learner will be able to describe the effects of the emotion on an individual. 3 3 Given a sensory stimulus in contrasting environments, the learner will be able to identify how his responses differed in each environment and to explain why this happened. 1,2,3,5,6 4 Given a description of an individual's response to a sensory stimulus in the presence of others, the learner will be able to describe the effects of his response on his relationships with other people. 3	**Behavioral Objectives** 1 Given a list of statements concerning the physical appearance, action, use, and misuse of assimilated substances, the learner will be able to discriminate between those statements which are based upon verifiable evidence and those which have no known factual basis. 2,4 2 Given the stages of habituation to a specific drug, the learner will be able to describe conditions that modify the progression from one stage to another in either direction. 2,3,4,6 3 Given an assimilated substance and a number of social forces such as family, community, and religion, the learner will be able to describe the process by which each force attempts to control an individual's use of the substance. 2,3,4 4 Given a list of foods representative of a variety of cultures and ethnic groups, the learner will be able to plan a balanced diet. 1,2,4 5 Given a social force such as occupation, fashion, or family, and an assimilated substance, the learner will be able to explain how the social force may affect an individual's use, non-use, and misuse of the assimilated substance. 2,3,4 6 Given a list of the ways in which peer groups use an assimilated substance, the learner will be able to identify those practices which are beneficial and those which are detrimental to health and to explain why. 2,3,4,6	**Behavioral Objectives** 1 Given the stages in the reproductive cycle of human beings, the learner will be able to arrange these stages in sequence from conception to birth and to describe the processes that occur at each stage. 3,4 2 Given the genetically determined characteristics of parents, the learner will be able to predict the possible inherited characteristics in offspring and to cite data to support these predictions. 3,4 3 Given a human characteristic, the learner will be able to describe how it grows and develops during life and to explain the reasons for the changes from stage to stage. 1,2,3,4,5 4 Given a factor that influences growth and development, the learner will be able to describe ways in which this factor can be modified and to explain the effect of the modification upon individual growth and development. 1,2,3,4,5 5 Given a practice conducted in a social group, such as peer, family, or community, the learner will be able to explain how this practice affects an individual's maturation during puberty. 1,2,3,4,5
4 (9-12)	**Behavioral Objectives** 1 Given a sensory stimulus in a specific environment, the learner will be able to explain how the stimulus can be used to achieve an effective relationship with the environment. 1,2,3,5,6 2 Given a sensory stimulus in a specific environment, the learner will be able to list the possible responses an individual may make to it, and to explain the possible effect that each response may have on an individual's growth and development and on his relationships with other people. 1,2,3,5,6	**Behavioral Objectives** 1 Given an assimilated substance, the learner will be able to list its source and component parts and to describe its effects on the body. 1,2,4,6 2 Given an assimilated substance, the learner will be able to describe the physical and chemical processes which occur in the body from the entry point of the assimilated substance to its effective point of utilization. 2,4 3 Given the local, state, and/or federal laws regulating the use of assimilated substances, the learner will be able to list the potential benefits or harmful effects to an individual and/or community if the laws are disobeyed or changed. 1,3,4 4 Given an assimilated substance, the learner will be able to list social and economic factors that affect or are affected by the use of the substance and to explain how these effects are beneficial or harmful to individual and community health. 1,2,3,4 5 Given the social, economic, environmental, medical, and/or legal problems which are caused by or which result from the use of an assimilated substance, the learner will be able to develop a comprehensive plan of action designed to alleviate these problems. 1,2,3,4 6 Given the local, state, national, or international health problems associated with a specific assimilated substance, the learner will be able to list the roles that individuals and appropriate governmental agencies play in the solutions to these problems and to explain the effectiveness of each agency. 1,2,3,4,6 7 Given a situation involving the interaction of an individual with an assimilated substance, the learner will be able to describe the individual's action and to explain the reason for this action. 1,2,3,4,6	**Behavioral Objectives** 1 Given a description of an individual's characteristics and his family and environmental background, the learner will be able to identify those hereditary and environmental factors which appear to influence the individual's unique growth and development. 1,2,3,4,5 2 Given a problem concerning genetic perpetuation, the learner will be able to develop a plan which is designed to alleviate the problem. 1,2,3,4,5 3 Given a factor that influences human inheritance, the learner will be able to make a personal decision concerning human propagation and to explain how it improves the quality of life. 1,2,3,4,5

Figure 67 (Continued)

their support is selected, and methods of presentation are determined —all of this is done so that a pupil can develop his own concepts. As stated in the first paragraphs of this chapter, the ultimate objective of health education is to stimulate a pupil to think for himself, critically and objectively, when health knowledge, attitudes, and practices are concerned.

To accomplish this objective, one must also teach the student to distinguish between rational and irrational thinking on his part. Much of our philosophy of education has been based upon the premise that the human being will always be rational in his thinking, and this is not true. Therefore, time must be devoted to creating a rational appreciation of the concept while stimulating him to think for himself.

Contributions from the Sciences. A health education curriculum is as broad or as limited in its content as the knowledge provided by the sciences. Successful research on poliomyelitis and measles vaccines increased the subject content in the area of immunology. In time, research on cancer will produce the long-awaited explanation of its cause, prevention, and control. Such findings will alter the nation's health pattern most vitally. Cancer is the second leading cause of death in this country. Needless to say, health instruction on this subject will then be more positive and meaningful. Observations made by the scientists on the effects of smoking and dependence-producing drugs are pertinent to the health of each individual.

Contributions of Specialists in Health Education. The content of a health education program is broadened by the contributions of specialists in health education, child development, and school health education. Among their accomplishments are publications (health books for children, textbooks, and manuals) and services as consultants in curriculum planning, as well as contributions to workshops and conferences on various phases of school health. These specialists may represent any of the various agencies concerned with health: departments of health or education, natural bureaus involved with the same areas, teacher education institutions, voluntary groups, or private industry.

The Background and Experience of the Teacher. The background and preparation of a teacher will influence his selection of course content. His own knowledge, attitudes, and practices will determine his effectiveness in health instruction. Every teacher who discusses health problems should have a general background in anatomy, physiology, personal health, including mental health, family life education, community health problems, and health problems of children. These are obtained in undergraduate college courses, in personal readings, and from in-service classes. The biases and prejudices of teachers should not be inflicted upon pupils. Teachers must be sure not only that what they teach is accepted scientific fact, but that they do not omit necessary information. One who does not believe in the principles of immunology will either not present the subject or will do so only with faint encouragement.

Suggested Content

From an analysis of the considerations discussed in selection of content, a fairly universal agreement on major health areas is usually reached. The Curriculum Commission of the School Health Education Division, American Association for Health, Physical Education, and Recreation recognized the following topics in anticipation of the crucial health problems of the next decade: accident prevention, aging, alcohol, disaster preparedness, disease and disease control, economics of health care, environmental conditions (water supplies, food protection, occupational health, air pollution), ionizing radiation, evaluation of health information, family health, international health, mental health, nutrition, and smoking.

The curriculum proposed by the New York State Education Department, following the legislation of 1967 proposed STRANDS which should affect knowledge, attitudes, and behavior to produce optimal health:

Strand I. PHYSICAL HEALTH. Individual Health Status, Nutrition, Sensory Perception, Dental Health, Fitness and Body Dynamics.
Strand II. SOCIOLOGICAL HEALTH PROBLEMS. Smoking and Health, Alcohol Education, Drugs and Narcotic Education, Disease Prevention.
Strand III. MENTAL HEALTH. Personality Development, Sexuality, Family Life, Education.
Strand IV. ENVIRONMENTAL AND COMMUNITY HEALTH. Environmental Health, Public Health, World Health, Epidemiology, Ecology, Consumer Health.
Strand V. EDUCATION FOR SURVIVAL. Safety, First-Aid, Catastrophe Survival.[11]

Syllabi were published, covering these strands with curriculum guides from grades one to twelve.

The preceding curricula present a somewhat similar identification of broad health problems. Practically all state boards of education plan their own curriculum guides for use in their schools. The exact outline and wording of health concepts can vary. What is important is the provision of adequate information on crucial health problems and the stimulation to influence their health attitudes and practices in the promotion of good health for themselves, their families, and society.

The School Health Education Study found from its survey that certain topics were widely taught in elementary and secondary schools: accident prevention, cleanliness and grooming, dental health, food and nutrition, and exercise and relaxation. Neglected crucial problems were venereal diseases, international health, consumer education, noncommunicable diseases, and sex education.

---

[11]"Critical Health Problems Legislation." *J.O.H.P.E.R.* 39:12, 1968.

Curriculum Organization

A curriculum should be organized to assure continuity, sequence, and integration. Fodor and Dalis feel that the principles of curriculum organization should reflect a concern for the learner and for the subject matter being developed.[12] The material to be presented to any group must be selected with an understanding of physical maturation, stage of mental maturity, and level of comprehension. It must be based upon an appreciation of the physical, social, emotional, and intellectual needs of children in their various stages of growth and development, upon the concepts of health which they have acquired, and upon their basic curiosities and interests. The readiness of children to accept certain information and experiences will determine the grade levels where these will be given. Also, placement of a subject or problem may vary somewhat in correlated sources. Students may evince more curiosity in one course than in another, and discussion will come sooner.

Any curriculum planning must avoid duplication of material in various grades and departments. Repetition breeds a negative attitude and boredom. A child does not want to hear the same refrain on teeth year after year. He does not want to see the same films again and again. He may walk from a class in health education to one in biology, chemistry, or physiology and be handed the same information on vitamins, alcohol, tobacco, or drugs. Such repeat performances will militate against an enthusiastic reception of ideas or any change in attitudes or practices. As one college freshman complained: "Please don't discuss drugs. In high school I had to write a research paper for one class, get up and discuss the problem in another, and prepare posters for a third. I am sick and tired of the subject." The drug problem has been discussed in high schools in the following classes: physiology, biology, sociology, psychology, home economics, health education, home making, and government. Teachers in these classes apparently feel a responsibility to discuss the problem. Here is a specific instance in which these teachers should plan in advance the placements of content and exactly what contribution or approach need be made in each course to the overall problem of drug dependence and drug abuse.

In the primary grades children are more receptive to instruction which emphasizes healthful practices. In the fifth and sixth grades, even though practices are still stressed, the opportunity to develop a wholesome attitude is used to reinforce health education objectives. Junior high school students are a group whose idealism is important in furthering these objectives. More factual information may be introduced in health teaching. The students in senior high school have matured to the degree that comprehension of scientific knowledge should provide the basis of health practices.

---

[12]John T. Fodor and Gus T. Dalis: *Health Instructor: Theory and Application.* Second edition. Philadelphia: Lea & Febiger, 1974, pp. 92–93.

Sometimes a topic is taught at one level, then skipped for a time, only to be repeated on a more advanced level with a different emphasis or interpretation. This is done in order to emphasize content appropriate to a student's comprehension and changed interests. This point is illustrated later in the chapter with the schedule of health content and teaching emphasis in junior and senior high schools. In addition, health information should be available at many levels of comprehesion through different media to provide an opportunity for all students to find a means which is acceptable to them. Our best guide is always the student's interest.

Planning a health education curriculum should be continuous throughout the year and from year to year, with a coordinated program of defined scope in progressive sequence.

Health Education in Kindergarten and Primary Grades
(Building Habits and Practices)

How much should a child know about health by the time he finishes the third grade? What can we reasonably expect in the way of desirable attitudes and practices? How is health teaching planned in the first three grades in order to fulfill these expectations?

The measure of success in health instruction is its influence on the life of an individual. In primary grades the approach for this success is through developing favorable attitudes and practices. Just enough factual information is given so that a child can understand "why." This information should serve as a vehicle for learning experiences which, if properly planned, will lead him to formulate the intended concepts. These in turn should be translated into desirable habits and practices. Instructional emphasis requires that special effort be made to cooperate with the home and community.

A small child is primarily interested in his environment, in his activities, and in being comfortable. He is imitative, is interested in people, and is influenced by examples.

In primary grades the health teacher is the classroom teacher. He must have basic objectives or a basic plan clearly in mind, even though health teaching in these grades is largely incidental, and based upon everyday living. It is correlated with the day's living, either in topics discussed, experiences, environment, or services. A New York school district has developed a resource center for kindergarten children which ties health topics to a mock-up of a health office.[13] Health teaching is a daily affair in kindergarten and first grade. There will be work units in the second and third grades.

Common experiences of the school day are: travel to and from

---

[13]Lorraine Benngsohn, Ruth Stanley, and Eugene Kolack: "A Health Education Resource Center for Kindergarten." *J. Sch. Health 43*:2:128–130, February, 1973.

school, school lunch, health appraisal, absenteeism for illness, an episode of illness while at school, weighing and measuring, tests for vision and hearing, toileting, dressing for playground activity during inclement weather, injuries, immunizations, care of pets in the classroom, visiting a school nurse, physician, or dentist, rest, play, talking over the birth of a new baby in the family, making friends, and adjusting from the freedom of home to the routine of school life.

Suggested Content

Safety. At school, to and from school, and at home.

Care of Eyes, Nose, Ears, Teeth, Skin, Hair. Oral cleanliness, significance of earaches, defects of vision and hearing, visits to dentist and physician.

Exercise, Sleep, Rest, Posture. Importance of sleep. Rest alternating with exercise.

Cleanliness and Grooming. Responsibility for self-care, toileting practices.

Nutrition and Food Habits. Selection of wholesome foods, relationship to growth. Social practices.

Communicable Disease Control. Personal hygienic habits in handling common cold, immunizations, protection from diseases, appropriate care.

Problems of Weather and Dress. Appropriate clothing, avoidance of chilling and getting wet.

Local Community Relationships. Home, school, neighborhoods —their contributions to healthful, safe living.

Building a Foundation for Mental Health. Emotional adjustment to the school environment and to peer group.

It is necessary to promote those practices which are beneficial and correct the faulty ones brought from home. A child learns by precept; he learns from what he sees and does and somewhat from what he is told. At school he is exposed to a healthful way of life; his day revolves around healthful practices and elementary concepts about hygienic care of the body. He may need to be taught how to use the drinking fountain and the toilet room. In the first and second grades he also secures some basic information from primer readers.

Health knowledge should support practices substantially by the time a child enters the third grade. Readers should be provided which explore the area of health. By the end of the third grade children should be expected to appreciate growth as a sign of good health, the relationship of food to growth, the relationship between feeling well and a hygienic regimen, and standards of conduct for healthful living, including knowledge of the spread of communicable diseases. During these three or four years the health unit sequences must be progressive. This means cooperative planning of teachers in these grades.

Health Education in Intermediate Grades

The intermediate grades (fourth, fifth, and sixth) represent a transition during which emphasis is changed from "how" to do things to "why." The child must have an understanding of "why," i.e., why he should appreciate good health, why he should want good health, the advantages and disadvantages of good and poor health. Children are becoming more interested in others, so that units on community health and accident prevention are appropriate. Many problems of living can be examined in terms of their causes and the proper steps which may be taken towards their solution. Information gained from the teacher, the health reader, the encyclopedia, and various other educational media should serve as a basis from which pupils develop their own concepts. A child should be prepared to show his understanding in terms of action. He assumes responsibility for his own behavior and can be critical of the action of others.

In the intermediate grades the health instruction program should be planned with a definite amount of time allotted to subject matter. This time to be devoted to health problems is often specified by official regulations. The placement of health teaching in the daily schedule should be flexible. Health instruction may be integrated with science, language arts, nature study, or social studies. In most elementary schools teaching within a classroom is directed by a single instructor, who may present health information in one or many of these areas, alone or concurrently, whenever the teaching will be most effective and meaningful. Health topics are commonly interwoven with science. Blocks of time may be devoted to health education alone, followed by a space, then be tied in with the science and social studies programs. Organization varies.

The health education curriculum for these three grades stresses the need for more factual information, outlines what a child is expected to know in each grade, and suggests experiences which will enrich the program.

It is interesting to observe how far afield a discussion may wander from an original experience. Several children in a fourth-grade science class were watching a piece of crumpled tin foil which was floating on water in a basin. Why does it float? Because of air. One child comments, "That's what happens when I swim. I don't sink because I have air in me." Where is the air? In the lungs. How does it get there? Where are the lungs? What do they look like? The health readers will provide further information. The teacher may even buy a set of animal lungs with attached bronchial tubes and trachea from the market and bring them to school the next day. The lungs can be inflated with air.

In the intermediate grades health teaching continues the emphasis on health practices made in the primary grades and, in addition, provides factual information.

SUGGESTED CONTENT

Organs of the Human Body. Their functions and their care—eyes, ears, teeth, heart, lung, reproductive system, etc. An innovative curriculum where each unit is organized around a body system has been developed.[14] The response has been enthusiastic and the results excellent.

Nutrition and Growth.
Exercise, Rest, Posture.
Safety and First Aid.
Effects of Alcohol, Tobacco, and Drugs in the Human Body.
Disease Prevention in Individual and Community.
Health Services in the Community.
Emotional and Social Health Problems, Including Sex Education.

The fourth-grade child is much more mature than he was in the primary grades and assumes greater responsibility for his own activities at school, in the neighborhood, and at home. Based upon their understanding, fourth-grade children should be able to accept responsibility for the following: (1) acceptable toileting habits, (2) selection of food at meals and between meals, (3) rest and relaxation, (4) safety, both personal and in relation to others, (5) care of eyes, (6) sufficient sleep, (7) care of teeth, (8) prevention of overexposure to sun, wind, rain, and other elements, (9) selection of clothing in relation to weather conditions, and (10) doing his share in maintaining a clean home environment. A child should have such competencies as skill and strength in muscular activities and an acceptable vocabulary in regard to parts of the body and health topics.

The course of study for fifth and sixth grades continues these emphases. Because the menarche (onset of menstrual function) may occur at age ten or 11, girls of this age should have definite information on the physiology of the reproductive system. Safety education introduces the new problem of training in bicycle riding. More responsibilities for individual behavior can be imposed. A more scientific approach, more reason, more discussion, more use of teaching material, and a greater variety of presentations are possible. Health committees and health clubs may be organized. These encourage children to participate in planning the curriculum. They can search for health problems and proceed through the various steps of problem solving to better information, attitudes, and practices.

Here again, instructional emphasis focuses upon the development in each student of basic health attitudes and practices. Special effort is made to secure the cooperation of home and community.

Health Education in Junior High School

In the seventh, eighth, and ninth grades the objectives of health education and the criteria for the selection of content still dictate the

[14]Roy L. Davis: "Making Health Education Relevant and Exciting in Elementary and Junior High School." *Health Serv. Report* 88:2:99–105, February, 1973.

curriculum. Many schools are experimenting with a "middle school" concept which has sixth, seventh and eighth graders together. However, a number of other grade groupings are also being tried. Junior high school students gather from a number of neighborhoods so that there is a diversity of health cultural patterns. These students are confronted with problems related to growth, physical changes, sexual maturation, and emotional changes. New problems and anxieties arise—group acceptance, heterosexual relationships, grooming, acne vulgaris, home conflicts in the drive toward independence—coupled with highly emotional attitudes and concerns directed toward themselves and their peers.

Health education teachers in junior high school are most often the physical education teachers. Science teachers also fulfill this role. Occasionally, teachers from the related fields of homemaking and social studies teach health education. Fortunately, opportunities are being increased for teachers who have specialized in health education.

In the departmentalized junior high school, health subject matter may be taught in several areas. However, if health teaching is offered in this diffused fashion only, emphasis which will motivate desirable health outcomes will probably be lost, so there will be omissions of necessary health information and experiences. Although information continues to be given in various courses, a scheduled health education course (health instruction, health science instruction) should be required. Some authorities recommend a daily class for one year. Minimum recommended requirement is one semester in the seventh or eighth grade, approximately 90 hours of instruction.

Since students have had varied preparations in health education in elementary schools, it would be wise to conduct pretests before starting new working units in junior high school. In this way repetition may be avoided and more time made available for introducing new material. The health education teacher also consults with instructors in related areas to ascertain the content of their courses. (See the schedule which follows later in this chapter on subject matter correlation and teaching emphasis.)

In junior high school instructional emphasis is focused upon personal health. Basic medical information must be taught. Common misconceptions should be corrected. Here again, opportunities are planned for experiences which will utilize health and safety facts. There should be individualization of instruction as much as possible. Instruction and learning experiences should be varied sufficiently to meet a student's needs in order for him to reach the concepts desired.

Suggested Content (Personal Health)

Personal Health and Fitness. On a more advanced level than in elementary grades, with an understanding of the medical and scientific bases for health practices. Problems concerned with eyes, ears, reproductive systems, respiratory systems, and other parts of the body, fatigue, recreation, exercise.

Nutrition. Scientific facts, research, selection of well-balanced diet, food fallacies.

Communicable Diseases. Causes, methods of spread, prevention, immunizations, care.

Growing into Maturity. Explanation of physical and emotional changes of adolescence to allay anxieties and promote understanding. Social relationships.

Emotional and Mental Health. The nervous system and its function. Emotions. The healthy personality.

Alcohol, Tobacco, Narcotics, and other Drugs. Emotional, physical implications, cost of use, relation to delinquency.

Safety and First Aid. Safety in all aspects of living. First aid. Civil defense program.

Health Misconceptions. Common misconceptions.

Cooperative Community Health. Fluoridation of water, air pollution, water purification, sewage disposal, communicable disease control, care of milk, community health agencies.

Health Education in Senior High School

In senior high school the adolescent is more mature in intellectual judgment as well as in physical development. He needs education and guidance in making enlightened choices of health behavior, for both immediate and future needs.

Orientation in health education differs from that in junior high school. Assuming that a student has had basic information in personal health and has accepted responsibility for his own physical welfare, the emphasis in curriculum for the older adolescent shifts to consumer health and to health problems which will concern him when he moves into the adult world.

One semester is recommended in grades 10, 11, or 12—approximately 90 hours of instruction.

Suggested Content (Consumer Health)

"1. *Emotional and Mental Health* (emotions, being acceptable to others and to self, facing reality, individual differences, the mentally healthy, the mentally unhealthy)

2. *Tobacco and Health* (composition of tobacco smoke, physiological effects, smoking and disease, cost in lives, health and dollars, tobacco advertising, tobacco education programs in other countries)

3. *Alcohol and Health* (physiological effects, emotional and mental effects, alcoholism, alcoholic beverage advertising)

4. *Drugs and Health* (depressing and stimulating drugs, glue sniffing, etc.)

5. *Personal Health & Fitness* (vital organs and their care through-

out adult life, exercise and physical fitness, body mechanics and posture)

6. *Problems of Life Conservation* (degenerative diseases—cancer, heart disease, arthritis, strokes, etc., health problems of adult life)

7. *Myths and Truths About Nutrition and Weight* (problems of food fads, vitamin pills, diet supplements, problems of overweight, fraudulent reducing schemes, potions, devices, etc.)

8. *Preventing Disease* (family immunization programs, body defenses, common respiratory infections, some specific disease problems, drugs and medicines)

9. *Consumer Health* (choice of professional help, medical and health quackery, Food and Drug Act, Food and Drug Administration, health and advertising of so-called "health" products)

10. *Physical and Emotional Understanding of Sex* (emotional health aspects of sex, perpetuation of the race, health issues of pregnancy, venereal diseases, problems of illegitimacy."[15]

The following schedule[16] illustrates the teaching emphasis in health education and subject matter correlation between health education and other subjects in the secondary school curriculum. It was formulated by representatives from curriculum committees in homemaking, science, social studies, driver education, and health and physical education in a State Department of Education. Ten dominant health problems were analyzed for component topics. The selected major area for handling the topic is in italics. Note at which level information is introduced or emphasized.

---

[15]Reproduced with permission from Utah State Department of Education.

[16]Permission to reproduce granted by State Department of Education, State of Utah.

HEALTH EDUCATION CONTENT	"PERSONAL HEALTH" JUNIOR HIGH	"CONSUMER HEALTH" SENIOR HIGH
Personal Health and Fitness		
Skin care and cleanliness	*Health,* Homemaking	Homemaking
Care of eyes, ears, nose, throat, teeth	*Health,* Science	*Health*
Body systems	*Health,* Science	Physiology, Biology
Sleep and rest	*Health*	Homemaking
Exercise and fitness	*Health,* Physical Education	*Health,* Physical Education, Biology
Body mechanics and posture	*Health,* Physical Education	Physical Education, Biology, Physics
Nutrition		
Food utilization	*Health,* Science	
Basic foods	*Health,* Homemaking	Homemaking
Choosing a balanced diet	*Health,* Homemaking	Homemaking
Undernutrition and overnutrition	*Health,* Homemaking	Homemaking
Food fads and diet quackery		*Health,* Homemaking
Overweight		*Health,* Homemaking
Overweight frauds and quackery		*Health,* Homemaking
Food and drug laws; enforcement; violations		*Health,* Homemaking, Social Studies

(*Table continued on following page.*)

Health Education Content	"Personal Health" Junior High	"Consumer Health" Senior High
Emotional and Mental Health		
Emotions	*Health*, Science	*Health*, Social Studies
Nutritional needs of a healthy nervous system	*Health*	
How the nervous system works	*Health*, Science	Physiology
Individual differences	*Health*, Science	*Health*
Becoming acceptable to self	*Health*, Homemaking	*Health*, Social Studies
Becoming acceptable to others	*Health*, Homemaking	*Health*, Social Studies
Facing reality		*Health*, Social Studies
Characteristics of the mentally healthy		*Health*, Social Studies
Problems of mental ill health		*Health*, Social Studies
Preventing Disease		
Germ theory of disease	*Health*, Science	Biology
Types of infections	*Health*, Science	Biology
Immunization	*Health*, Science, Social Studies	*Health*, Biology
Body defenses	*Health*	*Health*, Biology
Specific disease problems	*Health*, Social Studies	*Health*, Biology
Drugs and medicines		*Health*, Biology
Maturation		
Endocrine glands	*Health*	Biology
Secondary sex characteristics	*Health*	
Attitude toward the opposite sex	*Health*, Social Studies, Homemaking	*Health*
Courtship, maturation and emotional health		*Health*, Homemaking, Social Studies
Perpetuation of the race		*Health*, Social Studies
Common health issues of pregnancy		*Health*, Homemaking
Venereal diseases	*Health*, Social Studies	*Health*, Social Studies
Consumer Health		
Common health misconceptions	*Health*	
Health related advertising	*Health*, Language Arts	*Health*
Choosing medical help		*Health*
Medical fraud and quackery		*Health*
Medical and physical exams		*Health*
Problems of Life Conservation		
Life expectancy		*Health*
Heart and circulatory diseases of adult life		*Health*
Cancer		*Health*
Tuberculosis		*Health*

(Table continued on opposite page.)

Methods in Health Education

Instruction in health education, as it recognizes the interests and goals of the individual and society, should be dynamic. Teaching in the area of health education should follow methods and educational philosophies similar to those in the other disciplines.

The Incidental Approach

The incidental approach embraces all of a child's experience in his daily living which should contribute to his education for health.

HEALTH EDUCATION CONTENT	"PERSONAL HEALTH" JUNIOR HIGH	"CONSUMER HEALTH" SENIOR HIGH
Diabetes		*Health*
Arthritis		*Health*
Health agencies		*Health*, Social Studies
Alcohol and Health		
Physiological effects	*Health*, Science	*Health*
Emotional and mental effects	*Health*	*Health*
Sociological problems of alcohol		Social Studies
Safety problems of alcohol		Driver Education
Alcoholism	*Health*	*Health*, Social Studies
Advertising and alcohol	*Health*	*Health*
Tobacco and Health		
Makeup of tobacco smoke	*Health*, Science	*Health*
Physiological effects	*Health*, Science	*Health*
Smoking and disease	*Health*	*Health*
Advertising and tobacco	*Health*, Language Arts	*Health*
Drugs and Health		
Depressant drugs	*Health*	*Health*
Stimulating drugs	*Health*	*Health*
Cooperative Community Health		
Air	*Health*, Science	Social Studies
Water	*Health*, Science	Social Studies
Food contamination	*Health*, Homemaking	Homemaking, Social Studies, Biology
Sewage	*Health*, Science	Social Studies
Garbage – collection and disposal	*Health*, Science	Social Studies
Milk	*Health*, Science	Social Studies
Pest control	*Health*, Science	Social Studies, Biology
Community voluntary and official agencies	*Health*, Social Studies	Social Studies
Safety and First Aid		
First aid	*Health*	
Medical self-help		*Health*
Civil defense	*Health*, Social Studies	Homemaking
Safety at home	*Health*, Homemaking	Homemaking
Safety on farm and in the yard	*Health*, Industrial Arts, Vocational Agriculture	Vocational Agriculture
Gun safety	*Health*, Industrial Arts	Physical Education
Outdoor safety	*Health*	

Teaching is done *at the time of the experience* or when an experience or health problem is mentioned.

The screening examinations for vision and hearing, the preparation for the health examination and the examination itself, the project of measuring height and weight, immunization procedures, service as a patrolman, service on health councils, the school lunch program – these are only a few of the experiences at school which influence health knowledge, attitudes, or conduct. "Incidental" health education is important; it goes on all of the time at school; it is a quiet way to influence a child's health. Every teacher in a school participates in this type of health education. It is impossible to avoid it because so many situations at school have health implications.

A child's experiences outside school which involve his health are also to be included in his total health education—activities, such as visits to the family physician or dentist, discussions of family health problems, first aid and safety education in Scout work, listening and learning from television and radio programs on health topics, reading about health problems in the newspapers and magazines, and observing and participating in community health projects. Individual health counseling or guidance is another example of incidental teaching. These experiences may prompt an informal type of educational situation, or they may be incorporated into well-planned units of instruction.

Incidental health education, however, is neither adequate nor comprehensive. This type of instruction may omit many important competencies. Not only will important aspects of health knowledge be missed, but it is quite possible that the information acquired will not be integrated into a way of life, as manifested by desirable attitudes and practices. Just to mention some incident or experience with health implications may leave a superficial impression. It must be tied in with serious study.

The Planned Approach

The planned, organized, direct approach to health teaching and curriculum development recognizes health education as a discipline, provides basic knowledge, and encourages the attitudes and practices essential for healthful living, for healthful living of the individual, the home, and the community. The health education curriculum should be a continuous, progressive program from kindergarten through high school.

In kindergarten and first grade health teaching is scheduled daily and tends to be incidental. In the second and third grades a work unit is presented, followed by a space in time and then by another work unit. In the intermediate grades a block of time is devoted to health education. Then blocks of time are tied in with the science program alternating with the social studies program. In junior high school and senior high school scheduled health courses are examples of direct instruction. Or, the health information organized into teaching units is utilized in related fields, after careful planning by the instructors involved.

A teacher chooses methods and techniques which will do the job best and ones with which he is comfortable. Successful teaching depends upon careful organization, with preferable use of teaching units and lesson plans. This is done ahead of time. Having planned the content for the semester or year, a teacher works out his own units or he uses and modifies those already prepared. He should know what audiovisual aids and literature are available, what authorities may be invited as guest speakers, what resources exist in the community, what experiences are common to many of the students, what experiences he should plan, and what materials may be used for demonstration purposes. Since the teacher's schedule should be flexible within a basic structure, he may present an immediate problem, pulled out of a previously planned sequence. For instance, it his class is scheduled to have audiometric tests on a certain day, he can start a unit on hearing, discuss the mechanics of hearing, the importance of good hearing, the significance of an earache as an emergency illness requiring skillful medical care, and the value of early detection of impaired hearing. If he is successful in his teaching, the youngsters and their parents will follow through with recommendations from the tests.

A *method* refers to the procedure to be used in presenting educational materials to students. Another way of defining a method is: a procedure used to provide the student with experiences which will create understandings and involve him in health issues and decisions. There is no best way of teaching. Each topic requires that the teacher select the most fitting method or combination of methods which will stimulate interests and promote effective health teaching. A teacher must appreciate the fact that health education, as a discipline, occupies a peculiar position. More than acquisition of knowledge is involved. The objective is not simply to acquire isolated facts on anatomy and physiology or fragments of health information. Rather, through the factual information received and the planned learning experiences, a child should formulate certain concepts and arrive at some meaningful conclusions. The difficult task may be to motivate him to react in such fashion that, if necessary, he can adopt changed attitudes and practices. This may mean a whole change in the family pattern of living, for opinions on health and health practices are deeply ingrained in a family. Or, an individual may be resistant to some acceptable health practices, in spite of parental nagging. He may resist eating certain foods or brushing his teeth. Such situations are challenges to teaching skills.

Uses of the following methods are suggested:

The Lecture Method. This method is probably the oldest method of teaching. Factual information and explanations can be made concisely and fairly quickly. The lecture should be the springboard for further exploration, discussion, decision-making, and formulation of concepts.

The Problem-Solving Method. This method is used in handling either individual or group health problems. Health teaching on an *individual* basis (health guidance) depends upon an understanding of the problem and working out the best method of handling it. A child with poor hearing is placed in the seat where he can hear best, and has extra attention paid to his assignments and written work. He is taught to adjust to his handicap.

Problem Solving in a Group Situation. This is a basic teaching skill, is highly effective, and includes other methods to be described. It involves the following steps:

> The problem is selected. It is presented to the class for discussion. Students themselves may bring up the problem as the result of their observations or experiences.
>
> The problem is defined clearly and concisely and even broken down into subordinate problems which are pertinent to local needs and interests. Goals are discussed. Participation in this discussion should stimulate all members of the group.
>
> Data are collected by such means as lecture, observation, reading, surveys, interviews, and experiments.
>
> The data are interpreted.
>
> The students should reach some conclusions concerning the problem.
>
> These conclusions may be followed through with appropriate activities.
>
> These activities may be in terms of self-improvement or in benefits derived by the group, school, or community.
>
> The results should be evaluated.

Some Examples of Problem Solving. Given a large number of accidents at an intersection near a school, a group of students will define a goal—which is to eliminate the accidents, if possible—and will accumulate the data on the incidence of accidents, investigate circumstances surrounding each incident, interpret their conclusions, and then make recommendations. Presented to the proper authorities, their efforts may well culminate in the installation of a traffic signal. Evaluation follows as a survey is made of accidents after the installation. Is there a decrease?

An English teacher may well employ a problem-solving technique in correlation of mental and social health with his class work: He can read about a situation which presents psycho-social difficulties, then ask, "What should Mary do?" Let the students write an answer and finish the story.

A problem may be an elaborate and complex one which will involve a unit for a whole semester, e.g., "Growing into Maturity."

Committee Action is an Approach. Pupils may be organized into committees with definite objectives, such as investigation of fire hazards or lighting in a classroom, or studying the menus in the school lunch program. The results of their efforts should contribute to the understanding of the health problem under consideration in class. This approach is another type of problem solving. Work load should be shared. When the children encounter new and unfamiliar aspects of the problem, the teacher should help the students locate pertinent information.

Use of Textbooks or Health Readers. Most states have a policy of multiple adoption of textbooks. This is a function usually relegated to state departments of public instruction. Periodically, individuals in particular areas of instruction are asked to evaluate the textbooks in the field with recommendations on adoption. An examining committee for health books may consist of elementary teachers and their supervisors, teachers of health subject matter in secondary schools, principals, school physicians, dentists, school nurses, and consultants from teacher education institutions as well as from professional and voluntary agencies.

The usual criteria for selection of textbooks prevail: the physical features of a book, suitability of content for educational level, attractiveness of illustrations, and interesting appeal of material. For health textbooks additional questions are asked. Is the author qualified to write a text on health? Is the material scientifically sound and up-to-date?

Readers and textbooks on health should be readily available and should be used. Children enjoy looking at pictures and reading books. Readers have been written for each school grade. In the elementary grades they have often been published in a series which provides a gradated progression that is appropriate for the comprehension and experiences of school children through these years.

Health books today are written by experts in medicine and education. They are most attractive. A school system may adopt one series and buy many copies but should have copies from other publishers for reference. Several years after a new series appears, some of the information included will be obsolete, e.g., techniques in artificial respiration. Medical science progresses rapidly. A teacher must be alert to detect the changes; perhaps a new series with more current information should be substituted. Or, if this proves too expensive, the errors in the older texts should be pointed out. A partial list of publishers and their books is given at the end of this chapter. No attempt is made to evaluate the health readers. The value of each series will change as the years pass. A series must be scrutinized before adoption and discontinued when health facts no longer are up-to-date.

Textbooks offer factual information principally. They can be referred to as source material; they may even be entertaining. Use of this method in health education should be combined with others for effective learning.

Discussion. Discussion as a method should not be considered as an end in itself. It is used as a means to achieve understanding and, possibly, action. Any health topics may be discussed. A recent report on the effects of smoking or drugs may be the subject. Or, there may be a debate about an impending referendum on fluoridation of the public water supply.

Panel discussions, forums, or debates are valuable at junior and senior high school levels. They should create enthusiasm and eager participation. Talks on health topics should encourage students to express themselves effectively and also provide opportunities to observe how various conflicting ideas can be studied and crystallized by the thinking of the group. Panel discussions are best used for life adjustment problems or for those problems which have many possible solutions.

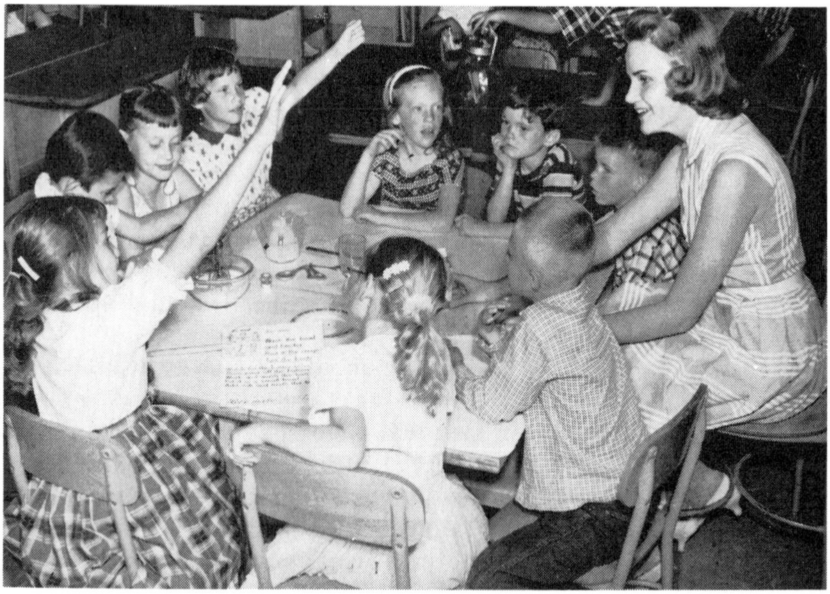

Figure 68 Discussion: student teacher and second-grade pupils discuss butter making. (Courtesy Utah Dairy Council.)

A class may divide into small groups in *buzz sessions*, for a short period of time, and discuss a health topic or subtopic; then the recorders of the group report the conclusions to the class as a whole. The role of the teacher in a discussion on health topics follows:

> Every effort must be made to keep the discussion in the area of scientific information. The teacher should help the students distinguish between authentic material and mere opinion.
>
> The teacher should encourage the class to challenge misconceptions or misunderstandings.
>
> The teacher should help students secure sound information and acquaint them with techniques for presenting it to the class for discussion.
>
> The discussion should make a positive contribution, enabling students to clarify ideas and formulate opinions.

Guest Speakers. Quite often an individual of specialized competence can add authority and detail to important areas in health instruction. Physicians, nurses, counselors, and consultants from professional organizations or voluntary agencies can make valuable contributions. It is important to have the class study the subject ahead of time so that the students can understand the speaker's vocabulary and feel free to ask questions. The teacher can give the class in advance the key ideas which may stem from the guest's talk. The class should know the position, importance, and name of the speaker. Later discussion in class can utilize the information provided by a speaker to emphasize new or important aspects of a problem.

Oral and Written Reports. The materials selected for pupil reports should be directly related to the health course or be timely. They should be assigned in advance so that students have sufficient time to prepare reports. Sometimes those participating in a study select their own topics. A teacher should use good judgment in suggesting subjects that are in keeping with an individual's ability and interests. Those who prepare oral or written reports learn as they collect data, and other children also learn by listening to these reports.

Demonstrations. The demonstration is invaluable in health instruction. In first aid, child care, and home nursing, many problems can best be understood in this manner. Important considerations include rehearsal prior to the class meeting and availability of equipment to be used. If the purpose is to develop skill, sufficient opportunity for the students to practice the skill should be provided.

Demonstrations should give a clear view of what a speaker is trying to explain and provide a long-lasting impression. Furthermore, they should add to the interest of a lecture and help motivate students. They may be used to teach a new subject, to add clarity to something not easily explained in words alone, or to point out misconceptions about subjects. They may be presented by teacher or students.

Projects in many classes may culminate in a demonstration. For instance, if the children are getting ready for a picnic, conversation will include the kinds of food to be taken. Sandwich fillings and bread can be brought to school and a demonstration be presented on preparation of sandwiches. Demonstrations can be used to emphasize basic facts in nutrition—a table can be set with a well-balanced lunch, children may demonstrate butter making, older students can put on showings before classes of younger children.

If possible, after a demonstration pupils should be offered the opportunity to develop their skills, e.g., preparing a sandwich, handling a doll to demonstrate bathing or diapering a baby.

Experiments. An experiment may include investigation of research facts, formulation of a problem, performing according to directions, drawing conclusions, and interpreting results. It may be used to observe physiological phenomena, as in watching the growth of laboratory animals, in growing bacteria, or in safety experiments.

This method is related to problem solving. The pupils themselves carry out the experiments, observations, and draw conclusions, some of which may apply to their personal lives.

Animal experiments are widely used in primary and intermediate grades. Observations may be made on growth, on nutritional values, on reproduction, on living habits. Teachers can make good use of this type of experimentation in discussing family relationships, good health, and good nutrition.

Penicillin molds can be grown on agar plates. Discussion can range far afield on uses of penicillin in acute infections. Some children may have been given such medication.

Use of vegetable coloring in detection of plaque deposited on teeth serves to emphasize the need for correct and regular brushing of teeth.

These are only a few examples of what can be done. Through ingenuity a teacher can plan quite a number of experiments with health implications. The latter need to be emphasized in the conclusions finally drawn.

Exhibits. Exhibits can have a definite educational value if they grow out of the interests and experience of the children. They may be prepared by a group or class or may be secured in many instances from health agencies. They may carry a dental health theme, or one on nutrition. By means of exhibits health instruction may be carried on as a school-wide project. If placed in a conspicuous location in the school building, they can make students aware of the health implications in many aspects of their daily living. Exhibits must be eye-catching, colorful, timely, and modern in design.

Health Museums, Health Fairs. An increasing number of museums devoted to health and physiology are being established. Other museums devote a section to health and medicine. Health fairs for the general population are being presented with a growing frequency in various cities, sometimes in conjunction with a medical meeting. Thousands of people and school children throng to these museums and fairs. In a permanent museum, such as the Hinsdale Health Museum, Hinsdale, Illinois, many lecture tours are scheduled for visiting classes of pupils.

People are fascinated by the displays on physiology and medicine. They particularly like animated portrayals. The talking lady model, plastic or glass, whose lifelike internal organs light up as she herself narrates how she functions, presents a lesson in physiology and stimulates children to take "better care of this wonderful house we live in." Highly entertaining portrayals make use of modern materials to present anatomic and health information in dynamic forms. Visits to displays of these types offer many opportunities for classroom discussion.

Field Trips. Field trips are organized visits which provide an impressive experience in seeing and learning about projects which have been discussed in class. There may be visits to dairies, hospitals, health museums, food centers, dental clinics, health departments, public health laboratories, pasteurization plants, water purification plants, and other health-oriented establishments. The school itself may be the object of an organized tour when topics such as safety, nutrition, hearing, or ventilation are being studied.

Visits to points of health interest demand sufficient preparation and follow-up. The teacher must determine the purpose of the trip, make arrangements, and know prior to the visit what is to be seen and explained. It would be wise for him to ascertain whether the students have had previous field trips to such a place. Too much repetition is to be avoided.

A field trip must have educational value. It should contribute to

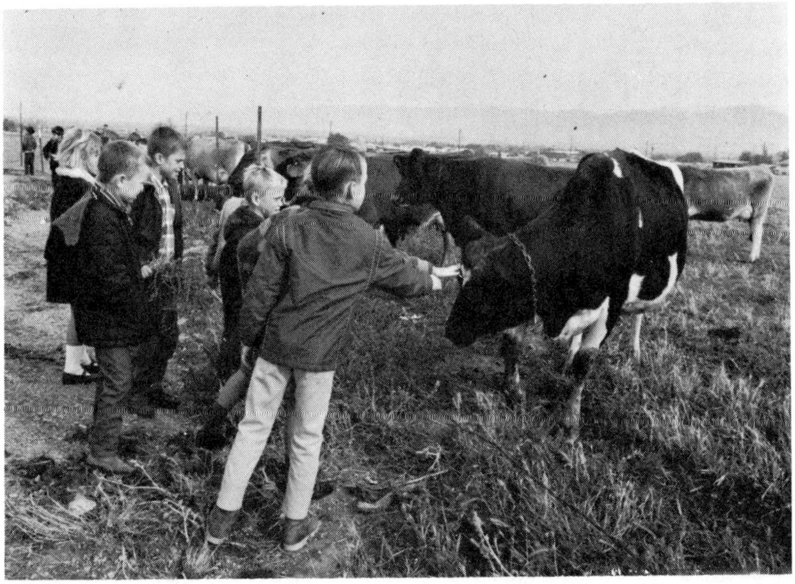

Figure 69 Field trip: second grade pupils visit a dairy. (This series of photographs by courtesy of Utah Dairy Council.)

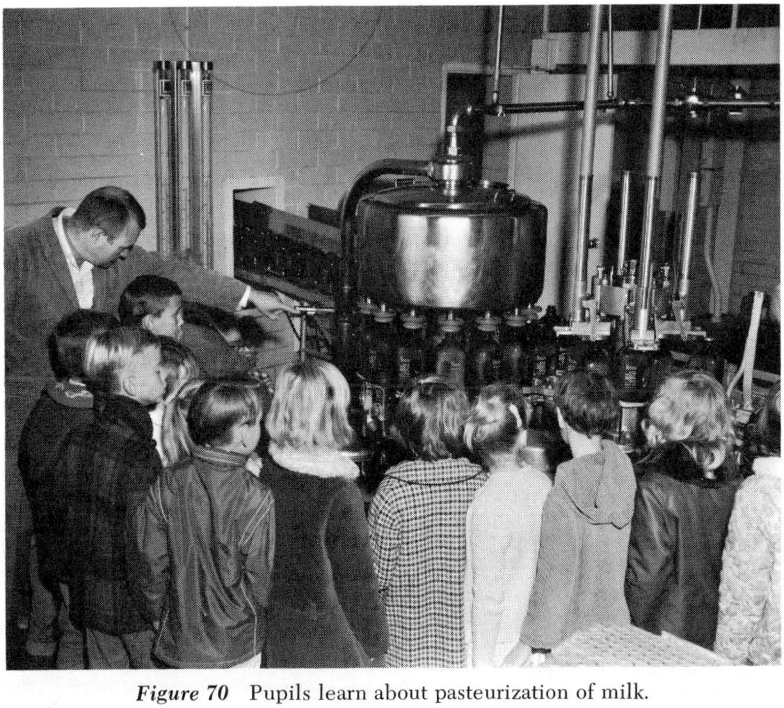

Figure 70 Pupils learn about pasteurization of milk.

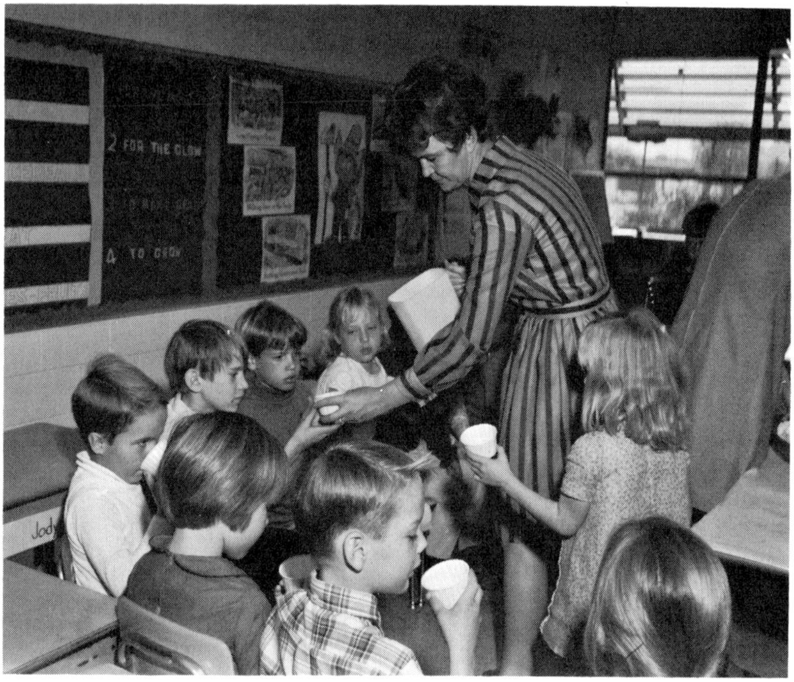

Figure 71 After the visit to the dairy farm, a unit on milk is discussed and milk is distributed.

the understanding of the health topic under consideration. Good teaching will relate the visit to the unit or problem of which it is a part, both prior to and upon completion of the trip. These trips are made by students at any age level.

Role-playing. Role-playing is used most effectively in a situation where a point needs clarification or where additional insight is desired. Role-playing, often referred to as sociodrama, is the spontaneous unrehearsed acting out of the situation by a group or by selected members of a group.

Each participant should understand that he is to act out a characterization as he feels it. If it is determined after discussion and evaluation that the drama should be re-enacted, the actors may play their roles over again, improving their interpretations in light of the suggestions they receive, or new actors may take over the roles to demonstrate other possible solutions. These re-enactments may suggest a variety of approaches for solving the basic problem. Role-playing is helpful in psychosocial areas; it helps anxious young people realize that the troubles affecting them occur also to other people. In this awareness a worried individual finds relief and assurance. For successful role-playing, the teacher must establish a warm, friendly relationship with the students so that the desired spontaneity can be achieved.

Each member of the listening group should be aroused sufficiently

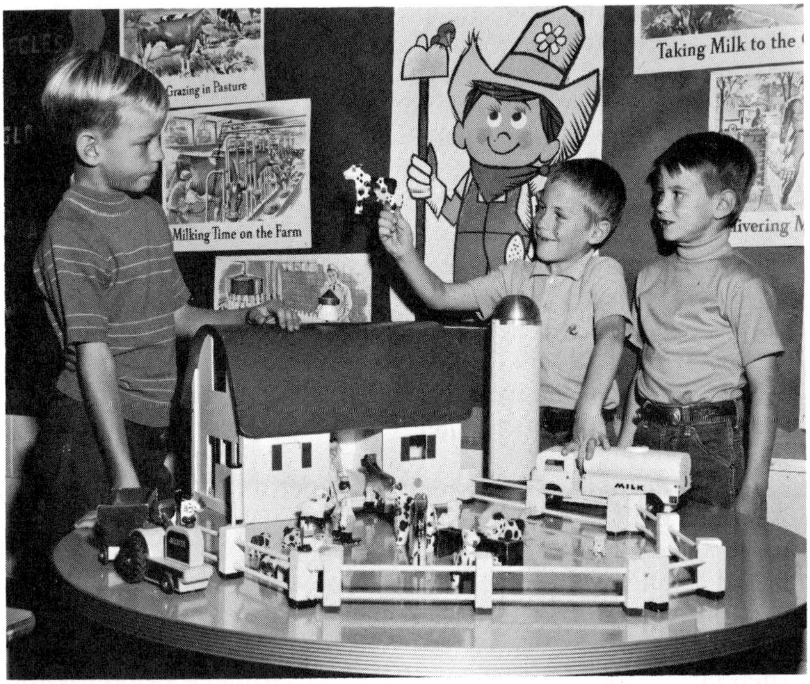

Figure 72 This is an exhibit prepared after the study of the dairy farm and plant.

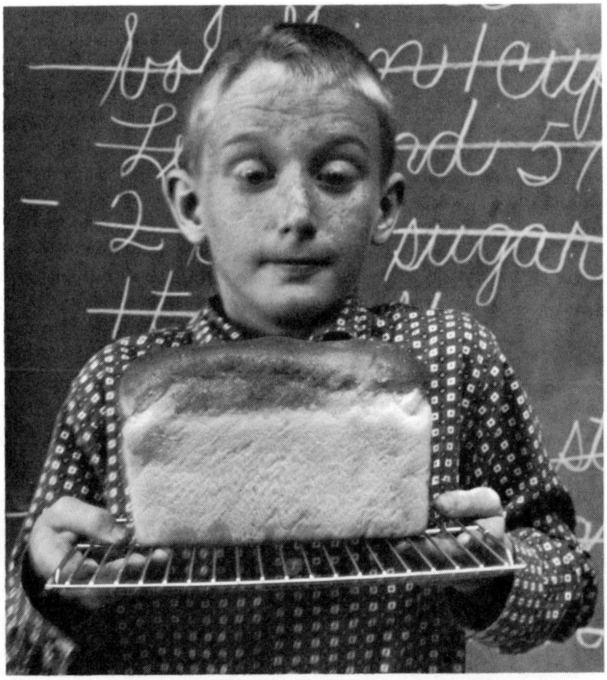

Figure 73 After the fifth grade visited a bakery, the children made their own bread at school. (Photograph courtesy National Dairy Council.)

to identify himself with the situation and realize that he may on occasion face a similar one. He should be interested in the outcome or solutions which may be worked through in the drama. Discussion and evaluation should follow enactment of the scene.

Children may act out many situations, possibly a scene in the cafeteria where food is being selected, a visit to the dentist, or complex problems involving honesty, respect, patriotism, self-confidence, or social adjustments.

Dramatizations. A planned enactment produced by the class for themselves or for performance before others can be a valuable health education experience. Simulated radio or television programs, puppet shows, pantomimes, skits, and plays have been used successfully. It is particularly important that attention is not distracted from the purposes of health instruction. The drama should be realistic and not based upon fantasy.

Student Participation. Children participate in many activities with health implications. These activities are usually of common occurrence and are based upon scientific principles. The significance of the health application concerned should always be understood by the student. Briefly, here are some activities:

- helping in the school lunchroom—observations in preparation and selection of foods, sanitation, cleanliness of environment.
- helping maintain a clean environment, inside and outside the building—picking up trash, checking or reporting unsafe playground apparatus—observations on safety, cleanliness, pride in one's environment.
- older students assisting the nurse or teacher in tuberculin testing and conducting screening procedures, such as measurements of height, weight, and vision.
- older girls working in a hospital as aides—sociological, psychological, and health implications.
- older children in a community youth-service organization teaching younger children to carry out resuscitation procedures, administer other first aid, identify poison ivy, plan well-balanced meals.

These merely suggest the opportunities which children of all ages have to participate in health activities—personal, group, and community.

The Teacher as an Example. Ordinarily one does not associate a teacher's behavior, appearance, or utterances with a method of instruction in health education. Nevertheless, the teacher who gets into line for a tuberculin test or places a well-balanced meal on a tray in the cafeteria is applying and teaching what he considers healthful precepts. One may cite grooming, selection of clothing, and conduct in public as matters to be observed by pupils. A teacher should never forget that he may be imitated.

New Classroom Strategies: Motivation and Involvement

The goal of the school and of the teacher is to arrange situations so that most, if not all, learners want to learn, are confident that they can learn what the school desires, and believe that what they learn is worthwhile for them. The key to this goal is motivation. Motivation may be seen as an inner striving condition, sometimes described as wishes, desires, needs, drives, and the like. A motive may be seen as an inner state that directs or channels behavior toward goals which result in appropriate behavior. The motivating conditions of an individual have three functions in the learning process: (1) they provide energy (2) they sustain the activity of the individual (3) they determine the behavior of the individual.

In the schools today there is a need to motivate for changed behavior, to impress upon the students the lessons of experience. Students need to realize that they can profit and learn through the experiences of others. We are in the middle of social and technological changes in knowledge, as well as in techniques for communicating this knowledge. We are faced with new and different objectives for and with the learner, varied means of reaching these objectives, kinds of experiences, content selection in relation to concepts, and ways of organizing educational experiences. We find that traditional methods fail to compete with the increasing variety of modern communication techniques to which students are exposed outside of school or even before they enter school. We need to apply the principles and understandings from research in concept learning, motivation, individual differences in needs, interests, attitudes, and problems to the teaching situation.

The classroom can be seen as a world in which events occur in rapid succession. In coping with the myriad details involved in a day's teaching, pressures may mount for the teacher, and he may focus primarily on the tasks, not on the children. The teacher may forget that his responses strongly influence the feelings and attitudes of the pupils. Teaching requires the teacher to treat the student as a human being who has dignity and respect. The teacher must bring the self of students into the classroom; he must be a facilitating person. The teacher must see himself as a helping person rather than as a driver or a pusher. He must search for ways in which students may find themselves experiencing success; he must create situations in which students can find themselves needed and wanted by others; and he must develop situations in which he can show each child that he matters and that he is accepted for himself or herself.

It is the nature of teaching to involve a positive personal relationship. However, in all areas of education, there is a real need for more successful communication in the teaching-learning situation. A positive teacher-student interpersonal relationship occurs when the teacher and the student engage in exchanges that seek to establish satisfactory generalizations, conclusions, or solutions. Thus, when people work together on a common issue, a positive interpersonal relationship is likely to result.[17] We need face-to-face encounters for this relationship. These encounters also give feedback to the teacher, which he needs in order to assess the effectiveness of his teaching.

We have advanced quite a distance from some of the early theories of teaching styles operative within the instructional setting. However, communication remains an extremely important factor in the teaching-learning process.

A characteristic of communication which creates a defensive climate is the taking on of the role of being the superior in the classroom by the teacher with the students as his subordinates (teacher toward pupil). To counteract this defensive climate, the teacher can develop a supportive climate instead by making the classroom situation one of equality. This will improve communication and make positive changes in interpersonal relationships. The teacher must attempt to create for himself, through his relations with others, a supportive or defense-reducing climate. This can be done through open and honest interaction with others. It is imperative that the teacher not become defensive. The students will learn to be open and honest only insofar as they are permitted to do so.

It should be evident that teaching-learning is dependent upon communication, and, in turn, good communication is dependent upon many factors. Communication is a two-way process, and, by definition, this process has not been completed until feedback has been brought about. Both teacher and student need to know that every point has been transmitted accurately.

One of the more interesting and dominant teaching strategies being employed today is that of operant conditioning, commonly known in education as behavior modification. The techniques of behavior modification are based mainly on the operant conditioning work of B. F. Skinner; they have a simple cause and effect basis that has been used with dramatic results in teaching, overcoming learning disabilities, behavioral research, and clinical psychology. Dennison states that operant conditioning is a process in which the frequency of an occurring voluntary behavior is modified by the consequences of the behavior.[18] Postively reinforced behaviors will occur more frequently than ignored behaviors, so that behaviors can be modified by systematically controlling reinforcement.

The goal of operant conditioning is the elimination of behavior excesses and/or the addition of new behaviors to correct personality deficiencies. This type of behavior modification is based on the belief that behaviors positively reinforced will occur more frequently than ignored behaviors.

Behavior excesses can be eliminated by two methods: (1) *extinc-*

---

[17]Ronald Hyman: *Ways of Teaching*, J. B. Lippincott Co., Philadelphia, 1970.

[18]Darwin Dennison: "Operant Conditioning Principles Applied to Health Instruction." *J. Sch. Health* 7:368–70, September, 1970.

tion procedures—no reinforcement of undesired behavior, or (2) *positive reinforcement*—reinforcement of a response that is antagonistic to the undesired behavior. Behavior deficits can also be eliminated by reinforcing behavior that the therapist wants the child to acquire.

Operant conditioning can be applied to a wide variety of situations, but it is limited to factors that can be observed, measured, and reproduced. For this reason not much interest is shown concerning the intrapsychic conflicts of the patient. One of the reasons for the growing popularity of operant conditioning, other than the fact that standard psychological therapy has not proved effective in some cases, is the fact that extensive study is not required to practice operant conditioning techniques.

In practice a teacher can use operant conditioning to solve a number of classroom problems. Recently released studies have shown operant conditioning to be effective in teaching children to attend quietly to studies, to cooperate with others, to listen closely to instructions, and to recite assignments. Studies have also shown that children who were massively, verbally reinforced have achieved more than children who were not reinforced.

For operant conditioning to be most effective the teacher employs the technique of "shaping." The teacher will start by reinforcing the child's positive behavior even though it may be far removed from the ultimate behavior the child should display. In the case of a hyperkinetic student who fails to complete his assignments the teacher would:

1. Reinforce the student for sitting in his seat;
2. Gradually lengthen the time to reinforcement until the student sits through the assignment period;
3. Reinforce the student for having needed materials on his desk;
4. Reinforce him each time he picks up a pencil and makes some effort toward working on the assignment;
5. Reinforce him when he has completed a problem;
6. Increase the number of problems completed before reinforcement is given until he finishes the assignment.

In studies done since 1960, operant conditioning has been shown to be effective in teaching children with hyperactivity, hyperaggressiveness, phobias, excessive anxiety, tantrums, social withdrawal, underachievement, short attention span, mutism, dyslexia, and stuttering. Short periods between the desired response and reinforcement have the greatest effect, but this creates the problem of selecting a reinforcement that does not lead to satiation. The most promising solution to this problem is the use of metal tokens that can be redeemed later for small gifts.

Another teaching strategy being employed today is that of the value theory. It is very evident that the values and attitudes of students are quite different today as compared with those of only a few years ago. Changes are coming more rapidly, and students ask more questions relating to their values and those of society. Schools are not doing much to help young people make sense out of the issues and appeals present today. Several kinds of problems seen at school and at home are caused by values or by a lack of values. The emphasis should be placed on valuing the process of achieving values, rather than on the values themselves. Values are seen as growing from a person's experiences. Different experiences can give rise to different values, and values can be modified as experiences accumulate and change. As guides to behavior, values evolve and mature as experiences evolve and mature. The conditions under which behavior is guided, in which values work, typically involve conflicting demands, and finally involve an action that reflects a multitude of forces. To help students develop values, one must assist the students in clarifying for themselves what they value, and not try to get them to accept a predetermined set of values.

One process for establishing the value theory in the classroom includes: (1) working toward a psychologically safe classroom climate, (2) working at eliminating tendencies to moralize, (3) starting slowly, but not too slowly, (4) keeping administrators and other teachers informed, (5) talking about the value-clarifying process in tentative terms, (6) preparing for some conflict, (7) making the ideas fit you, and (8) encouraging several colleagues to join you.[19]

Successful teachers, as a rule, are those who let some of their attitudes and values show but indicate in words and deeds that these are their own personal views and that students are expected to form their own attitudes and values based on class discussions, experiences, and self-analysis.[20] Values cannot be transmitted, but they can be learned. The teacher must raise issues, confront the student with inconsistencies, and get him to determine his own values. However, teachers should load the dice in favor of the values society wishes to perpetuate, and with so much ambiguity and conflict in our society at large, determining what values to teach is always a problem.

Another classroom strategy is that of reality instruction. Hawes summed up some of the problems of today which make the strategy of reality instruction necessary in the classroom.

> The technological and cultural forces of today seem to have a separating and depersonalizing effect. This situation causes people to experience the gnawing feelings of loneliness perhaps more frequently and more intensely than in the recent past. As authority, tradition, and conformity lose their potency to solve the problems of the day and to protect us from loneliness and uncertainty, self-esteem and the capacity to love become more necessary for human survival.[21]

---

[19]Louis Raths, Merrill Harmin, and Sidney Simon: *Values and Teaching.* Columbus: Charles E. Merrill Books, Inc., 1966.

[20]Josephine Rund: *Teaching for Changed Attitudes and Values.* 1971.

[21]Richard Hawes: "Reality Therapy," *Elementary School Guidance and Counseling.* December, 1969, pp. 121–127.

In order to combat loneliness and uncertainty we must learn ways to become more self-responsible (worthwhile) and socially responsible (the capacity to love). Mayshark feels that the professional educator has the responsibility of helping students to learn self-worth and the capacity to love and be loved. He states that before an individual can give and receive love, he must find someone to love and someone to love him.[22]

We cannot count on this needed love's being given at home, but teachers many times do not know how to react to this need of a student. At school the students need to learn to be responsible for each other, to care enough to help one another with the social and educational problems of the school. Educators appear to be more concerned about the need to feel worthwhile. It takes knowledge and the ability to think to achieve worthwhileness. In the process of achieving a feeling of self-worth, the student may gain the self-confidence necessary to give and receive love. A person's identity is usually acquired through either the home or school. If both are weak, the student may not have a chance. He may turn to delinquency and withdrawal if he cannot develop a success identity through love and self-worth. This results in a failure identity, an example of which is the drug culture which is dominated by individuals who feel little love.

In order to help students develop a success identity, the teachers must become involved. Too often we stand emotionally aloof. Education will flourish when teachers and students are involved together. We must learn how to ask questions rather than make statements, to try to make a "yes" out of a "no," to spend as little time as possible on classroom behavior problems, to spend time on open-end discussion sessions, to accentuate thinking rather than memory, and to accentuate practical, reasonable, and realistic solutions rather than reasons for behavior or fault finding. Eight guidelines for the application of reality therapy in the classroom follow: (1) the teacher must get personally involved with the student and let him know she is interested in him; (2) accentuate the present, do not reinforce past behavior by dwelling on it; (3) deal with behavior, help the child become aware of *what* he is doing, not *why*; (4) help the student make a value judgment about his own behavior; (5) help the child make a specific plan when he decides it is worthwhile to change his behavior, (6) encourage him to make a commitment to the plan, (7) eliminate punishment, and (8) do not reinforce excuses.[23] The atmosphere which the above guidelines will help create does much toward encouraging responsive behavior, successful identity, and the capacity to love.

The above instructional strategies are student centered, viable attempts to alter positively the teaching-learning process. Although their widespread effectiveness is not yet known, they deserve consideration and trial. Early evidence supports this use and evaluation.

---

[22]Cyrus Mayshark: "Can't Think. . .Can't Think. . .Can't Think." *Sch. Health Rev.* 3:12–13, May–June, 1972.

[23]*Op. cit.*, Hawes, Richard, pp. 121–27.

Schools and teachers must constantly be searching for and implementing dynamic teaching strategies in our ever-changing world.

Summary on Methods

Many techniques may be used in collecting and presenting data in health education. The decision as to the method or combinations of methods to be used depends upon many considerations: the needs and interests of children, their maturity and capabilities, their ages or grade levels, the proficiency of the teacher, and the facilities and teaching materials available.

In the elementary grades good use is made of such techniques as problem solving, reading health books, holding discussions, giving demonstrations, going on field trips, and carrying on experiments. The pupils themselves form committees to conduct surveys, make investigations, undertake projects, and make reports on their efforts. There may be visits from resource people in many health fields. Instructional materials described below, suitable to the age levels, are used to advantage.

In high school a wider variety of methods is used in health instruction. More detailed and advanced principles and concepts on a greater

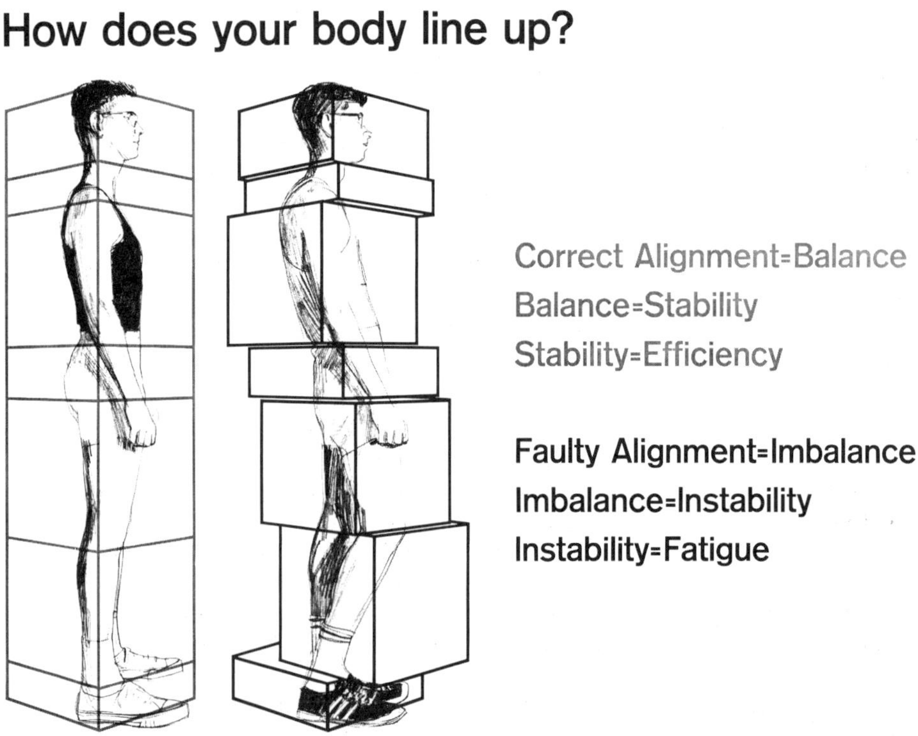

Figure 74 Use of a poster. (Photograph courtesy National Dairy Council.)

number of health problems should be presented in such ways as to evoke critical thinking and application.

Since the objective of health education is to provide learning experiences which will influence attitudes and practices, all of the techniques discussed above should be diverted towards that end. Thus, at the end of any presentation, the child should have not only a clear understanding of health problems but should personalize the information in such a way that he is aware of his own reactions and attitudes toward them. If the teaching is successful, he should then be prompted to adopt practices which are in keeping with acceptable health standards.

Educational Media

Criteria for Selection

Materials used in health teaching must contribute directly to the purpose of a unit or lesson plan. Above all, they must be current and authentic.

Recognition of the importance of health in our lives is mirrored in the wealth of source material available for teaching. Health touches upon every phase of living, and every medium of communication is concerned at some time with health subjects and problems. Sources of information will include books, magazines, films, pamphlets, newspapers, charts, models, posters, graphs, slides, transcriptions, recordings, radio and television programs. Scrapbooks, murals, and maps may be used. Audiovisual aids will often clarify the information the children receive from other sources. All of these materials offer great help in teaching because they create interest through variety and serve as additional attractive informative sources.

The criteria which are used to evaluate teaching aids selected for health education, regardless of resource, should include the following:

> The material shall be plainly identified as to its source in order to facilitate evaluation of bias, if any.
>
> It shall be free from advertising matter other than identification as above specified.
>
> It shall meet the criteria of scientific soundness in its field, both as to its content and as to omissions, if any.
>
> It shall meet the criteria of modern educational methodology.
>
> It shall not be associated directly or indirectly with advertising or the promotion of products, services, or concepts contrary to accepted good health principles and practices.[24]

The teacher should give considerable thought to the selection of the many types of materials that can be used for health education purposes. He should be aware that these materials can be used as sources

---

[24]American Association of School Administrators, National Education Association: *Health in School.* Washington: NEA, 1951, p. 435.

of information to arouse interest, motivate desirable behavior, and guide learning activities.

Resources

Health information supplies may be secured from many sources. The organizations from which one can secure them are usually classified under (1) official agencies, (2) professional associations, (3) voluntary groups, and (4) private industrial companies. These have been described in the chapter on Organization and Administration.

Teaching materials supplied by these resources are subject to the criteria stated above and act in complementary fashion to the teaching units in which they are to be used. Many resources are listed in Appendix A. The names of the agencies or companies will indicate in most cases the approaches to health in which they are most interested. This list is not exhaustive by any means. Its purpose is to indicate some of the sources of information for people who work in health education.

Films, Filmstrips, Slides, Television, Radio, Recordings, Teaching Machines. A teacher may use these to provide background knowledge, stimulate interest and appreciation, provide specific information or illustrations, review a unit, develop concepts and attitudes, summarize material, or as a means in testing. Their use is not a substitute for teaching but is an aid; just to present a movie as fulfilling the complete content of a topic is to be lazy and inept. Research has shown that students learn more effectively if an introduction or review precedes the showing. Ask them to look for something special, perhaps a mistake in fact, and their attention will be concentrated.

Use of some films is free; some are available for a nominal fee; some are available locally; some must be secured from a distance. A teacher should investigate every local source. He may visit a local health agency and inspect materials. These agencies are anxious to help teachers.

Effective use of slides, filmstrips, or films demands that the teacher be familiar with film catalogues and other film sources (Appendix A). He should become acquainted with the best resource material in the field. Popular films with their descriptions are listed at the end of each chapter on health problems in Part I. Desirable levels for their use are designated.

A recording of an interview with a health officer, a nutritionist, a physical educator, or some other important person may be played. These records can be stored and used repeatedly.

The best results are obtained from the use of these teaching devices when they have been *reviewed in advance.* How else can a teacher know that the material to be presented fits in with what he has already taught or what he wishes to teach? One cannot predict content from a title. He cannot be sure that the material is graded for his particular group or meets their interests. The vocabulary may be too technical or the approach inappropriate. A teacher should be able to apprise the children of specific aspects of the material before it is presented and build up to its presentation.

Not only do children see movies at school, but they watch television and listen to radio programs at home. Those on medical topics, usually sponsored by scientific organizations, ethical pharmaceutical companies, or by departments of instruction, may be regularly scheduled or be presented as occasional features on educational or commercial stations. Some are presented during the school day and may be shared by children at school and by their parents at home. Health problems which have been discussed on television and radio not only enlighten the public but should affect its attitudes and practices. The adjustments of a boy with a cleft palate should strike an understanding response. Discussions on headaches, crippling conditions, and surgical procedures have popular appeal.

Content of popular commercial programs which dramatize an incident, a physician, or a nurse is usually supervised by representatives of the medical profession for technical and scientific accuracy and for ethical interpretations. One must keep in mind, however, that the dramatization may be somewhat exaggerated. The primary objective of such a program is to entertain, not to teach.

Scientific reports presented dramatically on television concerning the value of a new vaccine or the conquest of a disease alert the whole nation. These can be discussed at school. On the other hand, this same public can be rather indiscriminate in its judgment; therefore, advertisements for laxatives, sedatives, analgesics, and such need to be interpreted in the light of scientific inquiry. Great emphasis should be placed upon the distinction between a scientific presentation on television and the many non-scientific commercialized advertisements. The school can assist in this interpretation. The field of television holds interesting possibilities in health education, both for the general public and in closed circuits for a local school or school system.

Graphic Materials. Visual aids in forms of charts, graphs, posters, cartoons, maps, diagrams, and tables facilitate teaching. Their use will accent points or facts to be stressed in a discussion or lecture. A picture is better than many words. Charts showing the structure and function of various organs of the body are indispensable in teaching physiology. Graphic materials may be used as a part of a display or serve as constant reminders if placed prominently in some part of a building and changed at intervals. A comical interpretation in chart form may be employed to attract attention. A simple listing chart or graph may be used to present statistics or to list topics which will be covered in a unit. They may present a grouping of newspaper or magazine clippings or cartoons. Various graphic materials can be part of an exhibit.

Visual aids are obtained from many sources. Many official and voluntary health agencies as well as commercial organizations have prepared them as part of their health education offerings.

Periodicals, Newspapers, and Illustrations. These may be used to provide current stories and news. The professional periodicals have a particular contribution to make in publishing latest health information, interpreting new trends in curriculum planning, and stimulating teachers to more extensive and improved teaching. A fairly complete list of reliable professional periodicals is included in Appendix A. Popular journals often contain authoritative articles on such subjects as nutrition, child care, sex education, and social adjustments, some of them original articles and some condensed reprints. Many people depend upon widely circulated lay journals for their health information.

If newspapers are used, the teacher should be concerned with the following questions: Are the facts correct? If the health material is presented in a syndicated article, what is the training and reputation of the author? Is his material authoritative? An article on a health topic may present one person's viewpoint, or the results of a recent experiment. How reliable is the information? Oftentimes it is difficult to know. One may have to check with an authoritative local source. Medical topics are even presented in comic strips. The same criticisms should hold.

IMPLEMENTING THE HEALTH EDUCATION PROGRAM

Implementing means putting into practice. It means that what has been presented in this chapter on health teaching should be translated into terms of action.

Regardless of the curriculum which may be planned, its adequacy at the local level to meet the needs of children and the objectives of health education depends upon (1) the attitude of the administration, (2) the attitude and professional preparation of teachers, (3) the progressiveness of both in keeping up-to-date on health information and techniques of teaching, and, finally, (4) upon the interrelationship of administration and teachers with the family and those agencies in the community and government interested in the health of the school child.

If a superintendent or principal does not consider health teaching very important, little stress or time will be given to this area at school. The administration is responsible for scheduling classes or units in health education. A teacher who is oblivious to the health needs of his community, or is indifferent to the whole subject of health, or is rigid in his beliefs and practices, or is blind to health defects in his pupils should not participate in a health education program. Moreover, a teacher should serve as an example of a healthy, emotionally stable individual.

The whole area of health information is dynamic, continually being changed by new discoveries in medicine and science, and a teacher must keep up-to-date on his knowledge and interpretation. Newer approaches and innovations for teaching should be studied and utilized. Finally, a health education curriculum must be under continuous scrutiny (evaluation) to determine whether the objectives of health education are being fulfilled.

The preceding discussion relates to implementation of a health education curriculum within a school or school system. However, health teaching is not solely the prerogative of a school. Nor are the experiences provided for health teaching by the school in promoting health education circumscribed and limited to the school. The child moves in a number of spheres. His health is the concern of the family, the community, voluntary and professional organizations, and government at all levels. This concern has been discussed at length in foregoing chapters. A great deal of excellent educational material is always being prepared by the organizations, with specific health problems in mind. The government also offers educational media through various boards and departments. Various legislative acts provide funds for purchase of teaching equipment to be used in schools, and for health examinations and medical care of children with health defects. The community offers opportunities for experiences which further understanding and appreciation of personal and public health problems. The family is intimately involved with health education in the school.

In implementation of a progressive health education curriculum all the resources and facilities beyond the school are utilized with an appreciable combined effort. Good school-community relations are essential for school health education.

EVALUATION OF SCHOOL HEALTH EDUCATION

See next chapter.

SUMMARY

School health education involves all of the health experiences to which a youth is exposed—his environment, the health services conducted, and health teaching. Its objective is to develop a health-minded individual who not only is capable of handling his own health problems but will appreciate and promote the good health of his family, community, and nation.

Health teaching should be presented in a well-planned, continuous, progressive health education curriculum from kindergarten through high school. Health education is considered a discipline in its own right, and should have blocks of time allotted to it. Content may be integrated or correlated with related subject matter areas in the intermediate grades and in junior and senior high school. In addition, junior and senior high schools usually include direct, organized teaching in health education courses.

DISCUSSION QUESTIONS AND ACTIVITIES

1. Define health education and school health education. How do they differ?

2. Summarize the evidence supporting the need for school health education.
3. What was the School Health Education Study (SHES)? What were some of its findings and conclusions? What are its implications?
4. Define curriculum and health curriculum. Describe the parameters of curriculum planning.
5. How is the selection of course content made? Indicate some suggested content for different grade levels.
6. On what bases are the scope and sequence of health instruction determined? Draw up a plan for a comprehensive health instruction from kindergarten through twelfth grade.
7. List some traditional methods of teaching. Illustrate a unique characteristic of each and analyze its effectiveness.
8. Why are motivation and involvement important to the learning process? What enhances and what inhibits the process?
9. How does operant conditioning and valuing apply to health instruction? Enumerate the underlying principles of these teaching strategies.
10. What criteria should be used for evaluation of the worth of health materials? Demonstrate the use of one or more resources that are available to the health teacher.
11. How would you go about the planning and implementation of a comprehensive health instruction program in an elementary school? A junior high or middle school? A senior high school?

READINGS

American Association for Health, Physical Education, and Recreation:
Health Packet for Elementary School
Health Packet for Secondary School
NEA–Publication Sales, NEA.

Association for Supervision and Curriculum Development: *Educational Accountability Beyond Behavioral Objectives.* The Association, 1972.

Association for Supervision and Curriculum Development: *The School of the Future.* The Association, 1972.

Journal of School Health. The following special issues:
"Growth patterns and sex education." 37:5a, 1967. A suggested program–kindergarten through grade twelve.
"Health instruction." Suggestions for teachers. Revised edition. 39:5a, 1969. Excellent.
"Mental health in the classroom." Revised edition. 38:5a, 1968.

National Science Supervisors Association: *Behavioral Objectives in the Affective Domain.* The Association, 1969.

Read, D. A., and Greene, W. H.: *Creative Teaching in Health.* New York: The Macmillan Co. 1971.

School Health Education Study: "Synthesis of research in selected areas of health instruction." 1963.
Available from NEA–Publication Sales, NEA.

Sch. Health Rev. January–February, 1973. The entire issue deals with health education in the elementary and junior high schools.

Yount, M. A. C.: "Review of research and studies related to health education practice (1961–1966)." *Health Ed. Monogr.* Society of Public Health Educators, 28, 1968.

Curriculum guides or manuals have been prepared by state departments of education. They outline a progressive curriculum for elementary and secondary schools and for each grade level. Teaching units have been prepared on many health topics.

Professional and voluntary health agencies distribute teaching units on subjects which command their particular interests. These agencies or resources are listed at the end of each chapter after the discussion of a health problem and in Appendix A (with addresses).

AUDIOVISUAL MATERIALS

Let's Talk About Films

18 min. Black and White National Film Board of Canada*

Presents a workshop meeting where group leaders discuss what was wrong when a leader elicited no response from the audience. Compares his experience with that of another leader who uses the same film and obtains a lively response. Stresses points which make for success—informal atmosphere, a leader who does not dominate the group, but centers discussion in the group.

The following colored films are to be used by teachers. They discuss *methods* in educational media:

From Indiana University, Audiovisual Department, Bloomington, Indiana 47401

"Wet Mounting Pictorial Material"	12 min.
"Handmade Materials for Projection"	20 min.
"Better Bulletin Boards"	13 min.

From Bailey Films

"Film and You—Using the Classroom Film"	13 min.
"Creating Cartoons"	11 min.
"Bulletin Boards: An Effective Teaching Device"	10 min.
"Torn Paper"	5 min.

PARTIAL LIST OF HEALTH BOOKS USED IN SCHOOLS

(Watch for new editions)

Primary and Intermediate Grades

The Healthful Living Program, Laidlaw Brothers, Inc., 1974.
Dimensions in Health Series, Lyons and Carnahan, 1967.
Basic Health and Safety Program Series, Scott, Foresman and Co., 1974.

Junior High School

Health and Growth Series
Health and Growth (7th grade)
Health and Growth (8th grade)
Chicago: Scott, Foresman and Co., 1972.
The Healthful Living Program
A Healthier You (7th grade)
Your Health and Your Future (8th grade)
River Forest, Illinois: Laidlaw Brothers, Inc., 1974.
Irwin, Leslie L., et al.:
Foundations for Fitness (7th grade)
Patterns for Living (8th grade)
Chicago: Lyons and Carnahan, 1967.

Senior High School

Diehl, Harold S., and Laton, Anita D.: *Health and Safety for You.* Third edition. New York: McGraw-Hill Company, Inc., 1969.

Gallagher, J. Roswell, Goldberger, J. H., Hallock, Grace T.: *Health for Life.* Palo Alto: Ginn and Co., 1964.

---

*See Appendix A for address of film company.

Jones, Evelyn G., Wright, Betty Lee, Behlmer, Reuben D.: *Living in Safety and Health.* Philadelphia: J. B. Lippincott Co., 1966.
Lawrence, Thomas Gordon, Clemensen, Jessie Williams, Burnett, R. Will: *Your Health and Safety.* Fifth edition. New York: Harcourt, Brace and World, Inc., 1963.
Meredith, Florence L., Irwin, Leslie W., Staton, Wesley M.: *Health and Fitness.* Fourth edition. Boston: D. C. Heath and Co., 1966.
Otto, James H., Julian, Cloyd, J., Tether, J. Edward: *Modern Health.* Revised edition. New York: Holt, Rinehart and Winston, Inc., 1971.

Resources (partial list)
American Association for Health, Physical Education, and Recreation
American School Health Association
American Social Health Association
Association Press—wealth of materials on many topics.
Child Study Association of America
National Council on Family Relations
Public Affairs Committee
Science Research Associates—many publications.
State Departments of Education

Chapter 21

EVALUATION OF THE SCHOOL HEALTH PROGRAM

An evaluation is a careful appraisal with specific standards or values in mind. An evaluation of the school health program measures the progress being made in achieving its objectives and consequently the objectives of its three component areas—school living, health services, and health education. Any dynamic operation needs to be evaluated at intervals so that it can keep alert, flexible, and incorporate indicated improvements. The purpose of a school health program is to promote and preserve the mental, physical, and social well-being of children, and procedures to achieve this end should be subject to appraisals. Are we achieving this purpose?

EVALUATION—BENEFITS, SCOPE, AND PROCEDURES

Benefits of Evaluation

1. The evaluation process should stimulate professional interest and arouse a desire for improving the school health program. Those in close contact with the school child—teachers, health counselors, principals, social workers, school nurses, and physicians—are in a position to watch the program in action from day to day. Nevertheless, their efforts should be evaluated more concretely. It is good to take stock periodically, weigh the strengths and weaknesses of a program, to appreciate the various roles, including one's own.

2. By use of evaluation instruments or guides, the appraisers can compare their own program and its activities with recommended standards and practices. Thus, the evaluation process itself is an educational experience.

3. The family and the child benefit from criticisms of the program. For instance, any improvement in procedures for detecting defects

and for referrals to private physicians and dentists should result in improved health of the children. If more emphasis on nutrition education is indicated, strengthening this aspect of health education should make an impression at home and upon the child.

4. The community will share in these appraisals. If the response of school children to a campaign for immunization has been gratifying, public health officials are stimulated to greater efforts and provision of more funds. If the health needs of children, such as need for a good mental health program, cannot be met by existing resources in a community, and if concrete statistics are presented to substantiate this need, leaders of a community may be moved to action. If the sanitarian makes specific recommendations for correction as a result of his annual inspection of food facilities, plumbing, and water supplies, not only the school and board of education but the parents and community may be involved if major changes are necessary. The same is true of recommendations made by building inspectors and firemen.

5. An evaluation is necessary in order to determine the effectiveness of health teaching and its benefits as measured in terms of improved personal health of children, efficient health services, and healthful school living. Evaluation goes on while a method of teaching is being implemented by students. In selecting a method or combination of methods a teacher is evaluating his own techniques in terms of desired outcomes.

6. An evaluation on a nation-wide basis may determine the status of health education. Is there a need? Where are the gaps? The impressive school health education study described in the preceding chapter was designed for this purpose. Surveys required two years. The conclusions reached point the way for action.

7. The results of the evaluation process should stimulate in-service studies and communication of ideas among those involved, thus promoting advancement of information and procedures which will improve a school health program.

Who Conducts the Evaluation?

Impetus for more or less formalized evaluations of the three aspects of a school health program depends upon the health consciousness of those most closely associated with the school child. Evaluation is a continuous process. Observations are constantly being made on such environmental factors as heat, lighting, and sanitation, upon handling the health problems of individual youngsters, and upon the results of health teaching. Even the custodian notices when children are eating too much candy.

Responsibility for organization and administration of the school health program and, to some extent, for the atttudes fostered towards health lies with the board of education and the administrators. At the school level, the principal, all school personnel, parents, and children should be involved in appraisals of progress. The school health council or a committee of children, sparked by a discussion of some health topic, may undertake an evaluation study. The PTA group may wish to investigate some aspect of the school health program. At times studies may be initiated by members of the community in cooperation with school personnel. If a deadlock exists between the local boards of health and education over payment of salaries to school nurses, the problem may be referred to a citizens' committee. In this instance, before formulating a recommendation, an evaluation of the contributions of the nurse would have to be a prime consideration.

Various health agencies often join efforts with the school to conduct a survey or study for evaluation purposes. The local tuberculosis association may request permission to participate in a tuberculosis-detection survey for appraisal of the health status of school-age children in a community. If the results of such a survey show that the per cent of positive tuberculin tests is very low, just how often should such surveys be conducted?

One school system[1] centered its intensive in-service evaluation around a School Health Education Evaluation Study, which lasted five and one-half years. A specialist in health education served as coordinator and consultant. Teachers, nurses, physicians, supervisors, and administrators from the schools were involved. Consultants from voluntary and official health agencies and other authorities were resource people.

The Scope of the Evaluation

Evaluation of the various phases of a school health program should not be spasmodic in character. Informal observation, of course, is continuous. Certain standardized procedures should be routine, including the annual inspection of plant facilities and the annual examination of food handlers. Timely surveys can also be made, possibly the response to a campaign for smallpox vaccinations. However, in order to avoid repetition and confusion, a long-term schedule of evaluation should be set up. Specific and different problems of the health program should be studied each year. The following general plan is a suggestion.

First Year:

1. The disease control program
2. The hearing testing program
3. The environment of the school in relation to health and safety

Second Year:

1. The vision testing program
2. The program of correlation of instruction
3. The dental hygiene program
4. The frequency and causes of absenteeism among students and staff

[1]Edward B. Johns: *School Health Education Evaluative Study.* Los Angeles area, 1954–1959. Los Angeles: University of California, 1960, 128 pp.

Third Year:
1. The effectiveness of the nursing and medical services, including the examinations
2. The growth and nutrition program, including the lunchroom
3. The psychological services and mental hygiene program
4. The program of direct teaching in health

Fourth Year:
1. The physical education program including the care of athletes and the program of athletics in relation to health
2. The emergency care program including first aid
3. Community relationships
4. The program of integrated instruction as it bears on health
5. The use of teaching aids in health instruction

Fifth Year:
1. The administrative and financial structure of the health program
2. The effectiveness of personnel
3. The relation of the school program to community practitioners and agencies
4. The school health education program as a functioning unit[2]

Procedures in Evaluation

The following steps may be undertaken in evaluation:

1. The objectives of the program must be defined and understood.

2. The present program should be appraised (according to techniques listed below) with attention paid to the adaptations which were made to meet the needs and problems of a particular school and community.

3. The findings are evaluated; possible beneficial changes should be recommended in the light of approved practices, with the local situation in mind.

4. Recommended changes should be planned (replanning).

5. There should be evaluation of the evaluation technique itself.

Such an evaluation will reveal the weaknesses and strengths of the health program. A word of caution should be included here. Any evaluation must be based upon the developmental or functional approach to education and to the school health program; namely, based upon our knowledge of the growth and development of school children, their characteristics, needs, and interests.

Techniques. Uses of the following techniques and evaluation instruments may be adopted by the examining individual or group in appraising the existing program:

Questionnaires may be submitted to parents, children, or other interested personnel.

The American Dietetic Association directed the following ques-

---

[2] Delbert Oberteuffer and Mary K. Beyrer: *School Health Education.* Fourth Edition. New York: Harper and Row, 1966, p. 517.

tions to nutritionists in an effort to understand the nutrition problems of teenagers: (1) What are some of the teenage problems in your community? (2) Why do you think these problems exist? (3) What has been done about these problems? (4) What do you think can be done about these problems? (5) Do you think a questionnaire concerning nutrition problems prepared for the teenagers would be helpful? Why?

The results of this questionnaire formed a good basis for improving the nutrition education program for adolescents at school (with specific suggestions), for improving school lunches and snacks, and for strengthening contacts with interested personnel in the school and in the community.

Questionnaires answered by students on the topics of smoking, use of alcohol, and use of dependency-producing drugs are widely used to assay their knowledge, attitudes, and practices. The responses give an idea as to current status of these practices and give clues for additional or improved techniques in teaching.

Surveys are particularly effective in appraising environment.

They are also used in contacting special interest groups. One significant study on smoking in teen-agers was conducted through telephone surveys. In Portland, Oregon such a survey[3] was made in 1967 of 315 boys, ages 12 through 18, and of an equal number of girls. The results, compared with a similar survey made ten years before, revealed an appreciable decrease in smoking. In 1957 the tabulation on a group of 17-year-old boys who smoked regularly (daily or weekly) was 34.7 per cent. Ten years later the estimate on the same group was 25.6 per cent. As for a comparable group of girls, the figures decreased from 25.5 to 15.7 per cent reported to be smoking in 1968.

Other implications from this survey were determined. For instance, attitudes toward smoking were voiced during the phone interviews. Behavior expectations were evaluated: Only 2.6 per cent of the total questioned expected to smoke at some future time; 45.1 per cent stated definitely that they did not expect to smoke. The survey also elicited the information that smoking among parents was on the decline – from 55 per cent to less than 50 per cent. Moreover, 91 per cent of these youngsters, especially the younger ones, believed that smoking is harmful to health.

Evaluations from specialists may be requested: fire inspectors, sanitarians, lunchroom supervisors, and health education consultants.

Check lists and score cards for covering many phases of the school health program are available. The lists are usually answered by "yes" or "no." Score cards allot points of evaluation for the various items presented. A study of these lists or cards will emphasize the fact that they portray the purposes and scope of the school health program; so findings can serve as a basis for changes or future planning. These findings should be used for these purposes and not remain as a mass of data.

---

[3]Daniel Horn: "Youthful Smoking in Decline." *Medical Bulletin on Tobacco*, June, 1968.

No check list is perfect or entirely adequate, nor will it meet all existing conditions. Manuals, guides, and check lists have been prepared by state and local departments of health and education, various health agencies, individual researchers or groups of educators, and by specialists in various fields (illumination engineers, school physicians). Textbooks describe the various phases of the school health program and elaborate on specific objectives and activities. From these and from the guides an individual or committee may formulate a check list which will fit the immediate school or school system.

Records should be studied. The wealth of information which should be available on a health record has already been discussed. It should contain the results of periodic health examinations and follow-ups, the observations of teachers and health personnel, data on immunizations, illnesses, operations and accidents, individual growth measurements, findings on vision and hearing tests, and the results of interviews with parents and children. These records evaluate the health status of the children, the progress of the health service program, and, to some extent, the effectiveness of teaching. A study of the accident records is important in safety education.

Observations on the benefits of a particular program are valuable. They may be checked off on a list or they may be subjective. If a child is more alert and happy and studies better after a daily, warm, well-balanced school lunch, such an observation may be subjective; but it is a good reflection upon the lunch program. If he makes better grades and gains weight, such findings can be tabulated. If children are motivated to keep the grounds clean of rubbish and to place lunch sacks in the proper containers, the cleanliness of the environment may be checked off on a list, but the attitudes engendered in the pride of children for their school cannot be measured as readily. Observations placed upon health records indicate an alertness on the part of teachers and health personnel.

The *response to "projects"* or campaigns measures their effectiveness. Health projects are undertaken throughout the year. There are "weeks" for dental health, safety, foods of various types, mental health, etc. Immunization campaigns and tuberculosis-detection programs are "musts." To achieve success with any project, health instruction should develop favorable attitudes which are translated into action. Dynamic steps—preparing exhibits and attractive bulletin boards or presenting skits, films, and programs in the auditorium—should produce the desired objective of a project. Such results can be evaluated, e.g., more trips to the dentists, more immunization permits signed by parents.

Photographs offer visual records of improvement. This is particularly true of environmental changes.

Tests and health questionnaires (inventories) measure health knowledge, attitudes, and practices of both the individual and family, provide information which can reflect upon health teaching, and serve

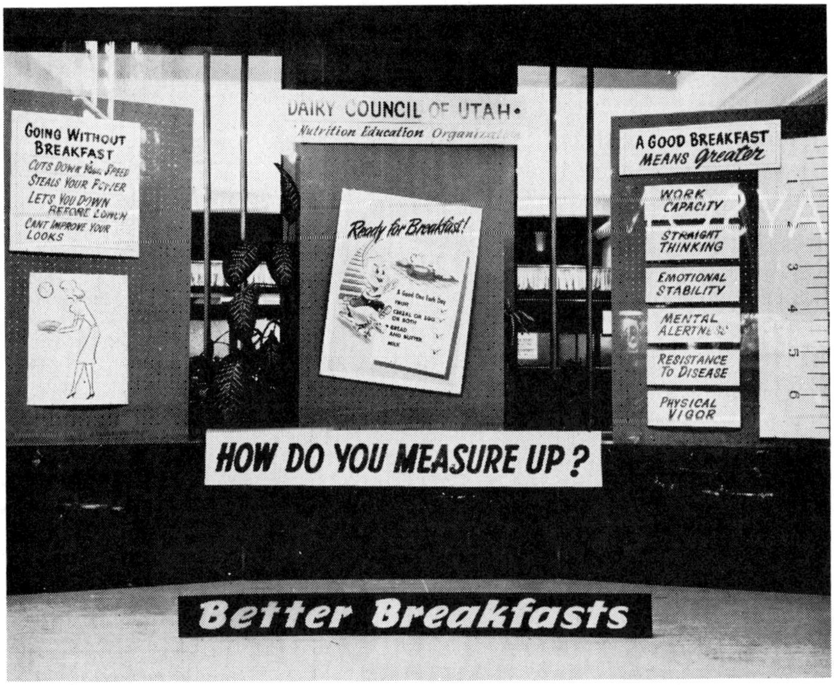

Figure 75

as a baseline for planning a comprehensive health education program or improving an existing one (see Appendix B for questionnaires). Tests should be brought up-to-date on current information and interests of students.

Self-inventories made by the children themselves (How am I doing?) in reference to the various phases of their health are effective in self-evaluation and will point up their needs (see Appendix C).

Interviews and discussions, both formal and informal, will bring forth definite information concerning various factors in the health program. These conversations may occur between teacher and pupil, teacher and parent, physician and parent, physician and pupil, physician and teacher, administrator and nurse, or in other relationships. One may learn that the girls or boys are dissatisfied with facilities in the toilet rooms. A mother may reveal a serious situation in a classroom where the children cower before a teacher who threatens to "knock their heads together." Interviews offer an effective method of ascertaining the emotional climate of a room.

Evaluation. Information from any of the preceding techniques or from combinations of them should be evaluated objectively and honestly. Such an evaluation takes time. The truth may not be palatable. Conversely, there will always be features which merit self-congratulations.

The results of the survey on smoking in teen-agers, mentioned earlier in this chapter, were especially gratifying. Education through the various media has definitely paid off.

No health program is all good or all bad. The findings of a study should be clearly stated, conclusions are drawn, and those concerned are ready to proceed toward improvement. Improvement may be in any of the areas of the school health program—environment, services, or health education.

Finally, while using the various preceding techniques in evaluation, the methods of evaluation themselves should be subject to critical review.

Replanning. Once the weaknesses are revealed, planned correction follows. Replanning requires objectivity and a basic knowledge of the factors involved in the school health program. Objectives should be kept in mind. A plan should be mapped out which seeks to fulfill these objectives. Specialists may be used as consultants. An in-service workshop may produce amazing results in understanding the roles of all members of the school health team. Better planned health education may be necessary. Promotion of better school-community relationships is always indicated. In the replanning, methods of implementing a program are outlined, and these plans should be put into effect. Replanning will probably require acceptance of new information, flexibility in attitudes, and a change in routine.

EVALUATION OF HEALTHFUL SCHOOL LIVING

The objectives: "provision of a safe and healthful environment, the organization of a healthful school day and the establishment of inter-personal relationships favorable to emotional, social, and physical health."

Manuals and guides prepared by state departments of health and education as joint projects or separately can be secured. These present standards and approved practices. Some contain suggested check lists.

Objective measurements are easy to make in evaluation of environmental factors. Building codes and health regulations are specific.

The check list for a healthful and safe school environment may be used:

1. In appraising the environment of school plants;
2. In discussing factors relating to a safe and healthful environment at in-service education meetings for school personnel;
3. In discussing the environment of school plants by members of health councils or committees and interested citizen groups, such as parent-teacher association study committees;
4. As a reference for use in collegiate courses for school administrators, teachers, and school nurse on both a preservice and in-service basis;
5. As an instructional aid for use by student groups in evaluating their school environment;

6. For study by members of governing boards of school districts, school administrators, teachers, school health personnel, custodians, school bus drivers, and others having responsibility for providing and maintaining a safe and healthful school environment;

7. In planning new school plants and in remodeling old ones.[4]

Any use of a check list or score card must be viewed realistically in light of the local situation. A small school without indoor plumbing or running water will have little use for ordinary standards. Criteria to fit its own local problems should be formulated. Such a school may aspire towards better facilities. Every school should strive for warmth, color, cleanliness, and a pleasant emotional atmosphere.

Once an evaluation of environment is made in specific terms, improvement should be made where indicated—elimination of fire hazards, better acoustics, safer playgrounds, removal of a despotic, unjust teacher.

EVALUATION OF SCHOOL HEALTH SERVICES

OBJECTIVES

1. To appraise the health status of pupils and school personnel;
2. To counsel pupils, teachers, parents, and others for the purpose of helping pupils obtain health care, and for arranging school programs in keeping with their needs;
3. To help prevent and control communicable disease;
4. To provide emergency care for injury or sudden illness;
5. To promote and provide optimum sanitary conditions and safe facilities;
6. To protect and promote the health of school personnel; and
7. To provide concurrent learning opportunities which are conducive to the maintenance and promotion of individual and community health.[5]

And in addition:

8. To maintain safety measures which will protect the health of pupils.
9. To plan services which will provide a healthful environment.

These objectives offer many approaches to evaluation. Moreover, health education and health services go hand-in-hand. An evaluation of one involves the other.

CONTINUOUS EVALUATION

An elementary teacher, after his working unit on teeth, will feel a deep sense of gratification when his charges bring back good reports

[4] Patricia J. Hill: "A Check List for a Healthful and Safe School Environment." Prepared for California State Department of Education. Sacramento. (1957).

[5] *Op. cit.*, Joint Committee on Health Education Terminology, 1973, p. 4.

from the dentist. His observations on the continued growth and happy dispositions of his children make him feel secure in his health teaching and in the emotional climate of his classroom. The health teacher feels a warm sense of reward at the response in immunizations to his discussion on tetanus. Statistical data often may be lacking, but an individual teacher should evaluate his health teaching performance constantly in terms of attitudes, practices, and good health of pupils. The health services offered at school provide an opportunity for evaluating this teaching. Talk to the nurse or physician. Adequacy of the services should be a matter of concern to all interested in teaching health education. The converse is also true. If health instruction is poor in quality or is absent, the demand for health services and co-operation with those in charge will be discouraging.

The nurse, physician, dentist, principal, and others associated with school health services are also measuring the values of the health service and striving for improvement. Day-to-day appraisals are inevitable.

Evaluation Studies

Since the area of health services comprises many activities, only a few evaluations should be run concurrently. A detailed check list will give an idea of the scope and organization of school health services and the type of questions asked in a survey.

EVALUATION OF SCHOOL HEALTH EDUCATION

School health education seeks to provide learning experiences which will favorably influence individual health behavior. Health behavior, that is, which has an influence on the individual, the family, and the community.

The basic needs, interests, and capacities of a child at each grade level are known. A curriculum is planned which seeks to achieve our objectives in health education through the developmental approach. How good a job has been done? What health information can a child be expected to know in each grade? What concepts and attitudes have been developed from health teaching? How has conduct been influenced? Which planned experiences were the most meaningful? The final evaluation of health education is not in lip-service but in an acceptable way of life, in healthful living. A favorable attitude aroused by instruction is translated into action.

Evaluation of health education is made in terms of scientific knowledge, desirable attitudes, and improved behavior (practices). Many evaluation instruments have been formulated in an attempt to judge these various aspects.

No one instrument or technique will elicit a clear-cut, selective evaluation of knowledge, attitude, or practice. Each will be measured and mirrored to a great extent by the other manifestations. For instance, the evaluation of a child's information and understanding and/or attitudes on nutrition can be determined by what he selects as he moves along the cafeteria line. Will it be the planned well-balanced lunch or a carbonated beverage and a piece of cake? Does he know the difference? Or, is it because he does not care? The answer may be quite complex, particularly on the health practice.

One word of warning on the use of any evaluation instrument. The expected response must be based upon current health or medical information. Information makes such quick changes. For instance, in the matter of health practices, one is not instructed today to go to bed with a common cold unless fever or severe malaise is present; yet old instruments expect the answer to be "bedrest." The correct answers to questions on immunizations need frequent alterations. The responses on an instrument only a few years old can well be obsolete.

Another factor must be considered—the background of the student, including his experiences and his vocabulary. A child who has never seen a grapefruit nor eaten a sweet potato or who has a limited vocabulary will fare poorly on a nutrition education test.

EVALUATION OF KNOWLEDGE

Health knowledge is not difficult to evaluate if clearly defined objectives were stated prior to the instructional experience. Some people have recommended the need for a broader range of objectives in the cognitive domain.[6] Thus, a modified evaluation strategy would need to be developed and implemented.

If a health instruction program has been well-organized and followed at school, a teacher knows what can be reasonably expected in information at a given grade. Oral and written tests will check this knowledge. At the same time the teacher should interpret knowledge in terms of understanding.

Essays, reports, notebooks, and similar writings on various topics may give some indication of what has been learned.

Tests have been formulated for various levels, elementary, secondary, and college. These are frequently objective in form, containing true-false, matching, multiple choice, or completion questions. Many areas of health information are covered. Questions should be pertinent and on current problems. In the selection of a standardized test, one must keep in mind that health interests of students do not remain the same over the years. Neither does the vocabulary. New

---

[6]Marian K. Solleder: "Evaluation in the Cognitive Domain," *J. Sch. Health 42*: 1:16, January, 1972.

research stimulates new interests. A health knowledge test must be kept up-to-date. If all of the students being tested live in the same locality, a standardized test can be modified to immediate concerns.

Preparation of these tests is not easy. Objective questions must be formulated carefully in order to avoid misinterpretation. Every person who teaches health education is limited by his own professional preparation in the area, by his interest and determined effort to keep up with current information, and by his emphasis on the various problems of health. A physical education teacher, a health educator, a biology, physiology, social studies, science, or home economics teacher—each of these will present a somewhat different approach and emphasis to this vital area of teaching. The individual who sits down to plan a standardized test is cognizant of these difficulties. In most instances a competent health teacher knows what he has taught and where he has placed his emphasis, and can formulate his own health knowledge test. Comparison of his own test against a standardized set of questions should provide interesting observations on what the experts consider pertinent background information.

A teacher may evaluate his own efficiency in teaching by giving a pretest. This is used as a baseline before presenting a unit or course. Gaps in information are determined. If the students are poorly prepared, basic facts must be given before advanced discussion is possible. A repeat of the pretest at the end of teaching should be revealing. How much more was learned? How efficient was the teaching?

Measurement of pure knowledge can be a sterile procedure, as far as health education is concerned. Knowing a fact is not enough. Did the pupil interpret the information in terms of its implications? Did he reach the concept which was desired?

> The manner in which short answer questions or essay type questions are phrased can either elicit a simple recall of information, or they can require the student to interpret, explain, or make reasoned judgments which indicate that he not only has a knowledge of the concept but he understands it.[7]

Another way to evaluate health knowledge is through the interpretations made by means of demonstrations, role-playing, planning of exhibits and posters, explanation of animal experiments, and other projects, through the observations he makes on field trips, and from other activities.

Check lists on health instruction are concerned with curriculum planning and methods utilized in instruction.

Evaluation of Attitudes

Health education is judged not only in terms of knowledge acquired, but in attitudes of students. It is difficult to evaluate attitudes.

[7]C. Harold Veenker: "Evaluating Health Practice and Understanding." *JOHPER* 37:31, 1966.

A student may parrot on a written examination what he has been taught and make an excellent grade. How does he really feel about a health problem? He has been exposed to several different viewpoints—those received from his peer group, his school, and his home.

Evaluation of attitudes may be made by:

1. Observation of health practices. An individual's behavior usually reflects his beliefs or attitudes. If a student acts favorably upon what he has been taught—eats a good breakfast, visits the dentist periodically, secures his immunizations—then he has achieved desirable attitudes.

2. Observation of improvement in health status. If corrections of defects have been made, noted by improvement in habits of eating and gain in weight, or the acquisition of glasses, health education and health services have influenced attitudes.

3. Answers to questions which are propounded with the early morning greeting, during informal discussions or interviews, or in filling out the health history forms. Consider the attitude and practice of a kindergartner who asks of his classmate as they plod toward school: "What will I tell her I had for breakfast this morning?"

One must be sure of the sincerity of the response. Do you personally approve of smallpox vaccinations? Wearing glasses? Do you use iodized salt for seasoning foods? Do you expect to smoke when you are older?

4. Comments expressed in written work, as in essays or autobiographies. A student's incidental comments may give a clue to his attitudes on various problems.

5. Tests. A standardized test to evaluate health attitudes is difficult to prepare. An attitude cannot be measured, except indirectly by the means described above. Research along these lines involves a close association with youth, gaining their confidence, appreciating their backgrounds of information, observing their conduct, judging sincerity, and posing informal questions.

Evaluation of Health Practices

Evaluation of health practices may be made by:

1. Observation of practices. A teacher may note the services which a student seeks, either at school or from the health resources of a community, the food he chooses, the response he makes to his environment, and any habits which have been altered after instruction or after having been offered experiences which have health implications.

2. Observation of improvement in health status. Corrections may be noted. A health examination may reveal improvement. A more alert and energetic child may evolve from altered eating habits and an increase in food intake. A more stable personality may follow visits to the mental health clinic.

3. Questionnaires, surveys, or inventories. A review of the

responses to a questionnaire or survey will be enlightening in an evaluation of health practices. Again, reference is made to the survey on smoking in teen-agers.

4. Information on health practices can be gleaned from autobiographies, pupils' diaries, and from direct parent-teacher conferences.

Self-inventories are personal and meaningful. How am I doing? How do I measure up? A student may prepare his own inventories in which he keeps an accurate account of his physical activites, his hours of sleep, the foods eaten. These can be compared against recommended practices, thus he can evaluate his own. See Appendix C.

A teacher must make sure that any evaluation of health practices is based upon current teaching, e.g., Do you stay home and rest when you have a cold? The response "No" is acceptable.

EVALUATION OF THE TOTAL SCHOOL HEALTH PROGRAM

The objective of the school health program is to maintain and improve the "health of pupils and school personnel, health services, health education and healthful living." This objective is extended to include the family, the community, and society.

Measurements of the health status of pupils and personnel can be done by health examinations and by evaluations of the three phases of the school health program. In addition, an evaluation should consider the organization and administration of the program.

The California State Department of Education prepared check lists or criteria for evaluating the elementary school health program and also the high school program. The large areas and their components to be evaluated are administration, health instruction, health services, and healthful school environment. Sample pages are reproduced in Appendix C.

SUMMARY

A program must be evaluated for its worth and for its future plans. Any program revolving around human beings is dynamic. Stock must be taken at frequent intervals. "It is important that what is being taught, how it is being taught, and the responses and reactions of pupils, parents, and the community in general be continually checked and appraised. The means available—observations, interviews, check lists, tests—are far from perfect, but in the absence of more precise methods they are helpful resources for the purpose. In the final analysis, evaluation is merely a stepping stone to improvement—a starting point for continued or redirected effort."[8]

[8]American Medical Association: "Report of the 8th National Conference on Physicians and Schools." Chicago, 1961, p. 76.

Our main concern should be the quality of the educational experience our youth are receiving. The school health program should do all that is possible to create and sustain an environment which will foster optimum health for students and teachers alike. Ultimately, the quality of the school health program will be evaluated in terms of the educational experience gained and the health status achieved.

DISCUSSION QUESTIONS AND ACTIVITIES

1. Discuss the reasons for evaluating the school health program. What should an evaluation reveal?
2. Find an evaluation chart for a school health program and make an assessment of the program of a local school.
3. Discuss how attitudes can be evaluated. Are these hard to measure? Why or why not?
4. Obtain a standard test of health knowledge and administer it to a class. What can these tests reveal?
5. Write to your state department of education and obtain an evaluation manual for school health environment.
6. Discuss the importance of establishing objectives for a program which can be related to evaluating that program.
7. Discuss your feelings on evaluation. Are you afraid of evaluation, or do you feel it can only help? What is the mentally healthy outlook on evaluation?
8. Make a list of persons you would consider qualified to evaluate your school health program. Why did you pick these people?
9. Discuss the significance of self-inventories. Can these be used constructively?
10. Discuss the significance that incidental observation has on evaluation. Can this be used as a part of a formal evaluation?

ADDITIONAL SOURCES OF INFORMATION

READINGS

Allen, R. E.: "Evaluating the conceptual approach to teaching health education—A summary." *J. Sch. Health* 42:118–9, February, 1972.

Allen, R. E.: "Evaluation of the conceptual approach to teaching health education." *J. Sch. Health* 43:293–4, May, 1973.

Evans, R. I.: "Research in the social psychology of persuasion and behavior modification: Relevant to school health education." *J. Sch. Health* 43:110–14, February, 1973.

Hastings, J. T.: "Evaluation in health education." *J. Sch. Health* 40:519–22, December, 1970.

Havighurst, R.: "Nuturing the cognitive skills in health." *J. Sch. Health* 42:73–6, February, 1972.
Joint Committee on Health Problems in Education of the National Education Association and the American Medical Association: Washington: NEA, *School Health Services.* Second edition. 1964, pp. 343–358.
Kilander, F.: *School Health Education.* New York: The Macmillan Co., 1968. Evaluation procedures.
Levin, A. L.: "Report of the school health education committee." *J. Sch. Health* 43: 200–1, April, 1973.
Lockwood, J.: "The effectiveness of health education programs for average and disadvantaged public school children." *J. Sch. Health* 40:15–6, January, 1970.
McAtee, P. A.: "Committee on evaluation in school nursing—One experience." *J. Sch. Health* 40:89–90, February, 1970.
Oberteuffer, D.: *School Health Education: A Textbook for Teachers, Nurses, and Other Professional Personnel.* New York: Harper & Row, 1972.
Seffin, J. R.: "A standardized achievement test of health education objectives in the cognitive domain." *J. Sch. Health* 42:43–6, January, 1972.
Solleder, M.: "Evaluation in the cognitive domain." *J. Sch. Health* 42:16–20, January, 1972.

EVALUATION INSTRUMENTS (partial list)

American Association of Health, Physical Education, and Recreation: "Evaluation Instruments in Health Education." Washington: The Association, 1969, 23 pp. Revised list compiled by Marian K. Solleder. A bibliography of tests of knowledge, attitudes, and practices for elementary, secondary, and college levels. A review of 135 instruments.
Appendix C, this text. Samples of check lists and self-inventories.
California State Department of Education, Sacramento:
"Check List for a Healthful and Safe School Environment." (1957), 51 pp.
"Criteria for Evaluating the Elementary School Health Program." (1962), 20 pp.
"Criteria for Evaluating the High School Health Program." (1962), 24 pp.
National Commission on Safety Education: "Checklist of Safety and Safety Education in Your School." Washington: NEA. 327 items to be checked.
National Dairy Council
"A Boy and His Physique." 1967, 34 pp. For teachers' use in senior high. Check list. Good for coaches and physical education teachers.
"A Girl and Her Figure." 1968, 36 pp. For teachers' use with "A Girl and Her Figure and You." 1967, 16 pp. For senior high girls. Self-evaluation.
"My Reflections." 1967, 21 pp. For junior high school girls. Check lists.
"Who—Me?" 1968, 24 pp. For junior high school boys. Check lists.

The following are NATIONAL HEALTH TESTS, available from McGraw-Hill, in black and white:

Part I	Communicable Diseases	30 min.
II	Reproduction and Birth	20 min.
III	Mental Health, Alcohol, Narcotics	11 min.
IV	Exercise, Nutrition, Diet	26 min.

References in footnotes in this chapter.
State and local departments of education can provide check lists.

APPENDICES

Appendix A

RESOURCES

RESOURCES FOR PRINTED MATERIAL

Below is a partial list of professional, official, voluntary, and industrial organizations who are interested in various health problems and have prepared materials for use in education. Pamphlets, reprints, charts, posters and exhibits may be available.

Many of these organizations maintain branches at district, state, or local levels. Anyone interested in health education should be familiar with the nearest agencies and utilize their services.

*Indicates that audiovisual materials are also available.

*Aetna Life Insurance and Affiliated Companies
Public Education Department
151 Farmington Avenue
Hartford, Connecticut 06115

Alexander Graham Bell Association for Deaf, Inc.
1537 35th Street, N.W.
Washington, D. C. 20007

Allergy Foundation of America
801 Second Avenue
New York, New York 10017

Allied Youth
1901 Fort Myer Drive
Arlington, Virginia 22209

American Academy of Pediatrics
1801 Hinman Avenue
Evanston, Illinois 60201

American Association for Health, Physical Education and Recreation
1201 Sixteenth Street, N.W.
Washington, D. C. 20036

American Association for the Study of Headache
5214 North Western Avenue
Chicago, Illinois 60625
Seymour Diamond, M.D., Secretary

American Association of Mental Deficiency
5201 Connecticut Avenue, N.W.
Washington, D. C. 20015

*American Automobile Association
1712 G Street, N.W.
Washington, D. C. 20006

American Baker's Association
20 North Wacker Drive
Chicago, Illinois 60606

*American Cancer Society
219 East 42nd Street
New York, New York 10017

American Cleft Palate Association
Mt. Royal and Guilford Avenues
Baltimore, Maryland 21202

American College of Allergists
145 East High Street
Springfield, Ohio 45502

*American Dental Association
211 East Chicago Avenue
Chicago, Illinois 60611

American Diabetes Association
8 East 48th Street
New York, New York 10017

American Dietetic Association
620 North Michigan Avenue
Chicago, Illinois 60611

American Dry Milk Institute
221 North LaSalle Street
Chicago, Illinois 60601

American Foundation for Allergic Diseases, Inc.
801 Second Avenue
New York, New York 10017

American Foundation for the Blind, Inc.
15 West 16th Street
New York, New York 10011

American Hearing Society
1537 35th Street, N.W.
Washington, D.C. 20007

*American Heart Association
44 East 23rd Street
New York, New York 10010

American Home Economics Association
1600 Twentieth Street, N.W.
Washington, D.C. 20009

American Hospital Association
840 North Lake Shore Drive
Chicago, Illinois 60611

American Institute of Baking
400 East Ontario Street
Chicago, Illinois 60611

American Institute of Family Relations
5287 Sunset Boulevard
Los Angeles, California 90027

American Meat Institute
59 East Van Buren Street
Chicago, Illinois 60605

American Medical Association
535 North Dearborn Street
Chicago, Illinois 60610

*American National Red Cross
17th and D Street, N.W.
Washington, D.C. 20006

American Nurses Association, Inc.
10 Columbus Circle
New York, New York 10019

American Otological Society, Inc.
525 East 68th Street
New York, New York 10021

American Public Health Association
1740 Broadway
New York, New York 10019

American School Health Association
515 East Main Street
Kent, Ohio 44240

American Seating Company
9th and Broadway
Grand Rapids, Michigan 49502

*American Social Health Association
1740 Broadway
New York, New York 10019

American Society of Dentistry for Children
7701 Fitzwater Road
Cleveland, Ohio 44141

American Speech and Hearing Association
1001 Connecticut Avenue, N.W.
Suite 532
Washington, D.C. 20036

Association for the Advancement of Instruction about Alcohol and Narcotics
155 East 44th Street
New York, New York 10017

Association for the Aid of Crippled Children
345 East 46th Street
New York, New York 10017

Association for Childhood Education International
1200 15th Street, N.W.
Washington, D.C. 20005

Bicycle Institute of America, Inc.
122 East 42nd Street
New York, New York 10017

Borden Company
Consumer Services
350 Madison Avenue
New York, New York 10017

Boy Scouts of America
New Brunswick, New Jersey 08901

Bristol-Myers Products Division
Education Service Department, UDH
45 Rockefeller Plaza
New York, New York 10020

Carnation Company
5045 Wilshire Boulevard
Los Angeles, California 90036

*Center for Mass Communication
Columbia University Press
1125 Amsterdam Avenue
New York, New York 10025

*Cereal Institute, Inc.
Home Economics Department
135 South LaSalle Street
Chicago, Illinois 60603

Child Study Association of America, Inc.
9 East 89th Street
New York, New York 10028

Cleveland Health Museum
8911 Euclid Avenue
Cleveland, Ohio 44106

Council for Exceptional Children, NEA
1201 Sixteenth Street, N.W.
Washington, D.C. 20036

Cream of Wheat Corporation
Minneapolis, Minnesota 55413

Epilepsy Foundation of America
1419 H Street, N.W.
Washington, D.C. 20005

Equitable Life Assurance Society
1285 Avenue of the Americas
New York, New York 10019

Family Service Association of America
44 East 23rd Street
New York, New York 10010

General Foods Corporation
Consumer Service Department
250 North Street
White Plains, New York 10605

General Mills, Inc.
9200 Woyzata Boulevard
Minneapolis, Minnesota 55413

Gerber Products Company
445 State Street
Fremont, Michigan 49412

Health Information Foundation
The University of Chicago
Chicago, Illinois 60637

Hinsdale Health Museum
40 South Clay Street
Hinsdale, Illinois 60521

Hogg Foundation for Mental Health
The University of Texas
Austin, Texas 78712

International Council on Exceptional Children
130 North Wells Street
Chicago, Illinois 60606

John Hancock Mutual Life Insurance Company
Health Education Service
200 Berkeley Street
Boston, Massachusetts 02117

John Tracy Clinic
806 West Adams Boulevard
Los Angeles, California 90007

Kellogg Company
Home Economics Service
Battle Creek, Michigan 49017

Kraft Foods Company
Consumer Services Department
500 Peshtigo Court
Chicago, Illinois 60690

Lerner Publications Company
Medical Books for Children
241 First Avenue North
Minneapolis, Minnesota 55401

Lever Brothers Company
390 Park Avenue
New York, New York 10022

Liberty Mutual Insurance Company
Loss Prevention Department
175 Berkeley Street
Boston, Massachusetts 02117

*Maternity Center Association, Inc.
48 East 92nd Street
New York, New York 10028

Medic-Alert Foundation International
Turlock, California 95380
Telephone 209-623-2371

*Mental Health Materials Center, Inc.
419 Park Avenue South
New York, New York 10016

*Metropolitan Life Insurance Company
Health and Welfare Division
1 Madison Avenue
New York, New York 10010

Muscular Dystrophy Association of America, Inc.
1740 Broadway
New York, New York 10019

National Academy of Sciences
National Research Council
2101 Constitution Avenue
Washington, D.C. 20037

*National Association for Mental Health, Inc.
10 Columbus Circle
New York, New York 10019

National Association of Ice Industries

Dept. N
810 18th Street, N.W.
Washington, D.C. 20006

National Association of Hearing and Speech Agencies
919 18th Street, N.W.
Washington, D.C. 20006

National Board of Fire Underwriters
465 California Street
San Francisco, California 94104

National Clearing House for Smoking and Health
U.S. Public Health Service
8600 Wisconsin Avenue
Bethesda, Maryland 20014

National Congress of Parents and Teachers
700 North Rush Street
Chicago, Illinois 60611

National Council on Alcoholism
2 Park Avenue
New York, New York 10016

*National Dairy Council
111 North Canal Street
Chicago, Illinois 60606

National Dairy Research Laboratories, Inc.
Oakdale, Long Island, New York 11769

National Education Association
1201 Sixteenth Street, N.W.
Washington, D.C. 20036

National Fire Protection Association
60 Batterymarch Street
Boston, Massachusetts 02110

National Foot Health Council, Inc.
321 Union Street
Rockland, Massachusetts 02370

*National Foundation
800 Second Avenue
New York, New York 10017

National Health Council
1740 Broadway
New York, New York 10019

National Institute for Child Health and Human Development
Department of Health, Education, and Welfare
Washington, D. C. 20201

National Institute of Mental Health
5454 Wisconsin Avenue
Chevy Chase, Maryland 20015

National Interagency Council on Smoking and Health
8600 Wisconsin Avenue
Bethesda, Maryland 20014

National League for Nursing, Inc.
10 Columbus Circle
New York, New York 10019

*National Livestock & Meat Board
36 South Wabash Avenue
Chicago, Illinois 60603

National Recreation Association
8 West Eighth Street
New York, New York 10011

National Research Council
Food and Nutrition Board
2101 Constitution Avenue
Washington, D.C. 20037

*National Safety Council
425 North Michigan Avenue
Chicago, Illinois 60611

*National Society for Crippled Children and Adults, Inc.
2023 West Ogden Avenue
Chicago, Illinois 60612

*National Society for the Prevention of Blindness
79 Madison Avenue
New York, New York 10016

*National Tuberculosis and Health Association
1740 Broadway
New York, New York 10019

Nutrition Foundation, Inc.
99 Park Avenue
New York, New York 10016

*Paper Cup and Container Institute
Public Health Committee
250 Park Avenue
New York, New York 10017

Personal Products Corporation
Education Department
Milltown, New Jersey 08850

Pet Milk Company
Home Economics Department
Research Division
Arcade Building
St. Louis, Missouri 63101

*Pharmaceutical Manufacturers Association
1155 15th Street, N.W.
Washington, D.C. 20005

Prudential Insurance Company of America
Public Relations & Advertising
Prudential Plaza
Newark, New Jersey 07101

Public Affairs Committee
381 Park Avenue
New York, New York 10022

Quaker Oats Company
Merchandise Mart Plaza
Chicago, Illinois 60654

Ralston Purina Company
Nutrition Service
Checkerboard Square
St. Louis, Missouri 63102

Research to Prevent Blindness, Inc.
598 Madison Avenue
New York, New York 10022

School Health Education Study
1507 M Street, N.W.
Room 800
Washington, D.C. 20005

Science Research Associates
259 East Erie Street
Chicago, Illinois 60611

Sunkist Growers
Consumer Service Division
Box 2706, Terminal Annex
Los Angeles, California 90054

Travelers Insurance Company
Public Information and Advertising Dept.
700 Main Street
Hartford, Connecticut 06115

UNESCO Publications Center
319 East 34th Street
New York, New York 10016

UNICEF
United States Committee
331 East 38th Street
New York, New York 10016

*United Cerebral Palsy Association, Inc.
321 West 44th Street
New York, New York 10036

United Nations
Department of Public Information
New York, New York 10017

*U.S. Department of Agriculture
Agricultural Research Service
Human Nutrition Research Branch
Home Economics Research Branch
Washington, D.C. 20250

U.S. Department of Health, Education, and Welfare
Washington, D.C. 20201

U.S. Government Printing Office
Superintendent of Documents
Washington, D.C. 20402

Volta Bureau
1537 35th Street, N.W.
Washington, D.C. 20007

Wheat Flour Institute
309 West Jackson Boulevard
Chicago, Illinois 60606

World Health Organization
Regional Office for the Americas
525 23rd Street, N.W.
Washington, D.C. 20037

RESOURCES FOR AUDIOVISUAL MATERIALS

Audiovisual materials may be obtained from (1) official agencies, such as health departments and state or local departments of education; (2) the film libraries of colleges, and universities; (3) voluntary agencies, either from national headquarters or their local branches; (4) professional groups; (5) commercial organizations; and (6) distributors which sell or rent films.

Films and filmstrips can be secured from many of these sources at little or no cost to the school. Many school systems purchase audiovisual materials and have established their own libraries.

Recommended audiovisual aids have been listed at the end of most of the chapters in this book. They may be used by teachers for their own information or for use in the classroom.

The agencies designated by an asterisk in the preceding section also supply films or filmstrips. The following is a partial list of the companies that have an excellent selection of current films on health subjects. Catalogs may be ordered from them.

Association Films, Inc.
347 Madison Avenue
New York, New York 10017

Audio Productions, Inc.
630 Ninth Avenue
New York, New York 10036

Avis Films, Inc.
P. O. Box 643
Burbank, California 91503

Bailey Films, Inc.
6509 DeLongpre Avenue
Hollywood, California 90028

Brandon Films, Inc.
221 West 57th Street
New York, New York 10019

Bray Studios
729 Seventh Avenue
New York, New York 10019

Campus Films Productions, Inc.
20 East 46th Street
New York, New York 10017

Carousel Films, Inc.
1501 Broadway
New York, New York 10036

Churchill Films
662 North Robertson Boulevard
Los Angeles, California 90069

Contemporary Films, Inc.
267 West 25th Street
New York, New York 10001

Coronet Instructional Films, Inc.
Coronet Building
Chicago, Illinois 60601

Encyclopaedia Britannica Educational Corporation
425 North Michigan Avenue
Chicago, Illinois 60611

Film Associates
11559 Santa Monica Boulevard
Los Angeles, California 90025

International Film Bureau
332 South Michigan Avenue
Chicago, Illinois 60604

Iowa State University
Audiovisual Department
Ames, Iowa 50010

McGraw-Hill Book Company
Text-Film Department
330 West 42nd Street
New York, New York 10036

Modern Talking Picture Service
3 East 54th Street
New York, New York 10022
(Excellent source for free films. Write for catalog)

National Educational Television
Indiana University
Bloomington, Indiana 47401

National Film Board of Canada
680 Fifth Avenue
Suite 819
New York, New York 10019

New York University Film Library
26 Washington Place
New York, New York 10003

Public Affairs Film Library
267 West 25th Street
New York, New York 10001

Psychological Cinema Center
Audiovisual Aids Library
Pennsylvania State University
University Park, Pennsylvania 16802

Roundtable Films, Inc.
275 South Beverly Drive
Beverly Hills, California 90212

Sterling Films, Inc.
316 West 57th Streeet
New York, New York 10019

Smart Foundation
65 East South Water Street
Chicago, Illinois 60601

Social Science Films, Inc.
4030 Chouteau
St. Louis, Missouri 63110

Universal Education and Visual Arts
221 Park Avenue South
New York, New York 10003

Walt Disney Productions
500 South Buena Vista Street
Burbank, California 91505

Special Catalogs on Health Topics

Council on Scientific Assembly, Motion Pictures, and Medical Television
"A List of Sources of Films on the Subject of Health." Chicago: The American Medical Association. Write for current catalog.

U.S. Department of Health, Education, and Welfare
Children's Bureau
"Selected Films on Child Life." (1962), 99 pp. A listing of 400 films on child health, family life, food and nutrition, mental health, safety, and sex education.
"Mental Health Motion Pictures." Write for current selective guide.

Public Health Service
Write for catalog on films dealing with health topics for general public. U.S. Government Printing Office, Washington, D.C.

Journals, Newsletters

The following journals or bulletins should be helpful as sources of accurate information on health. Where indicated, the agency sponsoring the journal is mentioned:

American Annals of the Deaf
Conference of Executives of American Schools for the Deaf
Gallaudet College
Washington, D.C. 20002

American Journal of Public Health and The Nation's Health
American Public Health Association
1740 Broadway
New York, New York 10019

California Journal of Elementary Education
California State Department of Education
Division of Textbooks and Publications
Sacramento, California 95814

Childhood Education
Association for Childhood Education
3615 Wisconsin Avenue, N.W.
Washington, D.C. 20016

Cleft Palate Bulletin (quarterly)
American Cleft Palate Association
Mt. Royal and Guilford Avenues
Baltimore, Maryland 21202

Crippled Child
National Society for Crippled Children and Adults
2023 West Ogden Avenue
Chicago, Illinois 60612

Diabetes
American Diabetes Association
18 East 48th Street
New York, New York 10017

Educational Leadership
Association for Supervision and Curriculum Development
National Education Association
1201 16th Street, N.W.
Washington, D.C. 20036

Elementary School Journal
University of Chicago Press
5750 Ellis Avenue
Chicago, Illinois 60637

Family Life
American Institute of Family Relations
5287 Sunset Boulevard
Los Angeles, California 90027

Food and Nutrition News
National Live Stock and Meat Board
36 South Wabash Avenue
Chicago, Illinois 60603

Health Bulletin for Teachers
Metropolitan Life Insurance Company
1 Madison Avenue
New York, New York 10010

Health Education Services for Schools and Colleges
American Medical Association
535 North Dearborn Street
Chicago, Illinois 60610

Hearing News
American Hearing Society
1537 35th Street, N.W.
Washington, D.C. 20007

Journal of American Association for Health, Physical Education and Recreation
1201 16th Street, N.W.
Washington, D.C. 20036

Journal of the American Dietetic Association
620 North Michigan Avenue
Chicago, Illinois 60611

Journal of School Health
American School Health Association
515 East Main Street
Kent, Ohio 44240

Journal of Speech and Hearing Disorders
American Speech and Hearing Association
1001 Connecticut Avenue, N.W.
Suite 532
Washington, D.C. 20036

Mental Retardation
American Association on Mental Deficiency
5201 Connecticut Avenue, N.W.
Washington, D.C. 20015

National Parent-Teacher
700 North Rush Street
Chicago, Illinois 60611

Nation's Schools
Modern Hospital Publishing Company, Inc.
Merchandise Mart
Chicago, Illinois 60654

NEA Journal
National Education Association
1201 16th Street, N.W.
Washington, D.C. 20036

Nutrition News
National Dairy Council
111 North Canal Street
Chicago, Illinois 60606

Public Health Reports
U.S. Public Health Service
Superintendent of Documents
Washington, D.C. 20402

Quarterly Journal of Studies on Alcohol
52 Hillhouse Avenue
Yale Station
New Haven, Connecticut 06520

School Health Review (Quarterly)
American Association for Health, Physical Education and Recreation
1201 16th Street
Washington, D.C. 20036

School Safety
(For elementary grades)
National Safety Council
425 North Michigan Avenue
Chicago, Illinois 60611

Social Health News
American Social Health Association
1740 Broadway
New York, New York 10019

The Child
U.S. Department of Health, Education, and Welfare
Children's Bureau
Washington, D.C. 20201

Today's Health
American Medical Association
535 North Dearborn Street
Chicago, Illinois 60210

Volta Review
Alexander Graham Bell Association for the Deaf, Inc.
1537 35th Street, N.W.
Washington, D.C. 20007

Appendix B

SCHOOL HEALTH RECORDS AND FORMS

WETZEL'S GRID

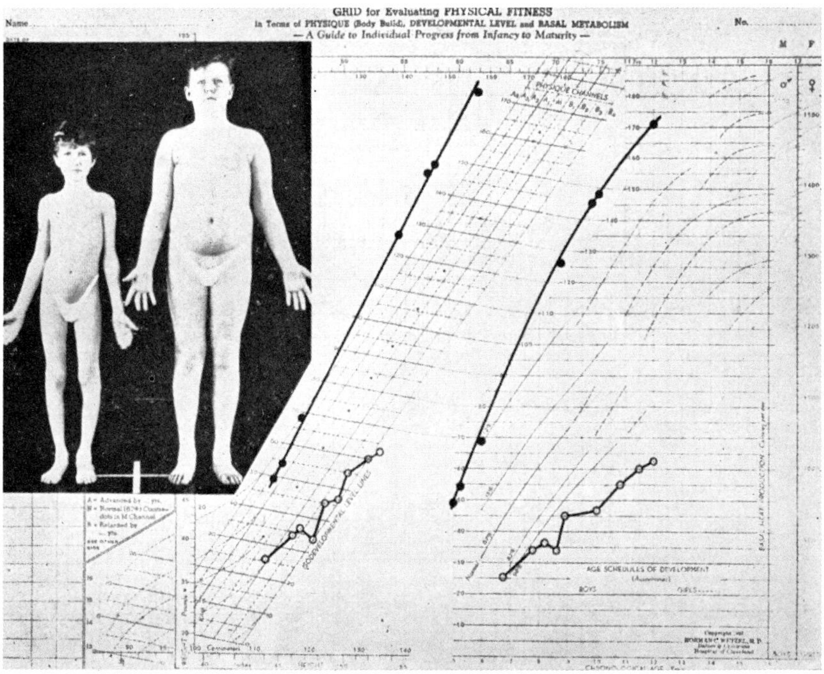

Figure 76 This illustration shows two opposite and quite obvious types of "undesirable growth progress" *i.e.*, "growth failure" over a period of 7 and 5¼ years, respectively. One boy proceeded from a moderately stocky build to obesity while advancing even more rapidly than the 2 per cent schedule or auxodrome calls for; the other, from a medium build in channel B_1 to the very slender physique channel B_4 and along a clearly "failing path" below (or behind) the 98 per cent standard.

The former subject gained 123 levels in 7 years (17.5 *lev./yr.* or 1.46 *lev./mo.*); the latter, only 38 levels in 5¼ years at 0.60 *lev./mo.* Between the two extremes is "the remaining 96 per cent of the population"—those with either *good*, or to some degree, *failing* growth records, all of which can be just as vividly displayed and individually evaluated as those shown here.

MEREDITH PHYSICAL GROWTH RECORDS

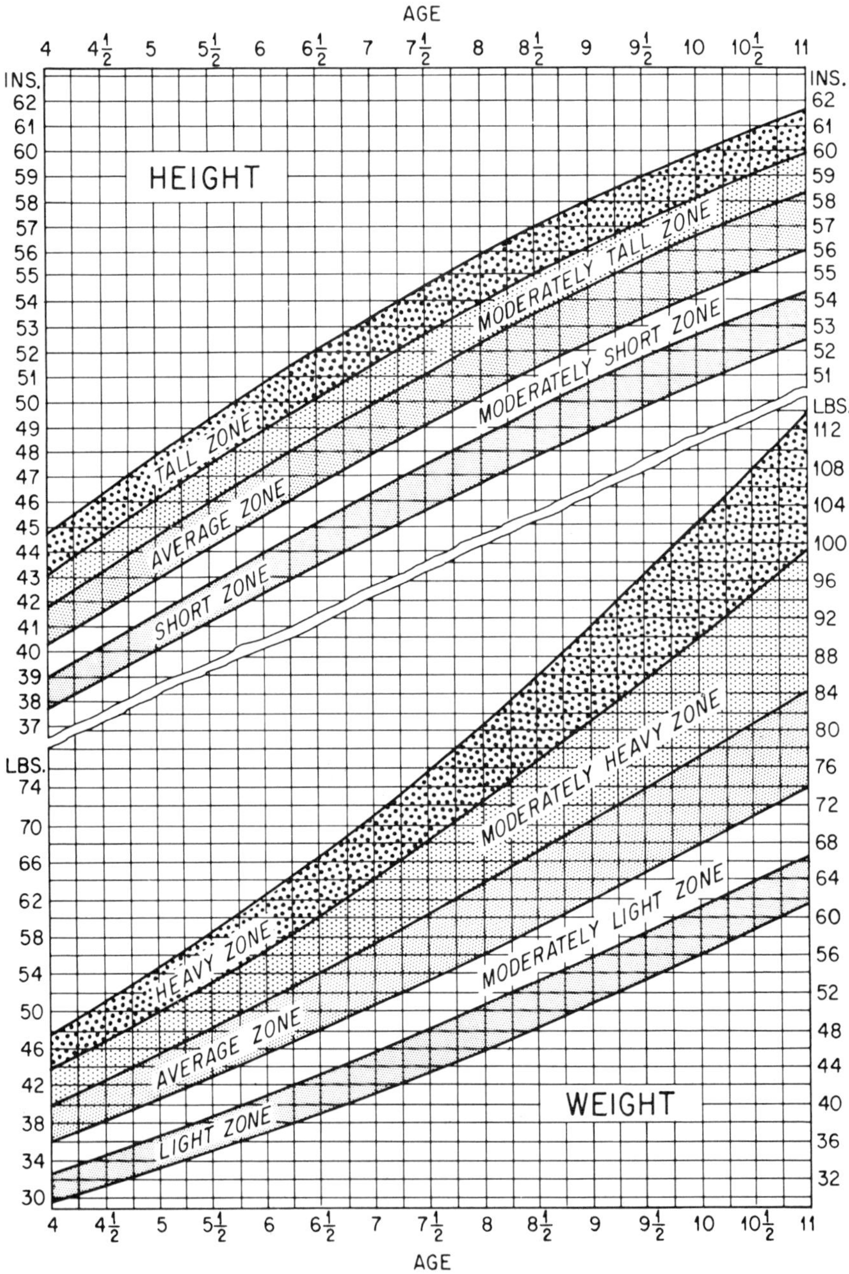

Figure 77 Boys, ages 4 to 11 years.

MEREDITH PHYSICAL GROWTH RECORDS *(Continued)*

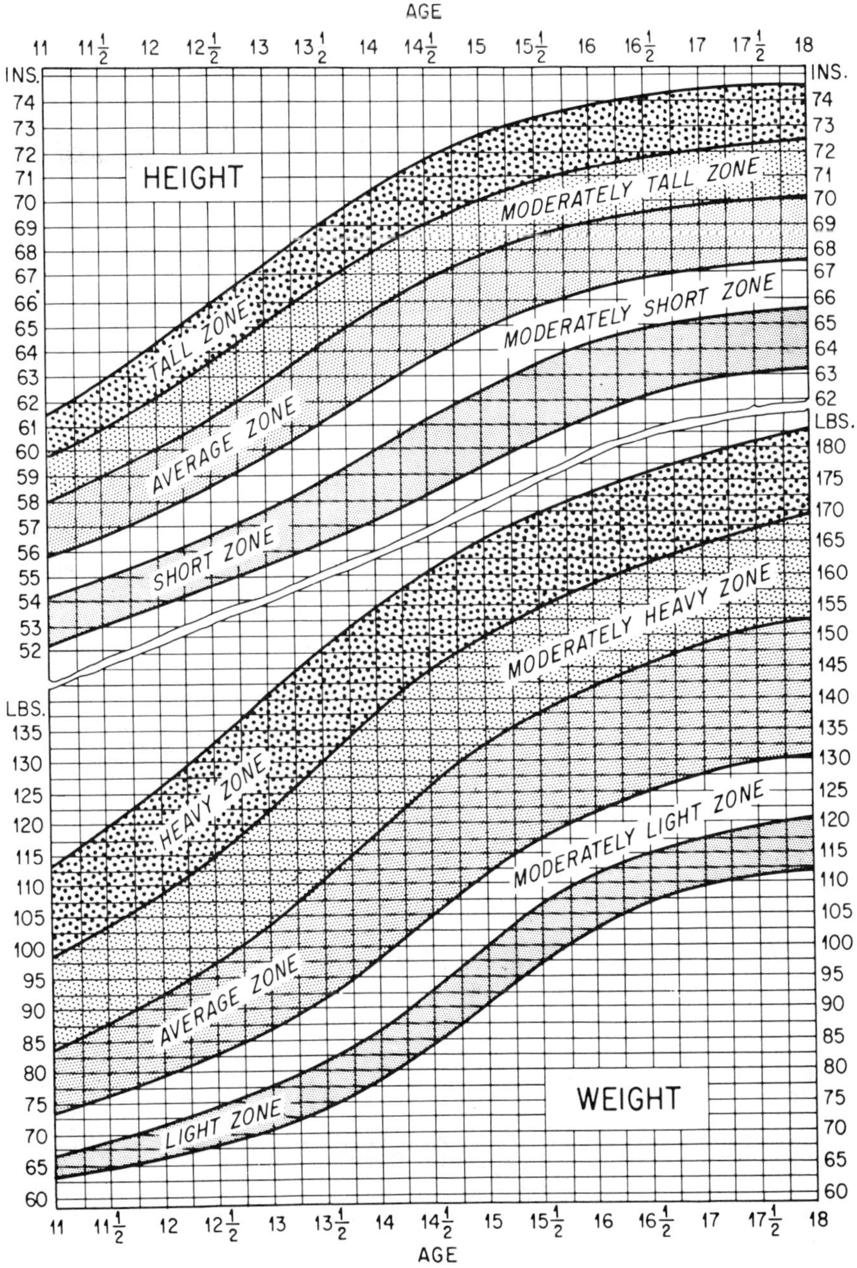

Figure 78 Boys, ages 11 to 18 years.

MEREDITH PHYSICAL GROWTH RECORDS* *(Continued)*

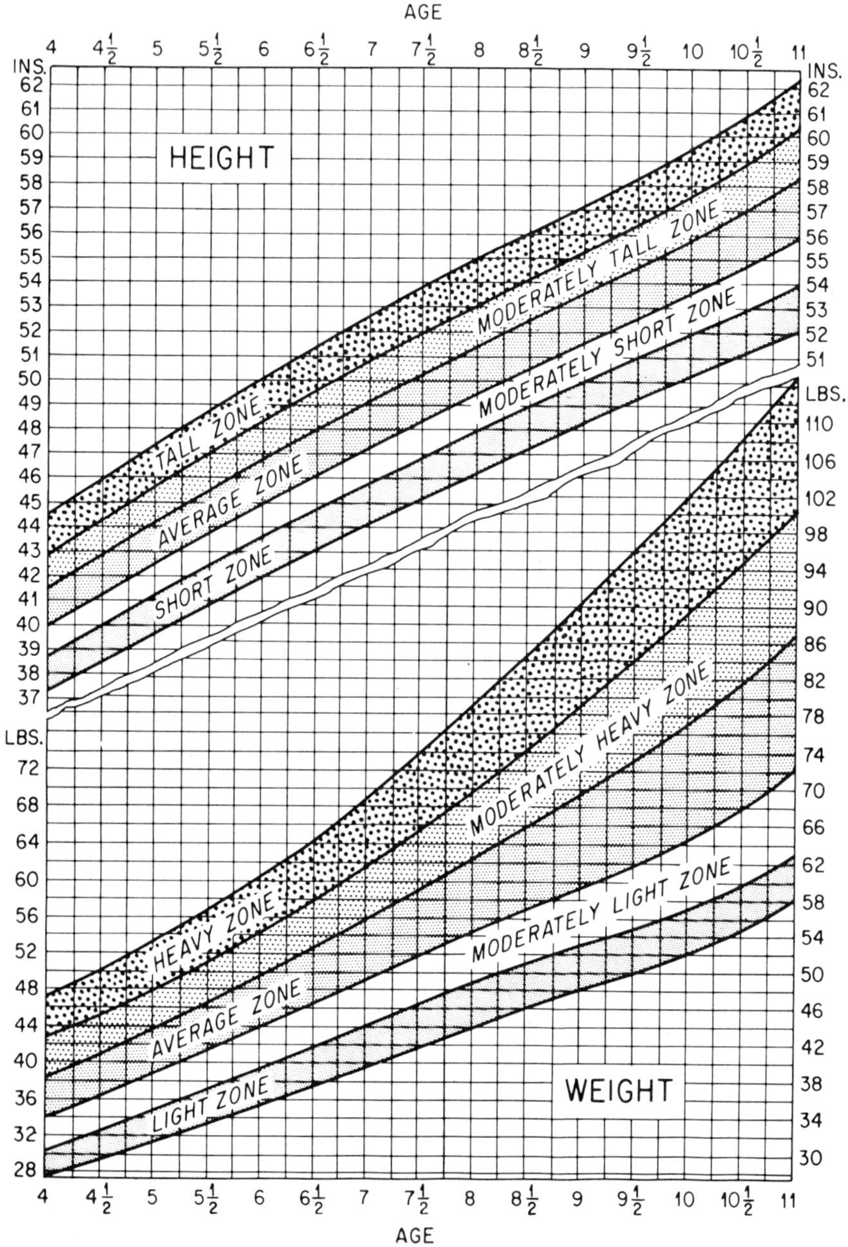

Figure 79 Girls, ages 4 to 11 years.

---

*Figs. 77–80 reproduced by courtesy of Howard V. Meredith and the Joint Committee on Health Problems in Education of the NEA and the AMA. Copies are available from either organization. Instructions for use are printed on forms. These forms have been adapted and simplified by school health services.

MEREDITH PHYSICAL GROWTH RECORDS* *(Continued)*

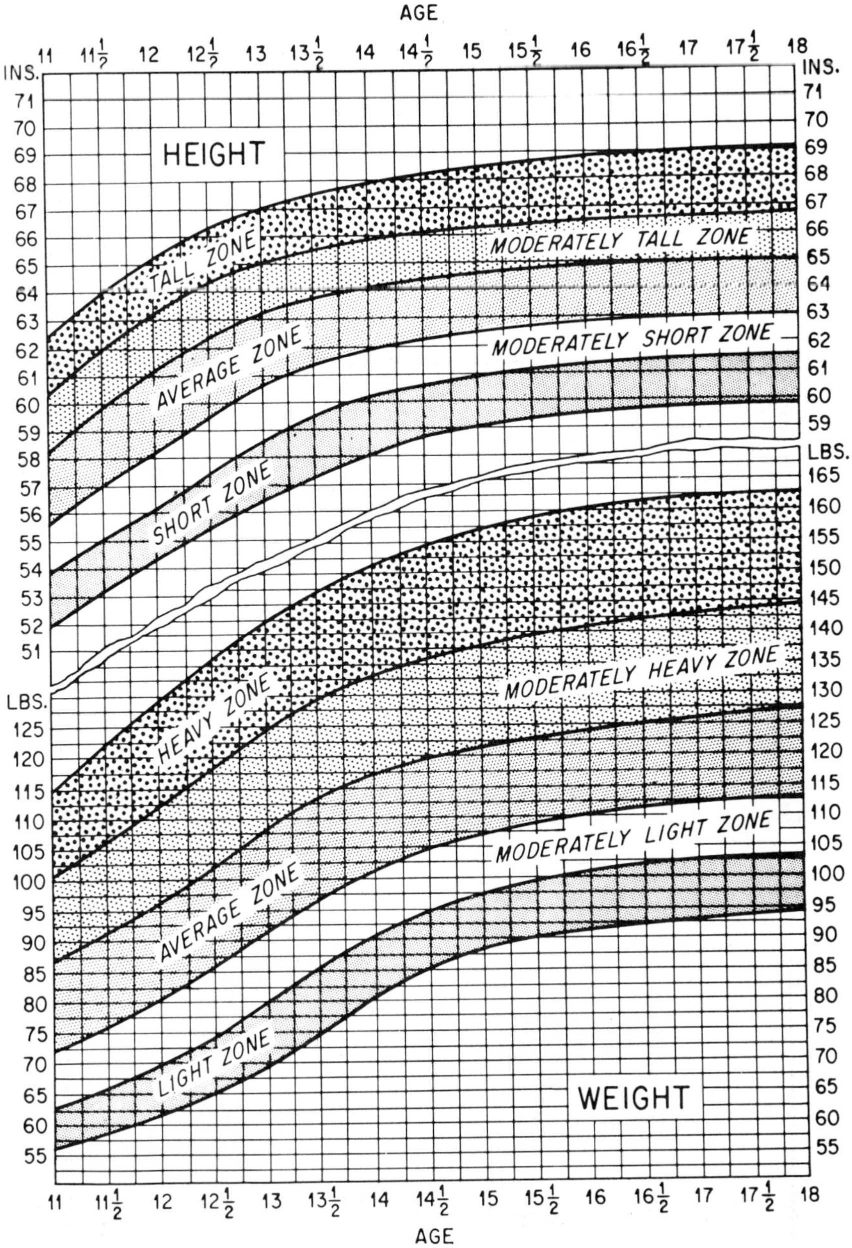

Figure 80 Girls, ages 11 to 18 years.

Child's
Name________________________________ Grade__________

School________________________________ Room No._______

DENVER PUBLIC SCHOOLS
Department of Health Service

NOTICE OF HEALTH APPRAISAL FOR ELEMENTARY PUPIL

The Denver Public School Health Service Department and the Denver County Medical Society encourage health appraisals of all children at regular intervals. The schools strongly recommend health appraisals of kindergarten or 1st graders, and 3rd, 6th, and 9th graders, plus pupils new to the schools, and those with health problems in any other grade. If it is possible for you to have your family doctor give this examination, we shall appreciate having him return the completed special health service examination blank which he has in his office.

For children whose physicians have not sent in this special health service examination blank, health appraisals by school physicians are offered at intervals during the school year.

A school doctor will be at your school some time in the near future. If you wish to have the school doctor give your child a health appraisal, will you please fill out the following blank and answer the questions on the back of this page?

We would like you to come to the school to talk with the physician. If you can plan to come, please be sure to check below and we will send you a definite appointment.

I desire the school health appraisal for my child Yes____ No____

I expect to be present at the appraisal Yes____ No____

Parent's signature________________________

Date________________

(Over)

STOCK NO. 10748
FORM 846 DSP 1-67-800 PADS E-207-58074

Please fill in the following and return to the school:

TUBERCULIN TEST AND IMMUNIZATIONS

(Check those your child has had with year last given)

YEAR LAST GIVEN

1. Tuberculin test and result: Negative ☐ Positive ☐ 19______
2. Immunizations against smallpox________________ 19______
3. Immunizations against diphtheria________________ 19______
4. Immunizations against whooping cough____________ 19______
5. Immunizations against tetanus________________ 19______
6. Immunizations against polio________________ 19______
7. Immunizations against measles________________ 19______

GENERAL HEALTH INFORMATION

1. Does your child have speech difficulties?________________
2. Is his eyesight normal?________________
3. Is his hearing normal?________________
4. Does your child seem to get along well with other boys and girls?

   Comment:________________

   ____
5. Does your child eat breakfast?________________
6. At what time does your child go to bed?________________
7. What particular health conditions such as serious illnesses, accidents, convulsions, tuberculosis, or diabetes has your child had?

   ____

   ____

   ____
8. What concerns do you have regarding your child's health?______

   ____

   ____

(Back of Form: Notice of Health Examination forElementary Pupils.)

HEALTH APPRAISAL REPORT FOR BOARD OF EDUCATION EMPLOYEES

THE BOARD OF EDUCATION OF SALT LAKE CITY

M. LYNN BENNION - SUPERINTENDENT OF SCHOOLS

OFFICE OF THE MEDICAL DIRECTOR

Daily association with school children and other employees makes it necessary for the employee to be free of communicable disease. Good health is desirable for all. Periodic health appraisals with attention to your physician's recommendations can prevent serious health problems. Carefully complete this confidential form.

TO BE FILLED IN BY EMPLOYEE:

Name .... (Last) (First) (Middle) .... Date of Birth Sex: Male ☐ Female ☐

.... Address .... Phone

Number and Ages of Children ....

Position Applied For .... Marital Status: Single, Married, Widowed, Divorced, Separated (Underline)

Please write X after each of the following conditions that you have or have-had; write 0 if you have not had them; Give dates; explain below:

Disease	Date	Disease	Date	Disease	Date
Tuberculosis - - ( )	....	Eczema - - - - ( )	....	Epilepsy - - - ( )	....
Hepatitis - - - ( )	....	Diabetes - - - ( )	....	Severe Injury - - ( )	....
Rheumatic Fever - ( )	....	Arthritis - - - ( )	....	Congenital Malformations - ( )	....
Nephritis - - - ( )	....	Thyroid Disease - ( )	....	Colitis - - - - ( )	....
Typhoid Fever - ( )	....	Other Glandular Disorders: .... - ( )	....	Tumor or Growth ( )	....
Dysentery - - - ( )	....	Difficulties with Pregnancy and/or Childbirth - - ( )	....	Mental Illness - - ( )	....
Malaria - - - - ( )	....	High Blood Pressure ( )	....	Other serious Conditions .... - ( )	....
Pneumonia - - - ( )	....	Ulcers of the digestive tract - ( )	....	Hernia - - - - ( )	....
Other serious infections: .... - ( )	....			Heart Disease - - ( )	....
Asthma - - - - ( )	....			Nervous Breakdown ( )	....
Hay Fever - - - ( )	....				

....

With whom do you live? ....

Do you now have: (write X or O, and give duration and part of body involved on line below).

Pain .... ( )	Mucus or pus discharge .... ( )	Skin discoloration .... ( )
Prolonged fatigue .... ( )	Numbness .... ( )	Nightmares .... ( )
Vomiting .... ( )	Lumps or swellings .... ( )	Chills .... ( )
Diarrhea .... ( )	Feeling of pressure .... ( )	Insomnia .... ( )
Bleeding .... ( )	Frequent Urination .... ( )	Depression .... ( )
Dizziness .... ( )	Other urinary disorders .... ( )	Nervousness .... ( )
Prolonged cough .... ( )	Fainting spells .... ( )	Paralysis .... ( )
Shortness of breath .... ( )	Rash .... ( )	Hungry nearly all the time .... ( )
Wheezing .... ( )	Skin Ulcers .... ( )	Poor appetite .... ( )
Weakness .... ( )	Fever .... ( )	Daily Use of Alcoholic Beverages .... ( )
Difficulty with sight .... ( )	Swollen Ankles .... ( )	Rapid or Irregular Heartbeat .... ( )
Difficulty with hearing .... ( )	Menstrual Disturbance .... ( )	

....

Have you ever had a surgical operation? (Explain) ....

Immunizations: (Give dates of last boosters or vaccinations)

Smallpox - - - - -	Diphtheria - - - -	Tetanus - - - - - ....
Typhoid - - - - -	Poliomyelitis - - -	Other - - - - - - ....

I certify that the above statements are true. Signed ....

Date ....

NOTICE TO PARENTS ABOUT HEALTH APPRAISALS FOR SECONDARY SCHOOL PUPILS

DENVER PUBLIC SCHOOLS

Department of Health Services

September 1967

Pupil's Name____________________________ Grade_______ Room_______

It is important for the school to have some information about every pupil's health. If possible, please have your family or clinic physician send a report of a recent examination to the schools. Will you ask him to send it on the special forms supplied by the schools?

If a recent health examination has not been performed by a private or clinic physician, please indicate your choice on the form below.

Health clearance is required periodically for participation in swimming classes, ROTC, and certain other school activities. In addition, annual medical appraisals are required for varsity sports.

In order to have health information of value to the school, we would appreciate your responses on the following:

1. Allergies________________
2. Convulsions or seizures________________
3. Diabetes________________
4. Frequent colds or sore throats________________
5. Frequent stomach-aches________________
6. Headaches________________
7. Heart trouble________________
8. Loss of time from school________________
9. Serious operations or accidents________________
10. Known exposure to tuberculosis Yes______ No______
11. Vision____________ Hearing____________
12. Other health problems, such as kidney trouble, ulcers, etc.________

____

____

HEALTH PRACTICES

1. *Eating*—Breakfast Yes______ No______ Between-meal snacks________________
2. *Rest and sleep*—Average hours________________
3. *Exercise and/or recreation outside of school*—Sports, clubs, music lessons, etc.________________

   ____
4. *Work activities outside of school*________________
5. *Emotional health*—Assuming responsibilities________________

   Getting along with others____________ Liking school____________

IMMUNIZATION RECORD AND TUBERCULIN TESTING (please state year last given)

Smallpox vaccination________________

Diphtheria-Tetanus________________

Polio: Number of Salk (shots) ________________

Types of Sabin (oral) doses I_______ II_______ III_______ Trivalent_______

Tuberculin test____________ Negative_______ Positive_______

PLEASE RETURN THIS SHEET PROMPTLY TO THE SCHOOL NURSE AFTER YOU SIGN BELOW

I will have our family or clinic physician give this examination. . . ________________
(Sign here)

I wish the school medical appraisal. . . . . ________________
(Sign here)

____
Date

STOCK NO. 10749
FORM 847 DSP 8-67-400 PADS E-969-59166

Name ______ Sex: M __ F __ Birth Date ______

LOS ANGELES CITY SCHOOLS – EXAMINATION BY PRIVATE PHYSICIAN (CONFIDENTIAL)
(To be retained as part of the Permanent School Health Record)

To the physician: Please complete both sides and return to the child's school in attached envelope.

Past Medical History:
Serious illnesses or injuries ______
______
Surgery ______
Allergic reactions ______
Birth History:
Pre-natal complications ______
Birth wt. ______ Delivery ______
Neo-natal complications ______
______ PKU ______
Immunizations (date completed or last booster):
Polio ______ DPT or ______
Measles ______ DT ______
Other ______ Smallpox ______

PARENTAL CONSENT: Consent is given for private physician's report to be sent to the school.

______
PARENT'S SIGNATURE

(**N** = normal. **O** = over for comment.)

	FUR. EXAM. REC.	UNDER R_x
Date of examination ______		
Wt ______ Ht. ______ B.P. ______		
Eyes ______ Vision ______ R:20/ L:20/		
Ears ______ Hearing ______		
Nose ______		
Mouth ______ Speech ______		
Throat ______ Tonsils ______		
Teeth ______ Orthodontia needed ______		
Heart ______		
Lungs ______		
Abdomen ______ Hernia ______		
G–U ______		
Neurologic ______		
Endocrine ______		
Menses: ______ abnormalities ______ menarche age ______		
Skin ______		
Posture ______ (Please indicate deviations from normal)		

Other orthopedic ______
Urine ______ Blood ______ (as indicated) Tuberculin Pos. ______ Neg. ______

(Over)

EXAMINATION BY PRIVATE PHYSICIAN (con't)

Does this child present:
Emotional problems ______
Behavioral problems ______
Other developmental problems ______

Has further investigation of above been undertaken:
Psychological testing ______
Neurological referral ______ EEG ______
Psychiatric referral ______
Other counseling ______
Medication ______

Physical Education (Required by State law):
Reg. ______ Limited or Corrective ______ (PLEASE STATE REASON)

Posture training ______

Recommendations and comments:

Signature ______ M.D.
______ M.D.
(PLEASE TYPE OR PRINT NAME)

Address ______
Phone ______ Date ______

LOS ANGELES CITY SCHOOLS
Health Services Branch – Auxiliary Services Division
(OVER)

33.171 2/68 100M

FORM 30B REV. 1-67

HEALTH APPRAISAL REPORT

SALT LAKE CITY BOARD OF EDUCATION
HEALTH SERVICES DEPARTMENT

THIS INFORMATION IS FOR OFFICIAL USE ONLY AND WILL NOT BE RELEASED TO UNAUTHORIZED PERSONS

NOTE TO PARENT: YOUR CHILD'S SUCCESS IN SCHOOL RESTS TO A VERY GREAT EXTENT ON HIS PHYSICAL WELL BEING. WITH THE CURRENT EMPHASIS ON PHYSICAL FITNESS, IT IS EVEN MORE IMPORTANT TO EXCLUDE IN EACH CHILD THE POSSIBILITY OF PHYSICAL HARM FROM ENGAGING IN STRENUOUS ACTIVITIES. THE IMPORTANCE OF THESE CONSIDERATIONS DEMANDS YOUR COOPERATION SO THAT ANY NECESSARY ADJUSTMENTS CAN BE MADE IN SCHOOL. THE EXAMINATIONS ARE COMPLETED BEFORE THE SCHOOL YEAR STARTS FOR GRADES OF **KINDERGARTEN, THIRD, SEVENTH** AND **TENTH.** ALSO ANY **NEW STUDENT** TO THE DISTRICT AND **ON ENTRANCE AND EVERY THREE YEARS FOR STUDENTS IN SPECIAL CLASSES.** TAKE YOUR CHILD TO THE MEDICAL DOCTOR OF YOUR CHOICE. YOU SHOULD TAKE WITH YOU A CLEAN FRESHLY VOIDED URINE SAMPLE. LABORATORY TESTS, IMMUNIZATIONS, A SKIN TEST FOR TB OR CHEST X-RAY MAY OR MAY NOT BE INDICATED AND THE SCHOOL RELIES ON YOUR PHYSICIAN'S RECOMMENDATION.

SECTION I OF THE FORM SHOULD BE COMPLETED BEFORE YOU REPORT FOR THE DOCTOR'S EXAMINATION. THE BACK OF THE FORM SHOULD THEN BE ADDRESSED TO THE SCHOOL PRINCIPAL AND A STAMP AFFIXED. YOUR DOCTOR WILL MAIL THE FORM DIRECTLY TO THE SCHOOL.

SECTION I

1. Last Name — First Name — Middle Name	2. Date of Birth	3. Age	4. Sex	5. School	6. Grade

7. Home Address	8. Phone	9. Father's Name	10. Mother's Name

11. **FAMILY HISTORY:** Has any blood relation of this child ever had any of the following? If yes note relationship at right.

Yes	No		Relationship:	Yes	No		Relationship:	Yes	No		Relationship:	Yes	No		Relationship:
		Tuberculosis				Epilepsy				High Blood Pressure				Cancer	
		Asthma				Hay Fever				Mental Disorder				Rheumatic Fever	
		Hives				Diabetes				Kidney Trouble				Rheumatism	

12. **Has child had or does child now have** (Please check at left of each item.)

YES	NO	(Check each item)	YES	NO	(Check each item)	YES	NO	(Check each item)	YES	NO	(Check each item)
		Scarlet Fever, Erysipelas			Hay Fever			Any Reaction to Serum, Drug or Medicine			Frequent Trouble Sleeping
		Diphtheria			Goiter or Thyroid Trouble			Tumor, Growth, Cyst, Cancer			Frequent or Terrifying Nightmares
		Meningitis			Sugar Diabetes			Rupture			Temper Tantrums
		Rheumatic Fever			Epilepsy or Seizures			Appendicitis			Depression or Excessive Worry
		St. Vitas Dance (chorea)			Tuberculosis			Piles or Rectal Disease			Loss of Memory or Amnesia
		Swollen or Painful Joints			Soaking Sweats			Frequent or Painful Urination			Speech Difficulties
		Mumps			Coughing of Blood			Kidney Stone or Blood in Urine			Bed Wetting
		Whooping Cough			Pneumonia			Kidney or Urinary Disease			Habit Spasm
		Frequent or Severe Headache			Asthma			Boils			Nervous Trouble of Any Sort
		Dizziness or Fainting Spells			Bronchitis or Chronic Cough			Venereal Disease			Poor Eating Habits
		Eye Trouble			Shortness of Breath			Recent Gain or Loss of Weight			Easy Bleeding or Bruising
		Eye Glasses			Pain or Pressure in Chest			Arthritis or Rheumatism			
		Ear, Nose, or Throat Trouble			Palpitation or Pounding Heart			Bone, Joint, or Other Deformity			
		Mouth Breathing			High or Low Blood Pressure			Lameness			
		Running Ears			Cramps in the Legs			Loss of Arm, Leg, Finger or Toe			
		Chronic or Frequent Colds			Frequent Indigestion			Foot Trouble			
		Severe Tooth or Gum Trouble			Stomach, Liver or Intestinal Trouble			Paralysis or Poliomyelitis			
		Sinusitis			Gall Bladder Trouble			Finger Sucking			
		Eczema			Jaundice			Nail Biting			

13. Has Child been immunized for:

Yes	No		If yes, list most recent year
		Tetanus	
		Diphtheria	
		Small Pox	
		Poliomyelitis	

14. Age at Walking	15. Age at Talking	16. Approx. gain in past 12 months lbs.	17. Is child ☐ right handed ☐ left handed	18. Date of last Dental Check

YES	NO	(Check each item Yes or No. Every item checked "Yes" must be fully explained in blank space on right.)	
		19. Does child take Medication? (If yes, give type, amount and reason)	
		20. Is there communicable disease or emotional illness in the home?	
		21. Do you know of any reason to limit child's physical activities?	
		22. Has child had a chest x-ray? (If yes, why, where, when and result)	
		23. Skin Test for Tuberculosis (If yes, give type, date and result)	
		24. Has child had difficulty with school studies or teachers? (If yes, give details)	
		25. Has child had or been advised to have any operations? (If yes, describe and give age at which occurred)	
		26. Has child ever had any illness or injury other than those already noted? (If yes, specify when, where, and give details)	

SECTION II

THIS SPACE FOR PHYSICIAN'S ELABORATION OF HISTORICAL DATA:

NOTE TO DOCTOR: WITH THE PRESENT EMPHASIS ON PHYSICAL FITNESS, THE MEDICAL EXAMINATION BECOMES EVEN MORE IMPORTANT. THE TEACHER REQUIRES PRECISE INFORMATION ON EACH PUPIL'S CAPABILITIES OR LIMITATIONS. YOUR SUPPORT IN SUPPLYING COMPLETE INFORMATION IS URGENTLY SOLICITED. KINDLY SEND THE COMPLETED FORM DIRECTLY TO THE SCHOOL.

PHYSICAL ACTIVITY CLASSIFICATION: (Information to be used in determining child's physical education and physical fitness program)

Check One or More (Use space at right for elaboration)	Comments:
☐ A. Full participation including competitive sports	
☐ B. Full participation excluding competitive sports	
☐ C. Restricted participation (Note restrictions)	
☐ D. No participation in sports	
☐ E. Limitation of ordinary activity. (Is stair climbing all right?)	
☐ F. Requires Rest Periods at school	
☐ G. Special Restrictions only (List)	

FOLD DOWN TO SEAL

BOARD OF EDUCATION
School Health Services Dept.
440 East First South
SALT LAKE CITY, UTAH 84111

PLACE
STAMP
HERE

Principal

.... School

....

Salt Lake City, Utah

SECOND FOLD TO HERE

MAKE FIRST FOLD HERE

SECTION II (Continued) **REPORT OF MEDICAL EXAMINATION** To be completed by Physician

1. Last Name — First Name — Middle Name

2. Height	3. Weight	4. Build ☐ Slender ☐ Medium ☐ Heavy ☐ Obese			5. Temperature	9. Hearing
6. Blood Pressure		7. Pulse		8. Distant Vision		Right WV /15 SV /15
Sitting	Sys	Sitting	After Exercise	2 Min. After	Right 20/ Corr. To 20/	
	Dias				Left 20/ Corr. To 20/	Left WV /15 SV /15

10. CLINICAL EVALUATION (Check each item)

	Normal	Not Done	Abnormal		Normal	Not Done	Abnormal		Normal	Not Done	Abnormal		Normal	Not Done	Abnormal
Nutrition				Oral Care				Heart				Genitalia			
Hygiene				Teeth				Abdomen				Hernia			
Eyes				Glands				Back				Speech			
E N T				Lungs				Extremities				Neurologic			

11. List any current medications

12. Are immunizations current? ☐ Yes ☐ No If not, list any deficits

13. Urinalysis: A. Specific Gravity		14. Hematocrit	15. Other Lab:
B. Albumin	D. Microscopic		
C. Sugar			

16. Summary of Defects and Diagnoses: (Complete Physical Activity Classification on reverse side.)

17. Recommendation for further Medical or Dental care:

18. Do you recommend that this child be considered for:

YES	NO	(Check each item)	YES	NO	(Check each item)	YES	NO	(Check each item)
		Speech Correction			Special Seating in Class			Special Class for the Motor Handicapped
		Lip Reading Instruction or Auditory Training			Home Instruction			Part-time Visual Resource Instruction
		Special Class for Emotionally Disturbed			Special Class for the Intellectually Handicapped			Psychological Evaluation

19. Typed or Printed Name, Address and Phone Number of Physician	20. Date of Examination	21. Signature
		M. D.

Sample Dental Card*

TO THE PARENT: Our school has a health program that is designed to improve, protect and promote the health of the child. As a part of this health program we strongly urge all parents to have their children visit their dentist at least once a year for a dental examination and whatever treatment may be necessary. In the interest of better dental health would you then have your child take this card to a dentist of your choice. When the examination and treatment are completed, the card should be returned to school.

____
Principal

(Front)

REPORT OF DENTAL EXAMINATION

This is to certify that I have examined the teeth of
______________________________ and:

- ☐ 1. All necessary dental treatment has been completed.
- ☐ 2. Treatment is in progress.
- ☐ 3. No dental treatment is nceessary at this time.

Further recomentations ______________________________

__________________ ________________________
Date Signature of Dentist

PLEASE RETURN THIS CARD TO THE TEACHER

(Back)

Sample Excusal Form

SCHOOL EXCUSE FORM FOR DENTAL APPOINTMENT

________________________ has an appointment for necessary
Name of Pupil

dental service on __________________ 19___ at__________ A.M. PM..

This service cannot be satisfactorily rendered outside of school hours. Therefore, it will be appreciated if this pupil may be permitted to keep the appointment as indicated above. Permission granted by:

________________________ ________________________
Signature of School Official Signature of Parent

________________________ was in my office from__________ A.M. P.M.
Name of Pupil

to________ A.M. P.M. on__________________ 19___ to have dental treatment.

____
Signature of Dentist

TO BE RETURNED TO THE SCHOOL TEACHER OR PRINCIPAL

(Front)

The Board of Education of________________________ and the ________________________ Dental Society are cooperating in a plan whereby public school children of________________________ may receive necessary dental care during school hours.
A permit from the school for such purpose, used judiciously, will enable school children to secure dental services that cannot be satisfactorily rendered during the hours school is not in session.
This permit is approved by the________________________ Board of Education and the________________________ Dental Society.

(Back)

*Sample forms recommended by the Study Committee on Dental Health of The American School Health Association. Report 1961–62. *J. School Health* 32:399–401, 1962.

DENVER PUBLIC SCHOOLS

Health Service Department

HEALTH EVALUATION OF PUPILS FOR PLACEMENT IN SPECIAL EDUCATION PROGRAMS

Name of child________________________ Date____________

Birthday of child____________ School attended (if any)____________

Address________________________ Phone____________

Parent, guardian, or other informant________________________

Reason for examination:________________________

		Date Last Seen
Name of clinics, hospitals, or doctors serving child	Clinic____________	____________
	Private M.D.____________	____________
	Specialist____________	____________

PAST AND FAMILY HISTORY: (Parent present ☐ or if not, nurse obtains data from home)

Birth: (type, weight, trauma, etc.)____________ Convulsions____________

Mother's health during this pregnancy________________________

Health, age, sex of siblings________________________

Child sat up________ Talked________ Walked________ Child's difficulty first noted____________

Diseases____________ Accidents____________

Operations: T&A____________ Others____________

PHYSICAL EXAMINATION: Height____________ Weight____________

Vision test (current) Rt.________ Lt.________ Comments____________

Hearing test (current) Rt.________ Lt.________ Comments____________

Check below (o) if essentially negative or (x) if abnormal and describe on back of sheet.

Mouth____	Glands____	Heart____	Genitalia____	Skin____	Coordination____
Teeth____	Eyes____	Abdomen____	Hernia____	Gait____	Skel. deform.____
Tonsils____	Ears____	Extremities____	Nutrition____	Allergies____	Toilet habits____

IMPRESSION OF CHILD AND MEDICAL RECOMMENDATIONS FOR EDUCATIONAL PROGRAM:

1. General physical condition is________________________
2. Health practices seem to be________________________
3. Family attitudes apparently are________________________
4. Specific health problems include: Vision ☐ Hearing ☐ Motor Incoordination ☐ Hyperactivity ☐
   Convulsive Disorder ☐ (on medication ☐ no medication ☐) Frequency of Episodes____________
   Date of last episode, etc.________________________
   Other:________________________
5. Recommendations:
   Further attention to________________________
   Placement in limited P.E. ☐ Regular P.E. ☐ Swimming ☐
   Other:________________________

____________ Date of Evaluation

____________ Signature of Physician

FORM 808

V______ DT______ P______

Name: Last First Middle Sex: M ☐ F ☐

LOS ANGELES CITY SCHOOLS
HEALTH RECORD

POLIO SABIN 1____ 2____ 3____
SALK 1____ 2____ 3____ E____
TRIVALENT 1____ 2____

Residence	Phone	School	Date Arr.	Birth Date Mo. Day Yr.
				Birthplace
				Arrived in Calif.
				Room Nos.

SYMBOLS ʌ NEEDS ATTENTION GRADE URGENCY 1, 2, 3, OR 4 **PHYSICAL EXAMINATION** A RECEIVED ATTENTION F FURTHER EXAM. NEEDED O OVER

Date of Examination	Name of Examiner	Grade	NUTRITION			EYES			EARS			NOSE & THROAT			TEETH				HEART		LUNGS	Orthopedic		Nervous System	Speech	Skin	Endocrine	Misc.
				Hgt.	Wgt.	Vision R	Vision L	Pathology	Hearing R	Hearing L	Pathology	Pathology	Tonsils	Adenoids	Decay	Cleaning	Gums	Orthodontia	Organic	Functional		Posture	Feet					

Rests: how long?
Assignment to Special Classes:
Corrective P. E.
Reg. Gym. Driver Training

FORM 34-EH-6 55M 8-67 (STK. NO. 815301) This card must be transferred with other record cards. Every child must have a health card or an "Excuse from Physical Education."

PERSONAL HISTORY Date Family Physician Address
Family Dentist Address

Asthma		Tbc—Child		Dental Decay		Convulsions		IMMUNIZATIONS	Years			HEALTH STATUS
Hayfever		Tbc—Family		Toothache		Fainting		Smallpox				Father
Eczema		Chickenpox		Freq. Colds		When?		Diph.				Mother
Diabetes		Measles		Freq. Sore Throats		Nose Bleeds		Wh. Cough				Bros. Ages
Heart Dis.		Ger. Measles		Freq. Coughs		Growing Pains		Tetanus				
Polio		Wh. Cough		Freq. Headaches		Operations		Polio				Sis. Ages
Pneumonia		Mumps		Wears Glasses								
Rheum. Fever		Hernia		Tires Easily		Accidents						
Scarlet Fever		Eye Difficulty		Recent Bed Wtg.		Other Ser. Ill.						

Appetite Milk Daily? Food Allergies?
Breakfast Bed time Rising Time

DENTAL RECORD						VISION SCREENING			Date	PHYSICIAN'S, DENTIST'S, OR NURSE'S NOTES
Date Examined	Name of Examiner	TEETH Decay	Cleaning	Gums	Orthodontia	Date	R	L		

Audiometer Date Date Date Date Date Mantoux Date
R.
L.

Health Appraisal Form: Cumulative Health Record. The results of the health appraisal are entered in the designated space on the permanent student record form.

DENVER PUBLIC SCHOOLS
HEALTH SERVICE DEPARTMENT

PARENT'S REQUEST FOR GIVING MEDICINE AT SCHOOL

I request the nurse or teacher to see that my child

______________________________ receives the medication
(Child's Name)

prescribed by ______________________________ for the period
(Physician's Name)

from ____________________ to ____________________.
(Date) (Date)

The medicine is to be furnished by me and is to be labeled with the name of the medicine, the amount to be given, time of day to be taken and the expected duration of treatment. The physician's name must be on the label.

Signature ______________________________
(Parent or Guardian)

Date ______________________________

School ______________________________

STOCK NO. 10721
FORM 821 DSP 7-61-100 PADS Y-556-50064

THE PHYSICAL EXAMINATION AND RECOMMENDATIONS INCLUDING A CHEST X-RAY MUST BE COMPLETED WITHIN THREE MONTHS PRIOR TO YOUR BEGINNING THE POSITION AND MUST BE PERFORMED BY A REGISTERED MEDICAL DOCTOR. THIS HEALTH APPRAISAL AND X-RAY REPORT MUST BE COMPLETED AND REPORTED NOT LESS THAN ONE WEEK BEFORE BEGINNING WORK.

TO BE FILLED IN BY PHYSICIAN OR PUBLIC HEALTH OFFICER:

Chest x-ray performed on .... Report ....
(Chest x-ray may be made by the Salt Lake City Board of Health for a charge of $1.00.)
If chest x-ray was made by the Board of Health, report may be sent directly to the School Health Director.

Date .... Signed, ..., M. D.

TO BE COMPLETED BY APPLICANT'S PHYSICIAN: Date of Examination ....

Name .... Age .... Height .... Weight ....

Vision without glasses: Lt. Rt. Hearing: Lt. Rt.
Vision with glasses: Lt. Rt.

Intradermal Tuberculin Test (P.P.D. Intermediate): Date .... Results ....

Urinalysis: Albumin .... Sugar .... Specific Gravity .... Microscopic ....

Blood: Hemoglobin .... gms. Other ....

Heart Rate .... Blood Pressure: systolic .... diastolic ....

Check Areas of Abnormality and Explain Below:

Head	( )	Glands	( )	Reflexes	( )
Eyes	( )	Thorax	( )	Extremeties	( )
Ears	( )	Lungs	( )	Posture	( )
Nose	( )	Heart	( )	Back	( )
Teeth	( )	Abdomen	( )	Feet	( )
Throat	( )	Hernia	( )	Attitude	( )
Neck	( )	Genitalia	( )	Emotional Status	( )

....

PERTINENT FINDINGS FROM HISTORY AND PHYSICAL EXAMINATION: ....

....

....

....

Is there communicable disease or emotional illness in the applicant's home? (Explain) ....

....

Do you think this person is emotionally and physically suited for work involving close contact with school-age children?

.... Explain: ....

....

Please give recommendations as to kind and hours of work. No limitations .... Limited (Explain) ....

.... How Long? ....

Is applicant now under treatment? .... Condition ....

How long is applicant expected to be under treatment? ....

What medicines is the applicant taking? ....

Next health appraisal advised ....

Date .... Signed ...., M.D.

State Medical License Number ....

Telephone .... Address ....

PHYSICIAN: Please send this confidential report directly to the HEALTH DIRECTOR OF THE BOARD OF EDUCATION OF SALT LAKE CITY, 440 East First South, Salt Lake City 11, Utah.

Appendix C

CHECK LISTS

The following *sample* pages from check lists are reproduced from "Criteria for Evaluating the Elementary School Health Program" and "Criteria for Evaluating the High School Health Program," criteria developed by a committee of the California Fitness Project and School Health Education Evaluative Study, Los Angeles Area, after a three-year study. (See Chapter 21.) Separate booklets for these two educational levels were published by the California State Department of Education in 1962. The privilege of using material from them is appreciated.

Preliminary introductory statements for both booklets observe that the criteria

> ... provide school personnel with a tool to use in making an evaluation of the school health program. The results of such an evaluation reveal the strengths and weaknesses of the program. Where weaknesses are revealed, the school health committee may act to bring all the available forces into action for the express purpose of securing strength in the program where weaknesses exist and for planning ways all other phases of the program may be kept strong....

The criteria in each set are organized into four divisions:

I—Administration, II—Health Instruction, III—Health Services, and IV—Healthful School Environment. The criteria are expressed in terms of desirable practices and presented in the left column. The evaluation should be made by a representative group of the faculty, including administrators, teachers, health service personnel, and others. The results should express judgments that are approved by the evaluation committee as a whole.

Provision is made for the quality of each *provision* or *practice* stated in the criteria to be judged on a four-point scale: *excellent, good, fair, poor.* If the provision is not made, the practice is not followed; or if the quality is fair or poor, there is space for listing changes needed. At the top of each section, space is provided for recording recommended steps to be taken in relation to the changes needed. Care should be taken to make recommendations that will not have an adverse effect on provisions or practices already judged excellent or good.

CRITERIA FOR EVALUATING THE ELEMENTARY SCHOOL HEALTH PROGRAM

Criteria	Quality of provision or practice: Excellent (near perfection)	Good (satisfactory)	Fair (slightly less than satisfactory)	Poor (unsatisfactory)	Provision not made or practice not followed	Changes needed
I. ADMINISTRATION A. The policies of the district's governing board provide for a school health program designed to help all pupils achieve the degree of health their potentialities permit through health instruction, health services, a healthful school environment—essentials of the program.	Recommended steps to be taken:					
1. The policies provide for a comprehensive and well-planned program of health instruction.						
2. The policies provide for essential health services.						
3. The policies provide for the maintenance of a healthful school environment.						
B. A written statement of the school district's point of view regarding the kind and quality of the school health program is available.	Recommended steps to be taken:					
1. The statement of point of view makes apparent the direction to be taken in providing health services.						
2. The statement of point of view makes apparent the direction to be taken in the program of health instruction.						
3. The statement of point of view makes apparent the direction to be taken in providing and maintaining a healthful school environment.						
C. Responsibility for planning, developing, and administering the district's school health program is delegated by the governing board of the district to the district superintendent of schools.	Recommended steps to be taken:					
1. A health committee with a membership that includes school personnel, representatives of community health services, and representatives of the other important segments of the community is assigned advisory responsibilities for the district's school health program.						
2. The superintendent has defined the duties of each person who has responsibility for providing health services.						
3. The superintendent has defined the duties of each person who has responsibility for health instruction.						
4. The superintendent has defined the duties of each person who has responsibility for the promotion and maintenance of a healthful school environment.						
5. The superintendent has defined for the principal his responsibility for the school health program.						
6. The superintendent and the principal have defined for the teachers and other members of the school staff their responsibilities for the school health program.						

CRITERIA FOR EVALUATING THE ELEMENTARY SCHOOL HEALTH PROGRAM

Criteria	Quality of provision or practice: Excellent (near perfection)	Good (satisfactory)	Fair (slightly less than satisfactory)	Poor (unsatisfactory)	Provision not made or practice not followed	Changes needed
F. Health personnel are adequate in number and specialization to provide needed services.	Recommended steps to be taken:					
1. School nurses are available in a ratio of one nurse for each 1,000 to 1,400 pupils. (Distances traveled to visit homes and type of terrain should be considered in determining the desired ratio.)						
2. Physicians are available for consultation and advice.						
3. Dentists are available for consultation and advice.						
4. Health service personnel serving the school are regularly credentialed.						
G. The professional library and the school library are well supplied with health materials.	Recommended steps to be taken:					
1. The professional library contains up-to-date books, courses of study, and periodicals on health.						
2. The materials in the professional library cover all phases of the school health program.						
3. The school library contains up-to-date books and periodicals on health.						
4. The books and periodicals in the school library are within the pupils' range of reading ability.						
5. The books and periodicals in the school library are adequate in number for the school population.						
H. Each classroom is supplied with the materials needed for use in health instruction.	Recommended steps to be taken:					
1. The classrooms for each grade are supplied with the basic textbooks in health that are supplied by the state.						
2. Each classroom is supplied with health materials, in addition to the state adopted textbooks, that cover each phase of health.						
3. The scope of the materials in each classroom is sufficient to provide for all the pupils, from the slowest to the fastest learner.						
I. The in-service education program for school personnel provides for health instruction to have the same emphasis as other areas of instruction.	Recommended steps to be taken:					
1. Sessions are devoted to presentation of current factual information about health.						

CRITERIA FOR EVALUATING THE ELEMENTARY SCHOOL HEALTH PROGRAM

Criteria	Quality of provision or practice				Provision not made or practice not followed	Changes needed
	Excellent (near perfection)	Good (satisfactory)	Fair (slightly less than satisfactory)	Poor (unsatisfactory)		
3. The scope of the content for the total program includes the following: a. Structure and function of the body.						
b. Food and nutrition.						
c. Physical activity and play.						
d. Rest, sleep, and relaxation.						
e. Mental health.						
f. Family health.						
g. Dental health.						
h. Disease prevention.						
i. Habit-forming substances.						
j. Safety and first aid.						
k. Consumer health.						
l. Community health.						
4. The sequence in which the content is introduced and developed is outlined for the total program.						
5. The scope of the content for each grade is outlined.						
6. The sequence in which the content is introduced and developed is outlined for each grade.						
7. The basic program of health instruction is developed through the use of units devoted primarily to health.						
8. Health instruction is enriched by making it a correlated phase of units in other subjects such as science, social studies, and homemaking.						
9. Pupils' interests and needs are utilized as motivation for learning.						
10. Health instruction is adapted to the pupils' abilities by employing the following methods separately or in combinations: a. Problem solving.						
b. Discussion.						
c. Demonstration.						
d. Reading.						
e. Recitation.						
f. Research.						
g. Construction.						

CRITERIA FOR EVALUATING THE ELEMENTARY SCHOOL HEALTH PROGRAM

Criteria	Quality of provision or practice: Excellent (near perfection)	Good (satisfactory)	Fair (slightly less than satisfactory)	Poor (unsatisfactory)	Provision not made or practice not followed	Changes needed
2. School personnel co-operate with representatives of the local health department in planning community immunization programs that are to be available to pupils.						
3. The school co-operates with local health agencies in conducting a tuberculosis case-finding program for pupils and school personnel.						
4. School health personnel report to the local health department the cases of diseases specified by the department.						
5. Parents are notified of in-school exposures to communicable diseases other than common colds.						
6. Pupils suspected of having communicable diseases are isolated while they are waiting to be removed from school.						
O. The health service program provides emergency service for injury and sudden illness and for disasters.	Recommended steps to be taken:					
1. Written policies and procedures for first aid and emergency care are provided to all school personnel.						
2. The policies and procedures pertaining to first aid and emergency care are approved by the local medical society or the health department.						
3. First aid is administered promptly to injured or ill pupils.						
4. Phone numbers of parents and of physicians to call in emergencies are on file for each pupil.						
5. Parents are notified immediately in instances of serious injury or illness.						
6. Teachers are prepared to render first aid.						
7. Periodic reviews of up-to-date first aid procedures are provided for all school personnel.						
8. First aid kits are available in each classroom and in the principal's office.						
9. The contents of first aid kits are replaced as required to maintain complete complements.						
10. The school nurse periodically inspects first aid kits and replenishes the supplies.						
11. First aid equipment, such as stretchers and blankets, is stored in readily accessible places.						
IV. HEALTHFUL SCHOOL ENVIRONMENT[1] A. The school environment is protected by employing personnel whose health is good, requiring all personnel to have regular health examinations, and providing measures that encourage good health practices.	Recommended steps to be taken:					
1. Pre-employment medical examinations are required of all personnel.						
2. Periodic medical examinations are required of all personnel.						

[1] Before this section is completed, study *Check List for a Healthful and Safe School Environment.* Sacramento: California State Department of Education, 1957.

CRITERIA FOR EVALUATING THE ELEMENTARY SCHOOL HEALTH PROGRAM

Criteria	Quality of provision or practice: Excellent (near perfection)	Good (satisfactory)	Fair (slightly less than satisfactory)	Poor (unsatisfactory)	Provision not made or practice not followed	Changes needed
2. Teachers with responsibility for providing instruction in health are supplied with up-to-date health materials to supplement text material.						
3. Up-to-date audio-visual materials on health are readily available to teachers.						
I. The in-service education program for school personnel provides for health instruction to have the same emphasis as other areas of instruction.	Recommended steps to be taken:					
1. Sessions are devoted to presentation of current factual information about health.						
2. Methods of health teaching to obtain changes in students' attitudes and practices are discussed and suggestions for improvements in instruction are presented.						
3. Evaluation of the school health program is discussed and suggestions for program improvements are presented.						
J. The in-service education program for school personnel provides for study of the school health services.	Recommended steps to be taken:					
1. The services provided by health personnel are reviewed in relation to their purpose.						
2. The procedures employed in providing health services are reviewed.						
3. Health services are studied in relation to all other phases of the school program.						
II. HEALTH INSTRUCTION A. A health instruction guide is provided by the school district or the office of the county superintendent of schools for use in the school.	Recommended steps to be taken:					
1. A health instruction guide is available in the school.						
2. The guide is designed to assist administrators, curriculum personnel, and teachers in developing and conducting the health instruction program.						
3. The guide provides for articulation of health instruction at the high school level with health instruction at the elementary and college levels.						
4. The guide includes a statement of basic beliefs about health instruction, specific objectives, scope and sequence of content, suggested student experiences, sources of materials, and suggestions for evaluation.						
B. Instruction in health is planned in accordance with specific objectives, covers basic health information in logical sequence, and is adapted to the students' needs and abilities.	Recommended steps to be taken:					

CRITERIA FOR EVALUATING THE ELEMENTARY SCHOOL HEALTH PROGRAM

Criteria	Quality of provision or practice: Excellent (near perfection)	Good (satisfactory)	Fair (slightly less than satisfactory)	Poor (unsatisfactory)	Provision not made or practice not followed	Changes needed
7. All teachers and health personnel participate in health counseling by helping students to solve their immediate problems and to develop skills in learning how to meet future concerns.						
E. There is a plan for evaluating health instruction in terms of student growth in health understandings, attitudes, and practices, and the results of the evaluations are utilized to improve the program.	Recommended steps to be taken:					
1. There is a planned program of evaluation to appraise the effectiveness of health instruction in terms of student growth in: a. Health understandings						
b. Attitudes about health and health practices						
c. Health behavior						
2. The results of evaluations are used to improve the health instruction program.						
III. HEALTH SERVICES A. A health services guide is provided by the school district or by the office of the county superintendent of schools.	Recommended steps to be taken:					
1. A health services guide provided by the school district or the office of the county superintendent of schools is available in the school.						
2. The guide contains the objectives for health services.						
3. The guide outlines the procedures employed in providing health services.						
4. The guide contains suggested ways health services can be adapted to meet special needs of individuals and of the total school population.						
B. A health service committee, preferably a subcommittee of the health council or committee, has advisory responsibility for health services.	Recommended steps to be taken:					
1. The health services committee has a membership representative of the school administration, teachers, school health personnel, and counselors.						
2. Consultation and advice of physicians, dentists, and other health specialists in the community are available, as needed, to the health services committee.						

CRITERIA FOR EVALUATING THE ELEMENTARY SCHOOL HEALTH PROGRAM

Criteria	Quality of provision or practice: Excellent (near perfection)	Good (satisfactory)	Fair (slightly less than satisfactory)	Poor (unsatisfactory)	Provision not made or practice not followed	Changes needed
O. The health service program provides emergency service for injury and sudden illness and for disasters.	Recommended steps to be taken:					
1. Written policies and procedures for first aid and emergency care are provided to all school personnel.						
2. The policies and procedures pertaining to first aid and emergency care are approved by the local medical society or the health department.						
3. First aid is administered promptly to injured or ill students.						
4. Phone numbers of parents and of physicians to call in emergencies are on file for each student.						
5. Parents are notified immediately in instances of serious injury or illness.						
6. Teachers are prepared to render first aid.						
7. Periodic reviews of up-to-date first aid procedures are provided for all school personnel.						
8. First aid kits are available in each building and in the central office.						
9. First aid kits with contents appropriate to the type of accidents that might occur are available in chemistry laboratories, homemaking departments, shops, gymnasiums, school kitchens and other areas where accidents are likely to occur.						
10. The contents of first aid kits are replaced as required to maintain complete complements.						
11. The school nurse periodically inspects first aid kits and replenishes the supplies.						
12. Rescue devices such as ring buoys, long poles, and knotted ropes are prominently displayed and readily accessible in each swimming pool area.						
13. First aid equipment, such as stretchers and blankets, is stored in readily accessible places.						
IV. HEALTHFUL SCHOOL ENVIRONMENT A. A committee, preferably a subcommittee of the health council or committee, has advisory responsibilities for the school environment.	Recommended steps to be taken:					
1. The environment committee has a membership representative of administration, faculty, cafeteria, and custodial staff.						
2. Consultation and advice of specialists such as physicians, public health sanitarians, safety engineers, and lighting specialists are available, as needed, to the environment committee.						

INDEX

Page numbers in *italics* indicate a figure. Page numbers followed by a (t) indicate a table.

Abdomen, injuries to, management of, 249
Accidents, causes, statistics on, 396(t), 397(t), 399(t)
  follow-up on, 440
  in school plant, 398
  outside school, 298
Acidosis, 271
Acoustics, in school plant, 385
Activities, extracurricular, regulation of, 395
Acne vulgaris, 240–243, *241*
  cause of, 241–243
  cleanliness and, 243
  counseling of adolescent, 244
  diet and, 242
  general health and, 243
  nervousness and, 244
Adenitis, 146
Adenoids, 136
Adolescence, emotional development in, 282
Alcott, William A., 346
Allergen(s), 221
  channels of entry of, 222
Allergic rhinitis, 223
Allergy(ies), 221–228
  effects of, 226
  incidence of, *221*
  management of, 226
  nasal, 223
  psychosomatic aspects of, 222
  school management of, 227
  skin, 225
Amblyopia, as result of strabismus, 89
Antitoxin, tetanus, 193
Appendicitis, clinical picture of, 248
Arthritis, 259
Articulation, defective, 148
Asthma, 223–225
  acute attack, 224
  effects of, 224
Astigmatism, *86*
  causes of, 87
"Athlete's foot," management of, 238
Audiogram, *118*, *119*
Audiometer, pure tone, 124, *125*
  speech, 125
Audiometer test, group pure tone, 124
  individual, 124
  limitations of, 124
Audiovisual materials, resources for, 531

Bacteria, dental caries and, 161
Battered child, 331–333
  laws regarding, 332
  parents of, 332
  school management of, 332
Behavior, "histrionic," 318
  suicidal, 287–290
Behavior patterns, common deviations of, 284–287
Blepharitis, 95
Blindness, color. See *Color perception, deficient.*
  in school, special services for, 106
  management of, 104–109
  special services for, history of, 105
  vocational guidance and, 108
Board of education, responsibilities of, 358
Body, growth and development of, 13–38
  and determining factors, 22–25
  definition, 14
  measurement of, 25–29
Body organs, normal growth of, *15*
Boils, 231
Bone(s), long, normal growth of, 21
  turbinate, 136
Botulism, cause of, 197
  control at school, 198
  description of, 197
  incubation period, 197
  transmission of, 197
Brain damage, hyperactivity and, 304
Breathing, obstructed, causes of, 137
Burns, emergency care of, 447
  floor, management of, 244
  minor, first aid procedures for, 447

Bus, school, safety requirements of, 392
Bus driver, 392

Calcium, in nutrition, 44
Cancer in children, mortality rates, 334(t)
school management of, 333–335
Canker sores, 142
Carbohydrates, in diet, 42
Carbuncles, 231
Carditis, 260
Caries, dental, bacteria and, 161
control and prevention of, 164–167
detection of, 164
factors influencing, 159–163
heredity and, 160
nutrition and, 160, 161
oral environment and, 160
preventive dentistry for, 164
prevention of, by flossing, 166
by fluoridation, 164
restorative dentistry for, 164
saliva and, 163
stages of, *162*, 163
systemic factors in, 159
Catarrhal jaundice. See *Hepatitis, infectious.*
Cerebral palsy, 319
Chickenpox, 198, *198*
Child abuse. See *Battered child.*
Chorea, 260
Classroom environment, 292, 405
Clubs, civic, 372
Cold, common, 199
Cold sore. See *Herpes simplex.*
Color blindness. See *Color perception, deficient.*
Color perception, deficient, 93–95
detection of, 94
Communicable diseases. See *Diseases, communicable.*
Communication, motivation strategies and, 496
Community health education, definition of, 5
Community-school relationship, 370–373
Conditioning, operant. See *Operant conditioning.*
Conjunctivitis, 95
bacterial. See *Conjunctivitis, epidemic.*
epidemic, 95
transmission of, 184
Convalescence, in communicable disease, 186
Counseling, health, and follow-up, 431–434
objectives of, 431
parents and, 433
school nurse and, 433
teacher's role in, 432
Counselor, responsibilities of, 364
health, responsibilities of, 432
Cumulative health record. See *Health record, cumulative.*
Curriculum, school, guidelines for, 395
Custodian, school, responsibilities of, 368, 390

Dandruff, 243
Deafness, conductive, 117
current facts, 132–134
hereditary, 122
neural, 117
sensorineural, 117
sensory, 117
types of, 117
Death in childhood, leading causes of, 335(t)
Decompensation, signs of, 262
Defects, dental detection of, 175–177
incidence of, 157, 158(t), 159(t)
Dental caries. See *Caries, dental.*
Dental health education, 177, *178*
Dental health program, objectives of, 175
Dental hygienist, school, responsibilities of, 366
Dentist, school, responsibilities of, 366
Depression, signs of, 288
Department of education, state, 357
Dermatitis, seborrheic, 244
Development, emotional, in adolescence, 282
in infancy, 278
of elementary school child, 279–281
of preschool child, 278
Developmental patterns, emotional, 278–283
Diabetes mellitus, 270–276
detection of, 272
physiology of, 270
school surveys for, 272
Diabetics, counseling for, 274
school management of, 273–275
Diet, acne vulgaris and, 243
well-balanced, 47, *48*
Digestive system, problems of, 247–253
emotional disturbances and, 248
Diphtheria, 199
Disease(s), communicable, 183–220. See also names of specific diseases.
acute stage of, 186
causes, 183
control of, history of, 342
convalescent stage of, 186
detection of, 188
in health examination program, 421
follow-up for, 189
gastrointestinal, 184
symptoms of, 189
health education and, 187, 195, 436
immunization and, 193–195
incubation period of, 185
isolation of patient in, 190
prodrome stage of, 185
progress of, 185
respiratory type, 184
symptoms of, 188
school health program for, 186–197
objectives of, 186–188
transmission of, 191
endemic, 192
heart. See *Heart, diseases of.*
periodontal, 167–169
venereal, 212–216
Driver education programs, 403

Droplet infection, 184
Droplet nuclei, 184
Dyslexia, 109–111
  detection of, 110
  management of, 110
  secondary, causes of, 110

E chart, as test for vision, *100*
Ear. See also *Hearing.*
  anatomy of, 116, *116*
  inner, disorders of, 121
  middle, infections of, 120
  outer, disorders of, 118
    foreign bodies in, 119
    infections of, 119
Eczema, 225
Education, special, funds for, 349
  state department of, 357
Elementary school, health education in, 477
  traffic safety and, 402
Elementary school child, emotional development of, 279–281
Elementary school teacher, responsibilities of, 4
Emmetriopia, 83, *84*
Emotional development, 29–36
  patterns of, 278–283
Emotional problems, 277–297
  detection of, 284–290
  follow-up for, 290–292
  learning disabilities and, 322
  mental retardation and, 321
  of physically handicapped, 298–338
  signs of, 285–287
Endocrine glands, malocclusion and, 173
  role in growth and development, 22
Environment, of classroom, 405
    emotional, 292
Epidemics, procedure during, 192
Epilepsy, 307–319
  causes of, 308
  detection of, 309–313
  differential diagnosis of, 318
  focal, 312
  follow-up program for, 313–316
  health education and, 316–318
  incidence of, 309
  psychomotor attacks in, 311
  school health program for, 309–318
  school management of, 313–315
  side effects of medication for, 314
  sociopsychological attitudes towards, 317
Eustachian tubes, 136
Extinction procedures, in operant conditioning, 496
Extracurricular activities, regulation of, 395
Eye(s). See also *Vision.*
  health problems of, 81–111
  health program for, 98–109
  infections of, 95. See also names of specific infections.
  injuries to, first aid for, 96
Eye(s) (*Continued*)
  problems of, detection of, 98–103
    follow-up for, 102
    incidence of, 101
  protection of, 97
  refractive errors of, 83–87, *84*, *86*
Eye safety, legislation for, 97

Fainting, 318
  causes of, 319
Farsightedness. See *Hyperopia.*
Fats in diet, 42
Feet, growth and development of, 76
Fever, glandular. See *Mononucleosis, infectious.*
  rheumatic, 258–261
  typhoid, 212
Fever blister. See *Herpes simplex.*
Fever sore. See *Herpes simplex.*
First aid, basic principles of, 445–448
  for burns, 447
  for eye injuries, 96
  for head injuries, 446
  for major injuries, 438
  for minor wounds, 438
  for skeletal injuries, 446
  for sudden illness, 448
  immediate care and, 439
  procedures for injuries, 438–440
First aid supplies, 440–442
Floor burns, management of, 244
Flossing, procedure for, 166
Fluoridation, 164
  in caries prevention, 164
Foods, groups of, *48*
Food poisoning, 250–252
  botulinus and, 251
  salmonella and, 251
  staphylococci and, 251
    preventive measures, 251
  symptoms of, 251
  typhoid-dysentery and, 251
Food rash, 225
Food services, in school, 61–65
Frenum, enlarged, 172

Gastroenteritis, 250
German Measles. See *Measles, German.*
Gifted child, 324
  management of, 325
Gingivitis, causes of, 167
  ulcerative necrotizing, 168
Glands, endocrine. See *Endocrine glands.*
Glands, "enlarged," 146
Glandular fever. See *Mononucleosis, infectious.*
Glasses, indicators for use, 91–93, 92
Gonorrhea, 214
Grand mal seizures, 310
  first aid for, 311

Growth and development, physical. See *Body, growth and development of.*
Growth chart, *26*

Handicapped child, 421
  definition of, 299
  emotional problems of, 298–338
  health services for, 435. See also name of specific handicap.
  responses to illness, 299
  teacher's role and, 300
Hay fever, 223
Head, injuries to, first aid for, 446
Headache, 325–331
  causes of, 326–331
  follow-up for, 330
  functional disorders and, 327–330
  migraine, 327–329
    characteristics of, 328
    emotional stress and, 328
    physiology of, 327
  muscle contraction, 330
  organic disorders and, 326
  vascular tension, 329
Health, definition of, 353
  department of, role in school health program, 371
  general, acne vulgaris and, 243
  in community, 354
  in home, 354
  in school, 355–370
Health, mental. See *Mental health.*
Health agencies, definition of, 7, 9
  private, role in school health program, 371
Health aides, school, responsibilities of, 368
Health appraisal, 413–430
  definition of, 413
  psychological tests for, 419
  screening tests for, 418
  special surveys for, 418
  teacher observation and, 415–418
Health attitudes, student, evaluation of, 520
Health coordinator, functions of, 362
Health councils, school, 359
Health counseling. See *Counseling, health.*
Health counselor. See *Counselor, health.*
Health education, community, definition of, 5
  definition of, 5
  dental, 177, *178*
Health education, school. See *School health education.*
Health educator, professional certification of, 362
  requirements for, 361
Health examination, parents and, 425
  procedure for, 426–430
    at school, 426
    in physician's office, 427
  time required for, 424
Health examination program, 419–427
  applications of, educational, 421
  objectives of, 419–422
  planning of, 422–426
Health facilities, in school plant, 387, *388*
Health history, necessary information for, 413–418
Health knowledge, student, evaluation of, 519–522
Health museums, school health education and, 490
Health practices, evaluation of, 521
Health program, dental, objectives of, 175
  for eyes, 98–109
  international, 350
  public, history and development of, 341–346
  school, administration of, basic patterns for, 358
    community participation in, 358–360
    current trends in, 348
    definition of, 8, 340(t)
    department of health and, 371
    development of, 341–352
    evaluation of, 509–524
      benefits of, 509
      by specialists, 513
      check lists for, 513, *552–559*
      responsibility for administration of, 510
      scope of, 511
      techniques for, 512–515
    federal legislation and, 356
    local administration of, 358
    medical centers and, 371
    organization and administration of, 353–375
    parents and, 369
    private health agencies and, 371
    private industry and, 372
    professional organizations and, 371
    public agencies and, 371
    replanning of, 516
    state legislation and, 357
    student participation in, 370
Health record, cumulative, 427–430, *429*
  uses of, 428–430
Health science, definition of, 5
Health services, for handicapped, 435. See also name of specific handicap.
  school. See *School health services.*
Health standards, for nonteaching personnel, 452
  for teacher candidates, 450
  for teachers, 450
Healthful school living, 376–411
  curriculum and, 394–396
  definition of, 376
  educational aspects of, 393
  evaluation of, 516
  school environment and, 376–393
Hearing, defective, classification of, 127, 127(t)
    detection of, 122–127
    incidence of, 126, 126(t), 127(t)
    management of, 128–131
    school health program for, 122–134
  group test for, 124
  health education and, 131–134

Hearing (*Continued*)
mechanics of, 116
multiple test for, 124
serviceable, definition of, 117
tests for, 123–127. See also names of specific tests.
Hearing conservation program, 131–134
in community, 131
in school, 131
parent participation in, 131
Heart, damage to, effects of, 255–257
diseases of, common causes of, 257–261
congenital, 258
detection of, 261–263
health examination and, 263
medical follow-up for, 263
physical education and, 265
public health and, 267
school health program for, 261–267
school management of, 264–267
teacher observation and, 262
vocational counseling and, 265
function of, normal, 254, *255*
growth of, 20, 254
Heart murmur, incidence of, 257
innocent, 256
organic, 257
Heart valves, damage to, 256
Heat, school plant and, 384
Height, changes with growth, 16, *17*, *18*, *19*, *20*
technique of measurement, 27, *28*
Hepatitis, infectious, 200
Heredity, and growth, 22
deafness and, 122
dental caries and, 160
malocclusion and, 170
Herpes simplex, 233
characteristics of, 234
Hives. See *Urticaria.*
Hyperactive child syndrome, 302
Hyperactivity, 301–307
due to brain damage, 304
management of, 304, 306
neurotic, 304
physiological, 303
Hypermetropia, *84*, 85
Hyperopia, *84*, 85
Hysterical conversion reaction, 318

Illness, and growth, 24
sudden, emergency procedures for, 448
Impetigo contagiosa, 231
Immunity, active, 193
"borrowed," 193
passive, 193
Immunization, communicable diseases and, 193–195
schedule for, 194
tetanus, 193
Infancy, developmental patterns in, 278
Infantile paralysis, 204
Infection(s), bacterial, 231
botulinus, 251
Infection(s) (*Continued*)
droplet, 184
fungal, 234–238
salmonella, 251
streptococcal, 207
viral, 232
Infectious hepatitis, 200
Infectious jaundice, 200
Infectious mononucleosis, 201
Influenza, 201
Injury(ies), abdominal, management of, 249
emergency care of, 437–448
head, first aid procedures for, 446
legal responsibility of teacher, 443–445
motor vehicle, 396
records and reports on, 442
skeletal, emergency care of, 446
Insulin reaction, 272
Insulin shock, 272
Insurance plans, 445
Invalids, management of, 266
Iodine, 44
sources of, 44
Iodine deficiency, effects of, 44
Iron, dietary sources of, 43
Iron deficiency, effects of, 43

Joint Committee on Health Education Technology, health definitions prepared by, 5–9
Junior high school, health education in, 478–479, 481(t)
traffic safety and, 403

Kwashiorkor, 54
Kyphosis, 71, 73

Lacerations, management of, 243
Learning disabilities, 322–324
causes of, 322
emotional implications of, 322
management of, 323
Legal responsibility, negligence and, 443
Lens(es), bifocal, 92
contact, indications for, 93
concave, as correction for myopia, 92
convex, as correction for hypermetropia, 92
corrective. See *Glasses.*
safety, types of, 92
Leukemia, 334
Library, design for, *383*
Lice. See also *Pediculosis.*
body, 239
crab, 240
head, 239, *239*
Lighting, engineering aspects of, 382
Lordosis, 71
Lunch program, school. See *School lunch program.*

Lymph nodes, cervical, 146, *147*
description of, 145
infection of, 145
Lymphatic system, anatomy of, 145

Manutrition, causes of, 50–53
effects of, 53–55
management of, 55
Malocclusion, 169–174, *171, 172*
causes of, 170–173
congenital defects and, 173
endocrine glands and, 173
enlarged frenum and, 172
enlarged tonsils and, 172
heredity and, 170
impacted teeth and, 173
mouth breathing and, 170, *171, 172*
oral habits and, 172
orthodontic correction of, 173
postural habits and, 172
prevention and treatment of, 173
results of, 173
Mann, Horace, 346
Maturation. See *Emotional problems.*
Measles, 202, *203*
German, 200
Media, educational, 501–504
evaluation of, 501
Medical centers, role in school health program, 371
Medication, anti-convulsant, side effects of, 314
Mental health, school responsibilities and, 292
Mental health education, school programs for, 283–293
Mental retardation, 320–322
behavior and, 321
emotional implications of, 321
Meredith's physical growth records, *536–539*
Minerals in diet, 43–45
Minor motor seizures, 312
Mononucleosis, infectious, 201
Motivation, communication and, 496
function in the learning process, 495
Mouth, examination of, 141
injuries to, 141
Mouth breathing, causes of, 137
detection of, 139
malocclusion and, 170
management of, 139
Mumps, 202, *203*
Myopia, *84*, 85, *86, 92*
causes of, 87
corrective lenses for, *92*

Nasopharynx, 136
examination of, 140
National Safety Council, 398
Nearsightedness. See *Myopia.*
Nervousness, acne vulgaris and, 244
Neurosis, hyperactivity and, 304
Niacin, 46
Nodes, lymph. See *Lymph nodes.*
Nonteaching employees, health of, 408
Nose, anatomy and physiology of, 134–137, *135*
injuries to, 138
Nosebleeds, causes of, 138
management of, 139
Nostrils, obstruction of, causes of, 137
chronic, results of, 137
Nuclei, droplet, 184
Nurse, school, responsibilities of, 366
Nutrition, 39–69
and growth, 24
calcium and, 44
carbohydrates and, 42
dental caries and, 160, 161
educational program for, 59
requirements, 39–49, 40(t)
standards for evaluating, 49, *49*

Obesity, causes and management of, 57–59
psychological factors in, 58
Occlusion. See also *Malocclusion.*
normal, *169*
Olfactory center, 136
Operant conditioning, extinction procedures in, 496
goal of, 496
use of, 497
Otitis media, causes of, 121
detection of, 120
Orthodontics, malocclusion and, 173
Overweight. See *Obesity.*

Pain, abdominal, school management of, 252
Palsy, cerebral, 319
Paralysis, infantile, 204
Parasitology, theory of, development of, 342
Parotitis, infectious, 202, *203*
Pasteur, Louis, 342
Pediculosis, 239
school management of, 240
Periodontal diseases, 167–169
Periodontitis, 168
Pertussis, 216
Petit mal seizures, 309
Pharynx. See *Throat.*
Physical education, heart diseases and, 265
Physical educator, responsibilities of, 363
Physician, school, responsibilities of, 364
Plaque, 160, *162*
Poliomyelitis, 204
Polyarthritis, 259
Positive reinforcement, 497
Posture, development during growth, 70–76
evaluation and measurement of, 72–74
good, promotion of, 74–76, *75, 76*
poor, causes of, 74

Presbyopia, bifocal lenses and, 92
Preschool child, emotional development in, 278
Private industry, role in school health program, 372
Problems, emotional. See *Emotional problems.*
Professional organizations, role in school health program, 371
Protein in diet, 41
Psychomotor attacks in epilepsy, 311
Psychosomatic problems, 290
Public health program. See *Health program, public.*
Pyorrhea, 168

Rabies, 204–206
Rash, food, 225
Reading disorder. See *Dyslexia.*
Reality instruction, 498
  guidelines for, 499
  teacher involvement and, 499
Records, school, use of, 400
"Red measles," 202, *203*
Rheumatism, 259
  inflammatory, 259
  juvenile, 259
Rhinitis, allergic, 223
Riboflavin, 46
"Running ear," 120
Rural areas, school health services for, 449
Rubella, 200
Rubeola, 202, 203

Safety, structural, school plant and, 386
  traffic, 402–404
Safety program, 396–404
  preventive, 398–404
    use of statistics in, 398–401
  school responsibilities and, 404
St. Vitus' dance, 260
Salmonellosis, 206
Sanitation, history of, 342
  in school plant, 389
Scabies, 238
Schools, elementary, organization of space in, 380
  secondary, organization of space in, 380
Schoolbuildings. See *School plant.*
School bus, safety requirements of, 392
Schoolgrounds. See *School plant.*
School health education, 457–508
  definition of, 7, 457
  demonstrations and, 489
  discussion method, 487, *488*
  dramatizations and, 494
  evaluation of, 518
  exhibits and, 490
School health education (*Continued*)
  experiments and, 489
  field trips and, 490, *491*, *492*
  graphic materials for, 503
  guest speakers and, 488
  health museums and, 490
  importance of, 458–460
  in communicable disease control, 187, 195, 136
  in intermediate grades, 477
    suggested content, 478
  in junior high school, 478–479, 481(t)
  in kindergarten and primary grades, 475–477
  in senior high, 480–482, 481(t)
  incidental approach to, 482–484
  lecture method for, 485
  legislation regarding, 462
  methods in, 482–494
  objectives of, 457, 469
  oral and written reports in, 489
  planned aporoach to, 484–494
  problem-solving method for, 485
  resources for, 502–504
    journals, 533
    printed material, 527–531
  role-playing and, 492
  state supervisors and, 462
  student participation in, 494
  studies regarding, 458–460
  textbooks and, 486
  use of basic health concepts in, 469–472, *470*, *471*
  use of motivation and involvement strategies in, 495–501
  use of periodicals in, 503
School health education curriculum, 461–504
  age level and, 468
  contents of, 464–475
  contributions of health education specialists, 472
  contributions from the sciences, 472
  determination of student needs, 465
  organization of, 474
  public health needs and, 468
  resources for, 461–464
  student experiences and, 467
  student interests and, 466
  suggested content of, 473
School health education program, implementation of, 504
School health educator, background of, 472
School health program. See *Health program, school.*
School health records and forms, *535–551*
School health services, definition of, 8
  evaluation of, 517, 518
  for personnel, 449–453
  for teachers, 450
  in rural areas, 449
  insurance plans and, 445
  objectives of, 412
  organization of, *414*
  preventive programs in, 448

School lunch program, 61, 63–65, 404
  facilities for, *63*
  federal, objectives of, 63
  supervision of, 61
School plant, accidents in, 398
  acoustical environment of, 385
  colors, 382
  community use of, 392
  custodian's responsibilities, 390
  design for, 378–389, *378, 381, 383, 391*
  environmental considerations, 380–385
  esthetic values, 382–384, 386
  fire safety and, 402
  floor plan for, *381*
  for elementary schools, 380
  health facilities for, 387, *388*
  lighting, 382
  modern, 376–389
    requirements for, 377
  old, 389
  operation and maintenance, 390
  organization of space in, 378–380, *378, 381*
  safety factors in, 386, 401, 402
  safety inspection of, 402
  sanitary facilities for, 389
  thermal environment of, 384
  visual environment of, 382–384
School principal, functions of, 360
Scoliosis, 71, *73*
Secondary school teacher, responsibilities of, 4
Seizures, epileptic, age distribution of, 312
  generalized motor. See *Grand mal.*
Senior high school, health education in, 480–482, 481(t)
  traffic safety and, 403
Shoes, proper fit of, 77
Sinuses, accessory nasal, 136
Sinusitis, 137
Skeleton, injuries to, emergency care of, 446
  normal growth of, 21
Skin, allergies of, 225
  cleanliness and, 230
  functions of, 230
  health problems of, 229–246
Skinner, B. F., 496
Smallpox, 207
Snellen test for vision, *99*
Social workers, school, responsibilities of, 367
Sores, canker, 142
Special education, funds for, 349
Speech, delayed, 149
Speech disorders, types of, 148–150
Staphylococci, food poisoning and, 251
Statistics, use of, in preventive safety program, 398–401
Stenosis, 256
"Stomach ache," significance of, 248
Strabismus, 88–91, *88*
  amblyopia and, 89
  causes of, 89
  convergent, 88, *88*
  corrective procedures for, 90
Strabismus (*Continued*)
  divergent, 88, *89*
  results of, 89
Stuttering, management of, 149
  mechanics of, 149
Sty, 95
"Sugar diabetes." See *Diabetes mellitus.*
Suicidal crisis, 288
Suicide, behavioral patterns in, 287–290
    teacher role and, 289
  incidence of, 287(t)
Superintendent of schools, functions of, 360
Supplies, first aid, 440–442
Syphilis, 215
System, lymphatic. See *Lymphatic system.*

Teacher(s), health of 406–408, 450
  responsibilities of, 1–9
Teacher candidates, health standards for, 450
Teaching aids. See *Media, educational.*
Teeth. See also *Dental.*
  anatomy and physiology of, 153, *154*
  deciduous, 154, *155*
  growth and development of, 153–157, *156, 157*
  impacted, malocclusion and, 173
  injuries to, 174
  permanent, *155*, 156
  primary, 154, *155*
Test(s), for hearing, 123–127
Tetanus, immunization against, 193
Tetanus antitoxin, 193
Tetanus toxoid, 193
Theory, value. See *Value theory.*
Thiamine, in nutrition, 46
"Three-day measles," 200
Throat, disorders of, detection of, 147
  examination of, 140, *142*
Tinea capitis, 234, *235*
Tinea cruris, 236
Tinea pedis, 236–238, *237*
  prevention of, 236
Tonsils, anatomy of, 143
  removal of, 143
Tonsillectomy, indications for, 143
Tonsillitis, 143
Toothbrushing, Bass method for, 178, *178*
Toxoid, tetanus, 193
Trachoma, 95
Traffic safety, in senior high school, 403
"Trench mouth," 168
Tuberculosis, 208–212
  health education for, 211
  school control of, 209
Tubes, eustachian, 136
Typhoid fever, 212

Ulcers, 249
Underweight, causes and management of, 56
Urticaria, 225

Value theory, 497
  establishment of, 498
Varicella, 198, *198*
Variola, 207
Verruca. See *Wart.*
Vision. See also *Eye(s).*
  accommodation in, 82
  acuity of, tests for, 99–103, *99, 100.* See also names of specific tests
    evaluation of, 101
  defective, definition of, 104
    management of, 104–109
    school programs for, 105–109
  development of, 84
  physiology of, 81–83, *82, 83*
Visual field loss, characteristics of, 104
  detection of, 104
Vitamin(s), in nutrition, 45
Vitamin A, in nutrition, 45
Vitamin B complex, in nutrition, 46
Vitamin C, 46
Vitamin D, 47
Vocational guidance, for blind, 108
Voice test for hearing, 123

Warts, 232, *233*
  treatment of, school program for, 233
Watch test for hearing, 123
Water, in diet, 41
Weight, changes with growth, 16, *16, 17, 18, 19, 20*
Wetzel's grid, 535
  use of, 27
Whisper test for hearing, 123
Whooping cough, 216
World War I, influence on public health program, 343–346

Youth groups, 372